Mosby's

REVIEW for the NBDE

Part 1

Mosby's

REVIEW for the NBDE

Part 1

Edited by

Frank Dowd, DDS, PhD

Professor and Past Chair
Department of Pharmacology
School of Dentistry
Creighton University
Omaha, Nebraska

MOSBY
ELSEVIER

MOSBY
ELSEVIER

11830 Westline Industrial Drive
St. Louis, Missouri 63146

ISBN-13: 978-0-323-02564-5
ISBN-10: 0-323-02564-1

MOSBY'S REVIEW FOR THE NBDE PART I

Notice

Knowledge and best practice in this field are constantly changing. As new research and experience broaden our knowledge, changes in practice, treatment and drug therapy may become necessary or appropriate. Readers are advised to check the most current information provided (i) on procedures featured or (ii) by the manufacturer of each product to be administered, to verify the recommended dose or formula, the method and duration of administration, and contraindications. It is the responsibility of the practitioner, relying on his or her own experience and knowledge of the patient, to make diagnoses, to determine dosages and the best treatment for each individual patient, and to take all appropriate safety precautions. To the fullest extent of the law, neither the Publisher nor the Editor assumes any liability for any injury and/or damage to persons or property arising out or related to any use of the material contained in this book.

The Publisher

ISBN-13: 978-0-323-02564-5
ISBN-10: 0-323-02564-1

Publishing Director: Linda Duncan
Senior Editor: John Dolan
Developmental Editor: John Dedeke
Editorial Assistant: Marcia Bunda
Publication Services Manager: Melissa Lastarria
Project Manager: Kelly E.M. Steinmann
Designer: Bill Drone

Printed in the United States of America.

Last digit is the print number: 9 8 7 6 5 4

Section Editors

Major M. Ash, Jr., DDS, MS
Marcus L. Ward Professor and Research Scientist, Emeritus
Department of Occlusion
University of Michigan
School of Dentistry
Ann Arbor, Michigan

Kenneth R. Etzel, PhD, MS
Associate Dean
School of Dental Medicine
University of Pittsburgh
Pittsburgh, Pennsylvania

Stanley J. Nelson, DDS, MS
Professor and Co-Chair
Department of Clinical Sciences
School of Dental Medicine
University of Nevada, Las Vegas
Las Vegas, Nevada

Joseph W. Robertson, DDS
Private Practice
Troy, Michigan

Jean Yang, DMD
Private Practice of Endodontics
Baltimore, Maryland
Dean's Faculty
Department of Endodontics
University of Maryland Dental School
Baltimore, Maryland

Contributors

Xia Lin, DMD
Private Practice
New York, New York

Grace Yang, DMD
Private Practice
New York, New York

Preface

How to Use This Text

Examinations are a means of strengthening our intellect. This text is a tool to help prepare students for taking the National Board Dental Exams and to point out strengths and weaknesses so they can better use their study time. This text is not meant to replace years of professional training or give away questions so that students may pass exams if they memorize the answers. Instead, this book will help direct students to the topic areas that they may need to review and strengthen knowledge and exam-taking skills.

Dental schools do well in preparing their students for practice and for board exams. In addition, for many colleges there is a good correlation between students who do well in their dental courses and those who score well on their board exams. Therefore to best prepare for board exams, students should focus on doing well in their courses. It is also in the best interest of students to focus more study time for their board exams on the areas in which they have not scored as well in their dental coursework. This is good news for students, since most are aware of their areas of weakness and therefore have the opportunity to focus more resources on these areas when studying for boards.

Board Examinations Are Like Marathons

Taking most board exams is similar to running a marathon; they take both mental and physical stamina, and one should prepare for them like one would prepare to partake in a long-endurance event. If one has never run a mile before, he or she cannot expect to prepare adequately in only one week for a 26-mile race. Therefore, preparation in advance is essential.

Helpful Hints for Preparing to Take Your Board Examinations

1. Know your weaknesses, and focus more of your resources on strengthening these areas. Look back at your grades from the courses that relate to the exam topics. These will indicate areas that need more attention. Also, use this book as a trial run to help point to content areas that may need more review.
2. Practice makes perfect. Just rereading old course notes may not be enough. The skill of taking an exam is more about pulling information from your brain, not stuffing more information into it. Therefore, when practicing to take board exams, practice retrieving information from your brain by taking practice exams. You can do this in several ways: study with others by asking each other questions; test yourself with flashcards or notes that are partially covered from view; or answer questions from this text. In each case, be sure to check your answer to find out whether you achieved the correct answer.
3. Practice answering examination questions in the same environment in which the test will be given. In other words, most board exams are not given in your living room with the TV or stereo blaring; therefore, do not practice in this environment. Consider practicing in an environment like the exam location and using the exam questions from this text.
4. If possible, eat and sleep well during the weeks before the exam. It is difficult to compete successfully in a marathon if one is malnourished or sleep deprived. Set regular bedtimes and eating schedules so that your routine stays as familiar and comfortable as possible.

5. If you have a regular exercise routine, stick to it. It will help you deal with the additional stress and provide consistency in your life.
6. Block off time for practice examinations, such as the review questions and sample exam in this text. Try to use the same amount of time and the same number of questions that will be given during the actual exam. This will help prepare you for the amount of pressure in the exam environment.
7. Stay away from naysayers and people who create hype around the board exams. Some of these people may have their own interests in mind. (Are they representing a board review company? Are they the type of person who makes themselves feel better by making others feel worse?) Instead, find people who are positive and demonstrate good study behaviors. Consider making a study group of people who are able to help the other members in the group stay positive.
8. If your school offers board reviews, consider taking them. These may assist you with building your confidence with what material you have already mastered and may help you focus on material that you need to spend more time studying.

Helpful Hints for Taking Practice Examinations and Full Exams

1. It is important to note that questions that are considered "good" questions by examination standards will have incorrect choices in their answer bank that are very close to the correct answer. These wrong choices are called "distracters" for a reason; they are meant to distract the test taker. Because of this, some test takers do better by reading the question and trying to guess the answer before looking at the answer bank. Therefore, consider trying to answer questions without looking at the answer bank.
2. Cross out answers that are obviously wrong. This will allow a better chance of picking the correct answer and reduce distraction from the wrong answers.
3. Only go back and change an answer if you are absolutely certain you were wrong with your previous choice, or a different question in the same exam provides you with the correct answer.
4. Read questions carefully. Circle or underline negative words in questions, such as "except," "not," and "false." If these words are missed when reading the question, it is nearly impossible to get the correct answer; marking these key words will make sure you do not miss them.
5. If you are stuck on one question, consider treating the answer bank like a series of true/false items relevant to the question. Most people consider true/false questions easier than multiple choice. At least if you can eliminate a few choices, you will have a better chance at selecting the correct answer from whatever is left.
6. Never leave blanks, unless the specific exam has a penalty for wrong answers. It is better to guess wrong than leave an item blank. Check with those giving the examination to find out whether there are penalties for marking the wrong answer.
7. Some people do better on exams by going through the exam and answering known questions first, and then returning to the more difficult questions later. This helps to build confidence during the exam. This also helps the test taker avoid spending too much time on a few questions and running out of time on easy questions that may be at the end.
8. Pace yourself on the exam. Figure out ahead of time how much time each question will take to answer. Do not rush, but do not spend too much time on one question. Sometimes it is better to move to the next question and come back to the difficult ones later, since a fresh look is sometimes helpful.
9. Bring appropriate supplies to the exam. If you get distracted by noise, consider bringing ear plugs. It is inevitable that someone will take the exam next to the guy in the squeaky chair, or the one with the sniffling runny nose. Most exams will provide you with instructions as to what you may or may not bring to the exam. Be sure to read these instructions in advance.
10. Some people find that they do better on exams by marking all of their answers on the test packet and then transferring answers to the actual test sheet or exam program. If you do this, be careful to fill in the answer that corresponds with the question.
11. Make sure that once you have completed the exam all questions are appropriately filled in. Find out how many questions there are for each section before taking the exam, to make sure you answer the correct number of questions.

Helpful Hints for the Post-Examination Period

It may be a good idea to think about what you will be doing after the exam.

1. Most people are exhausted after taking board exams. Some reasons for this exhaustion may

be the number of hours, the mental focus, and the anxiety that exams cause some people. Be aware that you may be tired, so avoid planning anything that one should not do when exhausted, such as driving across the country, operating heavy machinery or power tools, or studying for final exams. Instead, plan a day or two to recuperate before you tackle any heavier physical or mental tasks.

2. Consider a debriefing or "detoxification" meeting with your positive study partners after the exam. Talking about the exam afterwards may help reduce stress. However, remember that the feelings one has after an exam may not always match the exam score (e.g., someone who feels he did poorly may have done well, or someone who feels he did well may not have.)
3. Consider doing something nice for yourself. After all, you will have just completed a major exam. It is important to celebrate this accomplishment.

We wish you the very best with taking your exams and hope that this text provides you with an excellent training tool for your preparations.

Additional Resources

This review text is intended to aid the study and retention of dental sciences in preparation for the National Board Dental Examination. It is not intended to be a substitute for a complete dental education curriculum. For a truly comprehensive understanding of the basic dental sciences, please consult these supplemental texts.

Anatomical Basis of Dentistry, Second Edition
Bernard Liebgott

Anatomy of Orofacial Structures, Seventh Edition
Richard W. Brand, Donald E. Isselhard

Berne & Levy Princples of Physiology, Fourth Edition
Matthew N. Levy, Bruce M. Koeppen, Bruce A. Stanton

Biochemistry, Second Edition
David E. Metzler

Illustrated Anatomy of the Head and Neck, Third Edition
Margaret J. Fehrenbach, Susan W. Herring

Illustrated Dental Embryology, Histology and Anatomy, Second Edition
Mary Bath-Balough, Margaret J. Fehrenbach

Molecular Biology
David P. Clark

Oral Anatomy, Histology & Embryology, Third Edition
B. K. Berkovitz, G. R. Holland, B. J. Moxham

Physiology, Third Edition
Linda S. Costanzo

Rapid Review Gross and Developmental Anatomy
N. Anthony Moore, William A. Roy

Wheeler's Dental Anatomy, Physiology, and Occlusion, Eighth Edition
Major M. Ash and Stanley J. Nelson

Table of Contents

1

Anatomic Sciences

JEAN YANG, JOSEPH W. ROBERTSON

OUTLINE

The anatomic sciences portion of the National Dental Boards tests the following: gross anatomy, histology, and embryology. Gross anatomy encompasses a wide range of topics, including bones, muscles, fasciae, nerves, circulation, spaces, and cavities. Details and diagrams will focus on topics emphasized on the National Dental Boards. Since it is out of the scope of this book to cover every detail, it is recommended that you refer to past class notes, anatomy texts and atlases, and old exams for a more thorough understanding of the information discussed. Only a limited number of figures and diagrams are included in this text. It will be helpful to refer to other anatomy texts and atlases for more figures and diagrams.

1.0 GROSS ANATOMY

1.1 Head and Neck

1.1.1 Oral Cavity

Vascular supply

The main blood supply to the head and neck is from the subclavian and common carotid arteries. The origins of these arteries differ for the right and left sides. From the aorta, the brachiocephalic trunk branch off and bifurcate into the right subclavian and right common carotid artery. The left common carotid artery and left subclavian artery branch off separately from the arch of the aorta.

A. Subclavian artery
   1. Origin: the right subclavian artery arises from the brachiocephalic trunk. The left subclavian artery arises directly from the arch of the aorta.
   2. Important divisions:
      a. Vertebral artery—supplies the brain (refer to Internal Carotid section).
      b. Internal thoracic artery—descends to supply the diaphragm and terminates as the superior epigastric artery, which helps supply the abdominal wall.
      c. Thyrocervical or cervicothyroid trunk—divides into three arteries: the transverse cervical artery, suprascapular artery, and the inferior thyroid artery.
      d. Costocervical trunk—divides into two branches: the superior intercostals and deep cervical arteries, which supply muscles of intercostal spaces.
      e. Dorsal scapular artery—supplies the muscles of the scapular region.

B. Common carotid artery
   1. Origin: the right common carotid branches from the brachiocephalic trunk. The left common carotid branches from the arch of the aorta.
   2. The common carotid ascends within a fibrous sheath in the neck, known as the *carotid sheath*. This sheath also contains the internal jugular vein and the vagus nerve.

3. Major branches:
   a. Both the right and left common carotid arteries bifurcate into the internal and external carotid arteries.
   b. Note: the carotid sinus baroreceptors are located at this bifurcation. These baroreceptors help monitor systemic blood pressure and are innervated by cranial nerve (CN) IX.

C. Internal carotid artery
   1. Branches of the internal carotid artery, as well as the vertebral arteries, serve as the major blood supply for the brain.
   2. Origin: the internal carotid divides from the common carotid artery and continues in the carotid sheath into the cranium. Unlike the external carotid artery, it has no branches in the neck.
   3. Major branches:
      a. Anterior and middle cerebral arteries: the internal carotid terminates into these two arteries. These arteries will anastamose with the posterior and anterior communicating arteries to form the circle of Willis. The circle of Willis also communicates with the vertebral arteries via the basilar and posterior cerebral arteries (Figure 1–1).
      b. Pathology notes: berry aneurysms most commonly occur in the circle of Willis, particularly in the anterior communicating and anterior cerebral arteries. Strokes often occur from a diseased middle cerebral artery.
      c. Opthalamic artery—supplies the orbital area and lacrimal gland.

D. External carotid artery
   1. Branches of the external carotid artery supply tissues in the head and neck, including the oral cavity.
   2. Origin: the external carotid artery branches from the common carotid artery.
   3. Major branches (Figure 1–2):
      a. Superior thyroid artery
         (1) Origin: branches from the anterior side of the external carotid artery, just above the carotid bifurcation.
         (2) Major branches:
            (a) Infrahyoid artery—supplies the infrahyoid muscles.
            (b) Sternocleidomastoid artery—supplies the sternocleidomastoid (SCM) muscle.
            (c) Superior laryngeal artery—pierces through the thyrohyoid membrane, with the internal laryngeal nerve, as it travels to supply the muscles of the larynx.
            (d) Cricothyroid artery—supplies the thyroid gland.
      b. Ascending pharyngeal artery
         (1) Origin: branches from the anterior side of the external carotid artery, just above the superior thyroid artery.
         (2) Its branches supply the pharynx, soft palate, and meninges.
      c. Lingual artery
         (1) Origin: branches from the anterior side of the external carotid artery, near the hyoid bone. It often arises along with the facial artery, forming the lingualfacial trunk. It then travels

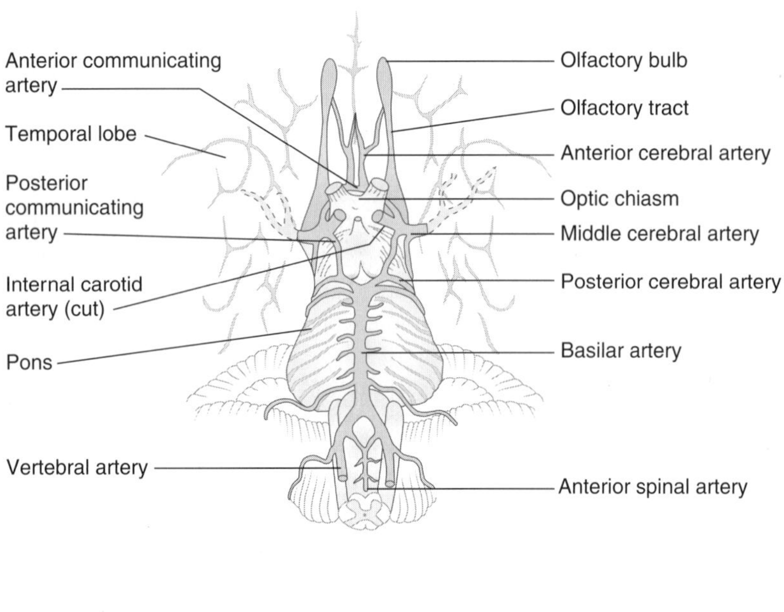

Figure 1–1. Inferior view of the brain: circle of Willis. (From Moore NA, Roy WA: Gross and Developmental Anatomy, St. Louis, Mosby, 2002.)

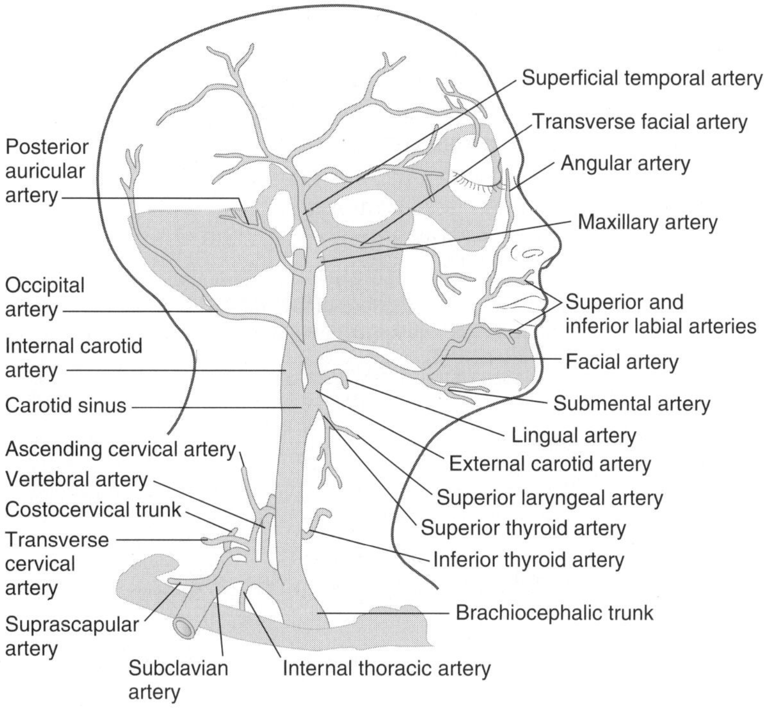

Figure 1–2. Lateral view of arteries of the neck and superficial head. (Modified from Moore NA, Roy WA: Gross and Developmental Anatomy, St. Louis, Mosby, 2002.)

anteriorly between the hyoglossus and middle pharyngeal constrictor muscles.

(2) Major branches:

(a) Suprahyoid artery—supplies the suprahyoid muscles.

(b) Dorsal lingual artery—supplies the tongue, tonsils, and soft palate.

(c) Sublingual artery—supplies the floor of the mouth, mylohyoid muscle, and sublingual gland.

(d) Deep lingual artery—supplies the tongue.

d. Facial artery

(1) Origin: branches from the anterior side, just above the lingual artery.

(2) Major branches and the structures they supply are listed in Table 1–1.

e. Occipital artery

(1) Origin: branches from the posterior side of the external carotid, close to CN XII.

(2) Branches of the occipital artery supply the sternocleidomastoid and suprahyoid muscles, dura mater, and meninges.

f. Posterior auricular artery

(1) Origin: branches from the posterior side of the external carotid, near the level of the styloid process and superior to the stylohyoid muscle.

(2) Branches supply the mastoid air cells, stapedius muscle, and internal ear.

g. Maxillary artery

(1) Origin: branches from the external carotid in the parotid gland and travels between the mandibular ramus and sphenomandibular ligament before reaching the infratemporal and pterygopalatine fossa. From there, the artery divides around the lateral pterygoid muscle into three major branches: the mandibular, pterygoid, and pterygopalatine divisions (Table 1–2).

Table 1–1. Major Branches of the Facial Artery and the Structures They Supply

BRANCHES	STRUCTURES SUPPLIED
Ascending palatine artery	Soft palate, tonsils, pharynx
Tonsillar artery	Tonsils, tongue
Glandular artery	Submandibular gland
Submental artery	Submandibular gland, mylohyoid and anterior digastric muscle
Inferior labial artery	Lower lip
Superior labial artery	Upper lip
Lateral nasal artery	Nose
Angular artery	Eyelids, nose

Table 1–2. Branches of the Three Major Divisions of the Maxillary Artery and the Structures They Supply

BRAN CHES OF THE THREE MAJOR DIVISIONS	STRUCTURES SUPPLIED
Mandibular division	
Inferior alveolar artery (IAA) branches	
Deep auricular artery	Tympanic membrane
Anterior tympanic artery	Tympanic membrane
IAA (dental branches)	Mandibular posterior teeth and surrounding tissues
Mylohyoid artery	Mylohyoid muscle, floor of mouth
Incisive artery	Anterior teeth and surrounding tissues
Mental artery	Chin, lower lip
Middle meningeal artery	Meninges of the brain, dura of bones in the skull
Pterygoid division	
Deep temporal arteries	Temporalis muscle
Pterygoid arteries	Pterygoid muscles
Masseteric artery	Masseter
Buccal artery	Buccinator, buccal mucosa
Pterygopalatine division	
Posterior superior alveolar artery	Maxillary posterior teeth, maxillary sinus
Infraorbital artery, including anterior and middle superior alveolar, orbital, and facial branches	Maxillary anterior teeth, orbital area and lacrimal gland
Greater palatine artery	Hard palate, lingual gingiva of maxillary posterior teeth
Lesser palatine artery	Soft palate, tonsils
Sphenopalatine artery	Nasal cavity

(2) Branches of the mandibular division:
   (a) Deep auricular artery and anterior tympanic artery—supplies the tympanic membrane.
   (b) Inferior alveolar artery (IAA): the IAA has the same branches and anatomic pathway as its corresponding nerve, the inferior aleveolar nerve, a branch of CN V_3, (refer to the inferior alveolar nerve [IAN] sensory pathway in the Cranial Nerves section).
   (c) Middle meningeal and accessory arteries—the middle meningeal artery will travel through the foramen spinosum to supply the meninges of the brain and dural lining of bones in the skull.

(3) Branches of the pterygoid division:
   (a) Deep temporal arteries—supply the temporalis muscle.
   (b) Pterygoid arteries—supply the pterygoid muscles.
   (c) Masseteric artery—supplies the masseter.
   (d) Buccal artery—supplies the buccinator and buccal mucosa.

(4) Branches of the pterygopalatine division:
   (a) The pterygopalatine division will follow the pterygomaxillary fissure into the pterygopalatine fossa, where the artery divides. Its major divisions include the posterior superior alveolar artery, the greater and lesser palatine arteries, and the infraorbital artery. All *of* these branches travel and divide with their corresponding nerves to the structures they vascularize. For their anatomic pathways, refer to the sensory pathways of their corresponding nerves in the Cranial Nerves section.
   (b) Posterior superior alveolar artery —supplies the maxillary sinus, molar, and premolar teeth as well as the neighboring gingiva.
   (c) Sphenopalatine artery—branches in the pterygopalatine fossa and travels to the nasal cavity, where it branches to supply surrounding structures. Note: it is most commonly associated with serious nose bleeds in the posterior nasal cavity.
   (d) Infraorbital artery—the termination point of the maxillary artery. Its branches supply the orbital region, facial tissues, and the maxillary sinus and maxillary anterior teeth (via the anterior superior alveolar artery).

Venous drainage

Deoxygenated blood from the head and neck is drained from the area by a network of veins that eventually terminate in the jugular veins. The blood from the jugular veins is ultimately returned to the heart via the subclavian and brachiocephalic veins, which join to form the superior vena cava.

A. Veins of the neck: jugular veins
   1. Internal jugular vein
      a. The internal jugular vein serves as the major source of venous drainage of deoxygenated blood from the head and neck region. This region consists of both extracranial tissues and intracranial structures, including the brain.
      b. Termination: the internal jugular vein travels down within the carotid sheath and joins the subclavian vein to form the brachiocephalic vein. The brachiocephalic vein terminates in the superior vena cava, which empties into the right atrium of the heart.
   2. External jugular vein
      a. The external jugular vein drains extracranial tissues from the head and face.
      b. Termination: the external jugular vein terminates into the subclavian vein.

B. Veins of the cranium: venous drainage of the brain
   1. Deoxygenated blood drains from the brain through a series of dural sinuses.
   2. Pathways of deoxygenated blood: blood from the superior sagittal sinus, inferior sagittal sinus (via the straight sinus), and the occipital sinuses drains at the confluence of sinuses, which is located in the posterior cranium. From here, the blood flows through the transverse sinuses to the sigmoid sinuses, which ultimately empty into the internal jugular vein. This pathway is illustrated in Figure 1–3.
   3. Note: cerebral spinal fluid is drained via reabsorption into the superior sagittal sinus.

C. Veins of the face: venous drainage of the face and oral cavity (Figure 1–4).
   1. Facial vein
      a. Serves as the major source of venous drainage for superficial facial structures, or the same areas that are supplied by the facial artery.
      b. Termination: the facial vein will join with the retromandibular vein to form the common facial vein, which drains into the internal jugular vein.
      c. Tributaries: supratrochlear, supraorbital, nasal, superior and inferior labial, muscular, submental, tonsillar, and submandibular veins.
      d. Dental significance: since the facial vein has no valves to maintain the direction of blood flow and it communicates with the cavernous sinus via the superior ophthalmic and deep facial vein, infection from the facial vein can travel to the cavernous sinus and cause severe medical problems (refer to cavernous sinus thrombosis, p. 6).
   2. Superior and inferior ophthalmic veins
      a. Drain tissues of the orbit.

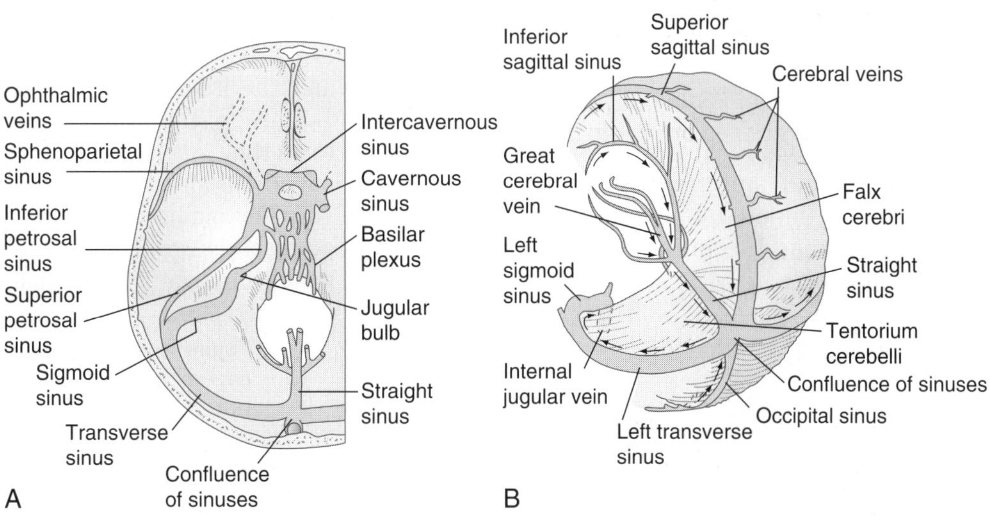

Figure 1–3. Dural venous sinuses. *Arrows note the direction of blood flow.* (From Moore NA, Roy WA: Gross and Developmental Anatomy, St. Louis, Mosby, 2002.)

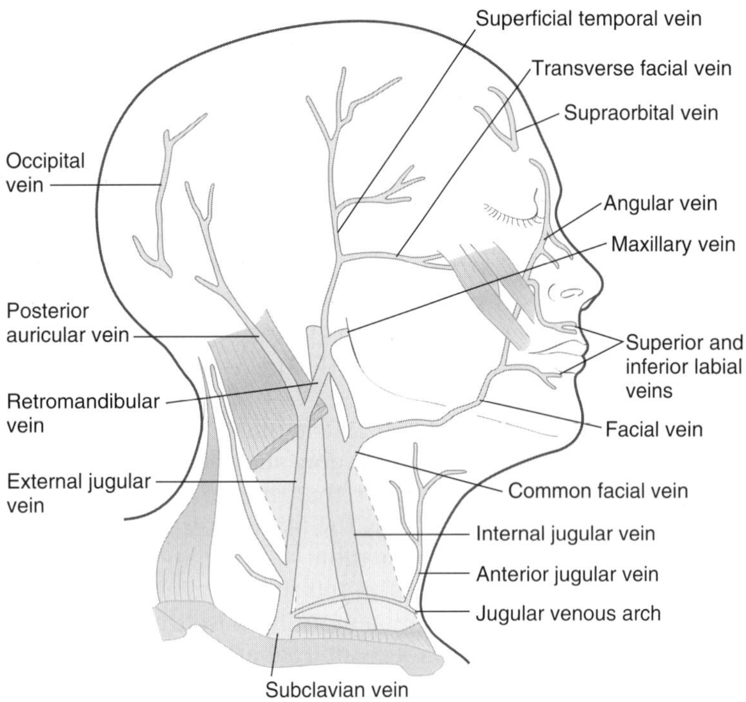

Figure 1–4. Lateral view of veins of the neck and superficial head. (From Moore NA, Roy WA: Gross and Developmental Anatomy, St. Louis, Mosby, 2002.)

b. Communicate with the facial vein via the supraorbital vein.
c. Termination: facial vein and cavernous sinus.

3. Retromandibular veins
   a. Formed by the joining of the maxillary and superficial temporal veins in the parotid gland.
   b. Termination: the retromandibular vein bifurcates into an anterior and posterior division. The anterior division descends and joins the facial vein to become the common facial vein, which terminates into the internal jugular vein. The posterior division terminates into the external jugular vein.
4. Pterygoid plexus
   a. A network of veins located at the level of the pterygoid muscles that drains deoxygenated blood from deep facial tissues, including the intraoral cavity, and the meninges.
   b. Termination: drains into the retromandibular vein via the maxillary veins.
   c. Tributaries include middle meningeal, infraorbital, sphenopalatine, muscular, buccal, palatine, inferior alveolar, and deep facial veins.
5. Cavernous sinuses
   a. Located on both sides of the sella turcica of the sphenoid bone. The right and left cavernous sinuses are joined by the intercavernous sinuses.
   b. Tributaries include the ophthalmic and external cerebral veins, the sphenoparietal sinuses, and the pterygoid plexuses.
   c. Structures running through the cavernous sinus include CN III, IV, V_1, V_2, VI, and the internal carotid artery (Figure 1–5). Note: these nerves and the structures they innervate can be affected by a cavernous sinus infection.
   d. Termination: the superior and inferior petrosal sinuses. The petrosal sinuses ultimately drain into the internal jugular vein.

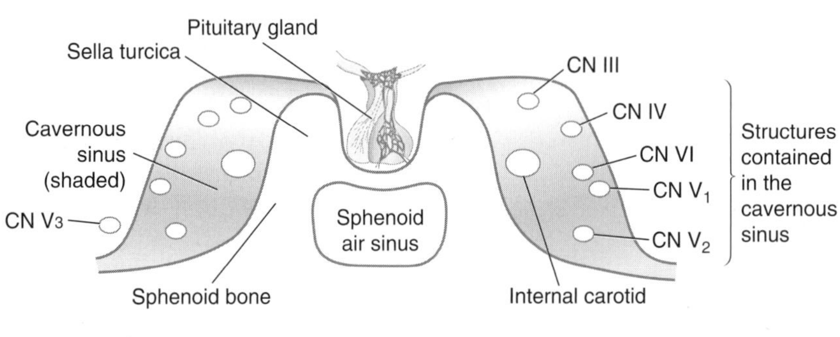

Figure 1–5. Coronal aspect of the cavernous sinus with its contents noted.

e. Cavernous sinus thrombosis: since blood flow in the cavernous sinus is slow-moving, dental or eye infections that spread to the cavernous sinuses can result in an infective blood clot, called *cavernous sinus thrombosis*. This can result in an urgent, and possibly fatal, medical emergency. The infection has the potential to spread as a result of certain venous communications with the cavernous sinus, including:
   (1) Superior ophthalmic vein—drains into the cavernous sinus. The superior ophthalmic vein can also act as a passageway for infection to spread from the facial vein to the cavernous sinus, since they are joined via the angular vein.
   (2) Deep facial vein—drains into the pterygoid plexus of veins, which in turn drains into the cavernous sinus. The deep facial vein is a tributary of the facial vein.

Lymphatic drainage

A. Lymphatic drainage of the head and neck is accomplished through a series of lymphatic vessels and lymph nodes. Lymph from a region is first drained into a primary lymph node, then a secondary lymph node, and ultimately ends up in the venous circulation.
   1. Superficial lymph nodes
      a. Submandibular nodes
         (1) Located beneath the angle of the mandible.
         (2) Secondary node: the submandibular nodes will drain into the deep cervical lymph nodes.
         (3) Tissues drained include the lower eyelids, nose, cheek, maxillary sinus, upper lip, palate, sublingual and submandibular glands, tongue body, all the maxillary teeth except the third molar, and all the mandibular teeth except the incisors.
      b. Submental nodes
         (1) Located beneath the chin.
         (2) Secondary node: lymph from the submental lymph nodes drains into the submandibular or deep cervical lymph nodes.
         (3) Tissues drained include the lower lip, mandibular incisors, floor of the mouth, the tongue apex, and the chin.
      c. Superficial parotid nodes
         (1) Located on the surface of the parotid gland.
         (2) Secondary node: deep cervical lymph nodes.
         (3) Tissues drained include the scalp, eyelids, external ear, and lacrimal gland.
      d. Retroauricular nodes
         (1) Located adjacent to the mastoid process.
         (2) Secondary node: deep cervical nodes.
         (3) Tissues drained include the scalp and external ear.
      e. Occipital nodes
         (1) Located at the occipital region of the skull.
         (2) Secondary node: deep cervical nodes.
         (3) Tissues drained include the scalp.

B. Deep lymph nodes
   1. Retropharyngeal nodes
      a. Located within the retropharyngeal space.
      b. Secondary node: superior deep cervical nodes.
      c. Tissues drained include the hard and soft palate, paranasal sinuses, nasopharynx, and the nasal cavity.
   2. Deep parotid nodes
      a. Located within the parotid gland.
      b. Secondary node: deep cervical nodes.
      c. Tissues drained include the parotid gland and middle ear.

C. Deep cervical nodes
   1. The chain of deep cervical nodes extends vertically down the entire length of the neck. They receive lymph from both superficial and deep lymph nodes.
   2. Termination
      a. The left deep cervical chains form the left jugular lymph trunk, which terminates in the thoracic duct.
      b. The right deep cervical chains form the right jugular lymph trunk, which terminates in the right lymphatic duct.

1.1.2 Cranial Nerves

Basic principles and definitions

A. Basic principles and definitions
   1. There are 12 cranial nerves; they are listed in Table 1–5.
   2. Function: cranial nerves function as sensory and/or motor neurons. Four cranial nerves (CN III, VII, IX, and X) also have parasympathetic functions (Table 1–5).

Table 1–3. Superficial Lymph Nodes

PRIMARY NODE	TISSUES DRAINED	SECONDARY NODE
Submandibular nodes	Lower eyelids Nose Cheek Maxillary sinus Upper lip Palate Sublingual gland Submandibular gland Maxillary teeth, except third molar Mandibular teeth, except incisors Tongue body	Deep cervical nodes
Submental nodes	Lower lip Mandibular incisors Floor of the mouth Tip of the tongue Chin	Submandibular or deep cervical nodes
Superficial parotid nodes	Scalp Eyelids External ear Lacrimal gland	Deep cervical nodes
Retroauricular nodes	Scalp External ear	Deep cervical nodes
Occipital nodes	Scalp	Deep cervical nodes

Table 1–4. Deep Lymph Nodes

	LOCATION	STRUCTURES DRAINED
Superior deep cervical lymph nodes	Inferior to the anterior border of the sternocleidomastoid muscles	Maxillary third molars Nasal cavity Palate Tongue
Deep parotid nodes	Middle ear Parotid gland	Deep cervical nodes
Retropharyngeal lymph nodes	Posterior pharynx, at the level of C1 vertebrae	Nasal cavity Palate Sinuses Pharynx

3. Foramen: a hole in bone. In this context, it specifically refers to the opening where a particular nerve passes through in the skull.
4. Ganglion: group of nerve cell bodies found outside the central nervous system (CNS).
5. Reflexes: cranial nerves also serve as afferent and efferent nerves for certain reflexes associated with the head and neck. These nerve reflexes are summarized in Table 1–6.

B. Cranial nerve pneumonics
   1. Cranial nerves: "Oh, Oh, Oh, To Touch and Feel Very Good, Very Awesome Humps."

Table 1–5. Summary of the Cranial Nerves

	NERVE	SENSORY	MOTOR	PARASYMPATHETIC
CN I	Olfactory	X	—	—
CN II	Optic	X	—	—
CN III	Oculomotor	—	X	X
CN IV	Trochlear	—	X	—
CN V	Trigeminal	X	X	—
CN VI	Abducens	—	X	—
CN VII	Facial	X	X	X
CN VIII	Vestibulocochlear	X	—	—
CN IX	Glossopharyngeal	X	X	X
CN X	Vagus	X	X	X
CN XI	Accessory	—	X	—
CN XII	Hypoglossal	—	X	—

TABLE 1–6. REFLEXES

	AFFERENT	EFFERENT
Corneal (blink) reflex	CN V_1	CN VII
Gag reflex	CN IX	CN X
Jaw jerk	CN V_3	CN V_3
Oculocardiac relex	CN V_1	CN X

2. Function: "Some Say Marry Money, But My Brother Says Big Brains Matter More." For example: CN I is Sensory, CN II is Sensory, CN III is Motor, CN IV is Motor, CN V is Both sensory and motor, and so forth.

Cranial nerve nuclei

A. Cranial nerve nuclei
   1. Nucleus: a group of nerve cell bodies in the CNS.
   2. Brainstem organization
      a. The brainstem plays a major role in transmitting information from the cranial nerves to and from the brain. The brainstem can be divided into three parts: the midbrain, pons, and medulla.
      b. Cell bodies of cranial nerves that share common functions are grouped into different clusters or nuclei. These motor and sensory nuclei are scattered throughout the brainstem and cervical spinal cord.
      c. The cranial nerve nuclei are listed in Tables 1–7 and 1–8.

Cranial nerves

A. CN I: olfactory nerve
   1. Foramen: cribriform plate of ethmoid bone.
   2. Sensory function: smell.
   3. Anatomic pathway: from the nasal epithelium, olfactory nerves cross the cribriform plate to join the olfactory bulb in the brain.

B. CN II: optic nerve
   1. Foramen: optic canal.
   2. Sensory distribution: vision.
   3. Anatomic pathway: there are two optic nerves. Each optic nerve consists of medial (nasal) and lateral (temporal) processes. When the right optic nerve leaves the retina, its medial process crosses over the midline at the optic chiasm and joins the lateral process from the left side, forming the left optic tract. The right lateral process remains on the right side, and together with the left medial process forms the right optic tract. The optic tract continues to the lateral geniculate nucleus of the thalamus (Figure 1–6).
   4. Note: the central artery of the retina, a branch of the ophthalmic artery, courses through the optic nerve.

C. CN III: oculomotor nerve
   1. Foramen: superior orbital fissure.
   2. Motor distribution: superior, medial, and inferior rectus muscles, inferior oblique muscle (Figure 1–7), and levator palpebrae superioris, which raises the eyelid.
   3. Parasympathetic distribution: lacrimal gland, sphincter pupillae, and ciliary lens muscles. The last two control the papillary light reflex (constricts pupil) and

TABLE 1–7. CRANIAL NERVE MOTOR NUCLEI

	CRANIAL NERVES	LOCATION: MIDBRAIN	PONS	MEDULLA	FUNCTION
Oculomotor nuclei	CN III	X	—	—	Motor
Edinger-Westphal nucleus	CN III	X	—	—	Autonomic (parasympathetic)
Trochlear nucleus	CN IV	X	—	—	Motor
Trigeminal motor nucleus	CN V	—	X	—	Motor
Abducens nucleus	CN VI	—	X	—	Motor
Facial (motor) nucleus	CN VII	—	X	—	Motor
Superior salivatory nucleus	CN VII	—	X	—	Motor (secretory)
Nucleus ambiguus	CN IX, X, and XI	—	—	X	Motor
Dorsal motor nucleus of the vagus	CN X	—	—	X	Motor and autonomic (parasympathetic)
Hypoglossal nucleus	CN XII	—	—	X	Motor
Accessory nucleus	CN XI	*Located in the cervical spinal cord*			Motor

TABLE 1–8. CRANIAL NERVE SENSORY NUCLEI

	CRANIAL NERVES	LOCATION Midbrain	Pons	Medulla	FUNCTION
Mesencephalic nucleus	CN V	X	X	—	Proprioception, jaw jerk reflex, including periodontal ligament fibers involved in the reflex
Trigeminal main (chief) sensory nuclei, or descending tract of CN V	CN V	—	X	—	Sensory function of CN V, including touch on the face Blink reflex
Cochlear nucleus	CN VIII	—	X	—	Sensory function of CN VIII, including hearing
Vestibular nucleus	CN VIII	—	X	X	Sensory function of CN VIII, including body positioning and equilibrium
Spinal trigeminal nucleus	CN V	—	X	X	Sensory of CN V, including pain and temperature Contains fibers of primary sensory neurons
Nucleus of solitary tract, or solitary nucleus	CN VII, IX, and X	—	X	X	Sensory of CN VII, IX, and X, including taste

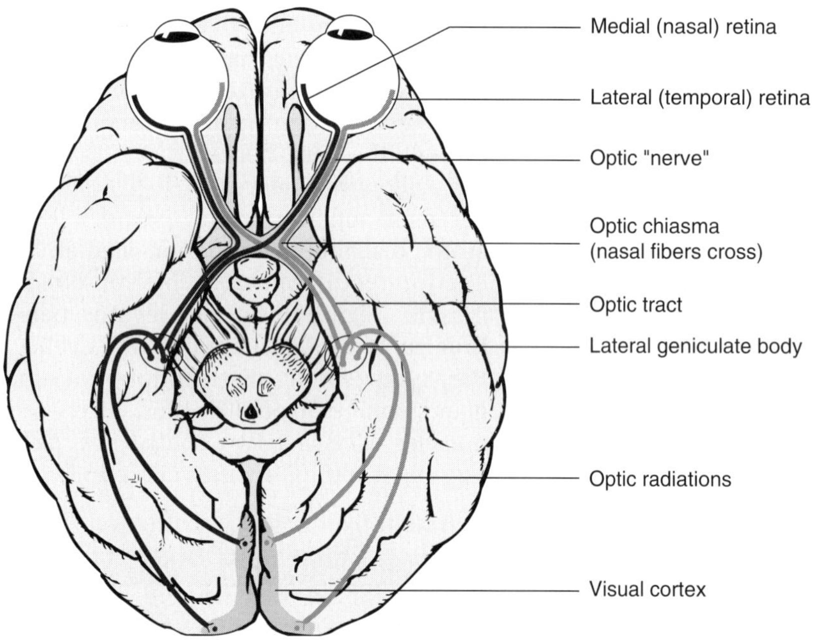

Figure 1–6. Optic pathway of CN II. (Modified from Liebgott B: The Anatomic Basis of Dentistry, ed 2, St. Louis, Mosby, 2001.)

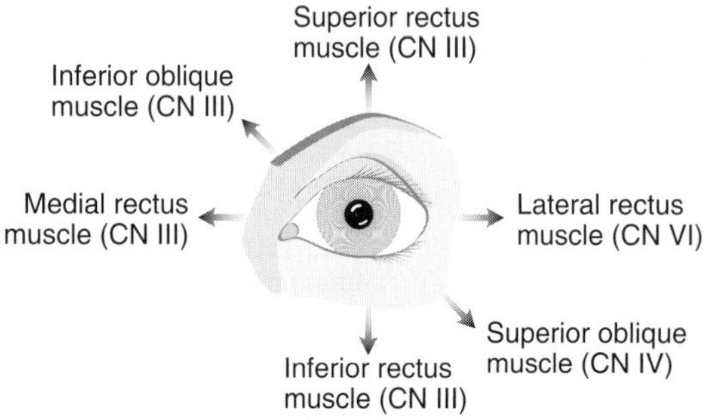

Figure 1–7. Muscles and nerves involved in the coordination of eye movements.

shape of the lens (constricts for near vision), respectively.

4. Motor pathway: oculomotor nerve fibers run through the oculomotor nucleus in the midbrain to the extrinsic eye muscles.
5. Parasympathetic pathway: preganglionic nerve fibers originate at the Edinger-Westphal nucleus in the midbrain and are carried by the oculomotor nerve to the ciliary ganglion, where postganglionic neurons extend to the lacrimal gland and eye (Figure 1–8).

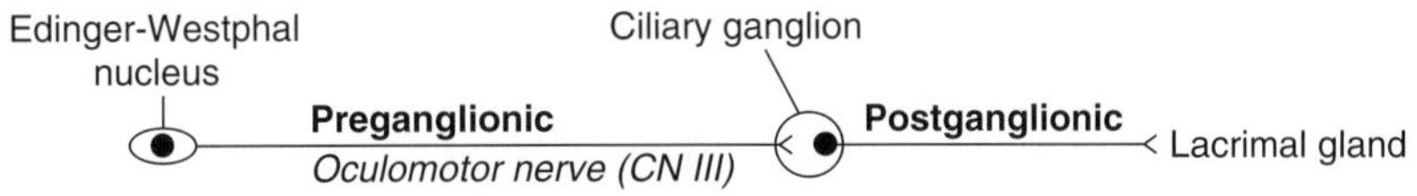

Figure 1–8. Scheme of parasympathetic nerve fibers of CN III.

6. Pneumonic: all eye muscles are innervated by CN III (oculomotor) except SO_4LR_6 (i.e., the superior oblique is innervated by CN IV and lateral rectus is innervated by CN VI).

D. CN IV: Trochlear nerve
   1. Foramen: superior orbital fissure.
   2. Motor distribution: superior oblique muscle, which moves the eyeball laterally and downward.

E. CN V: Trigeminal nerve
   1. Three divisions:
      a. V_1—ophthalmic nerve.
      b. V_2—maxillary nerve.
      c. V_3—mandibular nerve.
   2. V_1—ophthalmic nerve
      a. Foramen: superior orbital fissure.
      b. Sensory distribution: cornea, eyes, nose, forehead, and paranasal sinuses (Figure 1–9).
      c. Sensory pathway: the ophthalmic nerve branches from the trigeminal ganglion and exits the skull via the superior orbital fissure. It then divides into three major nerves: the frontal, lacrimal, and nasociliary nerves.
   3. V_2—maxillary nerve
      a. Foramen: foramen rotundum.

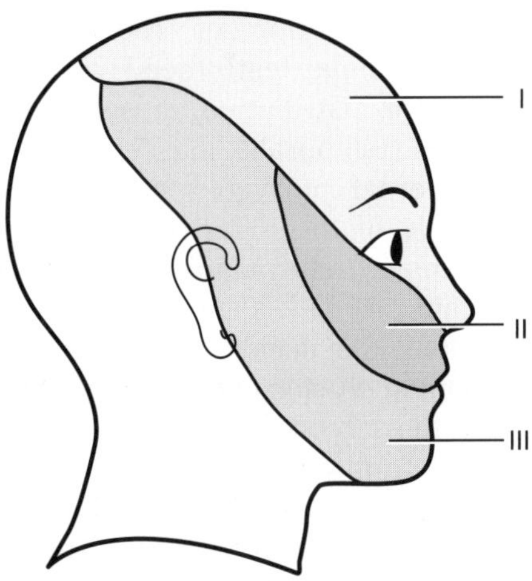

Figure 1–9. Sensory distribution for the three divisions of the trigeminal nerve. (Modified from Fehrenbach M, Herring S: Illustrated Anatomy of the Head and Neck, ed 2, Philadelphia, WB Saunders, 2002.)

      b. Sensory distribution: cheek, lower eyelid, upper lip, nasopharynx, tonsils, palate, and maxillary teeth (Figure 1–9).
      c. Sensory pathway: the maxillary nerve branches from the trigeminal ganglion and exits the skull through the foramen rotundum. It then passes through the pterygopalatine fossa, where it communicates with the pterygopalatine ganglion and terminates as the infraorbital and zygomatic nerves (Figure 1–10, Table 1–9).
      d. Pterygopalatine ganglion: branches of the pterygopalatine ganglion consist of sensory, sympathetic, and parasympathetic fibers and include nerves traveling to the lacrimal gland, oral cavity, upper pharynx, and nasal cavity.
      e. Infraorbital nerve: the posterior superior alveolar nerve branches off the infraorbital nerve in the pterygopalatine fossa. The infraorbital nerve then passes through the inferior orbital fissure to enter the orbit floor, coursing along the infraorbital groove toward the infraorbital canal. In the canal, the middle superior and anterior superior alveolar nerves branch off. The infraorbital nerve then exits the maxilla via the infraorbital foramen.
      f. Zygomatic nerve: after branching from the maxillary nerve, the zygomatic nerve passes through the orbit after entering from the superior orbital fissure. A nerve branches off to the lacrimal gland, carrying with it parasympathetic fibers from the pterygopalatine ganglion (CN VII). The zygomatic nerve continues into the zygomatic canal, where it divides into the zygomaticofacial and zygomaticotemporal nerves. It also travels to the lacrimal gland.
      g. Greater and lesser palatine nerves: the palatine nerves branch from the pterygopalatine ganglion and descend down the pterygopalatine canal toward the posterior palate.

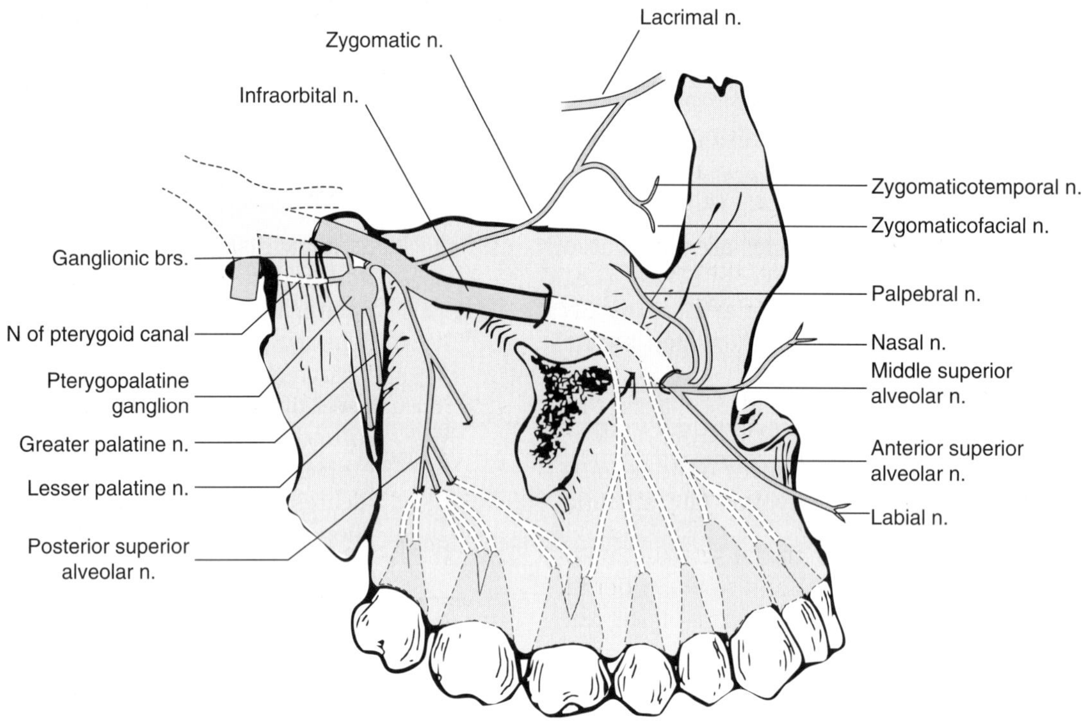

Figure 1–10. Branches of the maxillary nerve (CN V_2). (Modified from Liebgott B: The Anatomic Basis of Dentistry, ed 2, St. Louis, Mosby, 2001.)

TABLE 1–9. BRANCHES OF THE MAXILLARY NERVE (CN V_2)

V_2 BRANCH	FUNCTION	DISTRIBUTION
Posterior superior alveolar nerve	Sensory	Maxillary second and third molars Maxillary first molar: palatal and distobuccal root Maxillary sinus
Middle superior alveolar nerve	Sensory	Maxillary first and second premolars Maxillary first molar: mesiobuccal root
Anterior superior alveolar nerve	Sensory	Maxillary anterior teeth
Greater palatine nerve	Sensory	Posterior hard palate Lingual gingiva of maxillary posterior teeth
Lesser palatine nerve	Sensory	Soft palate Tonsils
Nasopalatine nerve	Sensory	Anterior hard palate Lingual gingiva of maxillary anterior teeth

h. Nasal branches: lateral nasal branches divide from the pterygopalatine ganglion toward the posterior nasal cavity. One of these branches, the nasopalatine nerve, extends past the septum, through the nasopalatine canal, and enters through the palate via the nasopalatine foramen. It also connects with the greater palatine nerve near the canine region.

4. V_3—mandibular nerve
   a. Foramen: foramen ovale.
   b. Sensory distribution: lower cheek, external auditory meatus, the temporomandibular joint (TMJ), chin, lower lip, tongue, floor of the mouth, and mandibular teeth (see Figure 1–9).
   c. Motor distribution: muscles of mastication (temporalis, masseter, internal and external pterygoid muscles), anterior belly of the digastric, tensor tympani, tensor veli palatine, and mylohyoid muscle.
   d. Note: the mandibular nerve (V_3) is the largest division of the trigeminal nerve and is the only one with motor function.
   e. Anatomic pathway: both motor and sensory fibers of the mandibular nerve exit the skull through the foramen ovale, where they form the mandibular trunk. The trunk then divides into an anterior and posterior division in the infratemporal fossa. The anterior trunk

further divides into the buccal (or long buccal), masseteric, lateral pterygoid, and deep temporal nerves. Divisions of the posterior trunk include the lingual, inferior alveolar, and auriculotemporal nerves (Figure 1–11, Table 1–10).

f. Inferior alveolar nerve (IAN): the IAN descends lateral to the lingual nerve and medial pterygoid muscle toward the mandibular foramen. It stays medial to the sphenomandibular ligament and lateral to the neck of the mandible within the pterygomandibular space. Before entering the foramen, the mylohyoid nerve branches off. The IAN then passes through the mandibular foramen into the mandibular canal, where it travels with the inferior alveolar artery and vein and forms a dental plexus, providing innervation to the mandibular posterior teeth. The IAN then divides into the mental nerve and the incisive nerve. The mental nerve exits the mandible via the mental foramen, which is usually located around the apex of the second mandibular premolar. The incisive

TABLE 1–10. BRANCHES OF THE MANDIBULAR DIVISION OF THE TRIGEMINAL NERVE (CN V_3)

V_3 BRANCH	FUNCTION	DISTRIBUTION
Long buccal nerve	Sensory	Cheek Buccal gingiva of posterior mandibular teeth Posterior buccal mucosa
Lingual nerve	Sensory	Lingual gingiva of mandibular teeth Floor of mouth
Inferior alveolar nerve	Sensory	Mandibular posterior teeth
Mental nerve	Sensory	Chin Lower lip Anterior labial mucosa
Incisive nerve	Sensory	Mandibular anterior teeth
Auriculotemporal nerve	Sensory	TMJ External auditory meatus Auricle
Deep temporal nerves, anterior and posterior	Motor	Temporalis muscle
Masseteric nerve	Motor	Masseter muscle
Lateral pterygoid nerve	Motor	Lateral pterygoid muscle

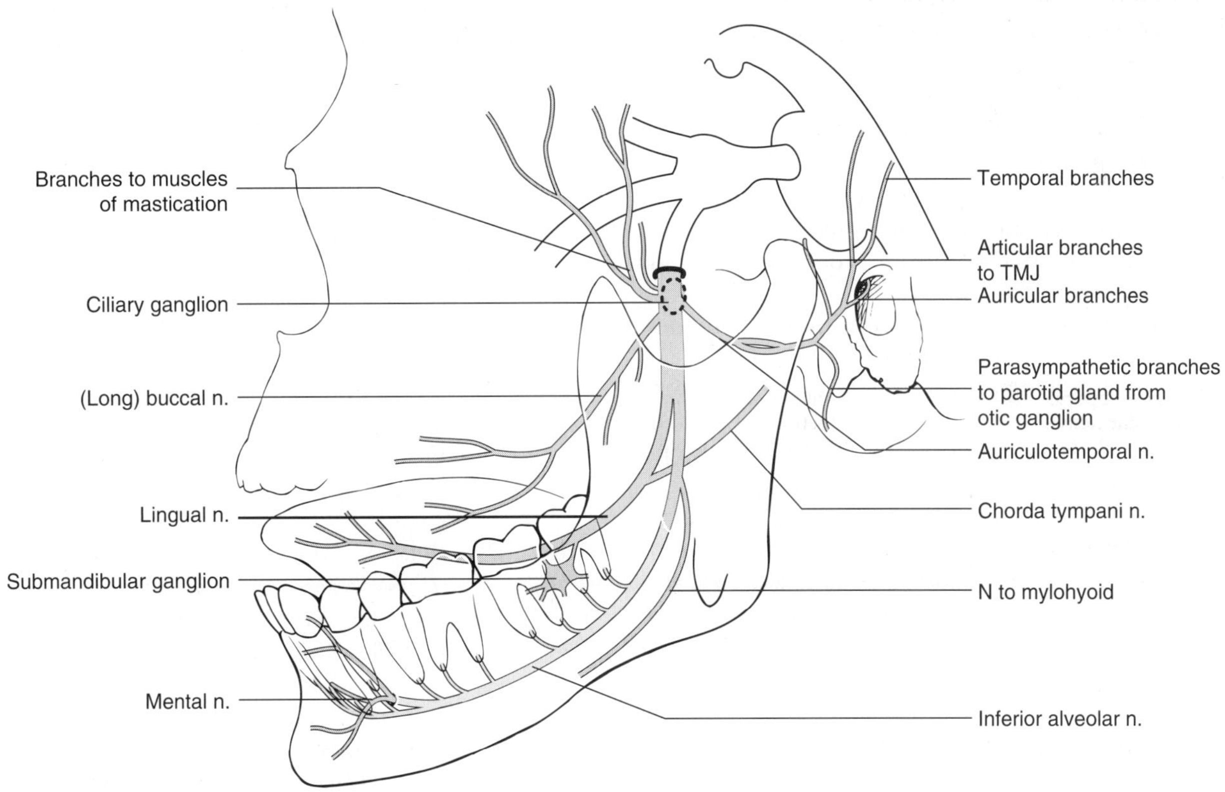

Figure 1–11. Branches of the mandibular division of the trigeminal nerve (CN V_3). (Modified from Liebgott B: The Anatomic Basis of Dentistry, ed 2, St. Louis, Mosby, 2001.)

nerve continues toward the mandibular anterior teeth.

g. Lingual nerve: the lingual nerve descends toward the base of the tongue, coursing between the medial pterygoid muscle and the mandible. It remains medial to the IAN. The chorda tympani (a branch from CN VII, containing parasympathetic fibers) joins it before it meets the submandibular ganglion, where it continues toward the submandibular and sublingual glands. The lingual nerve continues toward the tip of the tongue, crossing medially under the submandibular duct.

h. Auriculotemporal nerve: the auriculotemporal nerve travels posteriorly and encircles the middle meningeal artery remaining posterior and medial to the condyle. It continues up toward the TMJ, external ear, and temporal region, passing through the parotid gland and traveling with the superficial temporal artery and vein. Postganglionic parasympathetic nervous system fibers from the lesser petrosal branch, a branch from CN IX, join the auriculotemporal nerve to the parotid gland.

F. CN VI: Abducens nerve
1. Foramen: superior orbital fissure.
2. Motor distribution: lateral rectus muscle, which moves the eyeball laterally (i.e., abducts the eye) (Figure 1–7).

G. CN VII: Facial nerve
1. Sensory distribution: taste for the anterior two-thirds of the tongue.
2. Motor distribution: muscles of facial expression.
3. Parasympathetic distribution: sublingual, submandibular, and lacrimal glands.
4. Anatomic pathway: the facial nerve enters the internal acoustic meatus, located in the temporal bone. In the bone, the facial nerve communicates with the geniculate ganglion and the chorda tympani nerve branches off. The facial nerve then continues and descends to exit the skull via the stylomastoid foramen. The auricular nerve and nerves to the posterior belly of the digastric and stylohyoid muscles branch off before the facial nerve divides into five main branches: temporal, zygomatic, buccal, mandibular, and cervical branches (Figure 1–12). These nerves innervate the muscles of facial expression.
5. Greater petrosal nerve: the greater petrosal nerve branches from the geniculate ganglion, carrying preganglionic parasympathetic fibers in it, and travels through the foramen lacerum. It is then joined by the deep petrosal nerve (which contains sympathetic fibers from the carotid plexus) before it enters the pterygoid canal. It emerges as the nerve of the pterygoid canal. The nerve of the pterygoid canal continues toward the pterygopalatine fossa in the sphenoid bone, where it meets the pterygopalantine ganglion (Figure 1–13). Postganglionic parasympathetic fibers emerge from the ganglion and continue toward the lacrimal gland (along the zygomatic nerve, a branch of CN V_2), and smaller glands in the nasal cavity, upper pharynx, and palate (Figure 1–14).
6. Chorda tympani: the chorda tympani branches from the facial nerve, carrying both sensory fibers for taste and preganglionic parasympathetic fibers. It exits from of the temporal bone via the petrotympanic fissure and joins the lingual nerve (a branch of CN V_3) as it courses inferiorly toward the submandibular ganglion (see Figure 1–13). Postganglionic parasympathetic fibers emerge from the ganglion and continue toward the sublingual and submandibular glands (see Figure 1–14). Sensory fibers also branch from the nerve and provide taste sensation to the anterior two thirds of the tongue.

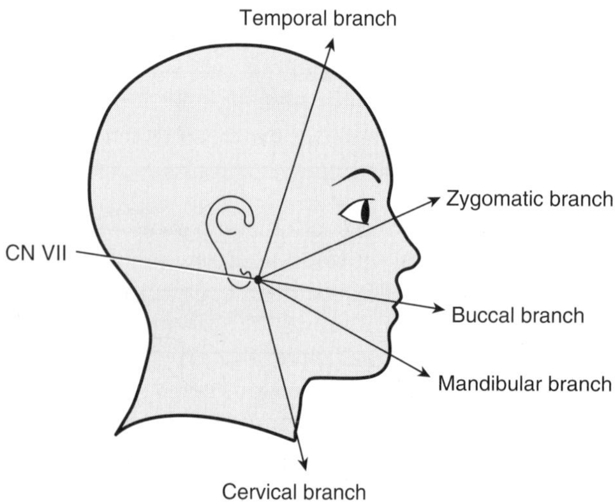

Figure 1–12. Facial nerve (CN VII): motor branches to the muscles of facial expression. (Modified from Fehrenbach M, Herring S: Illustrated Anatomy of the Head and Neck, ed 2, Philadelphia, W. B. Saunders, 2002.)

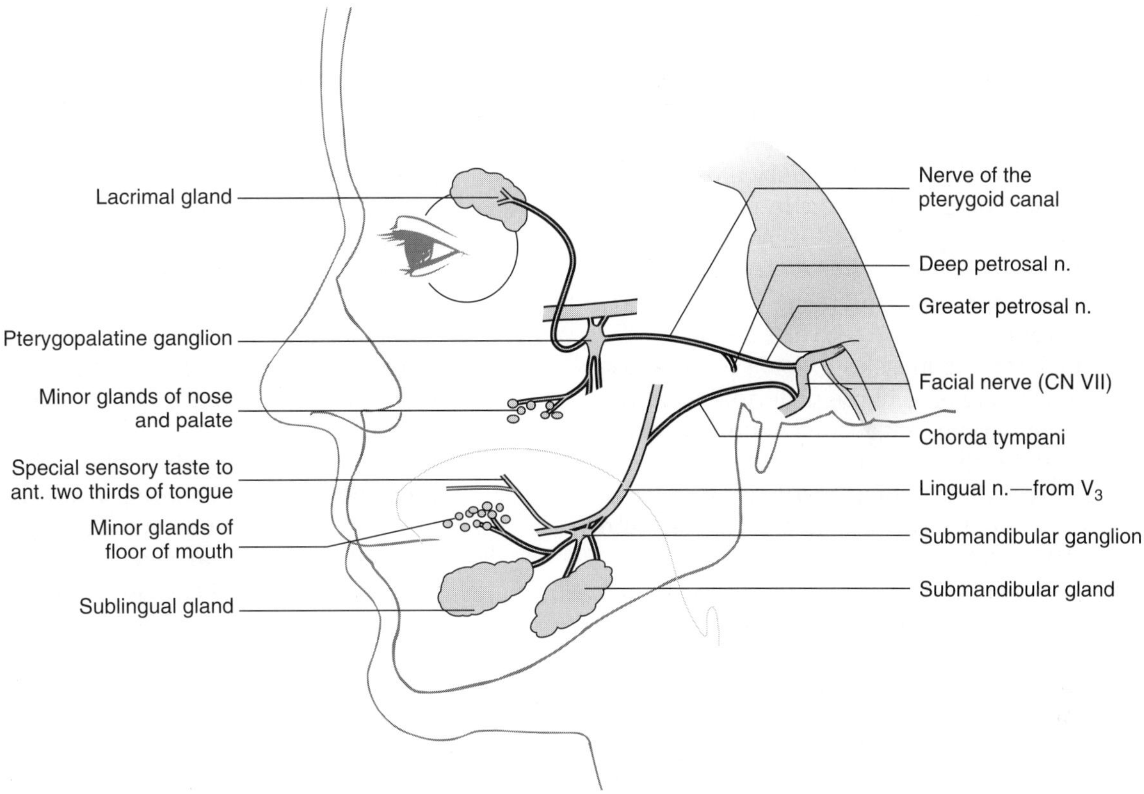

Figure 1–13. Facial nerve (CN VII) branches: greater petrosal nerve and chorda tympani. (Modified from Liebgott B: The Anatomic Basis of Dentistry, ed 2, St. Louis, Mosby, 2001.)

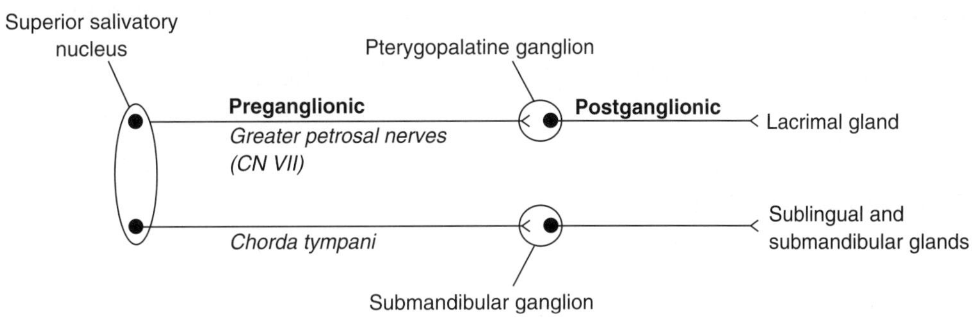

Figure 1–14. Scheme of parasympathetic nerve fibers of CN VII.

H. CN VIII: Vestibulocochlear nerve
   1. Foramen: internal auditory meatus.
   2. Sensory distribution: equilibrium, balance, and hearing.

I. CN IX: Glossopharyngeal nerve
   1. Foramen: jugular foramen.
   2. Sensory distribution: posterior one-third of the tongue (taste), pharynx, tonsils, middle ear, carotid sinus.
   3. Parasympathetic distribution: parotid gland.
   4. Motor and sensory pathways: the glossopharyngeal nerve exits the skull via the jugular foramen. It descends to the superior and inferior ganglion of CN IX, where the tympanic nerve of Jacobson (or tympanic nerve) branches off. Both ganglia contain sensory and motor cell bodies. The glossopharyngeal nerve then continues inferiorly to provide sensory and motor function to the posterior tongue, middle ear, pharynx, stylopharyngeus muscle, and carotid sinus.
   5. Parasympathetic pathway: the tympanic nerve carries preganglionic parasympathetic fibers toward the tympanic cavity

and plexus. It continues from there as the lesser petrosal nerve toward the otic ganglion, located behind the mandibular nerve (CN V_3). Postganglionic parasympathetic fibers emerge from the ganglion and travel along the auriculotemporal branch from CN V_3 to the parotid gland (Figure 1–15).

J. CN X: vagus nerve
   1. Foramen: jugular foramen.
   2. Motor distribution (with fibers from CN XI): the laryngeal muscles (phonation, swallowing), all muscles of the pharynx except the stylopharyngeus, and all muscles of the palate except the tensor veli palatine.
   3. Sensory distribution: posterior one third of the tongue (taste), heart, lungs, and abdominal organs.
   4. Parasympathetic distribution: heart, lungs, abdominal organs.
   5. Anatomic pathway: the vagus nerve exits the skull via the jugular foramen at the medulla. It descends through the superior and inferior ganglion of the vagus nerve, giving off branches in the pharynx and larynx. The vagus nerve descends and is accompanied by the carotid artery and jugular vein within the carotid sheath as it enters the thoracic area. In the thorax, the right and left vagus nerves then give off the right and left recurrent laryngeal nerves, respectively, which both travel back up to into the neck. The two vagus nerves meet to form the esophageal plexus. Past the diaphragm, the joined vagus nerves (esophageal plexus) divide into the anterior and posterior vagal trunks.
   6. Pharyngeal branches: the pharyngeal nerves branch from the inferior ganglion of the vagus nerve and travel to provide motor function to muscles of the pharynx.
   7. Superior laryngeal branches: branch from the vagus nerve just below the inferior ganglion. They divide into external and internal laryngeal branches.
      a. The external laryngeal nerve provides motor innervation to the cricothyroid muscle and inferior pharyngeal constrictor muscles.
      b. The internal laryngeal nerve travels with the superior laryngeal artery and pierce through the thyrohyoid membrane to provide sensory innervation to mucous membranes from the base of the tongue to the vocal folds. The internal laryngeal nerve also carries parasympathetic fibers.
   8. Recurrent laryngeal branches: the right recurrent laryngeal nerve ascends back to the neck around the subclavian artery. The left recurrent laryngeal nerve passes around the arch of the aorta or ligamentum arteriosum, before traveling up between the trachea and esophagus. As they ascend, the nerves provide sensory and parasympathetic innervation to mucous membranes and structures up to the vocal cords. The nerves then continue as the inferior laryngeal nerves in the larynx, providing motor innervation to all the muscles of the larynx, except the cricothyroid muscle. A motor branch also provides innervation to the inferior pharyngeal constrictor muscle.

K. CN XI: Accessory nerve
   1. Foramen: jugular foramen.
   2. Sensory distribution: sternocleidomastoid and trapezius muscles. Also joins with CN X in supplying motor function to palatal, laryngeal, and pharyngeal muscles.

L. CN XII: Hypoglossal nerve
   1. Foramen: hypoglossal canal.
   2. Motor distribution: intrinsic muscles of the tongue, genioglossus, hyoglossus, and styloglossus muscles.

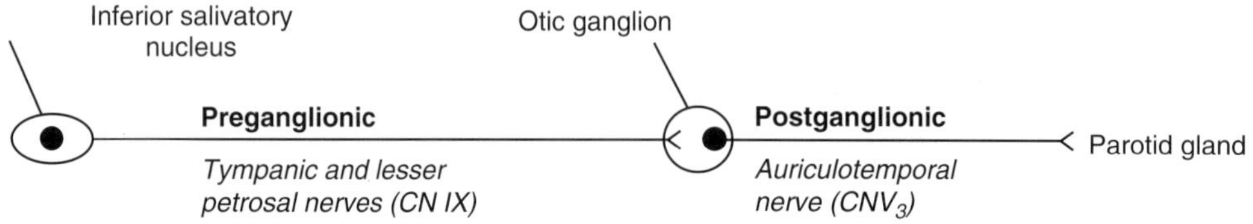

Figure 1–15. Scheme of parasympathetic nerve fibers of CN IX.

Spaces and cavities of the head and neck

Potential spaces, or fascial spaces, of the head and neck region are important for a dentist to know because many of these spaces communicate with the oral cavity. Odontogenic infections can therefore spread to these areas.

A. Spaces of the maxillary region
 1. Vestibular space of the maxilla
  a. Location: between the buccinator muscle and oral mucosa. It is inferior to the alveolar process.
  b. Potential odontogenic source of infection: maxillary molars.
 2. Canine fossa
  a. Location: positioned just posteriorly and superiorly to the roots of the maxillary canines. It remains inferior to the orbicularis oculi muscle, posterior to the levator muscles, and anterior to the buccinator muscle.
  b. Potential odontogenic source of infection: maxillary canines and first premolars.
 3. Canine space
  a. Location: situated within the superficial fascia over the canine fossa. It is posterior to the orbicularis oris muscle and anterior to the levator anguli oris muscle.
  b. Communications: buccal space.
 4. Buccal space
  a. Location: between the buccinator and masseter muscles.
  b. Consists of the buccal fat pad.
  c. Communications: canine and pterygomandibular spaces and space of the body of the mandible.

B. Spaces of the mandibular region
 1. Vestibular space of the mandible
  a. Location: between the buccinator muscle and oral mucosa. It is inferior to the alveolar process.
  b. Potential odontogenic source of infection: mandibular posterior teeth and canines.
 2. Space of the body of the mandible
  a. Location: between the body of the mandible and its periosteum.
  b. Potential odontogenic source of infection: all mandibular teeth.
  c. Communications: buccal, submental, submandibular and sublingual spaces, and the vestibular space of the mandible.
 3. Masticator space—includes four spaces:
  a. Temporal space
   (1) Location: between the temporalis muscle and its fascia.
   (2) Communications: infratemporal and submasseteric spaces.
  b. Infratemporal space
   (1) Location: laterally, it is bordered by the mandible and temporalis muscle. Medially, it is bordered by the lateral pterygoid plate and pharynx. It is inferior to the greater wing of the sphenoid bone.
   (2) Contents: maxillary artery and its branches, mandibular nerve and its branches, and the pterygoid plexus.
   (3) Infections of the infratemporal space are considered dangerous due to the potential of spread of infection to the cavernous sinus via the pterygoid plexus.
   (4) Potential odontogenic source of infection: maxillary third molars and infectious anesthetic needles.
  c. Submasseteric space
   (1) Location: between the masseter muscle and mandibular ramus.
   (2) Potential odontogenic source of infection: mandibular third molars (rare).
   (3) Communications: temporal and infratemporal spaces.
  d. Pterygomandibular space
   (1) Location: between the medial pterygoid muscle and mandibular ramus. It is inferior to the lateral pterygoid muscle.
   (2) Contains the inferior alveolar nerve and artery, lingual nerve, and chorda tympani.
   (3) This is the site for the inferior alveolar nerve anesthetic block.
   (4) Potential odontogenic source of infection: mandibular second and third molars. Also consider infectious anesthetic needles.
 4. Submental space
  a. Location: between the anterior bellies of the digastric muscles. It is superior to the suprahyoid muscles and inferior to the mylohyoid muscle.
  b. Contains the submental lymph nodes and anterior jugular vein.
  c. Potential odontogenic source of infection: mandibular central incisor, if the

apex of the incisor lies below the mylohyoid line. Note: Infection in this space causes swelling of the chin. If the infection spreads bilaterally to involve the sublingual and submandibular spaces, it is referred to as Ludwig's angina.
   d. Communications: space of the body of the mandible, submandibular and sublingual spaces.
5. Submandibular space
   a. Location: between the mylohyoid and platysma muscle. It is medial to the mandible and lateral to the anterior and posterior bellies of the digastric muscles.
   b. Contains the submandibular lymph nodes, submandibular salivary gland, and facial artery.
   c. Potential odontogenic source of infection: mandibular second and third molars.
   d. Communications: infratemporal, submental, sublingual and parapharyngeal spaces.
6. Sublingual space
   a. Location: between the tongue and its intrinsic muscles and the mandible. It is superior to the mylohyoid muscle and inferior to the sublingual oral mucosa.
   b. Contains the sublingual salivary gland, submandibular salivary gland duct, lingual nerve and artery, and CN XII.
   c. Potential odontogenic source of infection: mandibular anterior teeth, premolars, and mesial roots of the first molars, presuming that the apices of these teeth lie above the mylohyoid line.
   d. Communications: submental and submandibular spaces and the space of the body of the mandible.

C. Spaces of the neck
1. Parapharyngeal space
   a. Location: fascial space between the pharynx and medial pterygoid muscle, adjacent to the carotid sheath. It extends to the pterygomandibular raphe anteriorly, and around the pharynx posteriorly.
   b. Communications: masticator, submandibular, retropharyngeal, and previsceral spaces.
2. Retropharyngeal space
   a. Location: between the vertebral and visceral fasciae, just posterior to the pharynx. It extends from the base of the skull, posterior to the superior pharyngeal constrictor muscle, to the thorax.
   b. Because odontogenic infections can quickly spread down this space into the thorax, it is known as the *danger space*. For example, an untreated infection of a mandibular incisor, with an apex above the mylohyoid muscle, may spread along the following pathway: sublingual space → submandibular space → lateral pharyngeal or parapharyngeal space → retropharyngeal space → posterior mediastinum → possible death.
3. Pterygomandibular space
   a. Location: between the medial pterygoid muscle and mandibular ramus. It is inferior to the lateral pterygoid muscle.
   b. Contains the inferior alveolar nerve and artery, lingual nerve, and chorda tympani.
   c. This is the site for the inferior alveolar nerve anesthetic block.
   d. Potential odontogenic source of infection: mandibular third molars.
   e. Communications: parapharyngeal space.

1.1.3 Extraoral Structures

Ear

A. External ear
1. Includes the auricle and external auditory meatus (Figure 1–16).
2. The external auditory meatus (external ear) and tympanic cavity (middle ear) are separated by the tympanic membrane.
3. Tympanic membrane (eardrum)
   a. Its external surface is covered by epidermis (skin); its internal surface consists of a mucous membrane.
   b. It is transversed by the chorda tympani.
   c. Transfers sound vibrations from air to auditory ossicles.

B. Middle ear
1. Three bones: malleus, incus, and stapes (see Figure 1–16).
2. Loud sounds cause the tensor tympani (which attaches to the malleus) to contract, pulling the malleus and tympanic membrane inward to reduce vibrations and prevent damage.

C. Internal ear
1. Cochlea
   a. Senses hearing.

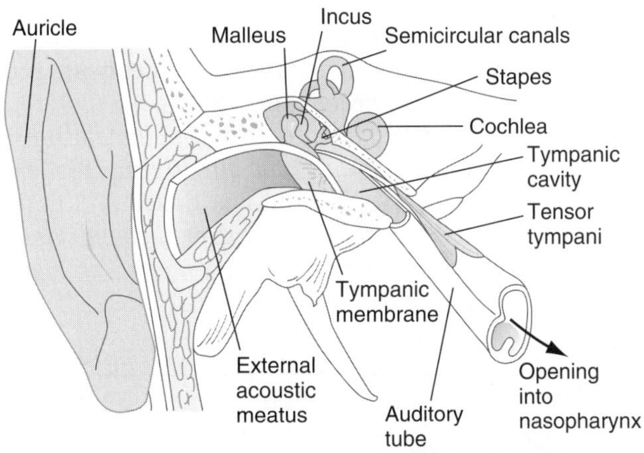

Figure 1–16. Right ear: external, middle, and inner ear. (Modified from Moore NA, Roy WA: Gross and Developmental Anatomy, St. Louis, Mosby, 2002.)

   b. Receptors (hair cells) for hearing are located in the organ of Corti. This spiral organ lies along the cochlear duct, over the basilar membrane.
2. Vestibule
   a. Senses equilibrium.
   b. Consists of the utricle and saccule.
3. Semicircular canals—sense balance and body position (see Figure 1–16).

Eye

Concentric layers or coats (Figure 1–17) and the lens

A. Fibrous layer
   1. Sclera—fibrous covering of the posterior five-sixths of the eyeball.
   2. Cornea—transparent, avascular layer that covers the center one sixth of the eyeball. It is more convex than the sclera and sticks out as a small lump.

B. Vascular coat
   1. Lies just behind the fibrous layer.
   2. Consists of the choroids, ciliary body, and iris.
   3. The center opening of the iris is the pupil. The size of the pupil is controlled by two muscles:
      a. Constrictor pupillae muscle—constricts the pupil. It is innervated by PNS fibers from CN III via the ciliary ganglion.
      b. Dilator pupillae muscle—dilates the pupil. It is innervated by sympathetic fibers.

C. Retina
   1. The inner lining of the eyeball.
   2. Photosensitive region.

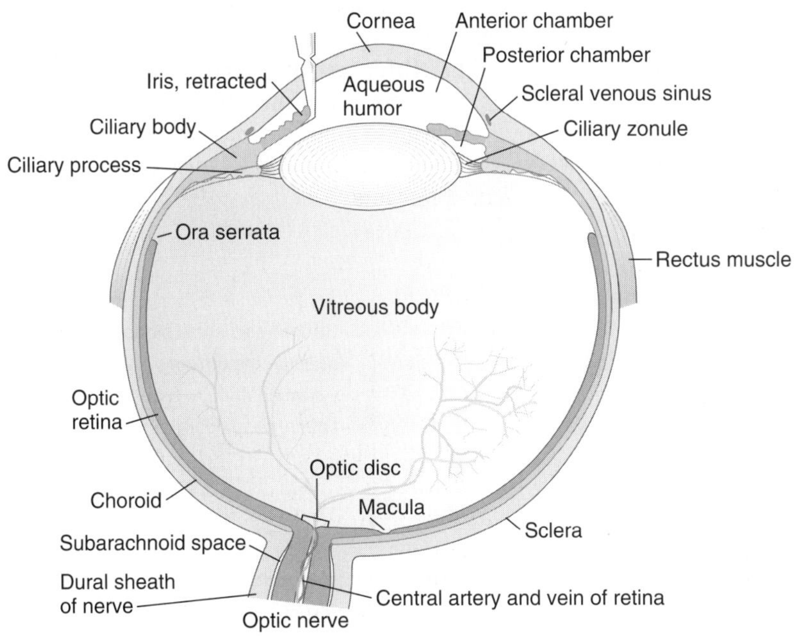

Figure 1–17. Right eyeball: superior view. (Modified from Moore NA, Roy WA: Gross and Developmental Anatomy, St. Louis, Mosby, 2002.)

a. Includes area posterior to the ora serrata.
b. Optic disc
   (1) Where the optic nerve exits.
   (2) Is void of photoreceptors (blind spot).
c. Fovea centralis
   (1) Located approximately 2.5 millimeters lateral to the optic disc in a yellow-pigmented area (macula luna).
   (2) Contains only cones. Vision is most acute from this area.
   (3) Note: as you move peripherally from this area, there is a decreasing number of cones and an increasing number of rods (see Figure 1–17).

3. Cells of the retina
   a. Epithelial cells
      (1) Comprise the pigment epithelium.
      (2) Change every 12 days.
   b. Photoreceptors—two types:
      (1) Rods
         (a) For nondiscriminative vision (low resolution). They are used for seeing in the dark and detecting motion.
         (b) Are highly convergent, making them very sensitive to light (Figure 1–18).
         (c) The density of rods increases toward the periphery of the eye. It decreases toward the center of the eye (macula and fovea centralis), where there are a greater number of cones.
      (2) Cones
         (a) For acute vision (high resolution). They are also used for color vision.
         (b) Are less convergent, which gives them higher resolution abilities.
         (c) Three types of cones: red, green, and blue.
         (d) The greatest concentration of cones is at the fovea. This area only contains cones and is the area with the highest visual acuity.

	CONES	RODS
Photopigment	Opsin	Rhodopsin
Convergence	Low	High
Sensitivity to light	Low	High
Resolution	High	Low

      (3) Photoreceptor membrane potentials
         (a) Low light (dark): a constant amount of cyclic guanosine monophosphate (cGMP) is released, causing sodium channels to open. This causes depolarization of the photoreceptor membrane, which results in the release of glutamate.
         (b) High light: causes decreased release of cGMP. This results in the closing of sodium channels, and the photoreceptor membrane hyperpolarizes.
   c. Bipolar cells—synapse with rods and cones.
   d. Ganglion cells—the axons of ganglion cells combine to form the optic nerve.
   e. Amacrine cells
      (1) Interneurons that connect bipolar and ganglion cells. May contribute

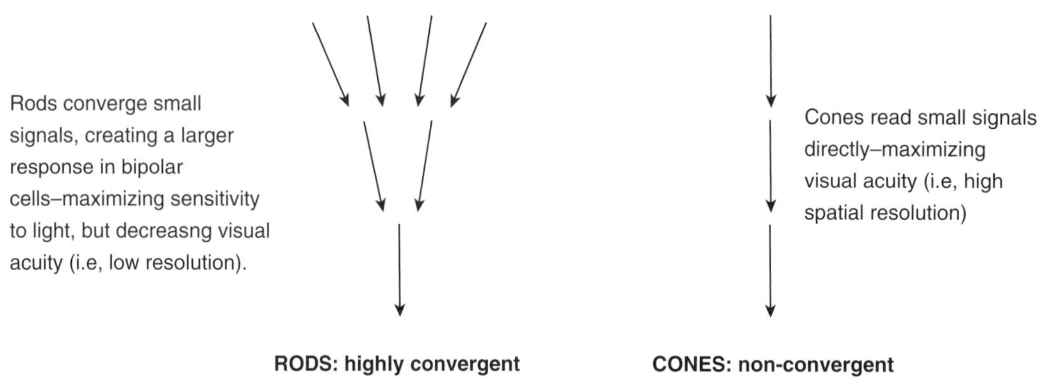

Figure 1–18. Photoreceptors: convergence.

to bidirectional communication between these two cells.

(2) May also play a role in detecting motion.

f. Horizontal cells

(1) Interneurons that connect rods and cones with each other and with bipolar cells.

(2) Axons aid in bidirectional communication between adjacent bipolar cells.

(3) Communication is via changes in membrane potential. No action potential is created.

D. Lens

The lens, by virtue of its shape, controls focusing for near or distant vision. The shape is controlled by:

1. Ciliary muscles. Contraction of these muscles leads to relaxation of:
   a. Fibers that suspend the lens, allowing it to become fatter and to focus for near vision.
   b. Stimulation of the parasympathetic nerve to the eye leads to contraction of the ciliary muscles and accommodation for near vision.

1.1.4 Osteology

Bones

A. The skull

1. There are a total of 22 cranial and facial bones in the skull (Figure 1–19). Note: some texts include the ossicles of the ears (total of six bones) in the total bone count, for a total of 28 bones in the skull.
   a. Cranial bones: ethmoid (1), frontal (1), occipital (1), parietal (2), sphenoid (1), temporal (2).
   b. Facial bones: inferior concha (2), lacrimal (2), mandible (1), maxilla (2), nasal (2), palatine (2), vomer (1), zygoma (2).
   c. Ossicles of the ears: malleus (2), incus (2), stapes (2).
2. Cranial sutures
   a. Coronal suture—joins the frontal and parietal bones (see Figure 1–19).
   b. Sagittal suture—joins the left and right parietal bones.
   c. Lambdoidal suture—joins the parietal and occipital bones (Figure 1–19).
   d. Squamosal suture—joins the parietal and temporal bones (Figure 1–19).

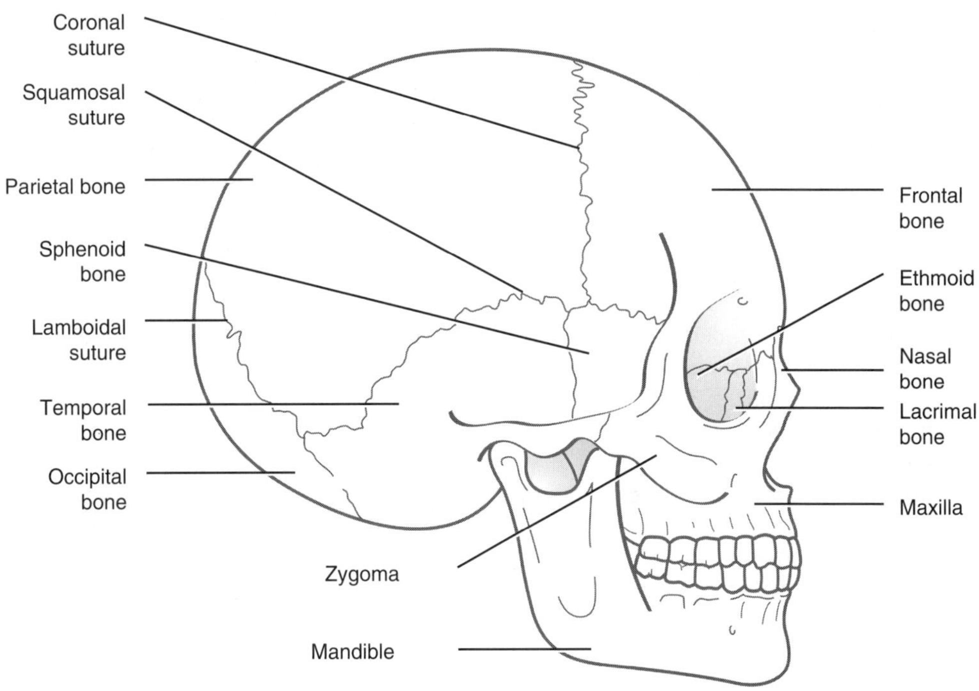

Figure 1–19. Lateral view of the skull: cranial bones and sutures. (Modified from Fehrenbach M, Herring S: Illustrated Anatomy of the Head and Neck, ed 2, Philadelphia, WB Saunders, 2002.)

e. Temporozygomatic suture—joins the zygomatic and temporal bones.
f. Medial palatine suture—joins the left and right palatine bones.
g. Transverse palatine suture—joins the maxilla and palatine bones.

3. Sphenoid bone
   a. The sphenoid bone is located along the midline of the cranium. It articulates with all the cranial bones and four facial bones: the maxilla, palatine bones, vomer, and zygoma.
   b. The sphenoid bone consists of a body, greater and lesser wings, and paired pterygoid processes.
      (1) The body contains the sphenoid sinuses.
      (2) The greater wing contributes to the roof of the infratemporal fossa and floor of the middle cranial fossa.
      (3) The lesser wing contains the optic canal, anterior clinoid process, and part of the superior orbital fissure.
      (4) The pterygoid process is composed of two thin plates: the medial and lateral pterygoid plates. The space between these two plates is the pterygoid fossa.
      (5) There is a space that forms between the pterygoid process and maxillae that is inferior and posterior to the orbit, called the *pterygopalatine fossa.*
   c. The sphenoid bone contains many foramina and fissures. This includes the foramen ovale, foramen rotundum and foramen spinosum, and the superior orbital fissure.
   d. Sella turcica—a cradle at the center of the bone that houses the pituitary gland.
4. Ethmoid bone
   a. The ethmoid bone is also located along the midline of the cranium. It articulates with the frontal, sphenoid, and lacrimal bones and the maxilla and vomer.
   b. Its structures include the cribriform plate, perpendicular plate, and the crista galli.
      (1) The cribriform plate serves as the roof of the nasal cavity and is pierced by olfactory nerves.
      (2) The perpendicular plate, along with the vomer and nasal septal cartilage, form the nasal septum.
   c. The ethmoid bone houses the ethmoid sinuses and forms the superior and middle nasal conchae.
5. Temporal bone
   a. The temporal bone forms the lateral walls of the skull. It articulates with the parietal, occipital, sphenoid, and zygomatic bones and the mandible.
   b. The temporal bone consists of three portions:
      (1) Squamous portion—includes the zygomatic process of the temporal bone. The inferior surface of the zygomatic process is the articular fossa. Anterior to this fossa is the articular eminence. This is where the TMJ articulates.
      (2) Petrous portion—includes the mastoid and styloid processes, the jugular and mastoid notches, inner and middle ear, and the carotid canal. Foramina include the stylomastoid foramen and the internal acoustic meatus.
      (3) Tympanic portion—includes the floor and anterior wall of the external acoustic meatus. It is separated from the petrous portion of the temporal bone via the petrotympanic fissure.
6. Maxilla
   a. The left and right maxilla fuse to form the maxillae. The maxillae articulates with the frontal, lacrimal, nasal, inferior nasal concha, vomer, zygoma, sphenoid, ethmoid, and palatine bones (Figure 1–20).
   b. Each maxilla consists of a body and four processes: the frontal, zygomatic, alveolar, and palatine processes.
      (1) The body contains the maxillary sinuses.
      (2) The frontal process:
         (a) Contains an orbital surface that is part of the inferior wall or floor of the orbit.
         (b) It also forms the medial orbital rim with the lacrimal bone.
         (c) A groove, or the infraorbital sulcus, is present on the floor of the orbit. It becomes the infraorbital canal and terminates at the infraorbital foramen.
         (d) The inferior orbital fissure separates the orbital surface from the sphenoid bone.

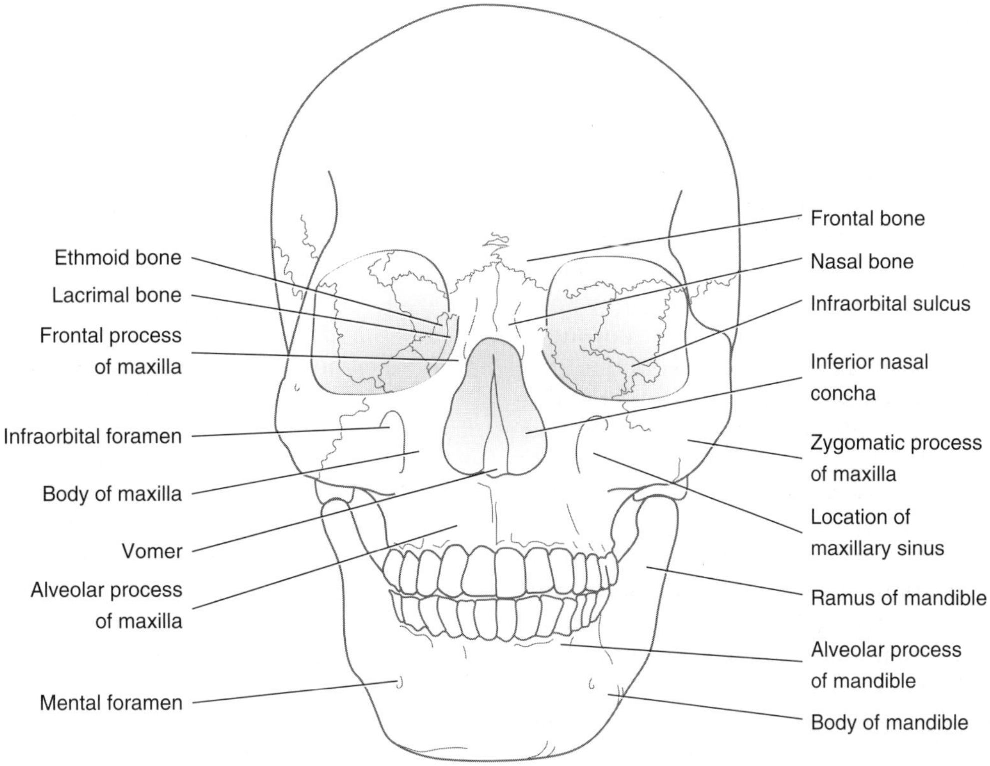

Figure 1–20. Anterior view of the skull: anterior aspect of the maxilla and mandible. (Modified from Fehrenbach M, Herring S: Illustrated Anatomy of the Head and Neck, ed 2, Philadelphia, WB Saunders, 2002.)

(3) The zygomatic process, along with the zygoma, forms the infraorbital rim.

(4) The alveolar process houses roots of the maxillary teeth. A bony prominence observed behind the upper third molar is known as the *maxillary tuberosity*.

(5) The right and left palatine processes, along with the palatine bones, fuse to form the hard palate (Figure 1–21). These two processes are separated by the median palatine suture. Anterior to this suture is the incisive foramen.

(6) Note: the posterior hard palate is covered by a fibrous, tendinous sheet called the *palatine aponeurosis*. The midline forms a ridge that is known as the *median palatine raphe*.

7. Mandible
   a. The mandible is a single bone that consists of two vertical rami, a horizontal

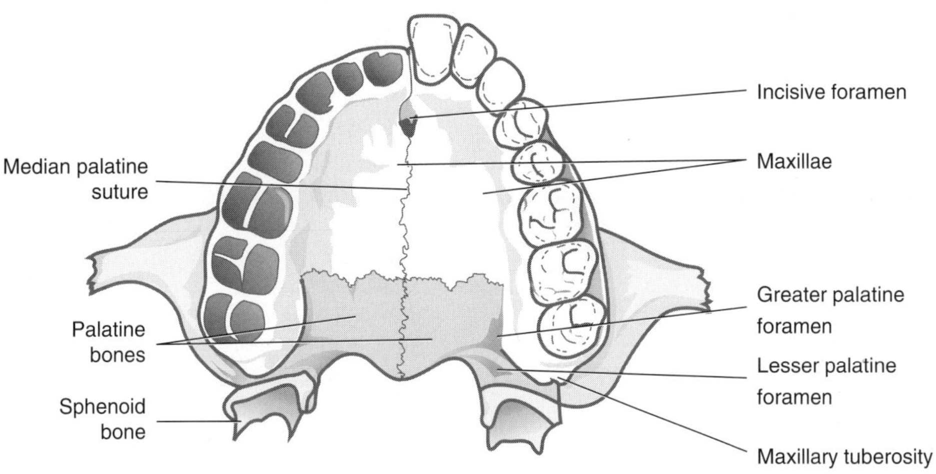

Figure 1–21. Inferior view of the hard palate. (Modified from Fehrenbach M, Herring S: Illustrated Anatomy of the Head and Neck, ed 2, Philadelphia, WB Saunders, 2002.)

body, and an alveolar process (see Figure 1–20).
(1) Each ramus includes a:
(a) Condyle—articulates with the mandibular fossa of the temporal bone to form the TMJ.
(b) Coronoid process—serves as an attachment for the temporal muscle.
(2) The anterior border of the ramus descends from the coronoid process to the external oblique line.
(3) The horizontal portion of the mandible consists of the body and alveolar process, which contain the roots of the lower teeth. If an imaginary horizontal line were drawn around the level of the mental foramen, it would separate the body from the alveolar process.
b. The mandible provides many surface landmarks.
(1) From the lateral aspect, important landmarks include the mental protuberance, the mental foramen, the external oblique line, the coronoid process, and the condyle (Figure 1–22, *A*).
(2) From the medial aspect, important landmarks include the mandibular foramen, lingula, the mylohyoid line and groove, the submandibular and sublingual fossa, and the retromolar triangle (Figure 1–22, *B*).
c. Mandibular growth takes place in several areas:
(1) The alveolar process and body increase in width and height.
(2) The mandibular arch is lengthened by adding bone to its posterior border of the ramus and removing bone from its anterior border.

B. Cranial openings
1. Cranial openings include foramina, canals, and meatus.
2. A summary of important cranial openings is presented in Table 1–11.

C. The orbit
1. The orbit is the cavity in the skull that houses and safeguards the eyeball. Seven cranial and facial bones make up the walls of each orbit, namely the frontal, sphenoid, zygomatic, palatine, ethmoid, maxilla, and lacrimal bones. A summary of these bones is presented in Table 1–12.
2. Bony openings of the orbit include the:
a. Optic canal—found at the apex of the orbit.
b. Inferior orbital fissure—separates the floor of the orbit from its lateral wall.
c. Superior orbital fissure—lies between the greater and lesser wings of the sphenoid bone.

D. The nasal cavity
1. The nasal cavity is divided into two parts by the nasal septum. Each side contains three conchae. The superior and middle

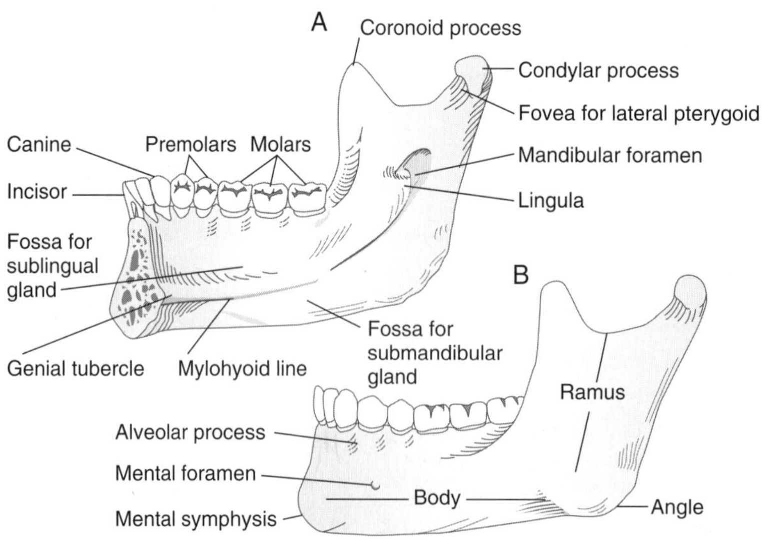

Figure 1–22. Landmarks of the mandible. A, Medial view. **B**, Lateral view. (Modified from Moore NA, Roy WA: Gross and Developmental Anatomy, St. Louis, Mosby, 2002.)

TABLE 1–11. CRANIAL OPENINGS, THEIR LOCATION, AND CONTENTS

FORAMEN	BONE	CONTENTS
Cribriform plate	Ethmoid	CN I
Foramen magnum	Occipital	CN XI and brainstem (medulla); vertebral and spinal arteries
Foramen ovale	Sphenoid	CN V_3
Foramen rotundum	Sphenoid	CN V_2
Foramen spinosum	Sphenoid	Middle meningeal vessels
Hypoglossal canal	Occipital bone	CN XII
Incisive foramen	Maxilla	Nasopalatine nerve
Inferior orbital fissure	Sphenoid, maxilla	CN V_2 (or infraorbital nerve) and zygomatic nerve; infraorbital artery, ophthalmic vein
Internal acoustic meatus	Temporal	CN VII and VIII
Jugular foramen	Occipital, temporal	CN IX, X, and XI; internal jugular vein
Optic canal	Sphenoid	CN II; ophthalmic artery
Stylomastoid foramen	Temporal	CN VII
Superior orbital fissure	Sphenoid	CN III, IV, V_1, and VI; ophthalmic veins

CN, cranial nerve; V_2 and V_3, second and third branch of CN V, respectively.

TABLE 1–12. SUMMARY OF THE CRANIAL AND FACIAL BONES THAT FORM THE ORBIT

ORBITAL STRUCTURE	BONES	COMMUNICATIONS
Roof or superior wall	Frontal bone—orbital plate Sphenoid bone—lesser wing	
Medial wall	Ethmoid bone—orbital plate	
Superior-medial wall	Lacrimal bone	
Inferior-medial wall	Frontal bone—orbital plates Maxilla—orbital plate	
Lateral wall	Zygomatic bone—frontal process Sphenoid bone—greater wing	Superior orbital fissure
Floor or inferior wall	Maxilla—orbital plate Zygomatic bone Palatine bone—orbital process	Inferior orbital fissure
Apex	Sphenoid bone—lesser wing Palatine bone	Optic canal

conchae are located in the ethmoid bone. The inferior conchae is a separate bone.

2. Between the conchae are small slit-like openings, or meatus, which allow communication between the nasal cavity and paranasal sinuses or the nasolacrimal duct. These openings include:
   a. Superior meatus—opens into the posterior ethmoid sinus.
   b. Middle meatus—consists of several openings, including the:
      (1) Semilunar hiatus—opens into the frontal, anterior ethmoid, and maxillary sinuses.
      (2) Ethmoid bulla—opens into the middle ethmoid sinus.
   c. Inferior meatus—communicates with the nasolacrimal duct, which drains tears from the eye.
   d. The sphenoid sinus directly communicates with the nasal cavity.
   e. Sphenopalatine foramen—opens into the pterygopalatine fossa.

E. Fossa

1. Pterygopalatine fossa
   a. Boundaries and communications of the pterygopalatine fossa are listed in Table 1–13.
   b. Communicates with the infratemporal fossa via the pterygomaxillary fissure.
   c. Contents: branches of the maxillary artery, branches of the maxillary nerve (CN V_2), and the pterygopalatine ganglion.
2. Infratemporal fossa
   a. Boundaries and communications of the infratemporal fossa are listed in Table 1–14.
   b. Contents: branches of the mandibular nerve (CN V_3), the chorda tympani, the otic ganglion, branches of the maxillary

TABLE 1–13. BOUNDARIES AND COMMUNICATIONS OF THE PTERYGOPALATINE FOSSA

AREA	BONES	COMMUNICATIONS
Roof	Sphenoid bone—body	—
Floor	Pterygopalatine canal	—
Anterior	Maxilla—tuberosity	Orbit via the inferior orbital fissure
Posterior	Sphenoid bone—pterygoid process	Pterygoid canal, foramen rotundum, and pharyngeal canal
Medial	Palatine bone—vertical plate	Nasal cavity via the sphenopalatine foramen
Lateral	Pterygomaxillary fissure	Infratemporal fossa via the pterygomaxillary fissure

TABLE 1–14. BOUNDARIES AND COMMUNICATIONS OF THE INFRATEMPORAL FOSSA

AREA	BONES	COMMUNICATIONS
Roof	Sphenoid bone—greater wing	Temporal fossa, foramen ovale, foramen spinosum
Floor	*Open*	—
Anterior	Maxilla—tuberosity	Orbit via the inferior orbital fissure
Posterior	*Open*	—
Medial	Sphenoid bone—lateral pterygoid plate	Pterygopalatine fossa via pterygomaxillary fissure
Lateral	Mandible—ramus, coronoid process	—

artery, the pterygoid venous plexus, the temporalis, and the lateral and medial pterygoid muscles.

1.1.5 Muscles

A. Muscles of facial expression: major muscles and their actions.
   1. Eyes and eyebrows
      a. Epicranius (occipitofrontalis) muscle—raises the eyebrows and forehead.
      b. Orbicularis oculi—closes the eyelid, blinking.
      c. Corrugator—depresses the eyebrows.
   2. Face
      a. Buccinator muscle—compresses the cheek against the teeth and aids in chewing.
         (1) Origin: buccal surface of the maxillary and mandibular alveolar processes and the pterygomandibular raphe.
         (2) Insertion: angle of the mouth/lip.
   3. Mouth
      a. Orbicularis oris—closes and protrudes upper and lower lips.
      b. Levator labii superioris—pulls lip up.
      c. Levator labii superioris alaque nasi—pulls lip up, flares nostrils.
      d. Mentalis—protrudes lower lip, tightens chin.
      e. Levator anguli oris—lifts the corner of the mouth.
      f. Zygomaticus major and minor—lift the corner of the mouth.

B. Muscles of mastication
   1. There are four primary muscles of mastication, including the temporalis, the masseter, and the medial and lateral pterygoid muscles.
      a. In general, the temporalis, masseter, and medial pterygoid muscles elevate the mandible or close the mouth.
      b. The lateral pterygoid muscle is involved in protrusion, depression, and lateral excursion of the mandible.
      c. The origins and insertions of these muscles are described in Table 1–15.
   2. The hyoid muscles assist the muscles of mastication in retruding and depressing the mandible.
   3. The muscles of mastication and hyoid muscles are involved in coordinating mandibular movements (Figure 1–23):
      a. Closing the mouth
         (1) Temporalis—anterior (vertical) and posterior fibers.
         (2) Masseter.
         (3) Medial pterygoid.
      b. Opening the mouth
         (1) Lateral pterygoid.
         (2) Assisting muscles:
            (a) Infrahyoid muscles—these muscles and the posterior belly of the digastric muscle will aid in depressing and stabilizing the hyoid bone, allowing the suprahyoid muscles to help pull down the mandible.
            (b) Suprahyoid muscles—especially anterior belly of the digastric muscle.
      c. Protrusion
         (1) Medial pterygoid.

TABLE 1–15. ORIGINS AND INSERTIONS OF THE MUSCLES OF MASTICATION

MUSCLE	ORIGIN	INSERTION
Temporalis	Temporal fossa	Coronoid process of mandible
Masseter		
Superficial head	Anterior two thirds of the inferior border of the zygomatic arch	Angle of mandible—lateral surface
Deep head	Posterior one third of the inferior border of the zygomatic arch	Ramus and body of mandible
Medial pterygoid		Angle of the mandible—medial surface
Superficial fibers	Pyramidal process of palatine bone, the pterygoid fossa of sphenoid bone and maxillary tuberosity	
Deep fibers	Pyramidal process of palatine bone and the medial surface of the lateral pterygoid plate of sphenoid bone	
Lateral pterygoid		Condyle of mandible—anterior surface
Superior head	Infratemporal crest of the greater wing of sphenoid bone	A few fibers insert into the anterior portion of the TMJ articular capsule
Inferior head	Lateral pterygoid plate of sphenoid bone	Condyle of the mandible—anterior surface

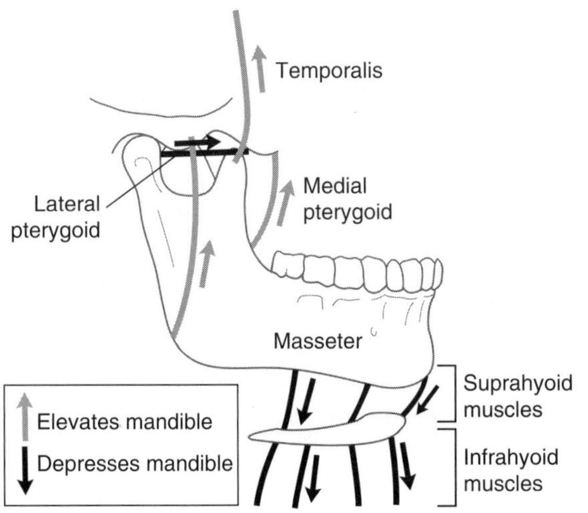

Figure 1–23. Role of muscles of mastication and hyoid muscles in mandibular movement.

(2) Lateral pterygoid—inferior head.

d. Retraction
   (1) Temporalis—posterior fibers.
   (2) Assisting muscles:
      (a) Suprahyoid muscles—especially both bellies of the digastric muscle.
      (b) Lateral pterygoid.

e. Lateral excursion
   (1) Lateral pterygoid—on the nonworking side (i.e., the opposite side of the direction of movement). Note: an injured lateral pterygoid will cause the jaw to shift to the same side of the injury.
   (2) Assisting muscle: temporalis, which acts as a stabilizer.

C. Hyoid muscles
1. The hyoid muscles are divided into two groups, depending on their location above or below the hyoid bone.
   a. The suprahyoid muscles are superior to the hyoid bone and include the anterior and posterior digastric muscles, the mylohyoid, geniohyoid, and stylohyoid. The mylohyoid muscle forms the floor of the mouth.
   b. The infrahyoid muscles are inferior to the hyoid bone and include the sternothyroid, sternohyoid, omohyoid, and thyrohyoid. A summary of these muscles is presented in Table 1–16.
2. Infrahyoid muscles
   a. Innervation: cervical nerves (C1–C3) via branches of ansa cervicalis.
   b. Major actions:
      (1) Assist the muscles of mastication in depressing or retruding the mandible.
      (2) Steady the hyoid bone and larynx when swallowing.
3. Suprahyoid muscles
   a. Innervation: refer to Table 1–16.
   b. Major actions:
      (1) Assist in pulling the mandible down during mouth opening.
      (2) Raise the hyoid bone and larynx when swallowing.

D. Neck muscles
1. The muscles in the neck include the platysma, the sternocleidomastoid (SCM), and the trapezius muscle. These muscles are summarized in Table 1–17.
2. Platysma—a thin layer of muscle found in the superficial fascia of the neck.

TABLE 1–16. ORIGINS, INSERTIONS AND INNERVATION OF THE HYOID MUSCLES

	INNERVATION	ORIGIN	INSERTION
Suprahyoid			
Digastric muscle			
Anterior belly	CN V_3	Digastric fossa	Intermediate tendon
Posterior belly	CN VII	Mastoid notch of temporal bone	Intermediate tendon
Mylohyoid	CN V_3	Mylohyoid line	Hyoid bone
Geniohyoid	C1* via CN XII	Genial tubercles	Hyoid bone
Stylohyoid	CN VII	Styloid process	Hyoid bone
Infrahyoid			
Omohyoid			
Superior belly	C1–C3	Intermediate tendon	Hyoid bone
Inferior belly	C1–C3	Scapula	Intermediate tendon
Sternohyoid	C1–C3	Sternum	Hyoid bone
Sternothyroid	C2–C3	Sternum	Thyroid cartilage
Thyrohyoid	C1 via CN XII	Thyroid cartilage	Hyoid bone

*C1, first cervical nerve.

TABLE 1–17. ORIGINS, INSERTIONS, AND INNERVATION OF THE NECK MUSCLES

	INNERVATION	ORIGIN	INSERTION
Platysma	CN VII	Fascia of the deltoids and pectoralis	Mandible
Sternocleido-mastoid	CN XI	Clavicle and sternum	Mastoid process of temporal bone
Trapezius	CN XI, C3–C4	Extends from the occipital bone to the cervical and thoracic vertebral column	Clavicle and spine of the scapula

3. Sternocleidomastoid
   a. A major landmark in the neck, dividing each side of the neck into anterior and posterior triangles (Figure 1–24). The anterior triangle can further be divided into the submandibular triangle and submental triangle. The posterior triangle can be divided into the occipital and subclavian triangle.
   b. Actions: contraction of one SCM will tilt the head laterally to that same side, while turning the face toward the opposite side. Contraction of both SCMs will flex the neck.
   c. The carotid pulse can be felt at the anterior-superior border of the SCM muscle, just posterior to the thyroid cartilage.

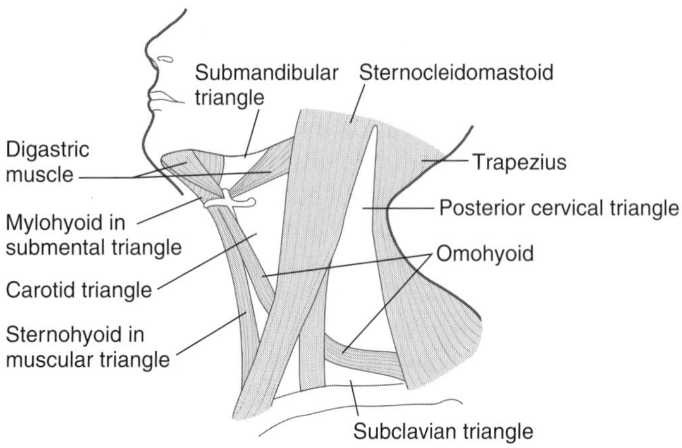

Figure 1–24. Neck triangles as viewed from the left side. (From Moore NA, Roy WA: Gross and Developmental Anatomy, St. Louis, Mosby, 2002.)

4. Trapezius
   a. Action: contraction of the trapezius elevates the clavicle and scapula (i.e, shrugging shoulders).

E. Muscles of the soft palate
1. Muscles of the soft palate include the palatoglossus, palatopharyngeus, levator veli palatine, tensor veli palatine, and uvula.
   a. The palatoglossus forms the anterior tonsillar pillar.
   b. The palatopharyngeus forms the posterior tonsillar pillar and also closes off the nasopharynx and larynx during swallowing.
   c. The tensor veli palatine wraps around the lateral side of the pterygoid hamulus and tenses the soft palate.
   d. A summary of these muscles is presented in Table 1–18.
2. Innvervation: refer to next page for innervation of muscles of the pharynx.

F. Muscles of the pharynx
1. The muscles of the pharynx include the superior, middle, and inferior constrictor muscles; the stylopharyngeus; and the salpingopharyngeus. The major action of these muscles is to move the pharynx and larynx during swallowing. A summary of their origins, insertions, and actions is presented in Table 1–19.
2. Innervation:
   a. Muscles of the soft palate and pharynx are all innervated via the pharyngeal plexus (CN IX, X, and XI), with the following three exceptions:
      (1) Tensor veli palatine—innervated by CN V_3.
      (2) Stylopharyngeus—innervated by CN IX.

Table 1–18. Origins, Insertions, and Actions of the Muscles of the Soft Palate

	ORIGIN	INSERTION	ACTION
Palatoglossus	Fascia of the soft palate	Tongue	Raises tongue, depresses soft palate
Palatopharyngeus	Soft palate	Thyroid cartilage, lateral wall of the pharynx	Moves palate down and back, moves pharynx up and forward, and raises and folds posterior wall of the larynx
Levator veli palatine	Petrous portion of temporal bone	Palatine aponeurosis	Raises soft palate
Tensor veli palatine	Medial pterygoid plate	Palatine aponeurosis	Tenses soft palate, opens auditory tube and eustachian tube
Uvula	Posterior nasal spine of the palatine bone and palatine aponeurosis		Contracts uvula

Table 1–19. Origins, Insertions, and Actions of the Muscles of the Pharynx

	ORIGIN	INSERTION	ACTION
Superior constrictor	Medial pterygoid plate, pterygoid hamulus, pterygomandibular raphe, mylohyoid line	Median pharyngeal raphe	Constricts pharynx to help push food down into the esophagus during swallowing. It also raises the larynx
Middle constrictor	Hyoid bone, stylohyoid ligament		
Inferior constrictor	Thyroid and cricoid cartilages		
Stylopharyngeus	Styloid process	Thyroid cartilage, lateral wall of the pharynx	Raise and dilates pharynx, helping food move through. It also raises the larynx
Salpingopharyngeus	Eustachian tube	Lateral wall of the pharynx	Raise and dilates pharynx, helping food move through

(3) Mucous membranes of the pharynx— innervated by CN V_2.

b. Motor function: CN XI via CN X nerve fibers.

c. Sensory function: CN IX.

G. Muscles of the larynx

1. The muscles of the larynx include the cricothyroid, oblique and transverse arytenoids, thyroarytenoid, and the lateral and posterior cricoarytenoids. A summary of these muscles and their actions is presented in Table 1–20.
2. Innervation: all muscles of the larynx are innervated by CN X via the recurrent laryngeal nerve except the cricothyroid, which is innervated by CN X via the external laryngeal nerve.

Tongue

A. Surface anatomy (Figure 1–25):

1. Dorsum of tongue—divided into two parts: the anterior two thirds of the tongue, which lies relatively freely in the oral cavity, and the posterior one third of the tongue, which covers the oral cavity and lies in the pharynx.
2. Sulcus terminalis—a V-shaped depression that divides the anterior two thirds from the posterior one third of the tongue. It is an embryologic remnant resulting from the fusion between the first and second pharyngeal arches.
3. Foramen cecum—a small pit located at the tip of the V of the sulcus terminalis. It

Table 1–20. Origins, Insertions, and Actions of the Muscles of the Larynx

	ORIGIN	INSERTION	ACTION
Cricothyroid	Cricoid cartilage	Thyroid cartilage	Raises cricoid cartilage, tenses vocal cords
Oblique arytenoid	Arytenoid cartilage	Arytenoid cartilage on the opposite side	Adducts vocal cords
Transverse arytenoid	Arytenoid cartilage	Arytenoid cartilage on the opposite side	Adducts vocal cords
Thyroarytenoid	Thyroid cartilage	Arytenoid cartilage	Adducts vocal cords
Lateral cricoarytenoid	Cricoid cartilage	Arytenoid cartilage	Adducts vocal cords
Posterior cricoarytenoid	Cricoid cartilage	Arytenoid cartilage	Adducts vocal cords

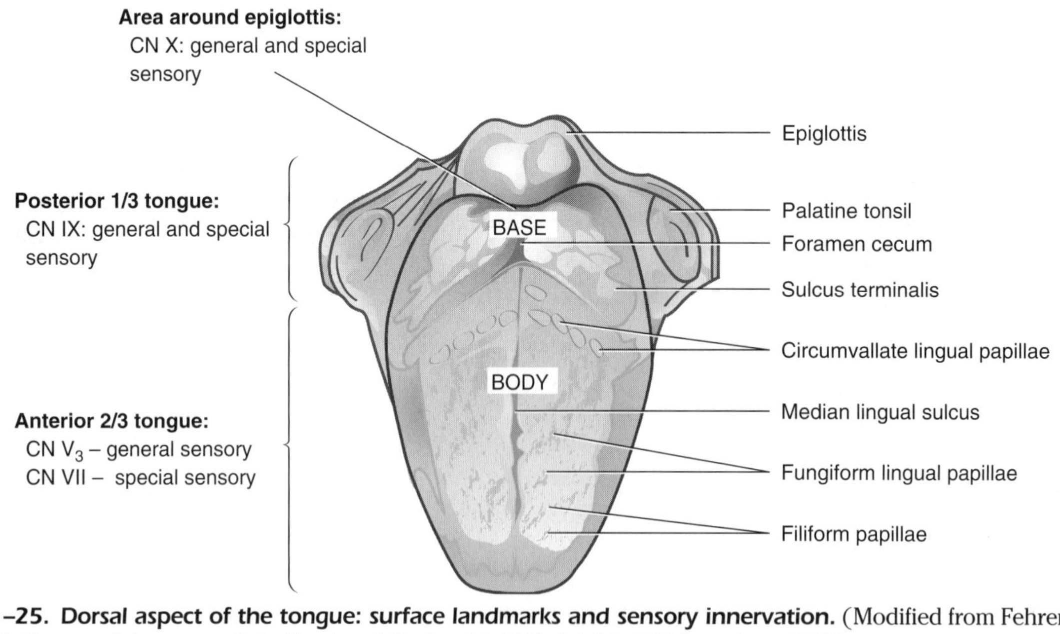

Figure 1–25. Dorsal aspect of the tongue: surface landmarks and sensory innervation. (Modified from Fehrenbach M, Herring S: Illustrated Anatomy of the Head and Neck, ed 2, Philadelphia, WB Saunders, 2002.)

is an embryologic remnant of the proximal opening of the thyroglossal duct.

4. Lingual papillae—elevated structures found on the surface of the tongue. There are four types:
   a. Filiform papillae
      (1) Thin, pointy projections that comprise the most numerous papillae and give the tongue's dorsal surface its characteristic rough texture.
      (2) Arrangement: in rows parallel with the sulcus terminalis.
      (3) Histologically show more keratinization than the other papillae.
      (4) Do not contain taste buds.
      (5) Note: an overgrowth of these papillae results in hairy tongue. A loss of filiform papillae results in glossitus.
   b. Fungiform papillae
      (1) Round, red spots that are less numerous than filiform papillae.
      (2) Histologically, they have a characteristic mushroom shape.
      (3) Contain taste buds.
   c. Circumvallate (vallate) papillae
      (1) The largest papillae and are 12 to 13 in number.
      (2) Arrangement: in a row parallel and just anterior to the sulcus terminalis.
      (3) Contain taste buds and small salivary glands known as *von Ebner's glands*.
   d. Foliate papillae
      (1) Vertical folds found posteriorly on the side of the tongue.
      (2) Contain taste buds.
   e. Note about taste buds: taste buds contain neuroepithelial (taste) cells. They can discriminate five taste sensations: salty, sweet, sour, bitter, and the recently described umami taste (taste of L-glutamate).

B. Muscles of the tongue
   1. Intrinsic muscles of the tongue—muscles found entirely within the tongue. Although they are not considered to be separate muscles, they can be divided into longitudinal, transverse, and vertical muscles. Their main function is to change the shape of the tongue.
   2. Extrinsic muscles of the tongue—there are three extrinsic muscles of the tongue, including the genioglossus, styloglossus, and hyoglossus (Note: some texts also include the palatoglossus). Although they all insert into the tongue, they originate from surrounding structures. A summary of their origins, insertions, and actions is presented in Table 1–21.
   3. Innervation:
      a. Motor function: motor innervation for all intrinsic and extrinsic muscles is from CN XII.
      b. Sensory function (see Figure 1–25):
         (1) For the anterior two thirds of the tongue:
            (a) General sensory—CN V_3 via the lingual nerve.
            (b) Special sensory (taste)—CN VII via the chorda tympani.
         (2) Posterior one third of the tongue: general and special sensation is innervated by CN IX.
         (3) Area around the epiglottis: innervated by CN X via the internal laryngeal nerve.
   4. Vascular supply—the blood supply is from branches of the lingual artery, including its terminal end, the deep lingual artery.

Triangles of the neck

The SCM divides each side of the neck into anterior and posterior triangles. These triangles can be subdivided into smaller triangles, as was described in Figure 1-24.

A. Anterior triangle
   1. Borders: anterior margin of the SCM, midline of the neck, and inferior border of the mandible.
   2. Subdivisions:

TABLE 1–21. ORIGINS, INSERTIONS, AND ACTIONS OF THE EXTRINSIC MUSCLES OF THE TONGUE

	ORIGIN	INSERTION	ACTION
Genioglossus	Genial tubercles on mandible	Tongue, hyoid bone	Protrudes and depresses tongue
Styloglossus	Styloid process of temporal bone	Tongue	Retracts tongue, curls up sides of tongue
Hyoglossus	Greater horn and body of hyoid bone	Tongue	Depresses tongue

a. Submandibular (digastric) triangles
   (1) Borders: upper margin of the anterior and posterior bellies of the digastric muscle, inferior border of the mandible.
   (2) Floor: mylohyoid and hyoglossus muscles.
   (3) Contents: submandibular gland, submandibular lymph nodes, lingual and facial arteries, CN XII, lingual nerve, and nerve to the mylohyoid muscle.

b. Submental triangle
   (1) Borders: between the right and left anterior bellies of the digastric muscle (beneath the chin) and body of the hyoid bone.
   (2) Floor: mylohyoid muscle.
   (3) Contents: submental lymph nodes.

c. Muscular triangles
   (1) Borders: inferior border of the superior belly of the omohyoid muscle, anterior border of the SCM, and the anterior midline of the neck.
   (2) Floor: sternohyoid and sternothyroid (infrahyoid) muscles.
   (3) Contents: anterior branches of the ansa cervicalis, infrahyoid strap muscles, and lymph nodes.

d. Carotid triangles
   (1) Borders: superior border of the superior belly of the omohyoid muscle, inferior border of the posterior belly of the digastric muscle, and the anterior border of the SCM.
   (2) Floor: inferior pharyngeal constrictor and thyrohyoid muscles.
   (3) Contents: common carotid artery (which bifurcates near the upper border of the thyroid cartilage) and its branches, the internal jugular vein and its tributaries, vagus nerve (CN X) including external and internal laryngeal nerves, CN IX (branch to carotid sinus), CN XI, CN XII, and branches of the cervical plexus.

B. Posterior triangle

1. Borders: posterior border of the SCM, anterior border of the trapezius and the clavicle.
2. Floor: splenius capitis, levator scapulae, posterior and middle scalene muscles.
3. Contents: external jugular and subclavian vein and their tributaries, subclavian artery and its branches (C3, C4), branches of the cervical plexus, CN XI, suprascapular artery and vein, nerves to the upper limb and muscles of the triangle floor, phrenic nerve, and the brachial plexus.
4. It is subdivided by the omohyoid muscle into the occipital triangle (above the omohyoid) and subclavian (supraclavicular) triangle (below the omohyoid).
   a. Subclavian (supraclavicular) triangle
      (1) Borders: inferior border of the inferior belly of the omohyoid, middle one-third of the clavicle, and posterior border of the SCM.
      (2) Contents: subclavian artery and vein, branchial plexus, cervical artery and vein, external jugular vein, scapular vein.
   b. Occipital triangle
      (1) Borders: superior border of the inferior belly of the omohyoid, posterior border of the SCM, and the anterior border of the trapezius.
      (2) Contents: accessory nerve.

1.2 Axilla, Shoulders, and Upper Extremities

The axilla is a space described as a pyramid, with a base composed of the skin and superficial fascia of the armpit. The apex rises to the level of the mid-clavicle. It contains the nerves and blood vessels supplying the upper limbs.

A. Axilla

1. Boundaries: the axilla is bounded by three skeletal and muscular walls.
   a. Anterior wall
      (1) Contains the clavicle superiorly and the pectoralis major and pectoralis minor muscles.
   b. Medial wall
      (1) The lateral thoracic wall covered by the serratus anterior muscle.
   c. Posterior wall
      (1) Formed primarily by the scapula and subscapularis muscle.
      (2) The teres major and latissimus dorsi muscles contribute to the inferior aspect of the posterior wall.
2. Contents:
   a. The axilla contains portions of the:
      (1) Brachial nerve plexus.
      (2) Axillary artery.
      (3) Axillary vein.

b. The axillary sheath encloses the artery, vein, and nerve as they pass through the axilla from the posterior triangle of the neck to the arm.

c. Axillary lymph nodes receiving lymph from the arm and breast travel through the axilla.

B. Shoulders and upper extremities

Limbs develop from outgrowths of the axial skeleton. The upper limb develops from body wall segments of the lower four cervical and first thoracic levels. Muscle, nerve, blood vessels, and lymphatic drainage arise concomitantly. The upper limb has four skeletal components: shoulder girdle, arm, forearm, and hand. Additional components include muscles, nerves, arterial supply and venous return, and lymphatic drainage.

1. The shoulder girdle consists of the scapula and clavicle.
   a. The scapula is a broad, flat, thin, triangular-shaped bone (Figure 1–26).
      (1) The concave anterior surface is anchored by muscles to the posterior surface of ribs two through seven.
      (2) Three sides:
         (a) A vertebral medial border paralleling the vertebral column.
         (b) An axillary lateral border facing the axilla.
         (c) A suprascapular superior border.
      (3) The spine of the scapula runs horizontally across the convex posterior surface and divides it into two fossae for muscle attachments.
         (a) The supraspinous fossa above the spine.
         (b) The infraspinous fossa below the spine.
      (4) The acromion articulates with the clavicle at the acromioclavicular joint. The suprascapular notch, on the superior border of the spine, is the site of transmission of the suprascapular nerve and vessels.
      (5) The coracoid process projects laterally and anteriorly from the superolateral border.
      (6) The glenoid fossa, just below the base of the coracoid process, articulates with the head of the humerus at the joint of the shoulder.
      (7) The subscapular fossa on the concave anterior surface fits against the convex surface of the adjacent ribs.
   b. The clavicle is an S-shaped bone commonly known as the *collarbone* (Figure 1–27).

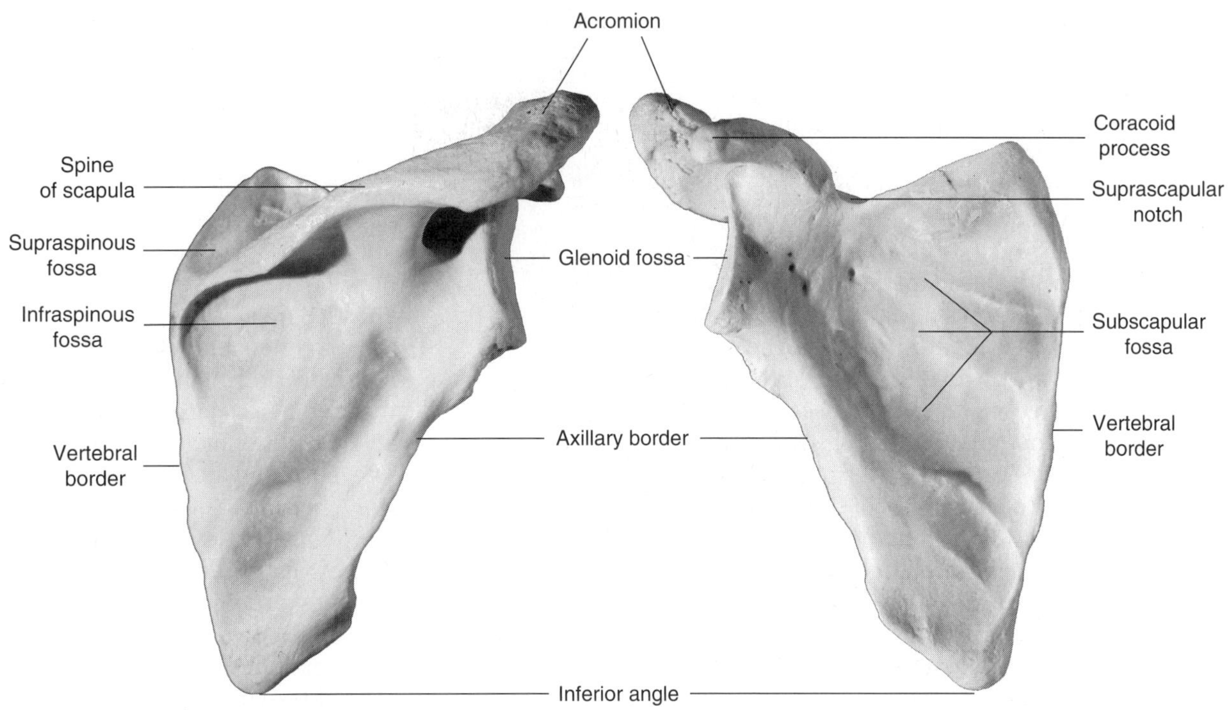

Figure 1–26. Right scapula. Posterior view *(left)* and anterior view *(right)*. (From Liebgott B: The Anatomic Basis of Dentistry, ed 2, St. Louis, Mosby, 2001.)

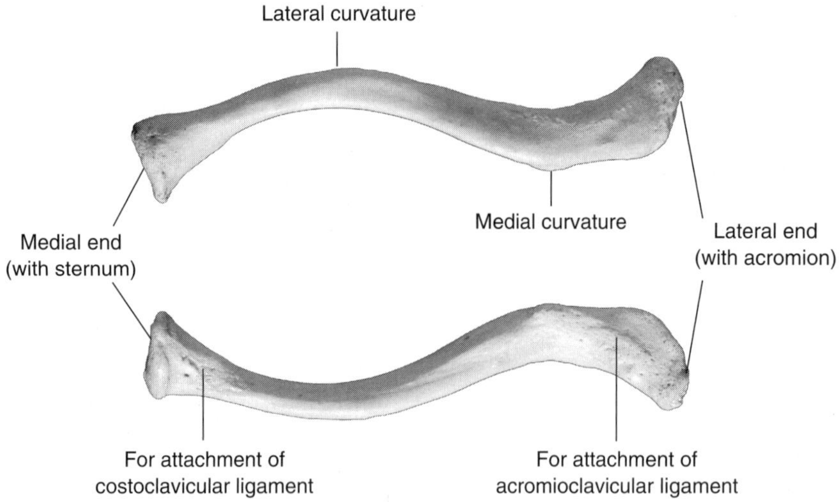

Figure 1–27. Right clavicle. Superior view *(top)* and inferior view *(bottom)*. (From Liebgott B: The Anatomic Basis of Dentistry, ed 2, St. Louis, Mosby, 2001.)

(1) The lateral end articulates at the acromioclavicular joint with the acromion of the scapula.
(2) The medial end articulates at the sternoclavicular joint with the manubrium.
(3) The medial half of the clavicle bends anteriorly, and the lateral half bends posteriorly.
(4) The inferior surface serves as the attachment for two ligaments.
   (a) The coraclavicular ligament binds the clavicle to the coracoid process.
   (b) The costoclavicular ligament binds the clavicle to the first rib.

2. The arm consists of the humerus bone (Figure 1–28).
   a. The humerus is the only bone of the arm.
      (1) The humerus articulates superiorly with the scapula and inferiorly with the radius and ulna of the forearm.
      (2) The rounded head on the superomedial aspect articulates with the glenoid fossa of the scapula.
      (3) The greater and lesser tubercles are on the anterior surface just below the head of the humerus and serve as attachments for muscles.
         (a) The greater tubercle is in the more lateral position.
         (b) The lesser tubercle is in the more anterior position.
      (4) The anatomical neck lies just below the head; a surgical neck where the shaft meets the upper portion of the humerus is often the site of fractures.
      (5) The intertubercular sulcus is occupied by the tendon of the long head of the biceps muscle; other muscles attach to the sides of the groove.
      (6) The deltoid tuberosity, an elevation located anterolaterally on the midshaft of the humerus, is the site of attachment of the deltoid muscle.
      (7) The trochlea, a spool-shaped process on the inferior surface, articulates with the ulna of the forearm.
      (8) The capitulum, a round area located laterally to the trochlea, articulates with the radius of the forearm.
      (9) The lateral epicondyle above the capitulum, and medial epicondyle above the trochlea, are prominences that serve as attachment sites for muscles.
      (10) The medial and lateral supracondylar ridges are located above the medial and lateral epicondyles and are attachments for muscles.
      (11) The coronoid fossa, on the anterior surface just superior to the trochlea, fits the coronoid process of the ulna of the forearm.
      (12) The olecranon fossa, on the posterior surface just superior to the trochlea, fits the olecranon of the ulna of the forearm.
3. The forearm consists of the radius and ulna (Figure 1–29).

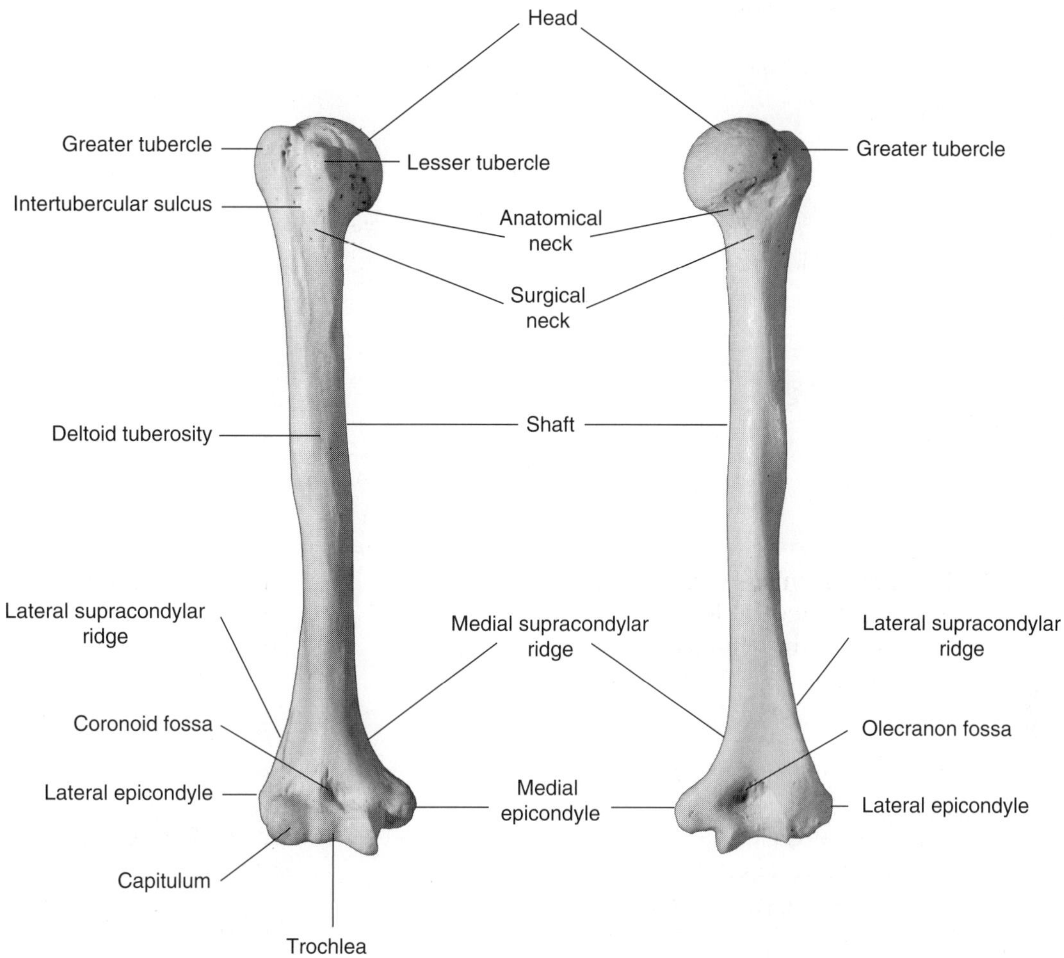

Figure 1–28. Right humerus. Anterior aspect *(left)* and posterior aspect *(right)*. (From Liebgott B: The Anatomic Basis of Dentistry, ed 2, St. Louis, Mosby, 2001.)

a. The radius is lateral to the ulna when in the anatomical position with palms facing forward or in the supine position.
   (1) The head of the radius is disc-shaped at the proximal end; it articulates superiorly with the capitulum of the humerus, and medially with the radial notch of the ulna.
   (2) The radial tuberosity, a projection just below the head on the medial surface, is a site of muscle attachment.
   (3) The lateral styloid process is the pointed, distal portion of the radius.
   (4) The ulnar notch, a shallow depression on the inferomedial aspect of the radius, serves as the articulation with the distal end of the ulna.

b. The ulna is lateral to the radius when in the pronated position with palms facing posteriorly.
   (1) The trochlear notch on the proximal end of the ulna curves around and articulates with the trochlea of the humerus.
   (2) The coronoid process extends in an anteroinferior direction from the trochlear notch.
   (3) The olecranon is formed from the superoposterior portion of the trochlear notch.
   (4) The medial styloid process is the distal projection of the ulna.

4. The wrist and hand consist of carpal bones, metacarpal bones, and phalanges.
   a. Carpal bones
      (1) There are eight short, cuboidal carpal bones in the wrist, each arranged in a proximal and distal row with four bones in each row.
         (a) Proximal bones—scaphoid, lunate, triquetral, pisiform.

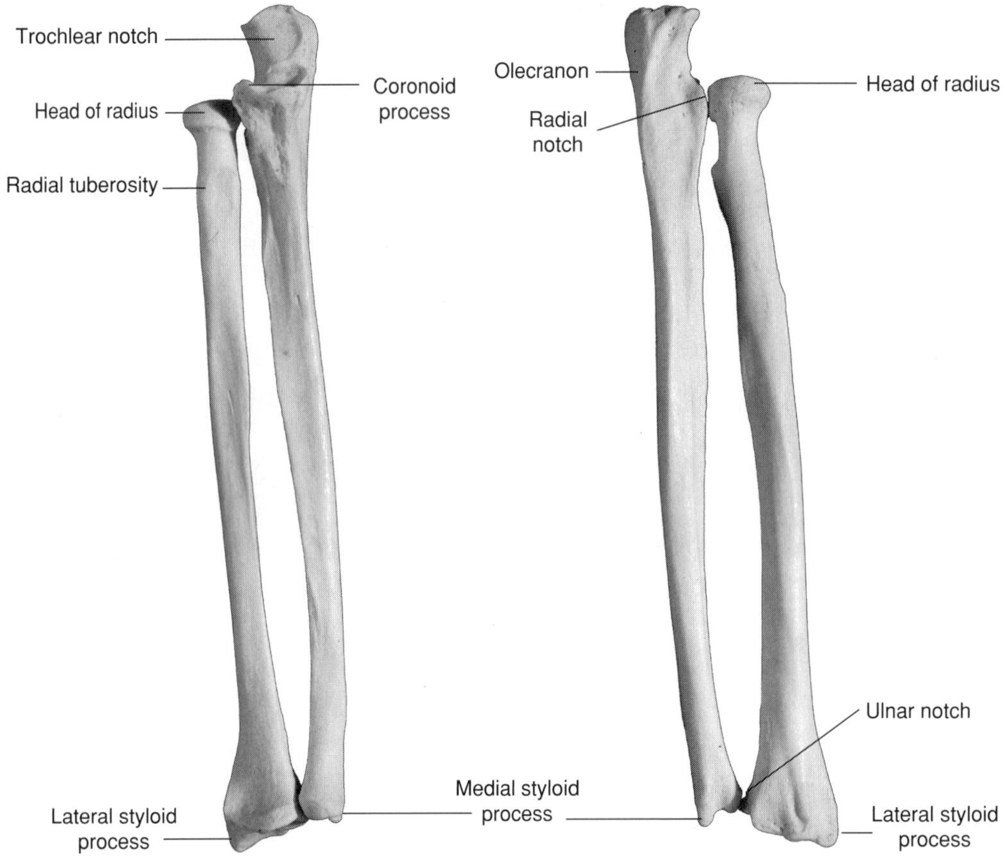

Figure 1–29. Ulna and radius of right forearm. Anterior view *(left)* and posterior view *(right)*. (From Liebgott B: The Anatomic Basis of Dentistry, ed 2, St. Louis, Mosby, 2001.)

(b) Distal bones—trapezium, trapezoid, capitate, hamate.

b. Metacarpal bones
   (1) These bones form the skeleton of the palm of the hand; each base articulates superiorly with the distal row of carpals and inferiorly with the phalanges.

c. Phalanges
   (1) Each finger has three phalanges: proximal, middle, and distal.
   (2) The thumb lacks a middle phalanx.

5. Muscles are grouped by region: pectoral, superficial back, shoulder, arm, forearm, and hand.
   a. Pectoral (Figure 1–30).
      (1) The pectoralis major muscle is a large, triangular muscle on the anterior chest wall arising from two heads (one from the clavicle and another from the sternum) and inserting into the humerus.
         (a) Can flex, medially rotate, and adduct the arm.
         (b) Supplied by the lateral and medial pectoral nerves.
      (2) The pectoralis minor muscle is a small, triangular muscle arising from the anterior chest wall deep to the pectoralis major muscle and inserting on the coracoid process of the scapula.
         (a) Protracts, depresses, and rotates the scapula laterally.
         (b) Supplied by the medial pectoral nerve.
      (3) The subclavius is a small muscle located below the clavicle.
         (a) Probably insignificant function.
         (b) Supplied by the nerve to subclavius.
      (4) The serratus anterior originates from the anterior chest wall and inserts into the vertebral border of the scapula.
         (a) Protracts the scapula and rotates it medially.
         (b) Supplied by the long thoracic nerve.

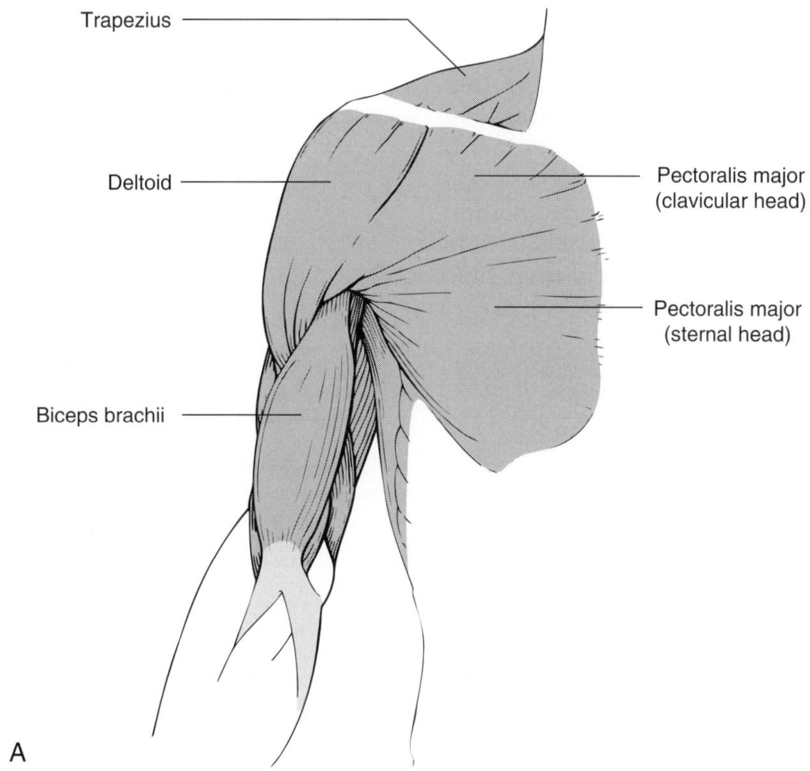

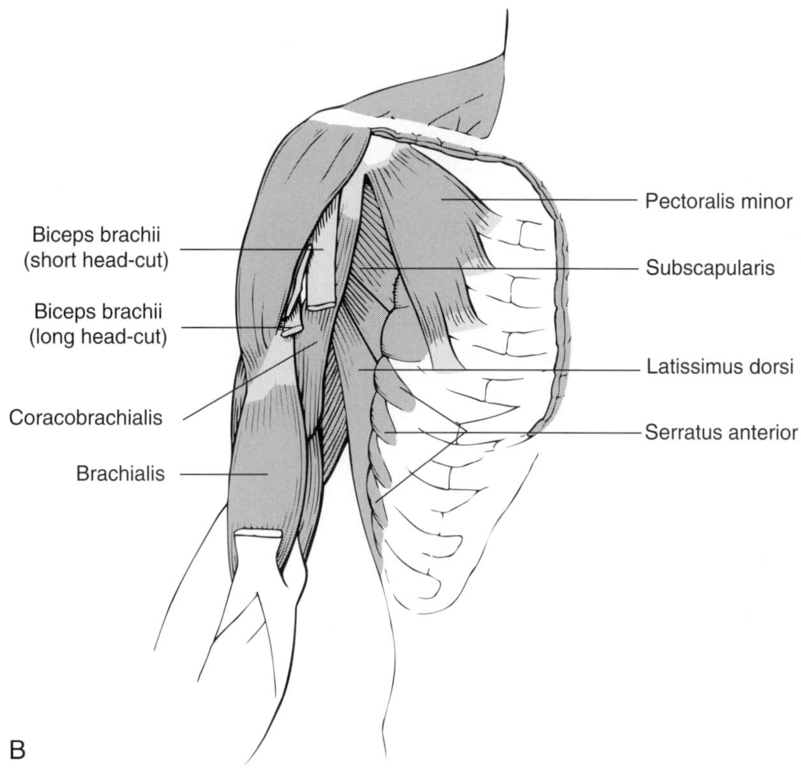

Figure 1–30. Muscles of pectoral region and anterior right arm. **A**, Superficial. **B**, Deep. (From Liebgott B: The Anatomic Basis of Dentistry, ed 2, St. Louis, Mosby, 2001.)

b. Superficial back (Figure 1–31, Table 1–22).
   (1) The trapezius muscle is large, thin, flat, and triangular; it covers the back of the neck and upper half of the trunk.
      (a) Superior fibers elevate and laterally rotate the scapula, inferior fibers depress the scapula, and middle fibers help to retract the scapula.
      (b) Supplied mainly by CN XI with a small supply from branches of the cervical plexus of nerves in the neck.
   (2) The latissimus dorsi is large, thin, and flat; it covers the lower half of the back, inserting into the humerus.
      (a) Adducts, extends, and medially rotates the arm.
      (b) Supplied by the thoracodorsal nerve.
   (3) The levator scapulae originates from the vertebrae to insert on the superior border of the scapula.
      (a) Elevates and medially rotates the scapula.
      (b) Supplied by the dorsal scapular nerve.
   (4) The major and minor rhomboid muscles originate from the vertebrae to insert into the vertebral border of the scapula.
      (a) Retracts and medially rotates the scapula.
      (b) Supplied by the dorsal scapular nerve.

c. Shoulder (see Figures 1–30 and 1–31, Table 1–23).
   (1) The deltoid muscle originates from bones of the pectoral girdle and inserts into the humerus, wrapping over the shoulder.
      (a) Anterior fibers flex and medially rotate the posterior fibers, and extend and laterally rotate the arm at the shoulder; middle fibers abduct the arm.
      (b) Supplied by the axillary nerve.
   (2) The teres major muscle originates from the scapula and inserts on the humerus.
      (a) Extends, medially rotates, and adducts the arm.
      (b) Supplied by the lower subscapular nerve.

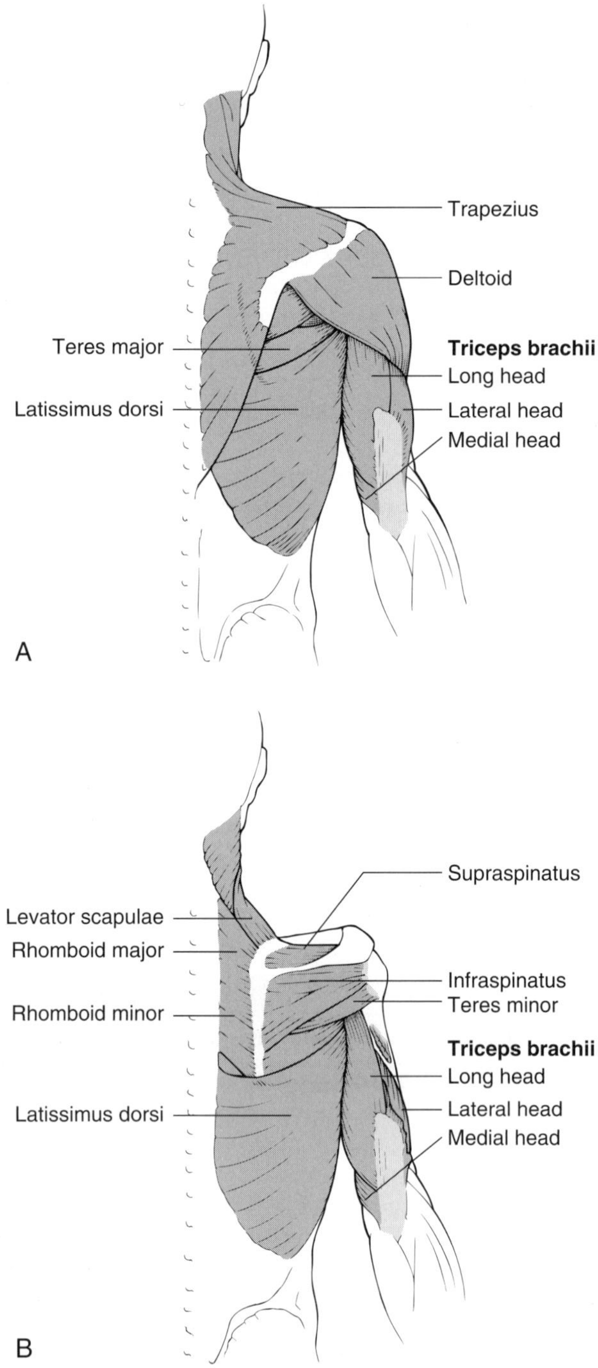

Figure 1–31. Posterior muscles of the right shoulder and arm. **A**, Superficial. **B**, Deep. (From Liebgott B: The Anatomic Basis of Dentistry, ed 2, St. Louis, Mosby, 2001.)

   (3) The rotator cuff muscles are four muscles (supraspinatus, infraspinatus, teres minor, and subscapularis) that originate from the scapula and insert into the upper humerus and joint capsule to hold the head of the humerus in the glenoid fossa.

TABLE 1-22. MUSCLES OF THE SUPERFICIAL BACK

MUSCLE	ORIGIN	INSERTION	ACTION(S)	NERVE
Trapezius	Vertebrae: all thoracic and cervical spines Ligamentum nuchae (membranous extension of cervical spines) Skull: superior nuchal line and inion	Scapula: spine and acromion Clavicle: superior lateral third	1. Upper fibers elevate scapula 2. Lower fibers depress scapula 3. Middle fibers retract scapula 4. Rotates laterally (glenoid fossa points up)	Cranial nerve XI: spinal accessory APR of C3-C4
Latissimus dorsi	Vertebrae: spines of T6 to T12 Os coxae: iliac crest Lumbodorsal fascia Ribs: lower three to four	Humerus: floor of intertubercular sulcus	1. Adducts arm 2. Extends arm 3. Rotates arm medially	Thoracodorsal nerve
Levator scapulae	Vertebrae: transverse processes of C1 to 4	Scapula: superior aspect of vertebral border	1. Elevates scapula 2. Rotates scapula medially (glenoid fossa down)	Dorsal scapular
Rhomboids	Vertebrae: spinous processes of C7 to T5	Scapula: vertebral border	1. Retracts scapula 2. Rotates scapula medially (glenoid fossa down)	Dorsal scapular

From Liebgott B: The Anatomic Basis of Dentistry, ed 2, St. Louis, Mosby, 2001, Table 9–2, p. 439.
APR, Anterior primary rami.

TABLE 1-23. MUSCLES OF THE SHOULDER

MUSCLE	ORIGIN	INSERTION	ACTION(S)	NERVE
Deltoid	Clavicle: inferior lateral third Scapula: acromion and spine	Humerus: deltoid tuberosity	1. Abducts arm 2. Flexes arm 3. Rotates arm medially (anterior fibers) 4. Extends arm (posterior fibers) 5. Rotates arm laterally (posterior fibers)	Axillary
Teres major	Scapula: inferior angle	Humerus: medial lip of intertubercular sulcus	1. Extends arm 2. Medially rotates arm 3. Adducts arm	Lower subscapular
Rotator cuff muscles				
Supraspinatus	Scapula: supraspinous fossa	Humerus: greater tubercle	1. Abducts arm 2. Stabilizes shoulder joint	Suprascapular
Infraspinatus	Scapula: infraspinous fossa	Humerus: greater tubercle	1. Rotates arm laterally 2. Adduction (slight) 3. Stabilizes shoulder joint	Suprascapular
Teres minor	Scapula: inferior lateral border	Humerus: greater tubercle	1. Rotates arm laterally 2. Extends arm 3. Adducts arm 4. Stabilizes arm at shoulder	Axillary
Subscapularis	Scapula: subscapular fossa	Humerus: lesser tubercle	1. Rotates arm medially 2. Stabilizes shoulder joint	Upper and lower subscapular

From Liebgott B: The Anatomic Basis of Dentistry, ed 2, St. Louis, Mosby, 2001, Table 9–3, p. 439.

(a) Supraspinatus muscle
(i) An abductor of the arm at the shoulder.
(ii) Supplied by the suprascapular nerve.
(b) Infraspinatus muscle
(i) Laterally rotates and slightly adducts the arm.
(ii) Supplied by the suprascapular nerve.
(c) Teres minor muscle
(i) Laterally rotates, extenses, and adducts the arm.
(ii) Supplied by the axillary nerve.
(d) Subscapularis muscle
(i) Medially rotates the arm.
(ii) Supplied by both the upper and lower subscapular nerves.

d. Arm muscles are divided into anterior flexors (biceps brachii, coracobrachialis, and brachialis) and posterior extensors (triceps brachii and anconeus) (see Figure 1–30, Table 1–24).
(1) Biceps brachii originates (the tendon of the long head) from the supraglenoid tubercle of the scapula and from the coracoid process of the scapula (the short head) and, along with the coracobrachialis, inserts into the upper forearm.
(a) Flexes the elbow.
(b) Supplied by the musculocutaneous nerve.
(2) Coracobrachialis originates from the coracoid process of the scapula and inserts on the humerus.
(a) Flexes and adducts the arm.
(b) Supplied by the musculocutaneous nerve.
(3) Brachialis originates from the humerus and inserts on the coronoid process of the ulna.
(a) Flexes the elbow.
(b) Supplied by the musculocutaneous nerve.
(4) Triceps brachii originates from three heads (one originates on the scapula and the other two on the humerus) and inserts into the ulna.
(a) Extends the arm.
(b) Supplied by the radial nerve.
(5) Anconeus arises from the lateral epicondyle of the humerus and inserts along with the triceps

TABLE 1-24. MUSCLES OF THE ARM

MUSCLE	ORIGIN	INSERTION	ACTION(S)	NERVE
Anterior (flexors)				
Biceps brachii	Scapula (short head): coracoid process Scapula (long head): supraglenoid tubercle	Radius: both heads blend into common tendon that inserts into radial tuberosity	1. Major flexor of forearm at elbow 2. Strong supinator of forearm at superior radioulnar joint 3. Weak flexor of arm at shoulder	Musculocutaneous
Coracobrachialis	Scapula: coracoid process	Humerus: medial aspect of mid shaft	1. Flexes arm 2. Adducts arm	Musculocutaneous
Brachialis	Humerus: anterior distal aspect	Ulna coronoid process	1. Major flexor of forearm at elbow	Musculocutaneous
Posterior (extensors)				
Triceps brachii	Scapula (long head): infraglenoid tubercle Humerus (lateral head): posterolateral surface Humerus (medial head): posterior surface below the radial groove	Ulna: all three heads blend into a single tendon that inserts into the olecranon	1. Extends forearm at elbow	Radial
Anconeus	Humerus: lateral epicondyle	Ulna: olecranon along with triceps	1. Extends forearm at elbow 2. Aids in pronation of forearm	Radial

From Liebgott B: The Anatomic Basis of Dentistry, ed 2, St. Louis, Mosby, 2001, Table 9–4, p. 440.

brachii on the olecranon of the ulna.
   (a) Considered by some to be a portion of triceps brachii.
   (b) Supplied by the radial nerve.

e. Forearm (and hand) muscles are divided into anterior (Figure 1–32, Table 1–25) and posterior (Figure 1–33, Table 1–26) groups, and then subdivided further into superficial, intermediate, and deep groups for anterior muscles, and superficial and deep groups for posterior muscles.
   (1) Anterior superficial group

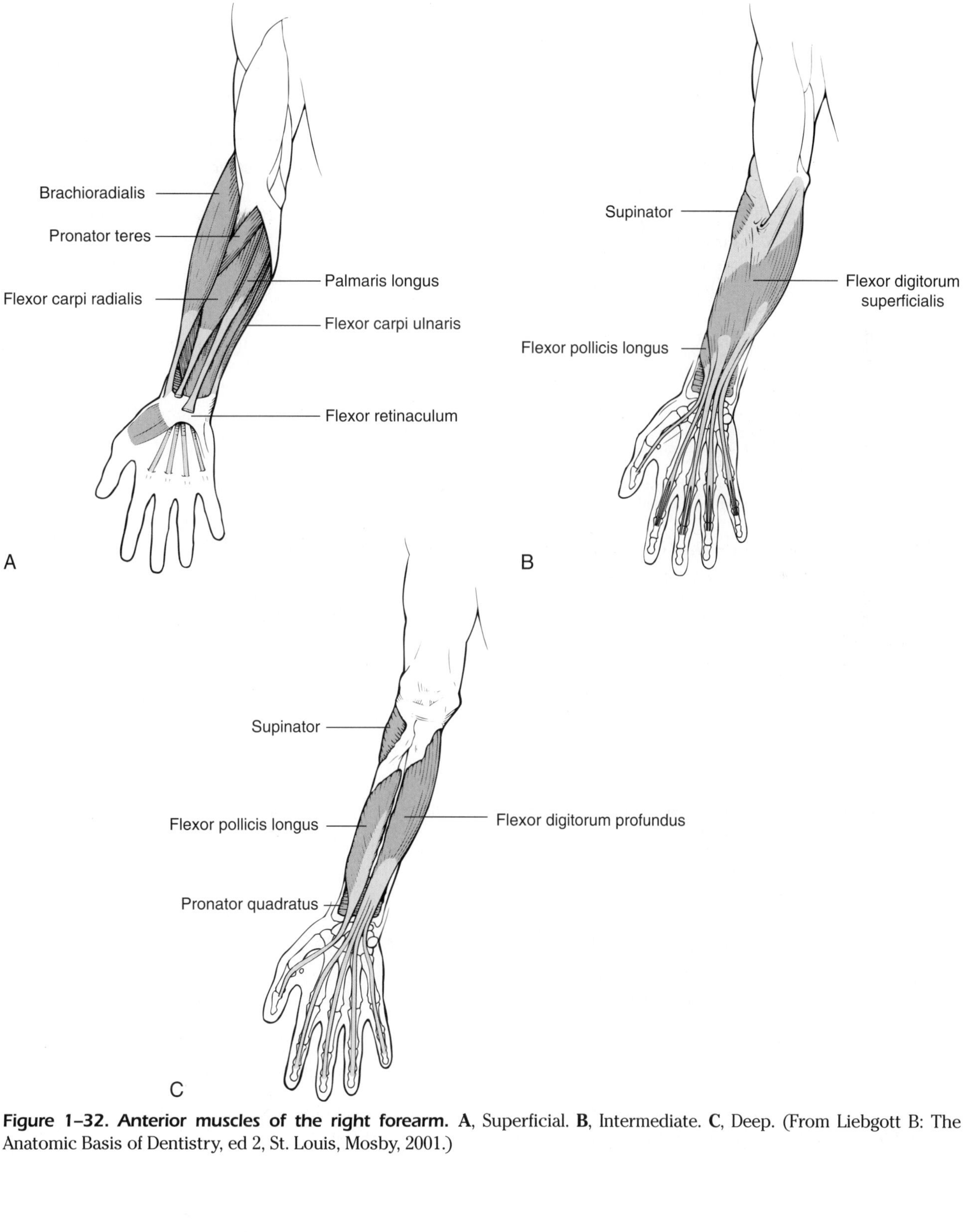

Figure 1–32. Anterior muscles of the right forearm. **A**, Superficial. **B**, Intermediate. **C**, Deep. (From Liebgott B: The Anatomic Basis of Dentistry, ed 2, St. Louis, Mosby, 2001.)

TABLE 1-25. MUSCLES OF THE ANTERIOR FOREARM COMPARTMENT

MUSCLE	ORIGIN	INSERTION	ACTION(S)	NERVE
Superficial				
Palmaris longus	Humerus: medial epicondyle via common flexor tendon	Palmar aponeurosis of hand Flexor retinaculum	1. Flexes hand at wrist	Median
Flexor carpi radialis	Humerus: medial epicondyle via common flexor tendon	Metacarpals: bases of 2nd and 3rd	1. Flexes hand at wrist 2. Abducts hand at wrist	Median
Flexor carpi ulnaris	Humerus: medial epicondyle via common flexor tendon Ulna: coronoid process	5th metacarpal, pisiform, and hamate bones	1. Flexes hand at wrist 2. Abducts hand at wrist	Ulnar
Pronator teres	Humeral head: medial epicondyle Ulnar head: coronoid process and medial aspect	Radius: lateral aspect of midshaft	1. Pronates forearm	Median
Intermediate				
Flexor digitorum superficialis	Humerus: medial epicondyle via common flexor tendon Radius: upper half of anterior shaft	Middle phalanges of all digits except thumb: palmar aspects	1. Flexes middle phalanges at proximal interphalangeal joints	Median
Deep				
Flexor pollicis longus	Ulna: coronoid process Interosseous membrane Radius: anterior surface of shaft	Distal phalanx of thumb: palmar side of base	1. Flexes thumb	Median
Pronator quadratus	Ulna: anterior distal surface of shaft	Radius: anterior distal aspect	1. Pronates forearm and provides power when pronating against resistance	Median
Flexor digitorum profundus	Ulna: medial and anterior aspect and adjacent interosseous membrane	Distal phalanges of all digits except thumb: bases	2. Flexes distal phalanges at distal interphalangeal joints	Ulnar and median

From Liebgott B: The Anatomic Basis of Dentistry, ed 2, St. Louis, Mosby, 2001, Table 9–5, p. 443.

(a) Pronator teres originates from the humerus and ulna to insert on the radius.
  (i) Pronates the forearm.
  (ii) Supplied by the median nerve.
(b) Palmaris longus originates from the medial epicondyle of the humerus and inserts into the palmar aponeurosis of the hand.
  (i) Flexes the hand at the wrist.
  (ii) Supplied by the median nerve.
(c) Flexor carpi radialis originates from the humerus and inserts into the bases of the second and third metacarpals.
  (i) A flexor and abductor of the wrist.
  (ii) Supplied by the median nerve.
(d) Flexor carpi ulnaris originates from the humerus and inserts into the fifth metacarpal, pisiform, and hamate bones.
  (i) Flexes and adducts the wrist.
  (ii) Supplied by the ulnar nerve.

(2) Anterior intermediate group
  (a) Flexor digitorum superficialis originates from the common flexor tendon of the medial epicondyle of the humerus and the upper one half of the radius, and inserts into the

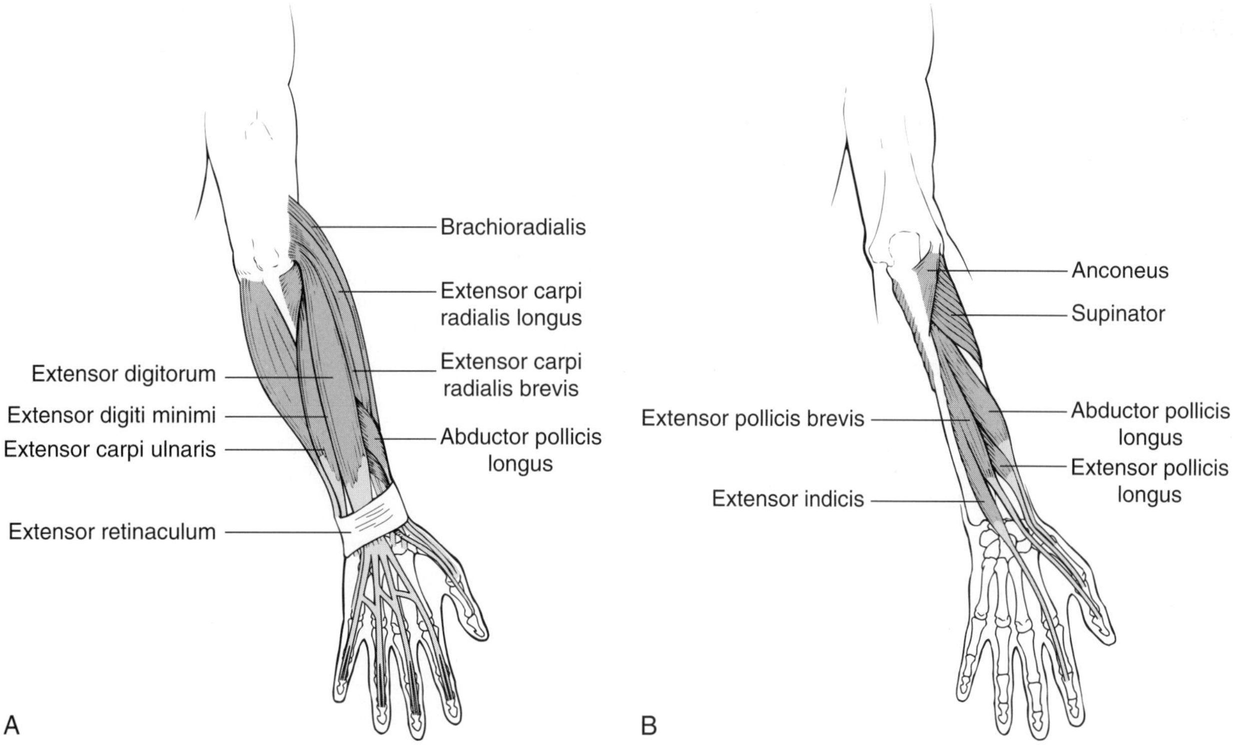

Figure 1–33. Posterior muscles of the right forearm. **A**, Superficial. **B**, Deep. (From Liebgott B: The Anatomic Basis of Dentistry, ed 2, St. Louis, Mosby, 2001.)

Table 1-26. Muscles of the Posterior Forearm Compartment

MUSCLE	ORIGIN	INSERTION	ACTION(S)	NERVE
Superficial				
Brachioradialis	Humerus: lateral epicondyle	Radius: styloid process	Flexes forearm at elbow: an exception	Radial
Extensor carpi radialis longus	Humerus: lateral supracondylar ridge and lateral epicondyle via common extensor tendon	2nd metacarpal: base	1. Extends hand at wrist 2. Abducts hand at wrist	Radial
Extensor carpi radialis brevis	Humerus: lateral epicondyle via common extensor tendon	3rd metacarpal: base	1. Extends hand at wrist 2. Abducts hand at wrist	Radial
Extensor carpi ulnaris	Humerus: lateral epicondyle via common extensor tendon Ulna: posterior border	5th metacarpal: base	1. Extends hand at wrist 2. Abducts hand at wrist	Radial
Extensor digitorum	Humerus: lateral epicondyle via common extensor tendon	Phalanges: lateral and dorsal aspects via extensor expansions	1. Extends the fingers 2. Aids in extending wrist	Radial
Extensor digiti minimi	Humerus: lateral epicondyle via common extensor tendon	Proximal phalanx of 5th (little) finger: dorsal aspect	Extends little finger	Radial
Deep				
Supinator	Humerus: lateral epicondyle Ulna: proximal aspect below the radial notch	Radius: lateral aspect of proximal end	Supinates forearm and turns palm forward in anatomical position, or up, as in accepting change when shoulder and/or elbow are flexed	Radial

(Continued)

TABLE 1-26. MUSCLES OF THE POSTERIOR FOREARM COMPARTMENT—CONT'D

MUSCLE	ORIGIN	INSERTION	ACTION(S)	NERVE
Abductor pollicis longus	Ulna: middle third of posterior aspect Radius: middle third of posterior aspect Interosseous membrane	1st metacarpal: radial side of base	1. Abducts thumb 2. Abducts wrist	Radial
Extensor pollicis longus	Ulna: middle third of posterior aspect Interosseous membrane	Distal phalanx of thumb: base	Extends distal phalanx of thumb	Radial
Extensor pollicis brevis	Radius: posterior aspect Interosseous membrane	Proximal phalanx of thumb: base	Extends proximal phalanx of thumb	Radial
Extensor indicis	Ulna: posterior aspect Interosseous membrane	Proximal phalanx of 1st (index) finger: dorsal aspect	Extends index finger	Radial

From Liebgott B: The Anatomic Basis of Dentistry, ed 2, St. Louis, Mosby, 2001, Table 9–6, p. 445.

middle phalanges of all four digits.
- (i) It is a flexor of proximal interphalangeal joints, metacarpophalangeal joints, and the wrist joint.
- (ii) Supplied by the median nerve.

(3) Deep anterior group
- (a) Flexor digitorum profundus originates from the anterior of the ulna and passes over the wrist as four tendons that insert into distal phalanges of the fingers.
  - (i) Flexes the distal phalanges and the wrist.
  - (ii) Supplied by the medial nerve on the radial aspect and the ulnar nerve on the ulnar aspect.
- (b) Flexor pollicis longus originates both ulna and radius and inserts into the distal phalanx of the thumb.
  - (i) Flexes the thumb.
  - (ii) Supplied by the median nerve.
- (c) Pronator quadratus muscle arises from the ulna and inserts on the radius.
  - (i) Pronates the forearm.
  - (ii) Supplied by the median nerve.

(4) Posterior superficial group
- (a) Brachioradialis arises from the lateral epicondyle of the humerus and inserts into the styloid process of the radius.
  - (i) Flexes the forearm at the elbow.
  - (ii) Supplied by the radial nerve.
- (b) Extensor carpi radialis longus muscle
- (c) Extensor carpi radialis brevis muscle
- (d) Extensor digitorum muscles
- (e) Extensor digiti minimi

(5) Posterior deep group
- (a) Supinator
- (b) Abductor pollicis longus
- (c) Extensor pollicis longus
- (d) Extensor pollicis brevis
- (e) Extensor indicis

6. Nerve supply
   a. The brachial plexus of nerves arises in the neck.
      (1) It passes downward over the first rib and under the clavicle to the axilla and then to the upper limb.
   b. The brachial plexus of nerves provides the entire motor and sensory nerve supply to the upper limb.
      (1) The plexus arises from five roots from the anterior primary rami of spinal nerves C5, C6, C7, C8, and T1.
      (2) The five roots unite to form three trunks:
         (a) The upper trunk forms from the roots of C5 and C6.
         (b) The middle trunk forms from C7.

(c) The lower trunk forms from C8 and T1.

(3) Each of the three trunks divides in two to form six divisions.

(4) The divisions reunite to form three cords:

(a) The lateral cord.

(b) The medial cord.

(c) The posterior cord.

(5) The cords divide to form five terminal branches.

c. The roots, trunks, and cords of the brachial plexus lead to several collateral branches; these supply some of the muscles of the neck, upper limb girdle, and arm; there also is a cutaneous nerve supply to the arm and forearm.

(1) The long thoracic nerve forms from the three upper roots of the anterior primary rami (C5, C6, and C7), runs inferiorly along the rib cage, and supplies the serratus anterior muscle.

(2) The dorsal scapular nerve forms from the most superior root of the anterior primary rami (C5) to supply the rhomboid muscles.

(3) The suprascapular nerve forms from the upper trunk, passes through the suprascapular notch of the scapula, supplies the subclavius muscle and infraspinatus muscle, and is sensory to the shoulder joint.

(4) The lateral pectoral nerve forms from the lateral cord and supplies most of the pectoralis major muscle.

(5) The medial pectoral nerve forms from the medial cord, supplies the pectoralis minor muscle, and helps supply the pectoralis major muscle.

(6) Three motor branches leave the posterior cord to supply muscles of the pectoral girdle; the upper subscapular nerve to the subscapularis muscle, the lower subscapular nerve to the subscapularis muscle and teres major muscle, and the thoracodorsal nerve to the latissimus dorsi muscle.

(7) The medial cutaneous nerves of the arm and forearm leave the distal end of the medial cord.

d. The six divisions of the brachial plexus join to form five terminal branches.

(1) The musculoskeletal nerve supplies the three large flexor muscles located on the anterior arm (biceps brachii, coracobrachialis, and brachialis) and then continues into the forearm as the lateral cutaneous nerve of the forearm.

(2) The median nerve supplies the flexors and pronators, which overlie the anterior of the forearm, and then ends as cutaneous fibers to the lateral portion of the palm and palmar aspects of the thumb, first finger, second finger, and lateral portion of the third finger.

(3) The ulnar nerve supplies smaller intrinsic muscles of the hand responsible for fine movement and also flexors and ends as cutaneous branches to the medial aspect of the hand.

(4) The radial nerve supplies all the extensor muscles of the upper limb and cutaneous branches to the skin of the posterior aspect of the arm, forearm, and the lateral aspect of the dorsum of the hand.

(5) The axillary nerve supplies the shoulder joint and the area of the deltoid muscle.

e. Cutaneous nerves of the upper limb form from both collateral and terminal branches of the brachial plexus (Figure 1–34).

7. Arterial supply (Figure 1–35)

a. The subclavian artery supplies blood to the entire upper limb.

(1) The right subclavian artery arises from the brachiocephalic artery and the left subclavian artery from the aortic arch; both loop upward and laterally through the root of the neck and descend over the first rib into the axilla.

(2) After crossing the first rib, the subclavian artery becomes the axillary artery.

(3) The axillary artery passes through the axilla and provides several collateral branches that follow collateral branches of the brachial plexus of nerves.

(a) The axillary artery crosses over the tendon of teres major

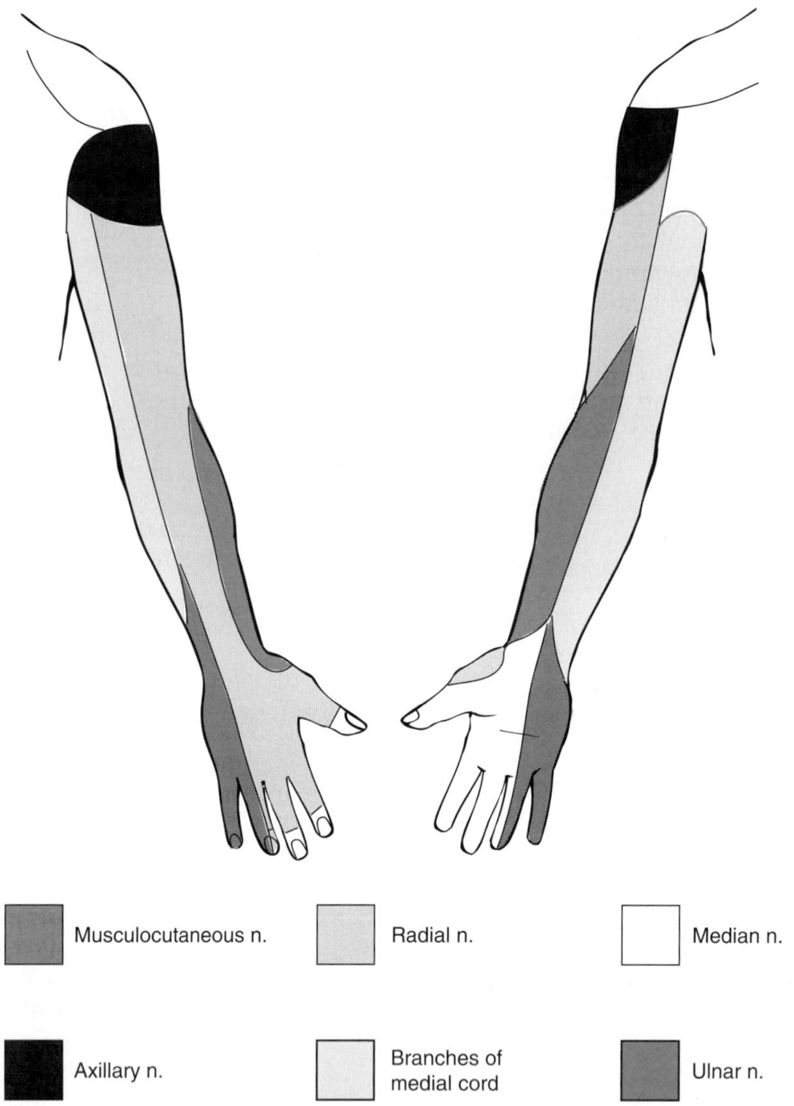

Figure 1–34. Cutaneous innervation of the upper limb. (From Liebgott B: The Anatomic Basis of Dentistry, ed 2, St. Louis, Mosby, 2001.)

muscle and enters the arm; at this point it is called the *brachial artery*.

(4) The brachial artery is positioned on the anterior aspect of the humerus at midlength after entering the arm from the medial aspect.
   (a) It provides several branches to muscles of the upper arm.
   (b) It descends to the cubital fossa on the anterior aspect of the elbow.

(5) The brachial artery splits into the radial and ulnar arteries below the elbow.

(6) The radial artery descends on the lateral surface of the front of the forearm; this is where the pulse is located on the wrist.
   (a) The radial artery enters the hand and loops medially as the deep palmar arch.
   (b) The deep palmar arch anastomoses medially with a branch of the ulnar artery.

(7) The ulnar artery descends on the medial surface of the front of the forearm.
   (a) The ulnar artery enters the hand and loops laterally as the superficial palmar arch.
   (b) The superficial palmar arch anastomoses medially with a branch of the radial artery.

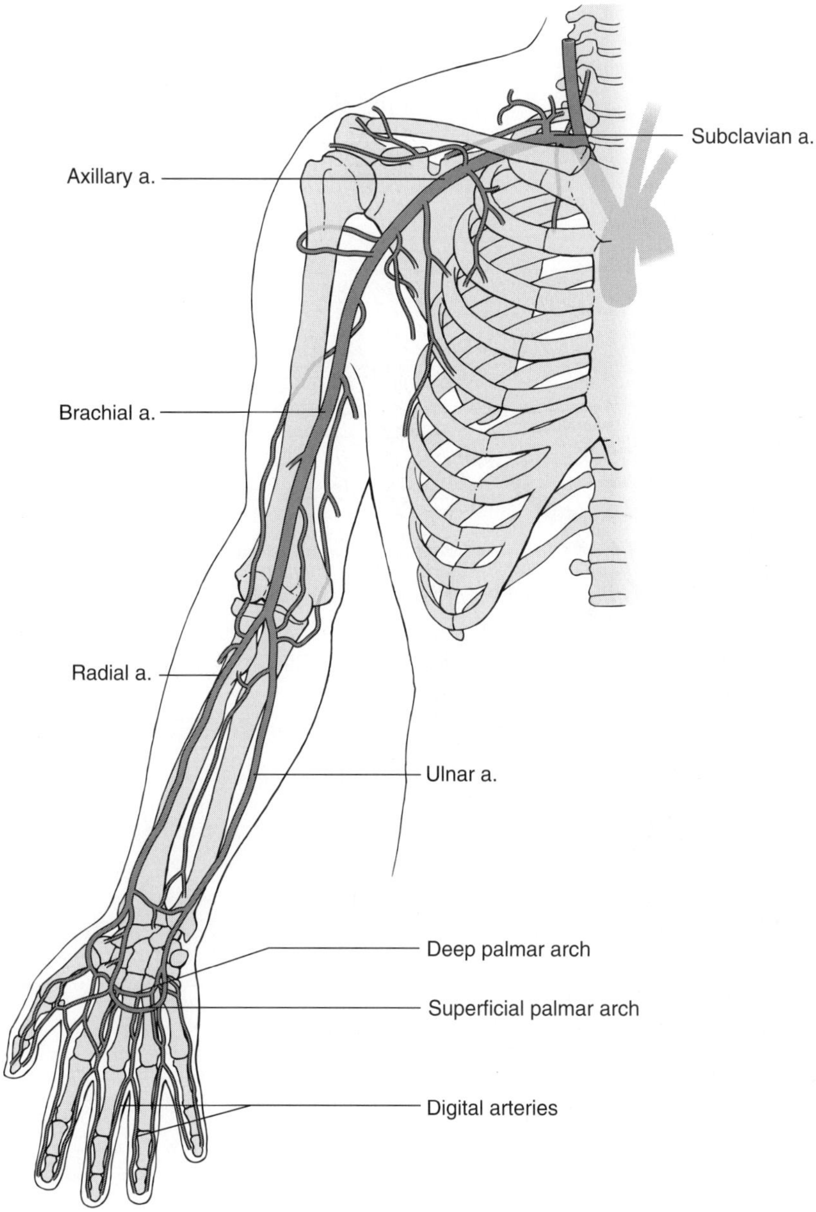

Figure 1–35. Arterial supply to the right upper limb. (From Liebgott B: The Anatomic Basis of Dentistry, ed 2, St. Louis, Mosby, 2001.)

   (8) Digital arteries arise from the palmar arches to supply the medial and lateral aspects of each finger.
8. Venous return (Figure 1–36)
   a. Deep veins
      (1) Deep veins of the upper limb share the names and parallel the deep arteries.
      (2) Deep veins collect as the axillary vein.
      (3) The axillary vein ascends over the first rib and is then called the *subclavian vein.*
   b. Superficial veins
      (1) The dorsal venous vein lies below the skin of the dorsum of the hand and receives tributaries from the fingers.
      (2) The cephalic vein drains the lateral aspect of the dorsal venous arch, spirals anteriorly at the wrist, and ascends on the lateral side of the arm and forearm.
      (3) The basilic vein drains the medial aspect of the dorsal venous arch and ascends on the medial side of the arm and forearm.
         (a) As the basilic vein traverses the cubital fossa, it receives blood from the cephalic vein through the median cubital vein and the median antebrachial vein.

(4) Near the midpoint of the arm, the basilic vein curves deeply and joins the axillary vein.

9. Lymphatic drainage (Figure 1–37)
   a. Deep lymph vessels
      (1) Deep lymph vessels follow radial, ulnar, brachial, and axillary veins to drain into axillary lymph nodes.
      (2) The axillary lymph nodes merge as the subclavian trunk.
      (3) The subclavian trunk drains upper limb lymph back into circulation at the confluence of the internal jugular and subclavian veins.

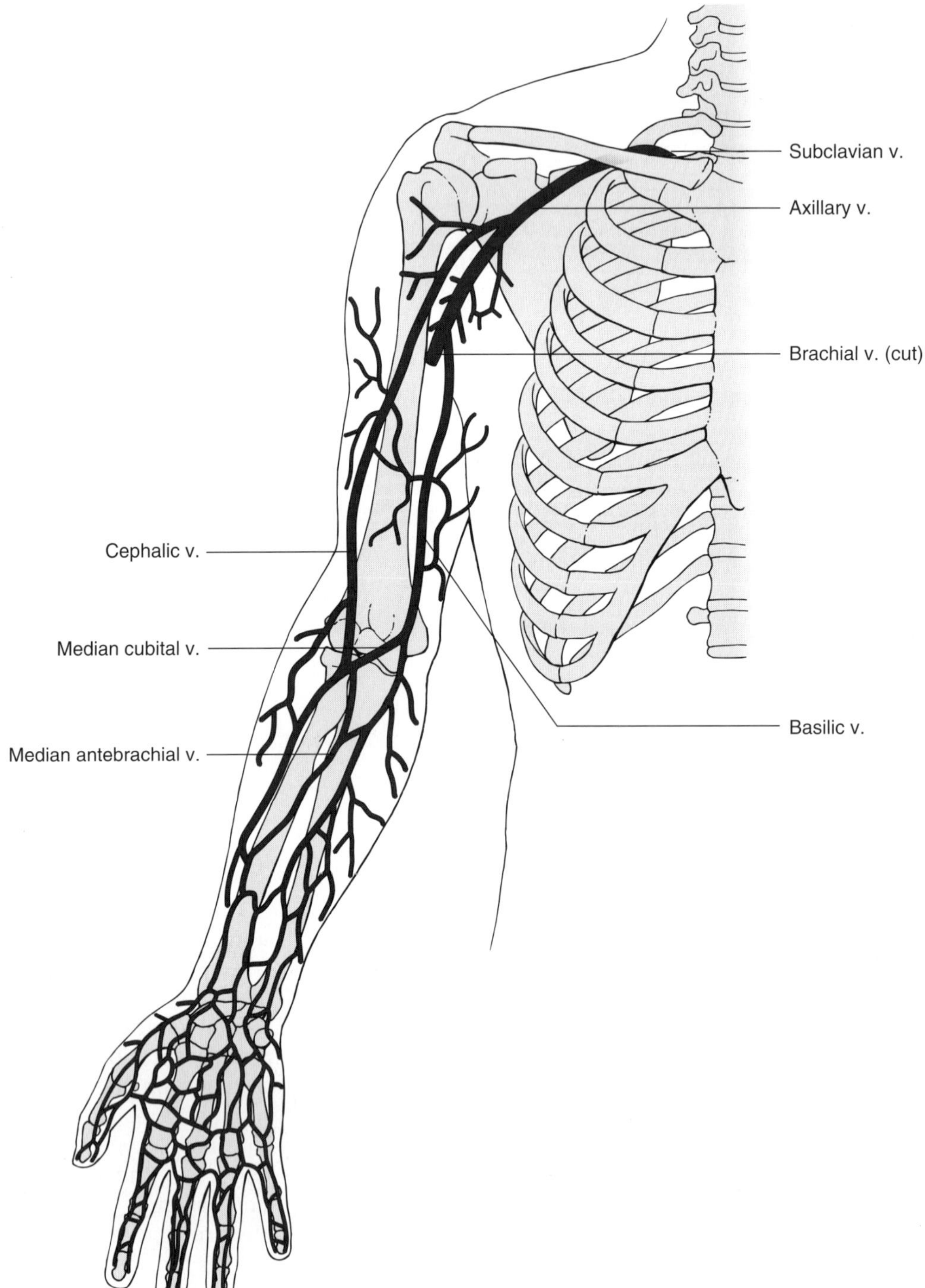

Figure 1–36. Venous return from the right upper limb. (From Liebgott B: The Anatomic Basis of Dentistry, ed 2, St. Louis, Mosby, 2001.)

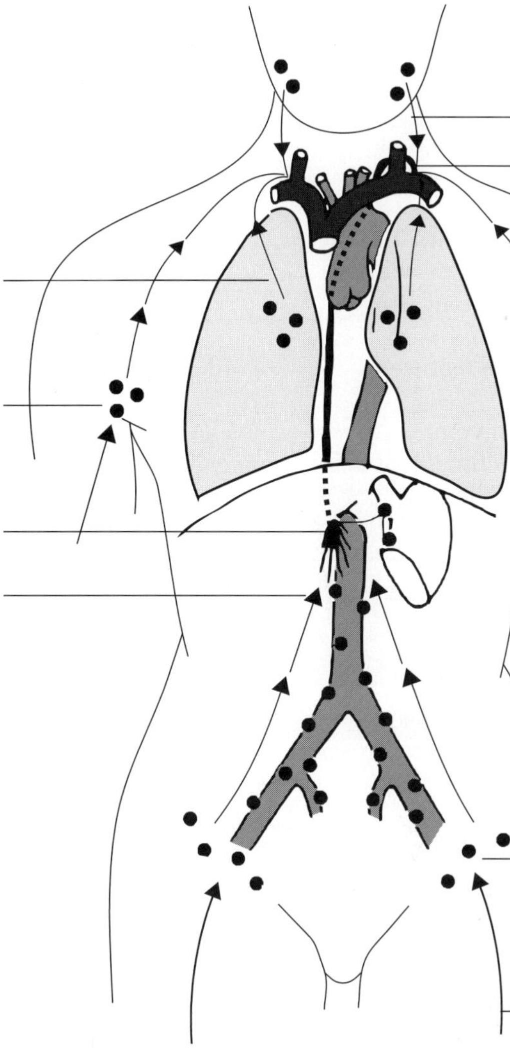

Figure 1–37. Major groups of lymph nodes and trunks showing scheme of the lymphatic flow back to venous system. (From Liebgott B: The Anatomic Basis of Dentistry, ed 2, St. Louis, Mosby, 2001.)

1.3 Thoracic Cavity

The thoracic cavity is surrounded by the thorax, a wall of muscle and bone. It extends from just superior to the first rib to the diaphragm. The diaphragm separates the thoracic cavity from the abdominal cavity.

A. The thoracic skeleton and its divisions: the thoracic skeleton is a round, cage-like structure consisting of the sternum, 12 pairs of ribs and associated costal cartilages, and 12 thoracic vertebrae.
   1. Sternum—composed of three portions:
      a. Manubrium
         (1) The midline jugular or suprasternal notch is palpated at the base of the anterior neck.
         (2) The lateral notches attach to the clavicles.
         (3) The lateral borders articulate with the costal cartilages of the first ribs.
      b. Body
         (1) Joins the manubrium through a symphysis at the sternal angle.
         (2) Costal cartilages of the second ribs articulate with the sternum at the junction of the manubrium and body.
      c. Xiphoid process
         (1) A small, inferior portion.
   2. Ribs—features:
      a. Head, which articulates with the body of a thoracic vertebra.
      b. Neck
      c. Tubercle, which articulates with the transverse process of a thoracic vertebra.
      d. Shaft
      e. Angle where the rib turns inferiorly and anteriorly.

f. Subcostal groove on the inferior internal surface that shelters the intercostal nerve and vessels.

3. Ribs—types:
   a. True ribs are the upper seven pairs that attach to the sternum via costal cartilages.
   b. False ribs are the lower five pairs of ribs that attach to the sternum via costal cartilages or, in the case of the last pair, not at all.
   c. The first rib has some unique features on the superior aspect area:
      (1) Groove for the subclavian vein.
      (2) Scalene tubercle for attachment of the scalenus anterior muscle.
      (3) Roughened area for attachment of the scalenus medius muscle.
4. Thoracic vertebrae—unique features include:
   a. Heart-shaped body.
   b. Long, slender spinous processes.
   c. The bodies and transverse processes have facets for articulation with ribs.
   d. Ribs 1, 10, 11, and 12 articulate with only a single vertebra.
   e. The others articulate with the body of their own vertebra and that of the vertebra above.
5. Joints
   a. In addition to joints between thoracic vertebrae, the remaining three types of joints allow for movement during inspiration.
      (1) Costovertebral joints are synovial joints between the heads of the ribs and vertebral bodies and between the tubercles of the ribs and transverse processes. They permit elevation and depression of the ribs.
      (2) Sternocostal joints are synovial joints between the costal cartilages of true ribs (exclusive of the costal cartilage of the first rib, which joins the first rib to the manubrium as a synchondrosis).
      (3) Costochondral joints are synchodroses between distal ends of ribs and their corresponding costal cartilages.

B. The thoracic wall—the thoracic (chest) wall includes surface features such as the breast and skeletal landmarks, muscles, and intercostal blood vessels and nerves.

1. The breast
   a. Arises as a modified sweat gland covered by skin within superficial fascia of the anterior chest wall.
   b. In women, the breast overlies the pectoralis muscle at the level of ribs 2 through 6. An axillary tail extends laterally and superiorly to the axillary region.
   c. Within the breast are 15 to 20 lobules of glandular tissue lying within fat of the superficial fascia.
   d. The ducts of the glands empty to the surface through the nipple. The nipple is surrounded by an areola containing areolar glands.
   e. The breast is supported through suspensory ligaments (of Cooper) that anchor it to underlying deep fascia.
   f. Arterial blood is supplied by mammary branches of the axillary artery, the internal thoracic artery, and intercostal arteries.
   g. The breast may be divided into quadrants. The two lateral quadrants drain to the superior nodes of the axilla. The two medial quadrants drain to the axillary nodes, the anterior chest wall, and the interior abdominal wall. They may even drain to the opposite breast across the midline. Malignancies may spread along lymphatic routes.
2. Skeletal landmarks
   a. The suprasternal or jugular notch at the base of the neck is important in locating the trachea.
   b. The costal margin, formed by the inferior aspects of costal cartilages 7 through 10, meets in the midline at the xiphoid process. This landmark may be used to help determine the correct position on the sternum for external compressions during cardiopulmonary resuscitation (CPR).
   c. The sternal angle between the manubrium and sternum marks the position of the second rib. From this location ribs can be counted externally, because the first rib cannot be palpated.
3. Muscles of the thorax—thoracic muscles stabilize the upper and lower ribs and elevate the remaining ribs during quiet inspiration. During forced inspiration, accessory muscles elevate the upper ribs to further increase thoracic volume.

a. The diaphragm is the most important muscle of respiration. When it contracts, it increases the size of the thorax by pulling the central tendon inferiorly. It is supplied by the right and left phrenic nerves, which are the anterior primary rami of C3, C4, and C5.

b. Extrinsic thoracic muscles are superficial muscles covering the chest wall that belong to other regions.
   (1) Upper limb muscles that originate from the thoracic skeleton include pectoralis major, pectoralis minor, serratus anterior, latissimus dorsi, rhomboid major, rhomboid minor, levator scapulae, and trapezius.
   (2) Muscles of the abdominal wall that attach to the thoracic skeleton include rectus abdominis, external oblique, internal oblique, and transversus abdominis.
   (3) Posterior muscles that attach to the thoracic skeleton include erector spinae and muscles of the back.

c. Accessory extrinsic muscles of respiration insert into the skeleton of the upper thorax and elevate the sternum and ribs during forced inspiration. These muscles of the neck region include sternomastoid, scalenus anterior, scalenus medius, and scalenus posterior.

d. Intercostal muscles of the thorax extend in several directions; from rib to rib, sternum to rib, and vertebra to rib. They are listed from the surface inward and are involved in the process of breathing. Intercostal nerves supply these muscles.
   (1) The external intercostal muscle runs from rib to rib in an anteroinferior direction. They elevate the ribs during inspiration.
   (2) The internal intercostal muscle extends from rib to rib in a posteroinferior direction perpendicular to the external intercostal muscle. It depresses the ribs during expiration.
   (3) The innermost intercostal muscles run parallel to the internal intercostal muscles. The intercostal nerves and vessels course between these two layers. Posterior fibers are called *subcostals*, and anterior fibers are called *transverses thoracis*. They are thought to depress ribs during expiration.

e. Levator costarum muscles are back muscles that participate in respiration. They originate from transverse processes C7 to T11, run down and laterally, and insert into an area between the tubercle and angle of the rib below. These muscles elevate ribs during inspiration. They are innervated by the posterior primary rami of thoracic spinal nerves.

f. The serratus posterior superior and inferior muscles are located on the posterior thoracic wall.
   (1) The superior muscle runs downward and laterally from the lower cervical and upper thoracic vertebral spines to the upper ribs. It elevates the ribs during inspiration.
   (2) The inferior muscle runs upward and laterally from the upper lumbar and lower thoracic vertebral spines and inserts into the lower ribs. It depresses or stabilizes the lower ribs.

4. Intercostal blood vessels and nerves are located between the internal and innermost intercostal muscles found between pairs of ribs. They run under the subcostal groove of the superior rib of the pair.
   a. Posterior intercostal arteries arise from the thoracic aorta in paired, segmented branches. They run laterally and anteriorly and supply the body wall.
   b. Anterior intercostal arteries arise from the internal thoracic artery. These supply the anterior body wall and anastomose with the posterior intercostal arteries. The internal thoracic artery divides into two terminal branches, the superior epigastric artery of the anterior abdominal wall and the musculophrenic artery of the diaphragm.
   c. Intercostal veins parallel the arteries. Anterior intercostal veins empty into the internal thoracic veins. Posterior intercostal veins empty into the azygos and hemiazygos veins. The superior intercostal veins empty into the brachiocephalic veins.
   d. Spinal nerves arise from the spinal cord in a paired, segmented manner. The anterior primary rami travel laterally and anteriorly along with the intercostal arteries and veins as intercostal nerves. Lateral cutaneous branches are given off laterally. As the nerves reach the

midline, anterior cutaneous branches are given off to the anterior chest wall.

C. The pleural cavities

The pleural cavities contain the lungs. The pleural cavity is lined with pleura, a serous membrane.

1. Parietal pleura lines the pleural cavity itself. Parietal pleura is subdivided by region.
   a. Costal pleura lines the inner aspect of the rib cage.
   b. Diaphragmatic pleura lines the superior aspect of the diaphragm.
   c. Mediastinal pleura covers the mediastinum.
   d. Cervical pleura (cupola) extends into the neck.
2. Visceral pleura lines the lungs.
   a. Both parietal and visceral pleura are continuous at the root of the lung.

D. Lungs

The pleural cavities contain the lungs. The functional site of the lungs are the alveoli, where the exchange of oxygen and carbon dioxide take place. The alveoli are supported by elastic tissue that tends to collapse and shrink the lung during expiration.

1. Surfaces of the lung
   a. The rounded, superior apex that bulges up through the thoracic inlet.
   b. The mediastinal surface that contacts the mediastinum.
   c. The convex costal surface that fits the ribs.
   d. The concave base or diaphragmatic surface resting on the diaphragm.
2. Borders of the lung
   a. The anterior border separates the costal surface from the mediastinal surface.
   b. The posterior border separates the costal surface from the mediastinal surface posteriorly.
   c. The lower circumferential border separates the diaphragmatic surface from the costal and mediastinal surfaces.
3. Fissures and lobes of the lung
   a. The lungs are divided into lobes by fissures. The right lung has three lobes, and the left lung has two. Although both lungs have an oblique fissure dividing them into a upper and lower lobes, the right lung has a second horizontal fissure that creates an additional middle lobe.
   b. The cardiac notch on the left lobe is a feature substituting for the lack of a third, middle lobe.
4. The hilum of the lung is the entrance and exit for the air tubes and blood vessels.
   a. The pulmonary artery carries unoxygenated blood from the right ventricle to the lungs, and the pulmonary vein carries oxygenated blood from the lungs.
   b. The bronchi arise from the midline trachea. They carry air to the lung through the hilum during inspiration and from the lung during expiration.
   c. The bronchial artery arises from the thoracic descending aorta and travels to the hilum to supply the lung.
   d. Autonomic nerves enter the lungs through the hilum.
   e. Lymphatic vessels enter and leave the lungs through the hilum.

E. Bronchi

The trachea is composed of cartilaginous rings connected with fibroelastic tissue. The rings are not complete; the posterior portion that lacks cartilage is covered with fibrous tissue and involuntary muscle.

The trachea descends along with but anterior to the esophagus from the neck. The isthmus of the thyroid gland crosses the second or third tracheal ring. The trachea enters the inlet of the thorax, deep to the sternum, and at vertebral level T5 it bifurcates at a midline cartilaginous ring called the *carina* into the right and left primary bronchus. The right primary bronchus is wider, shorter, and more directly in line with the trachea.

1. Right bronchus
   a. The right primary bronchus divides into three secondary bronchi, corresponding to the three lobes of the right lung. The secondary bronchus to the upper lobe separates before the primary bronchus passes through the hilum of the lung. The primary bronchus within the lobe divides and supplies secondary bronchi to the middle and lower lobes.
   b. Each secondary bronchus further divides into tertiary bronchi that continue to divide until they lose cartilaginous support.
   c. At this point the walls of the tubes are lined with smooth muscle and are called *bronchioles*. Bronchioles end as terminal bronchioles, with ductules that lead into alveoli.
   d. Alveoli are blind sacs that are one cell thick. They are the site of gas exchange.

e. Surrounding each alveolus are capillaries from arterioles supplied by pulmonary arteries. These capillaries anastomose with venules that course and unite as pulmonary veins.

2. Left bronchus

a. The structure of the left bronchial tree is similar to the right, with two exceptions. Because there are only two lobes in the left lung, there are only two rather than three bronchi that divide to create tertiary bronchi.

F. Blood supply

1. Bronchial arteries supply blood to the lungs. They branch from the descending aorta and course along with the bronchi and bronchioles to the parenchyma of the lung. Lymph vessels parallel the arterial vessels but drain in the opposite direction to the bronchomediastinal trunk.

G. Nerve supply

1. The lungs are controlled by the sympathetic and parasympathetic divisions of the autonomic nervous system.

a. Pulmonary branches of the vagus nerve (the tenth cranial nerve) function as parasympathetic efferent nerves. They are bronchoconstrictors and secretomotors.

b. Sympathetic efferents are derived mainly from the second, third, and fourth ganglia of the sympathetic trunk. They function as bronchodilators.

2. Both divisions form a pulmonary nerve plexus around the pulmonary vessels at the hilum of the lung. They surround and follow the vessels as they pass into the lung.

3. The phrenic nerve supplies pleura adjacent to the diaphragm and mediastinum. Costal pleura is supplied by intercostal nerves.

H. Mechanics of breathing

1. Air is inhaled during inspiration and exhaled during expiration.

a. Inspiration: the muscles involved in breathing enlarge the pleural cavity in three planes to increase the volume and decrease the pressure within the lungs.

(1) The transverse diameter increases when intercostal muscles raise the ribs at the costovertebral and costosternal joints and move them laterally.

(2) The anteroposterior diameter increases when the right and left rib pairs raise around the costovertebral joints and move the sternum anteriorly.

(3) The size of the vertical plane increases when the diaphragm contracts downward.

(4) During forced inspiration, additional muscles are called into action:

(a) Scalene muscles of the neck raise the first two ribs.

(b) The sternomastoid muscle raises the manubrium.

(c) Extremely labored breathing may include the pectoral muscles and the serratus anterior muscle.

b. Expiration: normal expiration is passive. Elastic recoil of the lungs forces air out when the muscles of respiration are relaxed.

(1) During forced expiration, abdominal muscles contract and raise intra-abdominal pressure while the diaphragm relaxes.

I. The mediastinum

The mediastinum separates the pleural cavities. It is a group of midline structures covered on the left and right surfaces with mediastinal pleura. The mediastinum contains the heart and associated great vessels, thoracic trachea and bronchi, the thoracic esophagus, the vagus nerves, phrenic nerves, and the thoracic duct. The mediastinum is divided into four areas: the middle mediastinum, anterior mediastinum, superior mediastinum, and posterior mediastinum (Figure 1–38).

Middle mediastinum

1. Contains the pericardial sac and enclosed heart.

a. Pericardial sac

(1) Pericardium is composed of a tough outer layer of fibrous tissue and an inner layer of serous membrane called *visceral pericardium* or *epicardium*.

(2) The outer layer is adherent to the diaphragm.

2. Heart

a. Shape and position—the heart is within the thorax, behind the sternum, and above the diaphragm. It is located closer to the anterior chest wall than the posterior chest wall.

(1) The superior border is at the level of the sternal angle.

(2) The inferior border passes to the left above the xiphoid process to a point

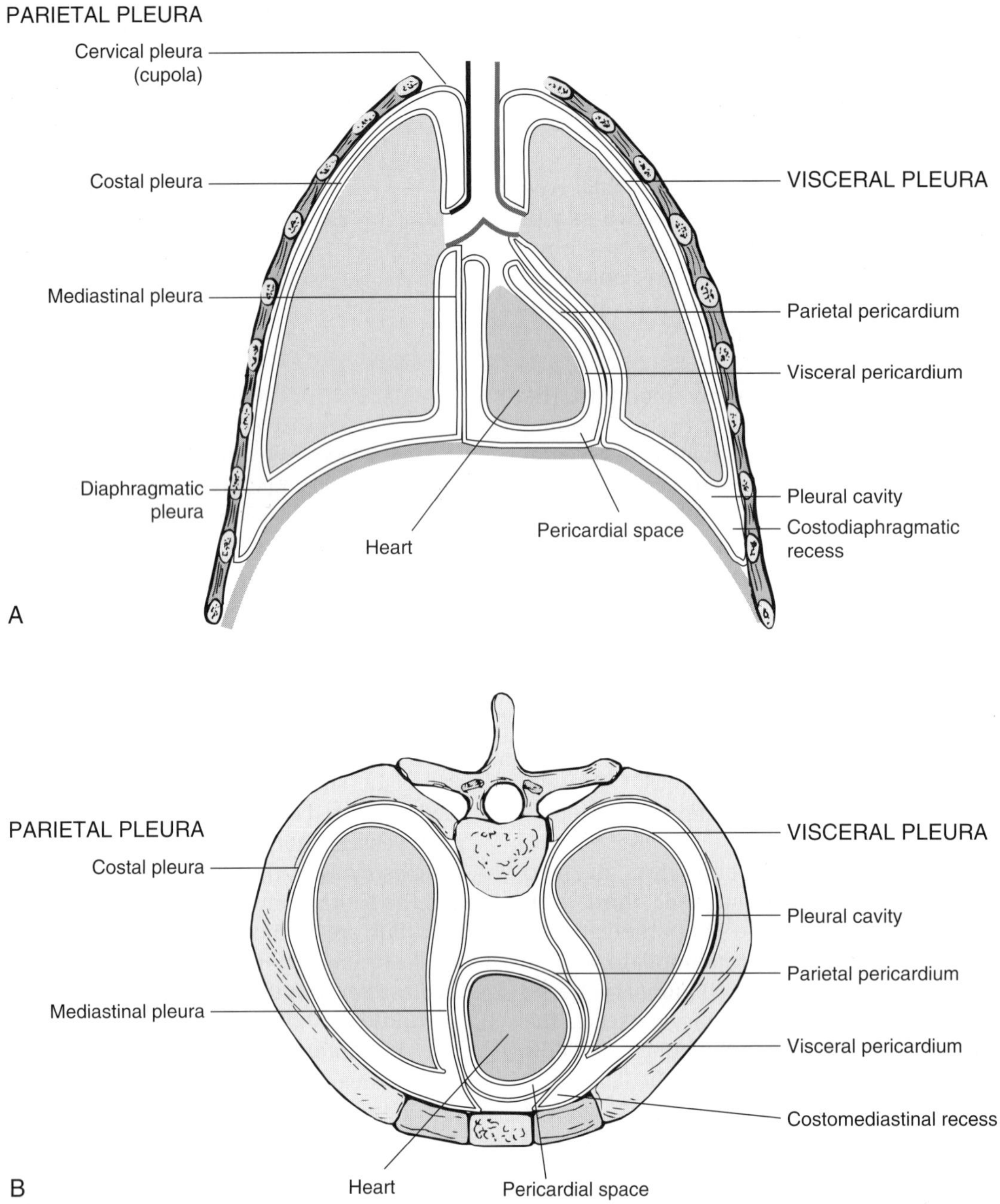

Figure 1–38. Sections through thorax to show pleural cavities, mediastinum, and coverings. A, Coronal section. **B**, Transverse section. (From Liebgott B: The Anatomic Basis of Dentistry, ed 2, St. Louis, Mosby, 2001.)

10 centimeters left of the midline. The inferior border ends to the left as the apex of the heart, at the fifth intercostal space or the sixth rib.

(3) The left border runs obliquely upward toward the sternal angle.

(4) The right border runs parallel to the right of the sternum inferiorly to the level of the 5th intercostal space.

b. Chambers

(1) The right atrium forms the entire right surface and border of the heart and about one-quarter of the anterior surface. The right auricle is an extension of the right atrium; it encircles the base of the aorta.

(2) The left atrium is on the posterior surface of the heart. The left auricle

encircles the base of the pulmonary trunk.

(3) The right ventricle forms two-thirds of the inferior border of the heart and most of the anterior surface.

(4) The left ventricle forms almost all of the left border of the heart and the apex, which is a small piece of the left inferior border.

c. Surface of the heart: the heart has three surfaces and an apex.

(1) The sternocostal surface is on the anterior surface of the heart. It is almost completely overlapped by the lungs.

(2) The diaphragmatic surface rests on the diaphragm.

(3) The posterior surface consists mostly of the left atrium and left ventricle.

(4) The apex of the heart may be observed beating in the left fifth intercostal space, about 10 cm from the midline.

d. Features of the heart—two grooves on the surface of the heart delineate underlying septa between chambers.

(1) The atrioventricular sulcus represents the septum separating the atria from ventricles.

(2) The interventricular sulcus represents the septum separating the right ventricle from left ventricle.

e. The heart wall—the heart consists of three layers.

(1) The epicardium (visceral pericardium) is a serous layer covering the external heart.

(2) The myocardium, a layer of cardiac involuntary muscle with the property of automaticity.

(3) The endocardium, an inner endothelial lining.

f. Entrances to and exits from the heart

(1) The superior and inferior venae cavae enter the right atrium carrying deoxygenated blood from the system. The superior vena cava carries returning blood from the head, upper limb, and thorax. The inferior vena cava carries returning blood from the lower limbs and abdomen.

g. Internal features of the right atrium—the right atrium of the heart receives blood from the superior and inferior venae cavae.

(1) The orifice of the superior vena cava lies superior to the orifice of the inferior vena cava. It does not have a valve.

(2) The orifice of the inferior vena cava lies inferior to the orifice of the superior vena cava. It has a small, albeit rudimentary, crescent-shaped valve.

(3) The crista terminalis is a ridge that runs vertically between orifices of the superior and inferior venae cavae. It represents the junction between the sinus venosus and the heart in the developing heart of the embryo.

(4) The pectinate muscles radiate out from the crista terminalis at right angles.

(5) The fossa ovalis, an oval depression above the valve of the inferior vena cava, represents the remnant of foramen ovale, the prenatal shunt from the right to the left atrium.

(6) The right auricle is an appendage of the right atrium.

(7) The left auricle is an appendage of the left atrium.

(8) The right atrioventricular valve leads to the right ventricle. It is called the *tricuspid valve* because it has three leaflets

(9) The coronary sinus opens into the right atrium just above the atrioventricular orifice. It returns blood from the heart walls.

(10) The sinoatrial and atrioventricular nodes are not visible upon gross inspection of the heart. The sinoatrial node is located at the junction of the superior vena cava and the right atrium. It is the pacemaker of the heart. The atrioventricular node is located above the opening of the coronary sinus. It relays the signal from the sinoatrial node.

h. Internal features of the left atrium—the left atrium receives blood from pulmonary veins from the lungs.

(1) Two right and two left pulmonary veins enter the heart through four separate orifices.

(2) The left atrium is drained through the left atrioventricular valve. This valve is called the *bicuspid* or *mitral valve* because it has two leaflets.

i. Internal features of the right ventricle—the right ventricle receives blood from the right atrium through the right atrioventricular valve. It has a thicker and more muscular wall than the right atrium because it is a pumping chamber.
   (1) Ridges of cardiac muscle called *trabeculae carneae* give the internal surface a roughened appearance.
   (2) The right atrioventricular or tricuspid valve has three leaflets. The bases of these are anchored to a tendinous ring around the orifice of the valve.
   (3) The chordae tendineae extend from the free edges of the cusps of the tricuspid valve to papillary muscles.
   (4) Papillary muscles anchor the chordae tendineae and cusps to the heart wall. These muscles contract as the ventricles contract, ensuring that the cusps of the valve seal the orifice but are not pushed back into the right atrium.
   (5) The pulmonary valve is a three-pocket valve. After the right ventricle contracts, the pockets of this valve fill with blood and prevent further backflow of blood into the right ventricle.
   (6) The septomarginal trabeculae contains cardiac fibers that conduct impulses from the interventricular septum to the anterior papillary muscle.

j. Internal features of the left ventricle—the left ventricle pumps blood to the whole body. The walls are thick and muscular.
   (1) The trabeculae carneae are ridges of cardiac muscle that roughen the surface as they do in the right ventricle.
   (2) The left atrioventricular valve has two valves. It is also known as the *mitral valve*.
   (3) The chordae tendinae prevent the valves from extending into the left atrium during ventricular contraction.
   (4) The aortic valve has three pockets. It prevents backflow of blood from the aorta back into the left ventricle following contraction.

k. Blood vessels—the right and left coronary arteries supply the heart muscle with oxygenated blood. They are the first pair of arteries to leave the aorta. They arise just above the aortic valve. The various cardiac veins of the heart drain into the coronary sinus, which is a single, large vein that enters the right atrium of the heart.
   (1) The right coronary artery passes inferiorly in the anterior atrioventricular sulcus and supplies blood to cardiac tissue. At the inferior margin of the heart it gives off the right marginal branch, then turns posteriorly and ascends into the posterior atrioventricular sulcus until it reaches the posterior interventricular groove. It divides into two branches, one of which continues posteriorly in the atrioventricular sulcus to anastomose with the circumflex artery. The other branch turns down toward the apex of the heart to anastomose with the anterior interventricular branch of the left coronary artery.
   (2) The left coronary artery, traveling between the left atrium and pulmonary trunk, reaches the atrioventricular or coronary sulcus. Here it gives off two branches. The anterior interventricular branch descends in the sulcus toward the apex of the heart. It curves posteriorly and anastomoses with the posterior interventricular branch of the right coronary artery. The circumflex branch travels around in the atrioventricular sulcus to the posterior of the heart. It descends obliquely to anastomose with the terminal part of the right coronary artery.
   (3) The great cardiac vein travels up the anterior interventricular sulcus and receives venous blood. It turns posterior and to the right as the coronary sinus. It receives two tributaries, the oblique vein from the left atrium and the posterior vein of the left ventricle. As the coronary sinus approaches the right atrium, it receives the middle cardiac vein

and small cardiac veins. Small cardiac veins of the right ventricle drain directly into the right atrium. A small amount of blood passes to and from the heart wall via small venae cordis minimae.

l. Innervation—intrinsic control of heartbeat. A specialized conduction system initiates the heartbeat and conducts the impulse to cardiac muscle.
   (1) The sinoatrial node initiates the heartbeat. It is located in the superior aspect of the crista terminalis at the junction of the superior vena cava and the right atrium. The initial impulse spreads out over atrial walls and causes them to contract and fill the ventricle.
   (2) The atrioventricular node is located in the atrioventricular septum just above the opening of the coronary sinus. It relays impulses from the atrial walls and relays them to the interventricular septum via the bundle of His.
   (3) The bundle of His divides into right and left segments, which descend in the interventricular septum to the right and left ventricular walls and cause them to contract.

m. Innervation—extrinsic modification of heartbeat.
   (1) Parasympathetic fibers from the vagus nerve (CN X) slow the heart rate.
   (2) Sympathetic fibers from the sympathetic trunk speed up the heart rate.
   (3) The cardiac plexus is found on the inferior aortic arch border anterior to the bifurcation of the trachea. It receives preganglionic vagal fibers and postganglionic sympathetic fibers; thus, it has both parasympathetic and sympathetic input. Efferent fibers from the cardiac plexus pass to the heart to modify the heartbeat.

n. Innervation—afferent or sensory cardiac nerves.
   (1) Afferent nerve fibers accompany sympathetic nerves and carry feedback from the viscera to the central nervous system. When cardiac muscle lacks oxygen, impulses may rise to a conscious, painful level as angina pectoris.

Anterior mediastinum

The anterior mediastinum contains connective tissue and fat, a small portion of the thymus gland, and a few lymph nodes.

Superior and posterior mediastinum

A. The trachea and bronchi are described in previous material about the lung.

B. The esophagus extends from the pharynx at vertebral level C6 to the abdomen at level T11.
   1. The esophagus has three components: a cervical, thoracic, and abdominal portion.
   2. The esophagus has four constrictions: the origin or pharyngeal end; where it passes the aortic arch; the superior mediastinum, at the bifurcation of the trachea; and where it passes through the diaphragm.
   3. The esophagus has a sphincter at both ends; the cricopharyngeus muscle prevents swallowing air at the pharyngeal end, and the cardiac sphincter prevents regurgitation of stomach contents at the abdominal end.
   4. The esophagus enters the thorax and superior mediastinum through the thoracic inlet. It is anterior to the vertebrae and posterior to the trachea. It descends into the posterior mediastinum. The aortic arch and descending aorta intervene between the vertebrae and the esophagus below the level of the heart. The esophagus turns anteriorly and slightly to the left as it passes through the diaphragm.
   5. In the cervical region, the esophagus receives branches from laryngeal arteries. In the thorax, it receives visceral branches from the aorta. In the abdomen, it receives branches from the short and left gastric arteries.
   6. The esophagus acquires autonomic nerves as it descends. In the cervical region, it receives sympathetic fibers from the cervical sympathetic ganglia and parasympathetic fibers from recurrent laryngeal branches of the vagus nerve. In the thorax and abdomen, it picks up sympathetic fibers from the sympathetic trunk.

The parasympathetic supply is from the vagus nerves. In the superior mediastinum, the right and left vagus nerves form a plexus around the esophagus and follow the esophagus into the posterior mediastinum and through the diaphragm. In the abdomen, the vagus nerves reconstitute as anterior and posterior vagal trunks.

C. Within the thorax, the aorta is divided into three parts: the ascending aorta, the aortic arch, and the descending aorta.
  1. The ascending aorta originates at the aortic orifice. It passes superiorly to the level of the second costal cartilage. Above the aortic valves, the ascending aorta bulges as the aortic sinus. The right and left coronary arteries arise from the right and left coronary sinuses.
  2. The aortic arch begins at the level of the second costal cartilage. It arches to the left, and its superior border lies at about the midpoint of the manubrium. It descends to level T4 and continues inferiorly as the descending aorta.
     a. The brachiocephalic artery is the first branch arising from the aortic arch. It arches up to the right sternoclavicular joint. At this level it divides into the right common carotid artery and the right subclavian artery.
     b. The left common carotid artery rises from the apex of the aortic arch posterior to the left sternoclavicular joint. It ascends through the left side of the neck.
     c. The left subclavian artery arises immediately distal to the left common carotid artery and passes to the left upper limb.
  3. The descending aorta descends from vertebral level T4. It descends through the posterior mediastinum and provides branches to thoracic viscera and the thoracic wall. It ends by passing through the diaphragm to become the abdominal aorta at vertebral level T12.
     a. Visceral branches supply the lungs, esophagus, pericardium, and diaphragm.
     b. Somatic branches consist of the lower nine posterior intercostal arteries and the subcostal artery.
  4. There are three main veins within the thorax, the inferior vena cava, the superior vena cava, and the azygos and hemiazygos systems of veins.
     a. The inferior vena cava drains the lower limbs and the abdomen. It pierces the diaphragm, rises in the thorax, and ends in the inferior aspect of the right atrium of the heart.
     b. The superior vena cava is formed by the right and left brachiocephalic veins at the level of the first costal cartilage behind the manubrium. It drains the upper limbs and the head and neck. The superior vena cava then descends behind the sternum and enters the right atrium of the heart at the level of the third costal cartilage. The brachiocephalic veins are formed by a union of the internal jugular veins and the subclavian veins at the root of the neck behind the sternoclavicular joints.
     c. The azygos and hemiazygos system of veins drains the thoracic wall. The right and left ascending lumbar veins ascend from the abdomen to the thorax.
        (1) The right ascending lumbar vein passes through the diaphragm and continues to rise as the azygos vein. The azygos vein empties into the superior vena cava.
        (2) The left ascending lumbar vein continues up into the thorax as the inferior hemiazygos vein and drains the lower intercostal veins. It ascends to approximately vertebral level T8 and then crosses the midline to join the azygos vein on the right side.
        (3) An accessory, or superior, hemiazygos vein drains the fourth, fifth, sixth, and seventh intercostal veins as it descends to the level of T8. At T8 it enters the azygos vein. The upper three intercostal veins join to form the superior intercostal vein, which ascends to drain to the left brachiocephalic vein.
  5. The thoracic duct begins in the abdomen as a small sac called *cisterna chyli*. Lymphatics drain into it from the lower extremities. Arising from cisterna chyli is the thoracic duct. It enters the thorax through the aortic opening in the diaphragm. Within the thorax it acquires lymphatic drainage through the bronchomediastinal trunk. As the duct approaches the neck, it empties its contents into the confluence of the left internal jugular and left subclavian veins.

6. Four types of nerves are found in the thorax: intercostal nerves, the sympathetic trunk and its branches, the phrenic nerve and its branches, and the vagus nerve.
   a. The intercostal nerves arise from the spinal cord as anterior primary rami of spinal nerves T1 through T12. These nerves supply the musculature of the thoracic walls and return cutaneous sensation from the skin of the chest wall and the upper abdominal wall.
   b. The sympathetic trunk and its branches run laterally to the thoracic vertebral bodies. Incoming white rami communicantes run from intercostal nerves in the ganglia of the sympathetic trunk. Outgoing postganglionic gray rami communicantes pass back to the intercostal nerves to be distributed along with the intercostal nerves.
      (1) Splanchnic nerves do not synapse in the sympathetic chain of ganglia.
   c. The phrenic nerve arises from the neck from anterior primary rami of spinal nerves C3, C4, and C5. It descends along the anterior surface of the scalenus anterior muscle, entering the thoracic inlet anterior to the subclavian artery. It descends along the lateral mediastinum to the diaphragm. It carries efferent and afferent fibers to and from the diaphragm.
   d. The vagus nerve exits the skull through the jugular foramina. It descends and enters the thoracic inlet anterior to the subclavian arteries. The right vagus nerve gives rise to the right recurrent laryngeal nerve. The left vagus nerve gives rise to the left recurrent laryngeal nerve. Both vagus nerves descend posteriorly to the root of the lung, where they provide pulmonary branches to the pulmonary plexus and branches to the cardiac plexus. The nerves descend through the thorax as a nerve plexus surrounding the esophagus, and then form again as anterior and posterior vagal trunks within the abdomen.
   e. The cardiac plexus is found below the aortic arch and anterior to the tracheal bifurcation. It receives sympathetic postganglionic fibers from the cervical sympathetic ganglia. It receives preganglionic parasympathetic fibers from the vagus nerves. Efferent fibers go to the heart.
   f. The pulmonary plexus surrounds pulmonary vessels at the root of the lungs. Sympathetic fibers come from the cardiac plexus. Parasympathetic fibers come from vagal nerves. Outgoing fibers go to the lung.
   g. The thymus gland is composed of lymphoid tissue. It produces T lymphocytes, shrinks following puberty, and is replaced by adipose tissue.

1.4 Abdominopelvic Cavity

The abdominopelvic cavity extends from the floor of the pelvis and rises to the level of the fifth intercostal space within the thoracic cage. The abdominal cavity is enclosed by the pelvic diaphragm below, the muscular anterolateral abdominal wall on the sides, and a muscular and bony posterior wall and the thoracic diaphragm above. The abdomen contains most of the digestive tract and the viscera of the genitourinary system.

A. Skeleton of the abdomen: the skeleton of the abdomen is divided into thoracic, vertebral, and pelvic components.
   1. Thoracic component: the abdominal cavity extends into the thoracic cage between the fifth intercostal space above and the costal margin below. The thoracic cavity has been discussed in Section 1.3.
   2. Vertebral component: the lower thoracic vertebrae, lumbar vertebrae, the sacrum, and the coccyx compose the vertebrae located in the abdomen.
      a. Thoracic vertebrae: there are 12 thoracic vertebrae. They have a number of features that distinguish them from the rest of the vertebrae in the spinal column.
         (1) The body is heart-shaped.
         (2) The body has an articulating facet for the head of a rib.
         (3) The transverse process has an articulating facet for the tubercle of a rib.
         (4) The spinous process is long and slender.
      b. Lumbar vertebrae: there are five lumbar vertebrae, distinguished by four features.
         (1) The body is large and bean-shaped.
         (2) There are no facets for ribs.
         (3) Transverse processes do not have transverse foramina.
         (4) The spinous processes are square.

c. The sacrum: the sacrum is a solid, triangular mass formed from five elements.
   (1) The posterior spinous processes are represented by a median crest.
   (2) Fused transverse processes form a lateral mass that terminates laterally as two ear-shaped articular surfaces.
   (3) The sacral promontory projects anteriorly.
   (4) The sacral canal continues the vertebral canal inferiorly from the lumbar region.
   (5) Four anterior and posterior pelvic foramina leave the sacral canal on either side. These transmit sacral anterior and posterior primary rami.
d. The coccyx: the coccyx is a triangular mass formed by the fusion of four segments.
   (1) Pelvic component
      (a) Os coxae: the ilium, ischium, and pubis bones fuse by about age 16 to form the os coxae. The right and left os coxae form the lower hip girdle. They join with the sacrum and coccyx to form the pelvic cavity, which surrounds and protects several pelvic viscera.
         (i) The ilium consists of a flared, flattened plate with a concave medial surface. It ends superiorly as the iliac crest. The iliac tubercle is a small, bony elevation on the superior lateral aspect of the iliac crest. The anterior inferior and anterior superior iliac spines are two small elevations on the anterior surface of the iliac crest.
         (ii) The inferior surface of the ischium (the ischial tuberosity) supports a person when sitting.
         (iii) The pubis on each side meets in the middle at the symphysis pubis. The pubic tubercle is lateral to the symphysis. The inguinal ligament connects the pubic tubercle to the anterior superior iliac spine.
         (iv) The pubis and ischium meet and form the obturator foramen.
         (v) The acetabulum serves as the receptacle for the femur.
         (vi) The ischial spine projects posteriorly from the ischium. It divides the posterior aspect of the bone into the greater sciatic notch above and the lesser sciatic notch below.
      (b) Pelvic cavity—is divided into an upper pelvis within the iliac crests, and a lower pelvis, which is surrounded by the right and left pubis, the ischium, and the sacrum. The sacrum extends into the lower pelvis as a promontory.

B. Divisions of the abdomen—the abdomen may be divided into regions according to two systems.
   1. One system divides the abdomen into four quadrants, based on the median sagittal plane in the abdomen intersecting with a transverse plane.
   2. The other system divides the abdomen into nine regions based on two sagittal and two transverse planes through the abdomen.
      a. The sagittal planes are located by a line joining the midclavicular point to the midpoint of the inguinal ligament.
      b. The transverse planes are located by a line joining the most inferior points of the costal margins, and a line joining the right and left iliac tubercles on the superior aspects of the iliac crests.

C. Abdominal walls—the abdominal cavity is enclosed by four walls. They are the anterolateral wall, the posterior wall, the superior wall formed by the thoracic diaphragm, and the inferior wall formed by the pelvic diaphragm.
   1. The anterolateral abdominal wall
      a. Surface features: several abdominal landmarks may be palpated, including the costal margins, xiphoid process, iliac crests, superior and inferior iliac spines, and pubic tubercles. The lateral limit of the rectus abdominis muscle is represented by linea semilunaris. Transverse bands running from the linea semilunaris and the midline repre-

sent underlying tendinous inserts of the rectus abdominis muscle. A slight crease from the anterior superior iliac spine runs toward the pubic tubercle, representing the position of the inguinal ligament.

b. Layers: the layers that comprise the anterolateral abdominal wall below the skin from superficial to deep are, in order: superficial fascia, deep fascia, muscles and aponeurosis, transversalis fascia, extraperitoneal layer, and the peritoneum.
   (1) Superficial fascia—also known as the *subcutaneous fatty layer*, it is usually divisible further into the more superficial Camper's fascia and the deeper Scarpa's fascia.
   (2) Deep fascia—this layer is more membranous than the more superficial fascia.
   (3) Muscles and aponeurosis (Table 1–27)—there are four pairs of bilateral muscles in the anterolateral abdominal wall. Three of the pairs are flat: the external oblique muscle, internal oblique muscle, and transverse abdominis muscle. The muscles are arranged in sheets with the fibers running in different directions for strength.
      (a) The external oblique muscle—the outermost muscle, which courses medially from the lower ribs. When the muscles run down and approach the midline, they merge with a membranous aponeurosis. Inferior fibers attach to the iliac crest. These fibers form a border called the *inguinal ligament.*
      (b) The internal oblique muscle—originates from the iliac crest. It runs upward and medially and inserts into the costal margin, the linea alba, and the pubis, along with transverse abdominis as a conjoint tendon.
      (c) The transversus abdominis muscle—originates from the lumbodorsal fascia, iliac crest, inguinal ligament, and lower costal cartilages. It runs medially, in a transverse direction, and inserts as an aponeurosis into the linea alba in the midline.
      (d) The rectus abdominis muscle—runs inferiorly from the costal margin and lower thoracic cage to the pubis, and is more like a belt or strap. This muscle is enclosed in a membranous

TABLE 1-27. MUSCLES OF THE ANTERIOR ABDOMINAL WALL

MUSCLE	ORIGIN	INSERTION	ACTION	NERVE
External oblique	External aspects of lower eight ribs	Iliac crest, aponeurosis of anterior abdominal wall at linea alba	Increase abdominal pressure	Segmented APR of thoracic spinal nerves
Internal oblique	Lumbodorsal fascia, iliac crest, inguinal ligament	Costal cartilages of last three ribs, linea alba of abdominal aponeurosis	Increase abdominal pressure	Segmented APR of thoracic spinal nerves
Transversus abdominis	Internal aspects of lower six costal cartilages, lumbodorsal fascia, iliac crest, inguinal ligament	Linea alba of abdominal aponeurosis	Increase abdominal pressure	Segmented APR of thoracic spinal nerves
Rectus abdominis	Pubic symphysis, pubic crest	Anterior aspect of xiphoid process, anterior aspects of costal cartilages 5, 6, and 7	Increase abdominal pressure, flex vertebral column	Segmented APR of thoracic spinal nerves

APR, Anterior primary rami.
From Liebgott B: The Anatomic Basis of Dentistry, ed 2, St. Louis, Mosby, 2001, Table 4–1, p.103.

sheath formed by the aponeurosis of the three flat muscles. The muscle inserts into the anterior wall of the membranous sheath.

In lower levels of the rectus sheath, all of the aponeuroses are superficial to the muscle. The arcuate line demarcates the limit of the aponeurotic layer in the posterior wall of the rectus sheath.

(4) Transversalis fascia—a layer of deep fascia is located just deep to the anterolateral abdominal muscles and the rectus sheath. The fibers run in a transverse direction.

(5) Extraperitoneal layer—located between transversalis fascia and the deeper peritoneum. It is a fatty layer of connective tissue.

(6) Peritoneum—is composed of organized connective tissue, in contrast to the extraperitoneal layer.

c. Blood and nerve supply

(1) The anterolateral abdominal wall is supplied by the lower six intercostal nerves of the thorax. From their origin, they stream downward and medially to the abdomen. Inferiorly, the abdominal wall is supplied by two branches of the first lumbar anterior primary ramus.

These branches (the iliohypogastric and ilioinguinal nerves) supply the skin and muscle of the lower portion of the anterolateral abdominal wall.

(2) Segmented branches of the aorta follow the spinal nerves in posterior areas. Segmented branches arise anteriorly from superior and inferior epigastric arteries in the bed of the rectus sheath.

2. Superior abdominal wall

The thoracic and abdominal cavities are separated by the diaphragm. Because the diaphragm projects upward as a dome, abdominal contents may be found within the thoracic rib cage and yet still be part of the abdominal cavity.

a. Origins of the thoracic diaphragm—muscular slips of the diaphragm originate from three sites of attachment.

(1) Sternal slips originate from the posterior aspect of the xiphoid process.

(2) Costal slips originate from internal surfaces of the lower six costal cartilages and the twelfth rib.

(3) Lumbar attachments arise as a right crus from the vertebral bodies and discs of L1, L2, and L3, and a left crus arising from the two vertebral bodies and discs of L1 and L2. The two crura cross to form the median arcuate ligament, which enters the abdominal aorta. Tendons from the crura to the transverse processes of L1 form medial arcuate ligaments. Tendons from the transverse processes of L1 to the midpoints of the twelfth ribs form lateral arcuate ligaments.

b. Insertion of the diaphragm

(1) Fibers of the diaphragm insert into the central tendon.

c. Structures passing through the diaphragm—several structures pass through the diaphragm on their way to or from the abdomen. Others pass between the diaphragm and the body wall.

(1) The aorta enters the abdomen through the median arch.

(2) The inferior vena cava passes out of the abdomen to the thorax through its own opening in the central tendon.

(3) The esophagus passes through its own opening.

(4) The thoracic duct passes through the median arch along with the aorta.

(5) The azygos vein passes through the right crus.

(6) The hemizygos vein passes through the left crus.

(7) The posterior and anterior vagal trunks pass into the abdomen, along with the esophagus, through the esophageal opening.

(8) The splanchnic nerves pass through the crura of the diaphragm.

(9) The sympathetic trunks pass behind the medial arcuate ligament to enter the abdomen.

(10) The superior epigastric arteries pass anteriorly between the sternal and costal origins of the diaphragm.

d. Functions of the diaphragm

(1) The main function is respiration.

(2) Another function is esophageal constriction to prevent gastric regurgitation during inspiration.

e. Nerve supply to the diaphragm

(1) The phrenic nerve is the motor and sensory supply. It arises in the neck from anterior primary rami of spinal nerves C3, C4, and C5.

(2) The phrenic nerve descends through the thoracic inlet and travels inferiorly on either side of the middle mediastinum to reach the diaphragm.

f. Blood supply of the diaphragm

(1) From the internal thoracic artery through the pericardiophrenic and musculophrenic arteries and from aortic branches through intercostal and phrenic arteries.

3. Posterior abdominal wall—consists of skin and fascia, bone, and three muscles.

a. The quadratus lumborum muscle is flat and runs from the twelfth rib and all the lumbar transverse processes down to the iliac crest.

b. Psoas major and iliacus muscles.

4. Inferior abdominal wall—is funnel-shaped.

a. Muscles

(1) Levator ani muscles originate along the internal aspects of the os coxae. The fibers run medially and inferiorly toward the rectum to blend with the longitudinal smooth muscle of the rectum.

(2) The coccygeus muscle is a portion of each levator ani muscle that runs from ischial tuberosity to the coccyx.

b. The perineum—is bound externally by the thighs and buttocks. On a deeper plane, it is bounded by the ischiopubic rami, which converge upon the symphysis pubis anteriorly, and sacrotuberous ligaments converging on the coccyx posteriorly.

D. Peritoneum and the peritoneal cavity

1. Nomenclature

a. Peritoneum is a lining tissue. Parietal peritoneum lines the inner abdominal body walls.

b. Visceral peritoneum covers viscera.

c. The peritoneal cavity is the space between the parietal and visceral layers. This space contains serous fluid, which lubricates the viscera.

d. Some abdominal organs in the peritoneal cavity are suspended by mesentery, which is a double-layered fold. Vessels and nerves pass to and from the viscera through the mesentery.

e. Retroperitoneal viscera organs lie within the extraperitoneal layer of the abdominal wall and do not possess a mesentery.

f. An omentum is a double-layered fold of peritoneum. It joins viscera.

g. Ligaments are specifically named folds of peritoneum that are parts of mesenteries or omenta.

E. Blood supply to the abdomen

1. Arterial supply: the abdominal aorta. The descending aorta of the thorax passes through the diaphragm and becomes the abdominal aorta. At vertebral level L4, it divides into the right and left common iliac arteries. These divide further into the right and left external iliac arteries, which descend to supply the lower limb and the right and left internal iliac arteries. The right and left internal iliac arteries supply pelvic structures.

a. Somatic branches

(1) Inferior phrenic arteries—arise from the aorta as it passes through the diaphragm. The right and left branches ascend to supply the inferior aspect of the diaphragm.

(2) Lumbar arteries—there are five lumbar arteries. The first four pairs arise from the aorta, but the fifth pair arises from the internal iliac arteries. The internal iliac arteries turn laterally to supply the lower abdominal wall. Anteriorly, segmented lumbar arteries anastomose with collateral branches of the superior and inferior epigastric arteries.

(3) Median sacral artery—the small median sacral artery continues from the bifurcation of the aorta and supplies the anterior aspect of the sacral area.

b. Unpaired branches to the gut and associated glands—three unpaired branches arise from the abdominal aorta to supply the gut and associated glands, the liver, the pancreas, and the spleen.

(1) Celiac trunk—arises as a short stem just below the diaphragm, at vertebral level T12, L1, and breaks

into three main branches. These branches supply the abdominal esophagus, stomach, duodenum, liver and gallbladder, part of the pancreas, and spleen.

(2) Superior mesenteric artery—arises immediately below the celiac trunk and supplies derivatives of the midgut, including the distal half of the duodenum, jejunum, ileum, caecum and appendix, ascending colon, and transverse colon.

(3) Inferior mesenteric artery—arises at vertebral level L3 and supplies derivatives of the hindgut distal to the left colic flexure.

c. Paired branches to the glands of the genitourinary system—three paired branches supply the glands of the genitourinary system; each originates from the aorta.

(1) Suprarenal arteries—arise either directly from the aorta or from the renal arteries.

(2) Renal arteries—originate from the aorta at vertebral level L1–L2. They pass laterally to supply the right and left kidneys.

(3) Testicular/ovarian arteries—travel inferiorly to supply the gonads.

2. Venous return: the inferior vena cava

The external iliac veins, which drain the lower limbs, and the internal iliac veins, which drain the pelvis, unite within the pelvis to form the right and left common iliac veins. These veins unite at vertebral level L5 to form the inferior vena cava. The vena cava acquires several tributaries as it passes up through the diaphragm. The vena cava leaves the abdomen when it passes through the diaphragm, enters the thorax, and drains into the right atrium.

a. Somatic branches

(1) Inferior phrenic veins—drain the inferior aspect of the diaphragm. They drain either to the superior aspect of the inferior vena cava or to the paired ascending lumbar veins.

(2) Lumbar veins—the body walls are drained by five lumbar veins. The first four drain to the inferior vena cava and the fifth to the common iliac vein. Ascending lumbar veins parallel the inferior vena cava on either side. These veins arise from common iliac veins, ascend on the posterior abdominal wall, and travel through the diaphragm to the thorax. Here they become the azygos and hemiazygos veins.

(3) Median sacral vein—drains the sacral region. It joins the left common iliac vein rather than the inferior vena cava.

b. Tributaries of genitourinary glands—the renal veins receive venous blood from the right and left kidneys. The suprarenal veins receive venous blood from the right and left suprarenal glands.

c. Tributaries of the gastrointestinal tract and associated glands—veins returning from the gut join to form the portal vein. The portal vein enters the liver and ultimately ends as a bed of capillaries. The portal capillary beds are drained by hepatic veins, which enter the vena cava as several hepatic veins.

F. Nerves of the abdomen

1. Somatic nerves

a. The anterior rami of the lower six thoracic spinal nerves and the first lumbar nerve supply the various layers of the anterolateral abdominal walls. Two branches of the anterior primary rami of L1, the iliohypogastric and ilioinguinal nerves, supply the lower portion of the abdominal wall.

b. The anterior primary rami of lumbar nerves L1 to L4 unite and divide within the substance of the psoas muscle to form the lumbar plexus.

c. The anterior primary rami of L4 and L5 and S1 through S4 unite to form the sacral plexus, branches of which provide motor and sensory nerves to the perineum and the remainder of the lower limb.

2. Autonomic nerves

a. Sympathetic nerves

(1) Greater, lesser, and least splanchnic nerves arise bilaterally from the thoracic sympathetic trunks. Without synapsing in the sympathetic trunk, they pass inferiorly through the diaphragm to the abdomen.

(2) Lumbar splanchnic nerves arise from the sympathetic portion of the sympathetic trunk.

(3) Within the abdomen are collections of secondary neurons. The largest

collection is the celiac ganglion and its plexus. The thoracic and lumbar splanchnic nerves synapse within these ganglia.

b. Parasympathetic nerves: parasympathetic innervation of abdominal viscera is shared by the vagus nerves and the pelvic splanchnic nerves.
   (1) Vagus nerves—the vagal plexus within the thorax regroups as anterior and posterior vagal trunks as the vagus nerve passes through the diaphragm. The anterior trunk supplies the liver and biliary apparatus, gastric pylorus, duodenum, and pancreas. The posterior vagal trunk supplies the remainder of the stomach and then joins the celiac plexus. Vagal and celiac plexus fibers are distributed to the gut and derivatives proximal to the left colic flexure.
   (2) Pelvic splanchnic nerves—within the pelvis, parasympathetic fibers from S2 through S4 join the inferior mesenteric plexus as pelvic splanchnic nerves and are distributed along with branches of the plexus. They supply the gut distal to the left colic flexure and the pelvic viscera.

   Parasympathetic fibers of the abdomen travel to their sites of innervation as preganglionic fibers and synapse with secondary neurons within the substance of the organ they supply.

G. Abdominal viscera—the gut wall consists of four layers—an outer layer of visceral peritoneum, a layer of smooth muscle, a submucosal layer, and an inner lining of mucous membrane.

1. The stomach—after passing through the diaphragm, the esophagus widens to form the stomach.
   a. Position: the stomach lies within the upper left quadrant. Its proximal end is immediately below the left dome of the diaphragm.
   b. Features
      (1) Cardiac portion—is adjacent to the cardiac orifice. The cardiac orifice is an area of circular muscle at the entrance to the stomach. Left of the cardiac orifice is the area where the stomach bulges upward, called the *fundus*.
      (2) Pylorus—toward the right, the stomach narrows, first to the pyloric antrum, and then the pyloric sphincter. The pyloric sphincter controls the release of gastric contents to the duodenum.
      (3) Body—the body of the stomach is located between the pylorus and cardiac portion.
      (4) Curvatures—the smaller, curved right superior border of the stomach is called the *lesser curvature*, and the larger, curved left inferior border is called the *greater curvature*.
      (5) Rugae—the mucosa within the stomach has a folded appearance due to the presence of rugae.
   c. Stomach wall—one important function of the stomach is to break up and mix ingested food. The stomach wall is composed of a thick and strong muscular wall for that purpose.
   d. Peritoneal coverings and attachments: the stomach is covered with visceral peritoneum. It is connected to other viscera by the greater and lesser omenta.
      (1) Lesser omentum: connects the lesser curvature of the stomach and the proximal 3 cm of duodenum to the liver above. The common bile duct, portal vein, and hepatic artery pass through the lesser omentum in this area. The lesser omentum ends as a free edge. Immediately posterior to the free edge is the epiploic foramen, which connects the greater and lesser sacs.
      (2) Greater omentum: connects the greater curvature of the stomach to three structures. The gastrocolic ligament, which runs down into the abdomen and then curves back upward and attaches to the transverse colon; the gastrosplenic ligament, which runs from the curvature of the spleen; and the gastrophrenic ligament, which becomes continuous with the parietal peritoneum of the diaphragm.
   e. Arterial supply: the blood supply to the stomach is derived from three branches of the celiac trunk.

(1) The left gastric artery passes to the left and runs superiorly to the level of the esophagus, and then turns along the lesser curvature to supply the stomach.

(2) The splenic artery passes to the left behind the stomach and the lesser sac along the superior border of the pancreas. It divides into the short gastric artery and the left gastro-omental artery. The short gastric artery runs superiorly along the greater curvature to the stomach. The left gastro-omental artery descends along the greater curvature to supply the stomach and the greater omentum.

(3) The common hepatic artery passes to the right of the celiac trunk and divides near the duodenum into two branches, the hepatic artery and the gastroduodenal artery. The hepatic artery ascends and supplies the liver with blood. On the way to the liver, it gives off the right gastric artery, which supplies the lesser curvature of the stomach, and then anatomoses with the left gastric artery. The hepatic artery continues superiorly, sends a cystic artery to the gallbladder, and then divides into right and left branches that supply the liver.

(4) The gastroduodenal artery passes inferiorly posterior to the duodenum and divides into two branches, the superior pancreaticoduodenal artery and the right gastro-omental artery. The superior pancreaticoduodenal artery supplies part of the pancreas and duodenum. The right gastro-omental artery runs to the left along the greater curvature of the stomach and anastomoses with the left gastro-omental artery. It supplies portions of the stomach and greater omentum.

f. Venous return

(1) The veins of the stomach parallel the arteries that supply the stomach. The right and left gastric veins drain directly into the portal vein. The short gastric vein and the left gastro-omental vein join the splenic vein, which drains to the portal vein. The right gastro-omental vein drains to the superior mesenteric vein, which joins the splenic vein to form the portal vein.

2. Duodenum—the first section of the small intestine.

a. Position: the duodenum has a semicircular shape like a C. It lies in front of the abdominal aorta and inferior vena cava and surrounds the head and neck of the pancreas.

b. Parts: the duodenum has four parts—a superior first part, descending second part, horizontal third part, and ascending fourth part.

c. Wall of the duodenum: the internal mucous membrane lining has many circular folds, the plicae circulares. Enzymes from the pancreas and bile from the liver are added in the second part at the major duodenal papilla. Above the major duodenal papilla is the minor duodenal papilla. It is the entrance of the accessory pancreatic duct into the duodenum.

d. Peritoneal attachments

(1) Most of the duodenum is retroperitoneal. As the fourth part of the duodenum ascends and curves anteriorly, the mesentery begins.

e. Arterial supply

(1) The blood supply to the duodenum is derived from the celiac trunk and the superior mesenteric artery. The superior pancreaticoduodenal artery arises indirectly from the celiac trunk. It follows the inner curve of the duodenum and supplies the superior portion of the pancreas and duodenum.

f. Venous return

(1) The superior and inferior pancreaticoduodenal veins transport the venous return from the duodenum to the portal vein via the superior mesenteric vein.

3. Jejunum and ileum

a. The fourth and ascending portion of the duodenum becomes the jejunum. The jejunum and ileum together form a more mobile portion of the small intestine because they have a mesentery.

b. The jejunum and ileum are located centrally in the abdominopelvic cavity and are framed by the large intestine. The greater omentum is draped anteriorly over the small intestine.

c. Peritoneum attachments
   (1) The root of the mesentery that attaches the jejunum and ileum to the posterior body wall runs diagonally from the duodenal to the iliocolic junction. Nerve and blood supply to the small intestine travels through the mesentery.

d. Small intestine wall
   (1) The mucous membrane of the surface of the small intestine has many folds covered by fingerlike projections called *villi*.

e. Arterial supply
   (1) The superior mesenteric artery supplies blood to the small intestine. This artery gives off intestinal branches that travel through the mesentery. At the small intestine, the arteries join as arcades. Vasa recti arise from the arcades and supply the gut itself.

f. Venous drainage—venous return drains to small intestinal tributaries of the superior mesenteric vein. The superior mesenteric vein joins the splenic vein to form the portal vein.

4. Colon—extends from the ileocolic junction to the anus.
   a. Position: the colon sits within the periphery of the abdomen, around the small intestine.
   b. Features and parts: the longitudinal muscle coat has three bands, called *teniae coli*. Contractions in teniae coli are called *haustra*. The outer peritoneal surface of the colon has appendices epiploicae, small bags of fat-filled peritoneum hanging from its surface. The large intestine has the caecum and appendix, ascending colon, transverse colon, descending colon, sigmoid colon, rectum, and anal canal.
      (1) Caecum and appendix
         (a) The ileum meets the colon at the ileocaecal orifice. The iliocaecal valve, located at the entrance to the orifice, prevents regurgitation back into the ileum. The vermiform appendix opens into the caecum below the ileocolic orifice.
      (2) Ascending colon
         (a) The ascending colon is attached to the posterior body wall. It is retroperitoneal and ascends and turns to the right as the right colic or hepatic flexure.
      (3) Transverse colon
         (a) The transverse colon has a mesentery. As it approaches the left side, it ascends to the level of the spleen and turns inferiorly. The flexure is the left colic or splenic flexure.
      (4) Descending colon
         (a) The descending colon is immobile. At the level of the left iliac crest, it turns medially as the sigmoid colon.
      (5) Sigmoid colon
         (a) The sigmoid colon once again acquires a mesentery and is mobile. It is S-shaped and, once in the middle of the sacrum, extends inferiorly as the rectum.
      (6) Rectum and anal canal
         (a) At the pelvic diaphragm, the rectum turns and becomes the anal canal. The involuntary internal sphincter ani and the voluntary external sphincter ani control the release of contents.
   c. Wall of the colon
      (1) The mucous membrane lining of the large gut does not contain any villi. The surface is designed for water absorption.
   d. Arterial supply: the colon is supplied by branches of superior and inferior mesenteric arteries.
      (1) Superior mesenteric artery
         (a) The iliocolic artery arises from the superior mesenteric artery and travels through the mesentery toward the iliocaecal junction. An ileal branch travels back to the ileum to supply the distal end of the ileum. An appendicular branch travels through the mesoappendix and supplies the appendix. Caecal branches supply the caecum, and colic branches ascend to supply the ascending colon.
         (b) The right colic artery arises from the superior mesenteric artery. It supplies the superior portion of the ascending colon.
         (c) The middle colic artery travels through the transverse meso-

colon to supply the transverse colon.

(2) Inferior mesenteric artery

(a) The inferior mesenteric artery arises from the abdominal aorta. It passes to the left and forms three terminal branches—the left colic artery; sigmoid arteries; and rectal branches to supply the descending colon, sigmoid colon, and rectum.

e. Venous return

(1) The caecum and ascending and transverse colon are drained by tributaries of the superior mesenteric vein. The descending colon, sigmoid colon, and rectum are drained by tributaries of the inferior mesenteric vein, which drains to the splenic vein. The superior and inferior mesenteric veins unite to form the portal vein.

H. The liver—sits under the diaphragm in the upper right quadrant. It is sheltered by the lower right ribs.

1. Surfaces and features

a. The liver has a smooth, diaphragmatic upper surface and an inferior visceral surface. It has four lobes. The right lobe lies to the right of the inferior vena cava and the gallbladder. The left lobe lies to the left of the ligamentum teres and the ligamentum venosum. The quadrate lobe lies between the gallbladder, the ligamentum teres, and the porta hepatis. The caudate lobe lies between the inferior vena cava, the ligamentum venosum, and the porta hepatis.

2. Peritoneal attachments

a. Coronary ligament—the visceral peritoneum that covers the liver reflects back onto the diaphragm as the diaphragmatic peritoneum. This area of reflection is called the *coronary ligament.*

b. Falciform ligament—The falciform ligament extends upward from the umbilicus to the liver. The free edge contains a thick ligament that is the remnant of the umbilical vein, called *ligamentum teres.*

c. Ligamentum venosum—the ligamentum venosum is the remnant of the ductus venosus, or umbilical vein that was the fetal bypass of the liver.

d. Lesser omentum—joins the liver to the stomach. The common bile duct, hepatic artery, and portal vein all course through the lesser omentum.

3. Blood flow to the liver—the blood flow to the liver is through the hepatic artery and portal vein.

a. Hepatic artery—arises from the common hepatic artery. It passes upward in the free edge of the lower omentum. It divides into left and right branches that supply the liver.

b. Portal vein—the inferior mesenteric vein unites with the splenic vein. The superior mesenteric vein joins the splenic vein to form the portal vein. The portal vein travels upward within the lesser omentum and divides into right and left branches to supply the liver.

4. Venous return—blood drains from the liver via hepatic veins to the inferior vena cava.

5. Structure

a. Liver tissue is separated into small functional units called *lobules* by fibrous septa. Each lobule consists of several sheets of epithelial cells radiating out from a central vein. Small branches of the hepatic artery, portal vein, and hepatic duct are located at the periphery of each lobule. The vessels empty their blood into spaces where exchange takes place between the epithelial cells and blood. The central vein of the lobules come together to form the hepatic vein.

6. Biliary apparatus

a. The bile canaliculi drain bile to interlobular ducts. The interlobular ducts form right and left hepatic ducts. These ducts join to form the common hepatic duct. The gallbladder arises from the common hepatic duct. A cystic duct joins the common hepatic duct to form the common bile duct. Bile is transported to the duodenum through the common bile duct.

I. Pancreas—lies transversely in the abdomen against the posterior body wall.

1. Features and parts

a. The pancreas is divided into three parts. The head is surrounded by the duodenum at vertebral level L1–L2. The body extends to the left and ends as the tail, which touches the hilum of the spleen.

2. Peritoneum—the pancreas is retroperitoneal. It is covered by the peritoneum anteriorly and provides a base for attachment of the transverse mesocolon.
3. Structure: the pancreas contains both an exocrine and endocrine portion.
   a. Exocrine portion
      (1) The lobules of the pancreas are drained by ductules, which drain into a main pancreatic duct. It empties its secretions, along with the common bile duct, into the ampulla of the duodenum.
   b. Endocrine portion
      (1) The pancreas contains clusters of cells called the islets of Langerhans, which produce insulin.
4. Arterial supply: the pancreas is supplied by branches of both the celiac trunk and superior mesenteric artery. The splenic artery arises from the celiac trunk and supplies the pancreas.
   a. The superior pancreaticoduodenal artery arises from the gastroduodenal branch and passes inferiorly to supply both the pancreas and duodenum.
   b. The inferior pancreaticoduodenal artery arises from the superior mesenteric artery and travels superiorly between the pancreatic head and duodenum to supply both structures.
5. Venous drainage—the splenic vein receives tributaries from the superior surface of the pancreas and courses to the left and takes part in formation of the portal vein. The superior and inferior pancreaticoduodenal veins drain directly to the portal vein.

J. Spleen—lies in the upper left quadrant of the abdomen, protected by ribs 9, 10, and 11.
1. Features
   a. The hilum of the spleen is located on the visceral surface. The tail of the pancreas contacts the hilum. Splenic vessels run to and from the hilum.
2. Peritoneum
   a. The spleen is attached to the stomach by the gastrosplenic ligament. The splenorenal ligament attaches the spleen to the left kidney.
3. Structure
   a. The spleen is divided by connective tissue septa into many compartments. Within the compartments are networks of cells surrounded by blood sinusoids.
4. Blood supply
   a. The spleen is supplied by the splenic artery and is drained by the splenic vein.

K. Kidneys—lie in the posterior body wall, with the medial border more anterior than the lateral border.
1. Features
   a. The lateral border is rounded, and the medial border is the concave hilum of the kidney, which contains a vertical slit called the *renal sinus* through which the ureter and renal vessels pass to and from the kidney.
2. Peritoneum
   a. The kidneys are retroperitoneal. A layer of fibrous renal fascia anchors the kidney to the posterior body wall. The left kidney is slightly higher than the right kidney and is joined to the spleen by the splenorenal ligament.
3. Structure
   a. The cortex is the pale, outer layer of the kidney. The medulla is the inner layer, which appears striped due to the renal pyramids. Medullary rays are composed of medullary tissue extending into the cortex from the base of the pyramids. The apex of a medullary pyramid is called the *renal papilla*. Minor calyces receive secretions from the renal papillae. Several minor calyces join to form a major calyx. The approximately three major calyces found in the kidney unite to form the renal pelvis. The renal pelvis is drained by the ureters to the bladder.
4. Blood supply
   a. The renal artery arises from the abdominal aorta, passes laterally, and enters the hilum of the kidney behind the inferior vena cava. The artery gives off a branch that passes superiorly to the suprarenal gland. Within the sinus of the kidney, the renal arteries end as interlobar arteries. They course through the renal columns to reach the cortex. In the cortex they bifurcate at right angles as arcuate arteries and anastomose with each other to form arcades.
   b. Veins leave the capillary beds and coalesce as renal veins. The right and left renal veins drain to the inferior vena cava.

L. Ureters—the ureter carries urine from the kidneys to the bladder. The ureters travel inferiorly just below the parietal peritoneum of the posterior body wall. They pass anterior to the common iliac arteries as they enter the pelvis.
   1. Blood supply
      a. Proximally, they receive branches from the renal arteries, midportions receive branches from testicular/ovarian arteries, and the distal portion receives branches from vesicular arteries.

M. The bladder—a receiving chamber for urine. The anterior border rests against the pubic bones. The superior aspect is covered with peritoneum.
   1. Entrances and exit
      a. The right and left ureters pass to the posterior of the bladder, converge inferiorly, and then enter the bladder about 2.5 cm apart. Along with the exit of the bladder, they form the trigone of the bladder.
   2. Structure
      a. The lumen of the bladder is lined with transitional epithelial mucosa. The walls contain smooth muscle fibers that, collectively, are called the *detrusor muscle.*
   3. Blood supply
      a. The superior and inferior vesical arteries arise from the internal iliac artery to supply the bladder. It is drained by veins of the same name that empty to the internal iliac vein.

N. Suprarenal glands—sit on top of the kidneys.
   1. Structure: the suprarenal glands have an outer cortex and inner medulla with distinct functions.
      a. The cortex is involved with production of steroid hormones.
      b. The medulla secretes epinephrine.

1.5 Cental Nervous System and Neuroanatomy

The human nervous system maintains homeostasis by regulating the internal environment. It also interprets and reacts to external stimuli. The response to external stimuli may be unconscious or conscious.

The nervous system consists of two kinds of cells: reactive cells called *neurons*, and supportive cells called *neuroglia*. It may be divided into central and peripheral components based on location, or somatic and autonomic divisions based on function.

A. The neuron—consists of cytoplasm and a nucleus surrounded by a plasma membrane. Neurons have the ability to communicate with one another at synapses through electrical impulses. Motor neurons transmit information, and sensory neurons receive information.
   1. Motor neuron
      a. The motor neuron consists of a cell body containing a nucleus, numerous dendrites that receive information, and a single axon that transmits information.
         (1) Dendrites are short, branching cellular extensions that conduct impulses toward the body.
         (2) Axons are long, cellular extensions that conduct impulses away from the body. Near its termination, each axon branches. Each branch ends as an axon terminal or bouton. Axon terminals of motor neurons synapse with muscle cells. Several extensions arise from the cell body of motor neurons; thus, they are termed *multipolar.*
   2. Sensory neuron
      a. The body of a sensory neuron has only one cellular extension and is classified as unipolar. The process is short and divides into two axons. One axon, called the *peripheral process*, continues to the periphery and either functions as a sensory receptor or synapses with a sensory receptor. Some authors refer to the branching component as *dendrites*. The other axon is called the *central process*; it extends into the central nervous system (CNS).
   3. Synapses
      a. Synapses are found either at the intercellular junctions of nerve processes or between nerve processes and the cells of effector organs. The presynaptic and postsynaptic cells membranes are separated by a synaptic cleft.
      b. Electrical impulses travel along the axon and cause the release of neurotransmitters from the terminus. The neurotransmitters diffuse across the synaptic cleft.
      c. The neurotransmitter may be excitatory or inhibitory. An excitatory transmitter depolarizes the postsynaptic membrane, and an inhibitory transmitter hyperpolarizes the postsynaptic membrane. Inhibitory and excitatory synapses may

be mixed; one site on the target neuron may receive input from only a few to as many as 1000 synapses with other neurons.

d. The net depolarization of the membrane will determine whether the target neuron propagates the impulse.

4. Neuroglia
   a. Neuroglia are supportive cells. They do not transmit impulses.
      (1) Neuroglia maintain homeostasis in the extracellular environment.
      (2) They electrically insulate nerve processes from one another.
      (3) They provide nutrition for neurons.

B. Definitions and terms
   1. Gray matter
      a. Neuronal bodies that are grouped together are called *gray matter*. It is located in the central part of the spinal cord surrounding the central canal; on the surfaces of the cerebrum and cerebellum of the cortex of the brain; and throughout the CNS as discrete, scattered, internal patches or nuclei.
   2. White matter
      a. Myelin speeds nerve conduction. Myelin has a shiny, white appearance, and myelinated nerves within the CNS cause nerve tissue to appear white.
   3. Peripheral nerve
      a. A peripheral nerve is composed of a bundle of myelinated axons traveling outside the CNS.
   4. Tract
      a. A tract is a group of myelinated axons traveling together in the CNS that share a common origin, destination, and function. Tracts run entirely within the brain and spinal cord.
   5. Nucleus
      a. A nucleus is a group of neuronal cell bodies in the CNS that are located in the same area and share the same function.
   6. Ganglion
      a. A ganglion is a collection of nerve cell bodies outside the CNS. The dorsal root ganglia and autonomic ganglia are examples. An exception is the basal ganglia of the cerebral hemispheres; they are nuclei by definition.
   7. Afferent fibers
      a. Afferent fibers are axons that carry nerve impulses toward the CNS or toward higher centers. They are also known as *sensory* or *ascending fibers*.
   8. Efferent fibers
      a. Efferent fibers are axons that carry impulses away from the CNS to muscles and glands. They are also known as *motor* or *descending fibers*.

C. Division based on location: the nervous system may be divided into the central nervous system containing the brain and spinal cord, and the peripheral nervous system consisting of the spinal and cranial nerves.
   1. Central nervous system
      a. Sensory component, in which incoming data are received at a conscious or unconscious level.
      b. A motor component, which is the origin of outgoing commands.
      c. An association component, which connects and coordinates various CNS centers.
   2. Peripheral nervous system: peripheral nerves consist of bundles of axons that convey information to and from the CNS.
      a. 31 pairs of spinal nerves from the spinal cord.
      b. 12 pairs of cranial nerves from the brain.

D. Division based on function
   1. Somatic nervous system
      a. The somatic nervous system controls the body's voluntary and reflex activities through somatic sensory and somatic motor components of both the central and peripheral nervous system.
   2. Autonomic nervous system
      a. The autonomic nervous system controls involuntary smooth muscle, cardiac muscle, and glandular tissue. It is not under voluntary or conscious control. It has a motor component that controls smooth muscle contractions of viscera and blood vessels and secretions of glands. It has a sensory component to provide feedback. The autonomic nervous system is also divided into a parasympathetic division and a sympathetic division.
         (1) The parasympathetic division of the autonomic nervous system is concerned with maintenance of day-to-day activity, which is also known as *vegetative function*. Examples of vegetative function include peristalsis and digestion, slowing the heart, and stimulating glandular secretions.

(2) The sympathetic division of the autonomic nervous system is antagonistic to the parasympathetic division and takes precedence during emergencies. It is also called the *fight-or-flight response*. During an emergency, blood is shunted to core muscles, hair stands on end, pupils dilate, the heart beats faster, respiration increases, and bronchioles dilate for more oxygenation of blood.

E. Peripheral nerves—located outside the CNS. Peripheral nerves share a common structure and function similarly; however, some have a somatic, voluntary function and others an autonomic function.

1. Structure
    a. The axon is the basic unit of a peripheral nerve. Each axon is covered by myelin-containing neurilemma, a fatty layer that acts as an insulator.
    b. The fibrous endoneurium covers each process and its coatings.
    c. The perineurium covers each bundle of processes.
    d. The epineurium is the final coating of the entire peripheral nerve.
2. Function
    a. Skeletal muscles form for movement and locomotion, and smooth muscle develops for peristalsis and emptying of contents.
    b. Both types of muscle have a motor (efferent) and sensory (afferent) nerve supply.
        (1) Somatic efferent to voluntary skeletal muscles.
        (2) Somatic afferent from skin and proprioception from endings in muscles, tendons, and joints.
        (3) Autonomic efferent to visceral smooth muscles and glands.
        (4) Autonomic afferent from organs and glands.
    c. Two additional modalities are found in the head, the special senses and branchial efferent nerves that supply skeletal muscles of the head and neck derived from branchial arches.
        (1) Special sensory for smell, vision, taste, hearing, and balance.
        (2) Branchial efferent for skeletal muscle in the head and neck that is derived from branchial arches.
3. Somatic peripheral nerves (CNS origins)
    a. Voluntary motor components (efferent somatic and branchial): motor pathways comprise two groups of neurons, upper and lower.
        (1) Upper motor neurons are located in the motor cortex of the cerebrum. These axons descend in tracts that cross the midline and synapse with lower motor neurons.
        (2) Lower motor neurons give rise to motor components of peripheral nerves.
            (a) Cranial nerves
                (i) Lower motor neurons are located in cranial nerve motor nuclei in the brainstem. The axons of these nerves leave the brainstem as motor components of cranial nerves.
                (ii) Cranial nerves III, IV, VI, and XII carry somatic efferent fibers. These nerves innervate skeletal muscle of the head that is derived from somites.
                (iii) Cranial nerves V, VII, IX, and X carry branchial efferent fibers that supply cranial muscles of branchial arch origin.
            (b) Spinal nerves
                (i) Lower motor neurons are located in the ventral horn of the spinal cord. Axons of these neurons leave the spinal cord as ventral roots that form the motor component of each of the 31 pairs of spinal nerves. These motor nerves supply all the skeletal muscles of the trunk and limbs.
    b. General sensory (sensory somatic)—general sensory pathways have three sets of neurons, which synapse with neurons in the sensory cortex of the brain.
        (1) Cranial nerves
            (a) Cell bodies of the primary neurons of cranial nerves are located near the brainstem within sensory ganglia. Peripheral processes pick up stimuli

from various regions of the head. The stimuli pass through the ganglia and central processes to sensory nuclei containing secondary neurons within the brainstem. Their axons cross the midline and rise to synapse with tertiary neurons in the thalamus. These, in turn, send axons up to the sensory cortex.

(2) Spinal nerves

(a) Cell bodies of the primary neurons of spinal nerves are contained in the dorsal root ganglia adjacent to the spinal cord. Their peripheral processes transmit impulses from sensory receptors in skin or proprioceptive receptors in muscles, tendons, and joints. Central processes pass through dorsal roots into the CNS and synapse with secondary neurons within the dorsal horn. Axons cross the midline and ascend to synapse with tertiary neurons in the thalamus of the brain. These neurons send axons up to synapse with the final set of neurons located in the sensory cortex of the brain.

c. Origins of autonomic nerves in the central nervous system—autonomic motor. The autonomic pathway consists of a two-neuron chain. The first neurons are in the autonomic motor nuclei in the CNS. Axons are sent that leave the CNS and synapse with a second set within an autonomic ganglia outside the CNS. The second neurons send out axons to the smooth muscle and glands of the viscera. This pathway has sympathetic and parasympathetic divisions.

(1) Parasympathetic division

(a) The parasympathetic division of the autonomic nervous system originates from the brain and sacral region of the spinal cord. The first neuron is found within parasympathetic motor nuclei.

(i) Cranial preganglionic fibers arise from parasympathetic motor nuclei within the brainstem and leave as components of cranial nerves III, VII, IX, and X. Cranial nerves III, VII, and IX supply cranial visceral elements. Cranial nerve X supplies the respiratory system, cardiac system, most of the gut, and associated glands up to the left colic flexure.

(ii) Sacral preganglionic fibers arise from parasympathetic motor nuclei in the ventral horns of the spinal cord at levels S2, S3, and S4 and leave through the ventral roots of pelvic spinal nerves. They then form pelvic splanchnic nerves that supply the distal portion of the gut and pelvic viscera.

(2) Sympathetic division

(a) The sympathetic division of the autonomic nervous system leaves the spinal cord at levels T1 to L2. The first neurons are located within the intermediolateral horns, which are found only in this region of the spinal cord. Preganglionic fibers leave the spinal cord along with the anterior spinal nerve roots. The fibers leave the nerve as myelinated white communicating rami.

(b) On either side of the vertebral column are a chain of cervical ganglia. These sympathetic trunks run the entire length of the vertebral column. Each vertebral level has an associated vertebral ganglia. The ganglia at levels C1 through C4 fuse to form the superior cervical ganglion. The ganglia at levels C5 and C6 fuse to form the middle cervical ganglion, and the ganglia at levels C7 and C8 fuse to form the inferior cervical ganglion. White communicating rami emerge from spinal levels T1 to L2 and run to the sympathetic trunk.

(c) Within the sympathetic trunk, preganglionic fibers may synapse with the neurons of the ganglion at that level, travel up or down to the sympathetic trunk to synapse in a ganglion at a higher or lower level, or leave the sympathetic trunk as splanchnic nerves. Splanchnic nerves extend into the abdomen and synapse in prevertebral ganglia. Postganglionic fibers in the first and second categories rejoin spinal nerves as unmyelinated gray communicating rami. Fourteen pairs of white communicating rami arise from spinal levels T1 to L2. Leaving the sympathetic trunk to join spinal nerves are 31 pairs of gray rami.

(3) Distribution of postganglionic sympathetic fibers

(a) Trunk and limbs

(i) Gray rami leave the sympathetic trunk at each spinal cord level to join each pair of spinal nerves. They are distributed along with the spinal nerves to the trunk and limbs where they supply smooth muscle of blood vessels. Sympathetic fibers also pass to the skin and supply sweat glands, and the arrector pili muscles that cause hair to stand on end.

(b) Head and neck

(i) Preganglionic fibers of the sympathetic trunk rise to the superior cervical ganglion. Here, the ganglionic fibers synapse with a second set of neurons.

(ii) Postganglionic fibers leave the ganglion and join the carotid arteries as the carotid periarterial plexus. The sympathetic postganglionic fibers are then distributed to visceral effector organs of the head by various branches of the external and internal carotid arteries.

(c) Thorax

(i) Postganglionic fibers of the three cervical sympathetic ganglia stream down the thorax to form the cardiac and pulmonary plexuses. These supply the heart and smooth muscle of the bronchial tree.

(d) Abdominal and pelvic viscera

(i) Preganglionic fibers leave the sympathetic trunk in the thorax as splanchnic nerves. These enter the abdomen and synapse in remote prevertebral ganglia.

(ii) Postganglionic fibers travel via branches of the abdominal aorta to the viscera of the abdomen. Thoracic splanchnic nerves supply derivatives of the foregut and midgut. Hindgut derivatives and urogenital pelvic viscera are supplied from lumbar splanchnic nerves from the sympathetic trunk of the lumbar region.

d. Origins of autonomic nerves in the central nervous system—autonomic sensory

(1) Visceral receptors monitor smooth muscle tone in viscera and vessels, blood chemistry, blood pressure, and the content volume in hollow organs. This information is relayed back to the CNS via sensory components of autonomic nerves. Afferent impulses carrying information such as a feeling of fullness, hunger, or nausea travel back to the CNS along parasympathetic nerves. The pathways for visceral or autonomic sensation within the CNS are the same as those for the somatic afferent nerve fibers. Feelings of pain or cramps travel back to the CNS along sympathetic nerves. The brain refers the pain to somatic sites that share the same spinal nerve innervation. The primary cell bodies are found in dorsal root ganglia of spinal nerves. Within the CNS, axons follow the same pathway as the somatic afferent fibers.

e. Nomenclature
   (1) Cranial nerves
      (a) The 12 cranial nerves originate from the brain. Each is assigned a Roman numeral. Some have one functional component, and others have more than one.
   (2) Spinal nerves
      (a) Spinal nerves exit through intervertebral foramina and break into two main rami.
         (i) Posterior primary rami supply mixed sensory and motor nerves to structures of the back, the back of the neck, and the back of the head.
         (ii) Anterior primary rami supply mixed sensory and motor fibers to the lateral and anterior aspects of the trunk and all the upper and lower limbs.
   (3) Nerve plexus
      (a) In certain areas of the spinal cord, anterior primary rami tend to join and divide in complex patterns called *nerve plexuses*.
         (i) The cervical plexus is formed by the anterior primary rami of spinal nerves C1 to C4. It supplies structures in the anterior and lateral regions of the neck.
         (ii) The brachial plexus is formed from the anterior primary rami of spinal nerves C5 through T1. It supplies all the structures of the upper limb.
         (iii) The lumbar plexus is formed by the anterior primary rami of spinal nerves L1 through L4 and supplies the pelvis and entire lower limb.
         (iv) The sacral plexus is formed by the anterior primary rami of spinal nerves L4 through S4 and supplies the perineum and lower limb.
         (v) The coccygeal plexus is formed by the anterior primary rami of spinal nerves S4 to Co 1 and supplies skin of the coccygeal area.

f. Cutaneous distribution
   (1) Most of the skin of the body is innervated by spinal nerves. The face and anterior scalp are innervated largely by cranial nerve V.

2.0 HISTOLOGY

2.1 Ultrastructure

2.1.1 The Cell

A. Cell (plasma) membrane
   1. Consists of a phospholipid bilayer (Figure 1–39). This bilayer contains proteins that are incorporated in the membrane (integral proteins) or attached to the inner or outer surface (peripheral proteins). Some of these proteins can move freely within the phospholipids bilayer. This model of the cell membrane was first described by the Fluid Mosaic Model.*
   2. Besides phospholipids, the membrane also contains other lipids, including cholesterols and glycolipids.
   3. The membrane proteins and lipids are held together via noncovalent interactions.

B. Cell organelles
   1. Nucleus
      a. Is surrounded by a nuclear envelope that consists of two (an inner and outer) membranes. This envelope contains many holes, or nuclear pores, that allow for the selective passage of molecules through it (Figure 1–40).
      b. Contains DNA and RNA.
         (1) In the nucleus, DNA appears as chromatin, which consists of a complex of DNA, histones, and proteins.
         (2) During cell division, chromatin condenses into chromosomes. Each chromosome consists of two parallel, spiral-like filaments (chromatids) that are joined together at the centromere. Sex chromatin: the male has one Y and one X chromosome. The female has two X chromosomes.
      c. Nucleolus—a circular-shaped structure found inside the nucleus that is the site of ribosomal RNA synthesis.
      d. Barr body—In some female nuclei, during interphase one of the X chromosomes becomes inactive and condenses

*Singer SJ: Early history of membrane biology. Annu Rev Physiol 66:1-27, 2004.

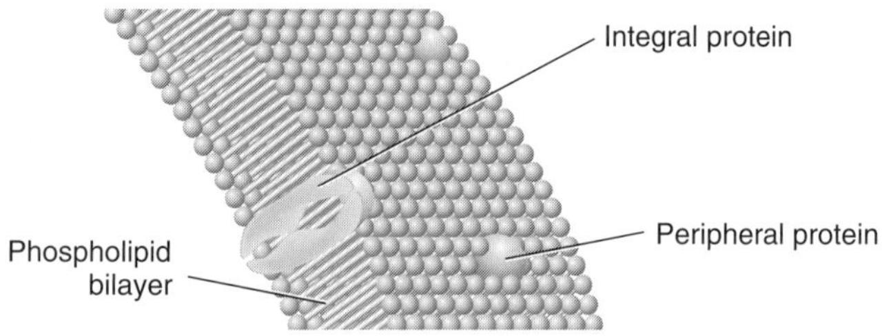

Figure 1–39. Plasma membrane. (Modified from Bath-Balogh M, Fehrenbach M: Illustrated Dental Embryology, Histology, and Anatomy, ed 2, Philadelphia, WB Saunders, 2006.)

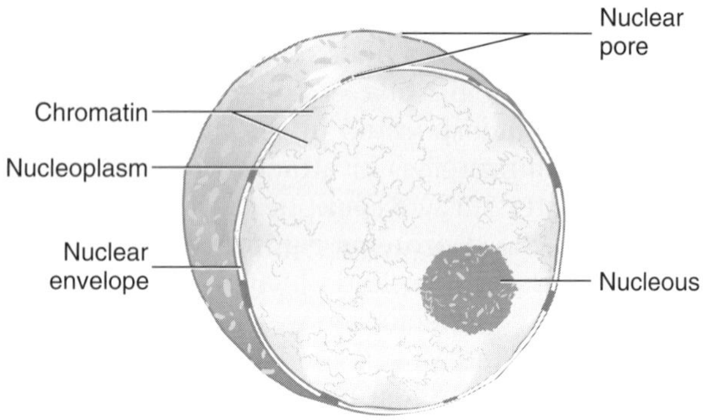

Figure 1–40. Nucleus. (Modified from Bath-Balogh M, Fehrenbach M: Illustrated Dental Embryology, Histology, and Anatomy, ed 2, Philadelphia, WB Saunders, 2006.)

to form a small, visible mass called the *Barr body*.

e. During apoptosis (programmed cell death), the nucleus undergoes the following changes:
   (1) Karyolysis—dissolution of the nucleus.
   (2) Pyknosis—the nucleus shrinks and the chromatin condenses.
   (3) Karyorrhexis—fragmentation of the nucleus, and the chromatin disintegrates.

2. Mitochondria
   a. The powerhouse of the cell, where adenosine triphosphate (ATP) is produced.
   b. Is surrounded by two (inner and outer) membranes. The inner membrane appears as folds that project into the inner matrix, called *cristae*.
   c. Contains circular DNA, which is similar to the genetic material found in bacteria.
3. Rough endoplasmic reticulum
   a. Consists of a network of tubules, vesicles, and flattened sacs.
   b. Ribosomes are bound to its surface, giving the endoplasmic reticulum a rough appearance.
4. Smooth endoplasmic reticulum
   a. Consists of a network of tubules and vesicles. No ribosomes are bound to its surface.
   b. In general, it is responsible for the synthesis of lipids. In the liver, it is involved in glycogen metabolism and detoxification of various drugs and alcohols. It also contains P450 enzymes. Cytochrome P450 enzymes are important in the detoxification process. In muscle, the smooth sarcoplasmic reticulum (equivalent to endoplasmic reticulum in other tissues) plays a major role in the storage of calcium.
5. Ribosomes
   a. Are responsible for protein synthesis.
   b. Are composed of RNA subunits that are made in the nucleolus.
6. Golgi apparatus
   a. Consists of a complex of layered, membrane-bound cisternae.
   b. Responsible for modifying and packaging proteins from the rough endoplasmic reticulum. Products are sent in vesicles to the plasma membrane, lysosomes, or secretory vesicles.
7. Lysosomes
   a. Are small, membrane-bound vesicles that contain many hydrolytic enzymes.
   b. Play an important role in the intracellular digestion of phagocytosed particles.
8. Centrosome
   a. Oval-shaped organelle located next to the nucleus. It plays a role in the formation of mitotic spindles during cell division (refer to Mitosis section)
   b. Contains a pair of centrioles and is composed of triplets of microtubules arranged in a cartwheel pattern.

9. Cytoplasmic inclusions
   a. Contain stored metabolites, such as fats and glycogen, pigments (melanin), or crystalline granules.
   b. May also contain residual materials such as spent lysosomes and digested materials.
10. Cilia and flagella
    a. Are motile processes that protrude from the cell membrane.
    b. Cilia are usually shorter then flagella. They are found in multiple numbers and are organized in parallel rows. They are present on the surface of respiratory epithelium and female reproductive tracts.
    c. Flagella are typically longer than cilia and do not occur in multiple numbers.
    d. A cilium is surrounded by plasma membrane. Its central core, the axoneme, consists of a central pair or two microtubules at the center. It is surrounded by nine peripheral doublets, or pairs of microtubules. The microtubule arrangement is therefore described as a "9 + 2 pattern." At the base of the axoneme is the basal body. The microtubule organization in the basal body consists of nine peripheral triplets (Figure 1–41).

C. Cell cycle and mitosis
   1. The cell cycle can be divided into four phases (Figure 1–42):
      a. G_1 (first gap) phase
         (1) Begins after mitosis and ends at the start of the S phase.
         (2) Cells grow and perform their usual functions.
         (3) This phase is typically longer than the other phases.
      b. S (synthesis) phase
         (1) DNA in the nucleus is replicated.

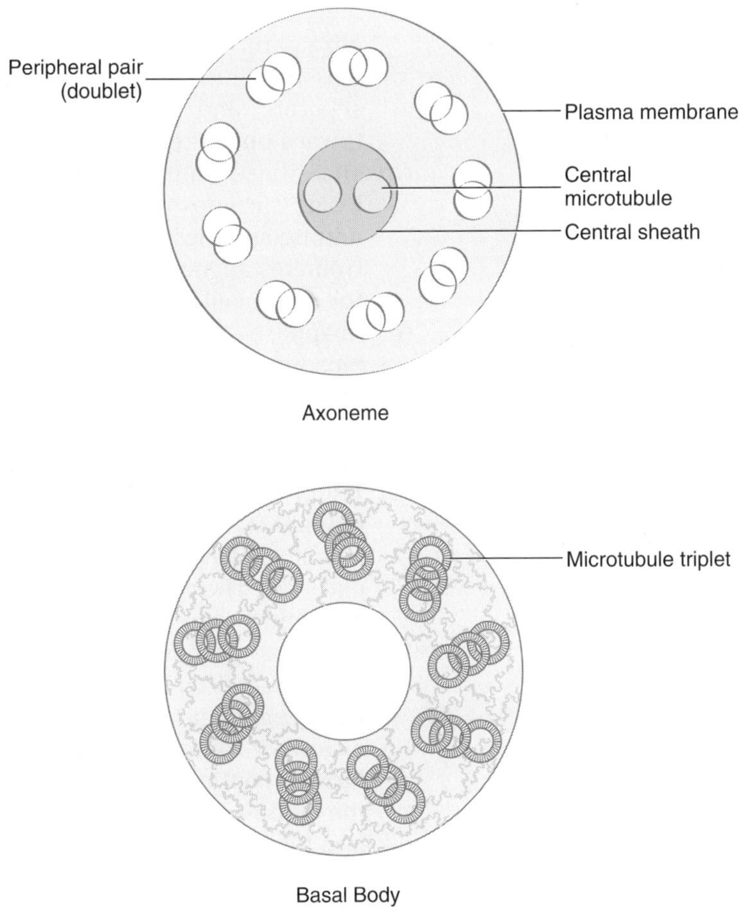

Figure 1–41. Cilium axoneme *(top)* and basal body *(bottom)*: cross-section. (Modified from Bath-Balogh M, Fehrenbach M: Illustrated Dental Embryology, Histology, and Anatomy, ed 2, Philadelphia, WB Saunders, 2006.)

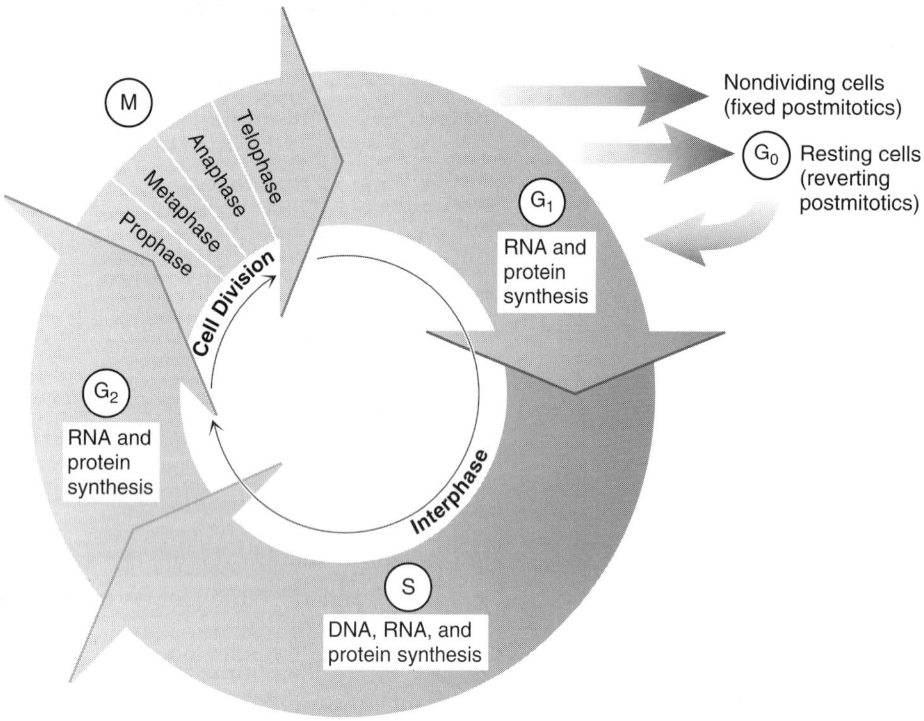

Figure 1–42. Cell cycle. (Modified from Burns ER, Cave MD: Histology and Cell Biology, St. Louis, Mosby, 2002.)

(2) The sections of chromatin that appear loosely coiled and lightly colored are actively synthesizing RNA and are known as *euchromatin*. In areas of no genetic activity, the chromatin appears in clumps and stains darkly; it is called *heterochromatin*.

c. G_2 (second gap) phase
   (1) Cells prepare for mitosis.
   (2) Includes the buildup of ATP and tubulin, which is needed for the formation of spindle fibers.

d. M—mitosis (Figure 1–43).
   (1) With the exception of sex cells, which divide via meiosis, somatic cells divide by mitotic division. This results in the production of two genetically identical daughter cells, formed from a single parent cell. Like the parent cell, each daughter cell carries the diploid number (46 in humans) of chromosomes.
   (2) Mitotic division can be divided into five phases:
      (a) Interphase—includes the G_1, S, and G_2 phases.
      (b) Prophase—nuclear membrane and nucleolus disintegrates; chromatin condenses; centrioles in centrosomes replicate, separate, and begin migrating toward opposite poles.
      (c) Metaphase—mitotic spindles form. Chromosomes attach to mitotic spindles with their centromeres aligned with the equator of the cell.
      (d) Anaphase—centromeres (chromosomes) split. The separated chromatids are pulled by the spindles to opposite poles in the cell.
      (e) Telophase—nuclear membrane reappears. The chromosomes uncoil and lengthen to their normal form. The cytoplasm begins to divide into two daughter cells, a process known as *cytokinesis*. This begins with the formation of a circumferential furrow, or cleavage furrow. This furrow continues to constrict the cytoplasm until it divides it into two daughter cells.

2. Cells that are nondividing or in the resting state are in the G_0 phase. If stimulated, they can enter the cell cycle.

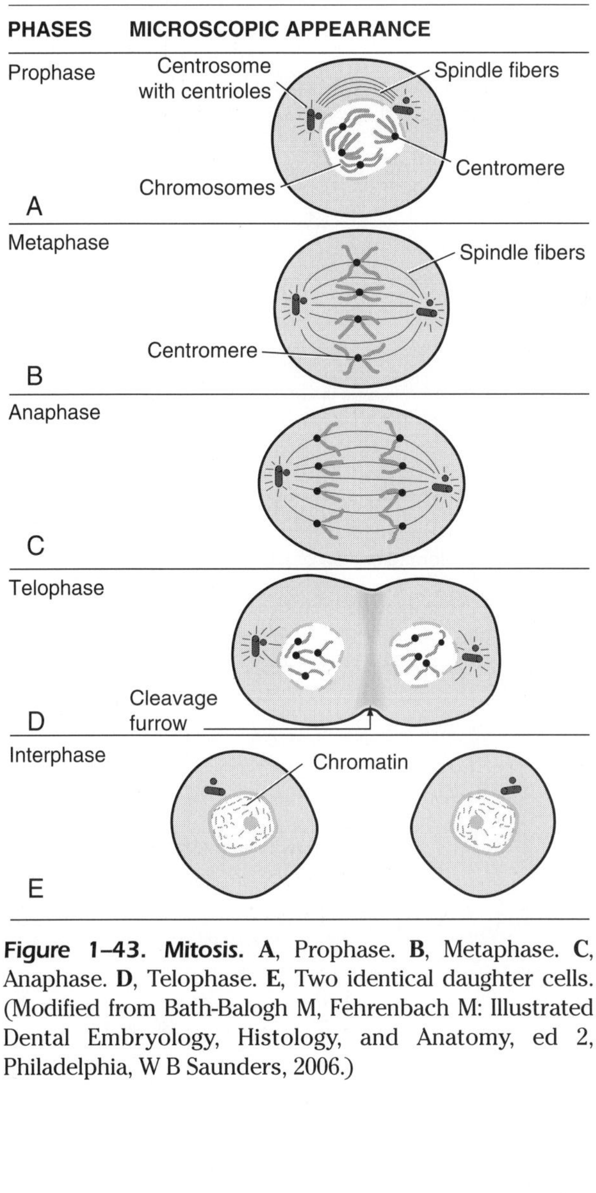

Figure 1–43. Mitosis. **A**, Prophase. **B**, Metaphase. **C**, Anaphase. **D**, Telophase. **E**, Two identical daughter cells. (Modified from Bath-Balogh M, Fehrenbach M: Illustrated Dental Embryology, Histology, and Anatomy, ed 2, Philadelphia, W B Saunders, 2006.)

D. Meiosis
  1. Meiosis is how sex cells divide. It differs from mitotic division in that there are two successive cycles of meiotic cell division (Figure 1–44). This results in the production of four genetically different daughter cells. Each daughter cell carries half of the diploid number (23 in humans) of chromosomes.
  2. Chiasmata formation—occurs only in meiosis, during the first meiotic division. This is when the duplicated chromosomes cross over and exchange alleles. This rearrangement results in genetically different gametes (chromosomes).

2.2 Basic Tissues

A. Epithelium
  1. The tissue that covers and lines all body surfaces.
  2. Classification of epithelia
     a. Number of cell layers
        (1) Simple epithelium—single layer of epithelial cells.
        (2) Pseudostratified epithelium—a single layer of epithelial cells, where every cell contacts the basal lamina, but not all cells reach the epithelial surface. It may appear as multilayered but is actually a single layer of cells.
        (3) Stratified epithelium—more than one layer of epithelial cells.
        (4) Transitional epithelium—a type of stratified epithelium. It is generally found only in the urinary tract and bladder. The epithelium appears transitional between stratified squamous (when the epithelium is stretched) and stratified cuboidal (when it is relaxed).
     b. Shape
        (1) Squamous—flattened cells.
        (2) Cuboidal—cube-shaped (square) cells.
        (3) Columnar—rectangular cells.
     c. Epithelium can also be classified by the presence of specialized surface structures. For example, ciliated versus nonciliated, and keratinized versus nonkeratinized epithelium.
  3. The distribution of epithelia found in the body is summarized in Table 1–28).
  4. Epithelial cell junctions
     a. Junctional complex—consists of the zonula occludens, zonula adherens and desmosomes.
        (1) Zonula occludens (tight junctions)—forms a seal between the plasma membrane of two adjacent cells. This seal prevents contents of the lumen from passing through.
        (2) Zonula adherens (adhering junctions)—found deep in the zonula occludens. It serves to bind the epithelial cells together and contains the glycoprotein E-cadherins.

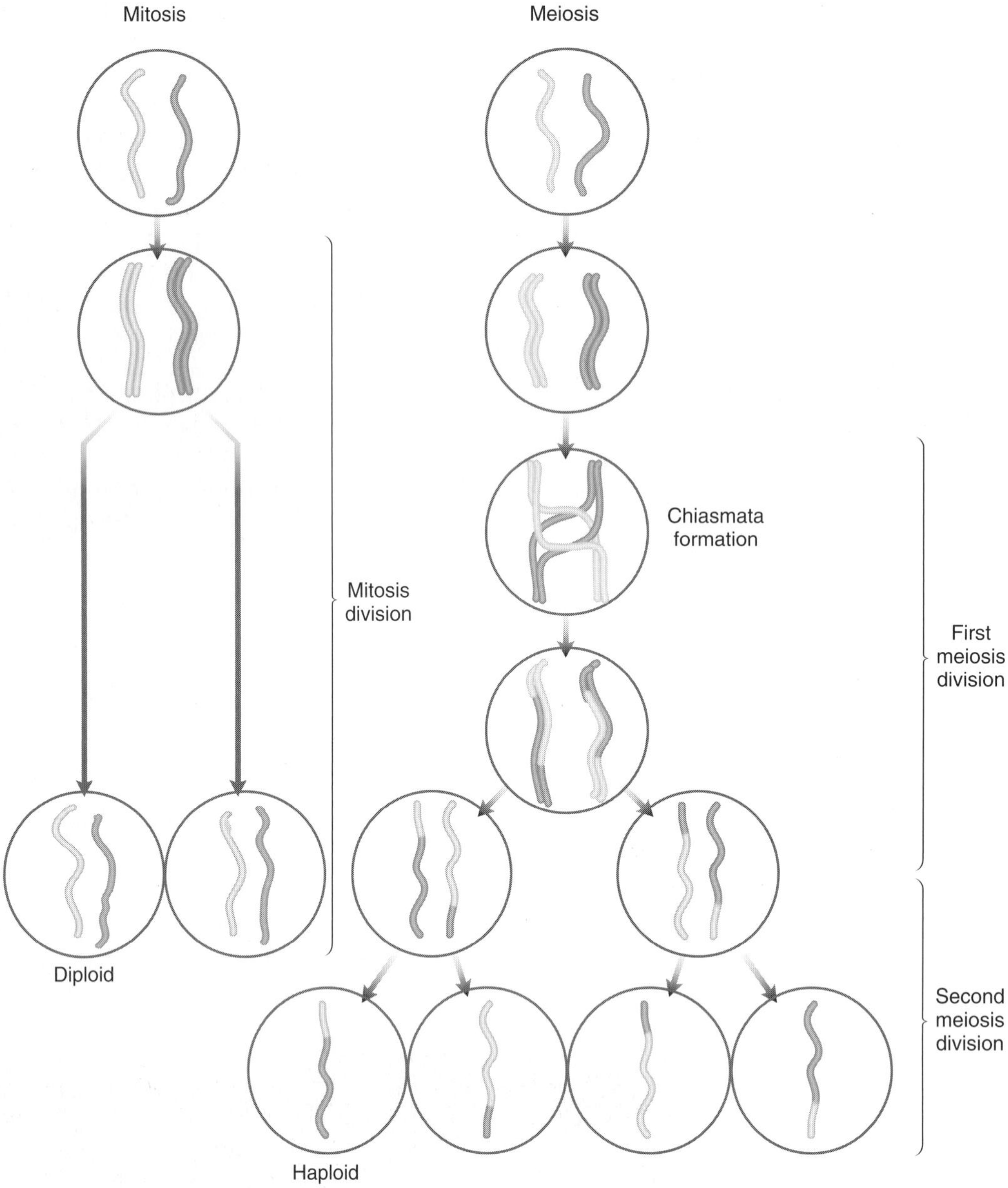

Figure 1–44. Comparison of mitosis and meiosis. (Modified from Burkitt HG, Young B, Heath J: Wheater's Functional Histology, ed 3, Churchill Livingston, 1993.)

(3) Desmosomes (macula densa)—small, circular patches deep in the zonula adherens. It serves to bind the epithelium together and contains the glycoprotein desmogleins.

b. Gap junctions—small pores found between adjacent cells that allow the passage of small molecules.

5. Epithelial surfaces
   a. Luminal surface—the surface of the lumen may contain specialized structures such as cilia, microvilli, or sterocilia.

6. Basal surface—contains hemidesmosomes, which help to anchor the epithelium to the basement membrane.

B. Basement membrane (lamina)
   1. An acellular, condensed layer that forms a barrier between the epithelium and connective tissues. It is composed of type IV collagen, fibronectin, laminin, entactin, and heparan sulfate.
   2. Attachment of the epithelium to the connective tissues involves a complex of hemidesmosomes and tonofilaments from the epithelium and anchoring collagen fibers from the connective tissues.

Table 1–28. Summary of the Three Types of Epithelia

NUMBER OF LAYERS	CELL SHAPE	FUNCTION	DISTRIBUTION
Simple	Squamous	Diffusion, filtration, and secretion	Blood vessels (endothelium) Body cavities (mesothelium) Pericardium Peritoneum Pleura
	Cuboidal	Secretion	Bronchioles Salivary glands acini Thyroid gland Ovary capsule
	Columnar	Secretion and absorption	Intestinal lining Gallbladder
Pseudostratified	Columnar—*ciliated*	Secretion	Respiratory tract (except bronchioles) Nasopharynx Paranasal sinuses Nasal cavity Eustachian tubes
	Columnar—*nonciliated*	Secretion	Salivary gland ducts Male urethra
Stratified	Squamous—*keratinized*	Protective barrier Prevent dehydration	Skin (epidermis)
	Squamous—*nonkeratinized*	Protective barrier Secretion	Oral cavity Oropharynx Laryngopharynx Esophagus Vaginal canal Anal canal
	Cuboidal	Protective barrier	Large ducts of several exocrine glands
	Transitional	Protective barrier	Bladder Urinary tract

C. Connective tissue

1. Connective tissues consist of an extracellular matrix and cells. The extracellular matrix is made up of amorphous ground substance, fibers, and glycoproteins.
   a. Amorphous ground substance
      (1) Has a semifluid, gel-like consistency that allows for the exchange of molecules and fluid between cells and the circulatory system.
      (2) Contains proteoglycans. Proteoglycans are proteins with covalently bound glycosaminoglycan chains (Figure 1–45).
      (3) Glycosaminoglycans (GAGs)
         (a) GAGs are made of repeating sulfated disaccharide units.
         (b) GAGs form hydrogen bonds with large amounts of water, forming a gel-like matrix.
         (c) Ground substance stains basophilical due to the presence of GAGs contained in sulfated proteoglycans.
         (d) Types of GAGs:
            (i) Chondroitin sulfate (chondroitin 4-sulfate, chondroitin 6-sulfate)—the most abundant GAG. It is found in cartilage.
            (ii) Keratan sulfate—found in cartilage and the cornea.
            (iii) Heparan sulfate—found in cell membranes and basement membranes.
            (iv) Dermatan sulfate—found in skin, blood vessels, and heart valves.
            (v) Hyaluronic acid.
         (e) Known as the "cement substance of tissue."
         (f) Found in bone, cartilage, tendons, synovial fluid, and the vitreous humor of the eye.
   b. Fibers
      (1) Collagen
         (a) Most abundant protein in the body, about 30% dry weight.

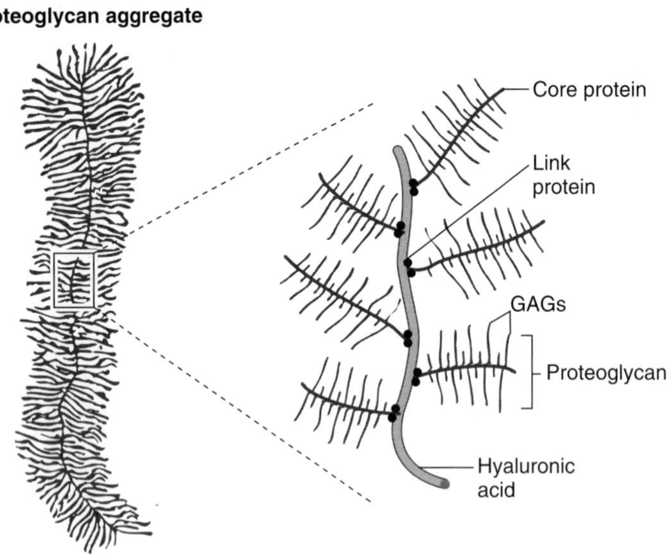

Figure 1–45. Proteoglycan aggregate. (Modified from Burns ER, Cave MD: Histology and Cell Biology, St. Louis, Mosby, 2002.)

(b) Is secreted as tropocollagen (a triple helix containing hydroxylysine and hydroxyproline), which polymerizes in the extracellular matrix to form collagen.
(c) Type I collagen—most abundant type of collagen. Found in connective tissues, tendons, ligaments, bone, teeth, and the dermis of the skin.
(d) Type II collagen—found in hyaline cartilage.
(e) Type III collagen—constitutes reticulin fibers. These fibers play a role in the structural component in the liver, bone marrow, and lymphoid organs.
(f) Type IV collagen—found in basement membranes. Does not form fibers or fibrils.

(2) Elastin—a flexible protein that is arranged into elastic fibers. These fibers also contain fibrillin.

c. Glycoproteins
(1) Glycoproteins are found in the extracellular matrix.
(2) Types of glycoproteins include:
(a) Fibrillin—plays a role in the deposition of elastic fibers.
(b) Fibronectin—plays a role in the deposition of collagen fibers. It also aids in the attachment of cells to collagen.
(c) Laminin—found in basement membranes.
(d) Entactin—binds laminin to type IV collagen in basement membranes.
(e) Tenascin—plays a role in the embryological development of nerve cells.

2. Some miscellaneous cells
a. Fibroblasts—produce collagenous, reticular, and elastic fibers.
b. Immune cells—includes macrophages, mast cells, plasma cells, and lymphocytes.
c. Adipocytes—fat cells that store and metabolize fat. Collectively, they form adipose tissue.

D. Muscle
1. There are three types of muscle: smooth, skeletal, and cardiac. Their histological characteristics are summarized in Table 1–29.
a. Smooth (visceral) muscle
(1) Smooth muscle is under autonomic or hormonal control, or involuntary control.
(2) Cells are capable of mitosis.
(3) Smooth muscle is found in the walls of blood vessels, organs, and visceral structures, including the gastrointestinal tract, the uterus, and the urinary bladder.
b. Skeletal muscle
(1) Skeletal muscle is under conscious or voluntary control.
(2) Cells are incapable of mitosis.

(3) Anatomical organization (Figure 1–46):
   (a) Skeletal muscle is covered by a dense collagenous tissue called the *epimysium*.
   (b) Muscle fibers are grouped into bundles (muscle fasciculi). The connective tissues covering the muscle fibers and fasciculi are known as *endomysium* and *perimysium*, respectively.
   (c) Histological staining (H&E staining) of a muscle fiber reveals A and I bands.
      (i) A band—dark bands with a light band (H band) in the center.
      (ii) I band—light bands with a thin band (Z line) bisecting it.
      (iii) The contractile unit of skeletal muscle, or sarcomere, is the area between two Z lines.
      (iv) Sarcomeres contain two types of filaments: thick and thin. Thick filaments consist mostly of myosin; thin filaments consist mostly of actin.

c. Cardiac muscle
   (1) Is incapable of mitosis.
   (2) Histological organization:
      (a) Consists of rows of myocardial cells connected in a series (Figure 1–47).
      (b) Myocardial cells are separated by intercalated discs, which consist of:
         (i) Gap junctions—areas of communication between the cells that allow electrical currents to travel through them.
         (ii) Desmosomes ("spot welds")—attach cells together.
   (3) Histological appearance, as compared to skeletal muscle:
      (a) Similarities:
         (i) Both are striated muscle.
         (ii) The contractile unit for both is sarcomere consisting of thin and thick filaments.

TABLE 1–29. SUMMARY OF THE THREE TYPES OF MUSCLE

	HISTOLOGICAL CHARACTERISTICS
Smooth muscle	Nonstriated muscle Spindle-shaped (fusiform) cells Gap junctions (nexi) Nucleus centered in *widest* part of cell
Skeletal muscle	Striated muscle Prominent A bands and I bands Multiple nuclei found at the cell periphery
Cardiac muscle	Striated muscle Specialized gap junctions (intercalated discs) and desmosomes Nucleus centered in cells

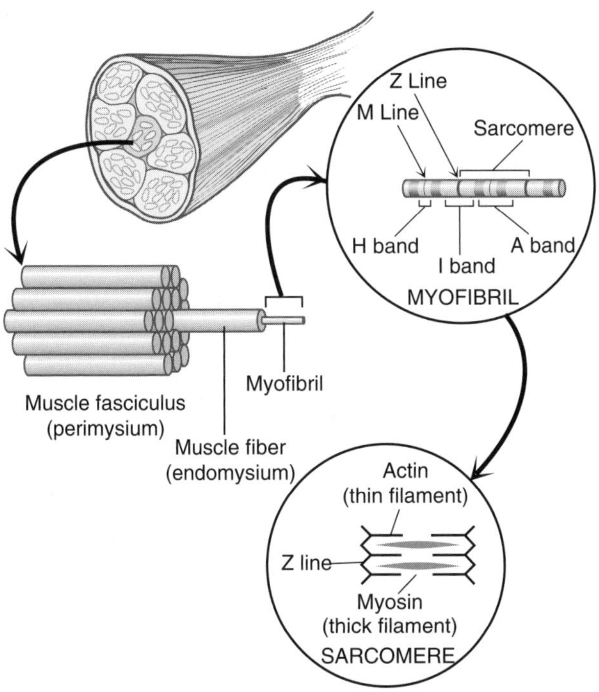

Figure 1–46. Anatomical organization of skeletal muscle.

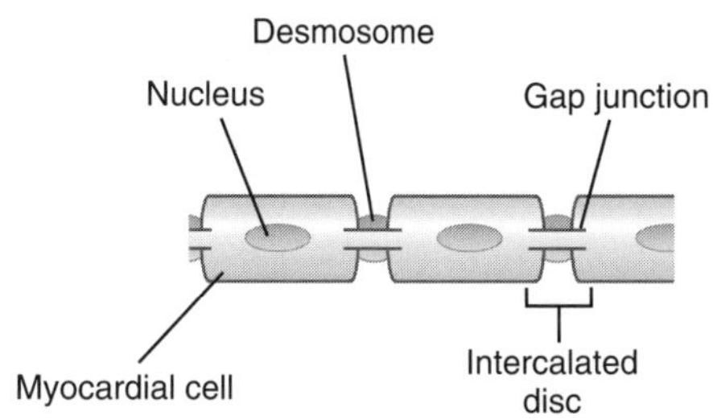

Figure 1–47. Diagram of my ocardial cells.

(b) Differences:
  (i) Cardiac muscles have larger T tubules and more mitochondria.
  (ii) Nuclei are centered in cells.
  (iii) Presence of intercalated discs between cells.

E. Nervous tissue
1. Neurons consist of a cell body, a single axon, and dendrite(s).
   a. Cell body—contains the nucleus and cell organelles.
   b. Dendrites
      (1) Receive and transmit information toward the cell body.
      (2) Are usually short and highly branched.
   c. Axon
      (1) Transmits impulses away from the cell body.
      (2) A long, uniform process that is usually surrounded by a myelin sheath. The myelin sheath consists of Schwann cells that are separated by spaces called *nodes of Ranvier*.
2. There are three types of neurons (Figure 1–48):
   a. Multipolar neurons—have dendrites extending directly from the cell body. Example: motor neurons.
   b. Bipolar neurons—have a single dendrite that extends from the cell body. Example: neurons that function in the senses of smell and sight or that coordinate balance.
   c. Pseudounipolar—have a single dendrite. The dendrite and the axon are joined. Example: most primary sensory neurons.
3. Glial cells
   a. Function as support cells to neurons and include Schwann cells and oligodendrocytes.
   b. Schwann cells—make up the myelin sheath around myelinated axons in the parasympathetic nervous system.
   c. Oligodendrocytes—make up the myelin sheath around myelinated axons in the central nervous system.
4. Synapse
   a. The site at which a nerve impulse (action potential) is passed from one nerve to another (i.e., nerve impulses are sent from one nerve's axon to the receiving nerve's dendrites) (Figure 1–49).

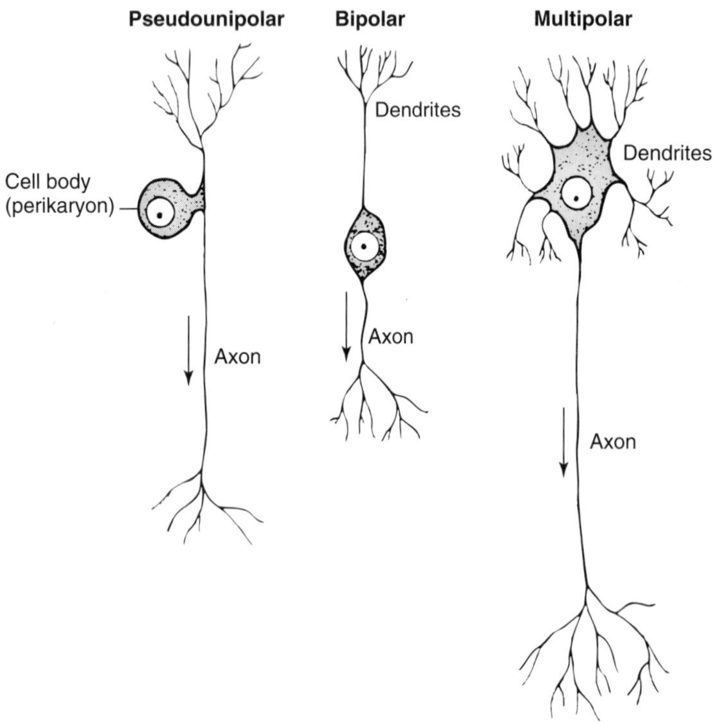

Figure 1–48. Three main types of neurons. *Arrows* indicate the direction of nerve impulse conduction. (From Burns ER, Cave MD: Histology and Cell Biology, St. Louis, Mosby, 2002.)

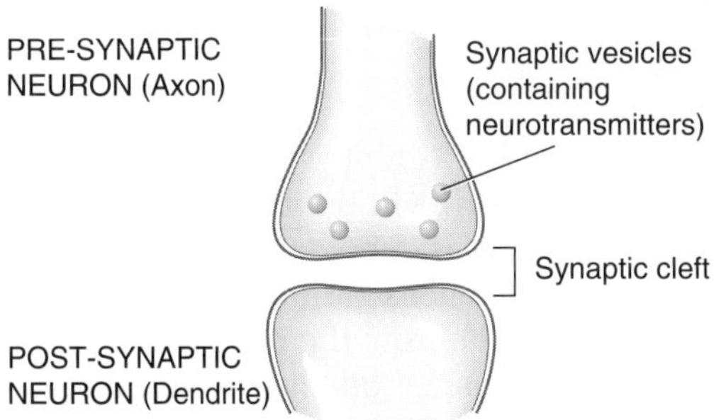

Figure 1–49. Nerve synapse.

b. Synaptic transmission: refer to Biochemistry/Physiology Review.

2.3 Bone, Cartilage, and Joints

2.3.1 Bone

A. General characteristics
1. Bone is constantly being remodeled throughout life. Bone plays many roles, including providing support against mechanical stresses, hematopoiesis, and calcium homeostasis (i.e., calcium storage).
2. Bone consists of:
a. A calcified (mineralized) matrix—contains inorganic substances consisting mostly of calcium hydroxyapatite. Osteogenin, a glycoprotein that binds calcium and collagen, is also present.
b. Extracellular matrix—contains organic substances including type I collagen and glycosaminoglycans (i.e., ground substance).
c. Cells, including osteoblasts, osteoclasts, osteocytes.
d. Note: during the calcification (mineralization) of bone, its inorganic content increases, and its water content decreases. The amount of collagen does not change.
e. Osteoid—bone that has not yet been calcified (i.e., contains no mineralized matrix).

B. Two types of bone
1. Cortical (compact) bone
a. 70% of bone in the body
b. Dense bone that consists of parallel cylinders tightly stacked together, called *Haversian systems* or *osteons* (Figure 1–50).

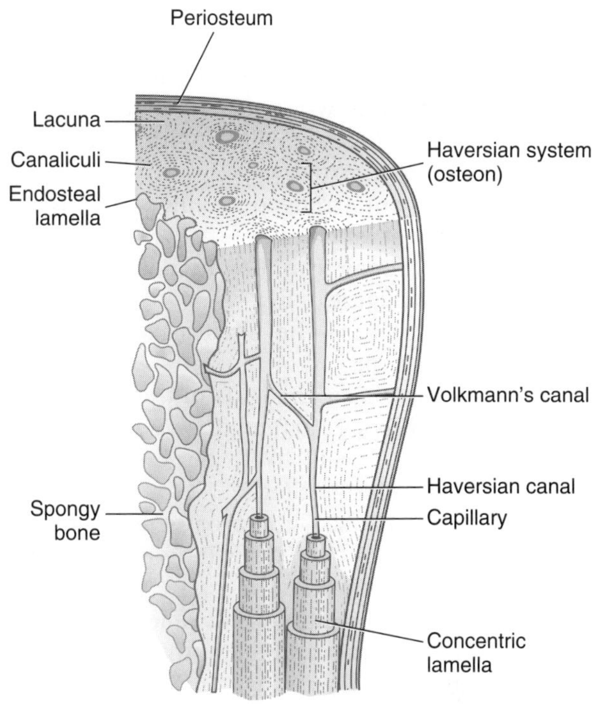

Figure 1–50. Compact bone. (Modified from Leeson CR, Leeson T, Papan A: Atlas of Histology, Philadelphia, WB Saunders, 1985.)

c. A Haversian system consists of layers of bone (lamellae) that are concentrically arranged, with the oldest layer near the periphery. The lamellae circumscribe a neurovascular canal (Haversian canal), which contains nerves, lymphatics, and blood vessels.
d. Haversian canals are interconnected by Volkmann's canals.
e. As the bone is laid down, osteocytes get trapped in spaces called *lacunae*. Lacunae have mini-canals known as *canaliculi*, which connect them with the central canal.
f. Cortical bone is covered by a thick, connective tissue called the *periosteum*. The periosteum attaches to the bone by Sharpey's fibers. Note: Sharpey's fibers also attach the periodontal ligament (PDL) to alveolar bone.
g. During bone apposition, resting lines will appear between the old and newly formed cortical bone.
2. Cancellous (trabecular, spongy) bone
a. Protected by an outer shell of cortical bone.

b. The major site for bone remodeling and metabolic activity.
c. Consists of a sponge-like structure with a network of bony plates (trabeculae) that are filled with pockets of bone marrow.
d. It is not arranged in concentric layers.

C. Anatomy of long bones
1. Long bones can be divided into three zones (Figure 1–51):
a. Diaphysis—the shaft (midportion) of the bone.
b. Epiphysis—the ends of the bone. If the epiphysis articulates with another bone, it will likely be surrounded by articular cartilage.
c. Metaphysis—the area where the bone narrows between the epiphysis and diaphysis.
2. Epiphyseal plate (physis)—found between the epiphysis and metaphysis in children who are still growing.

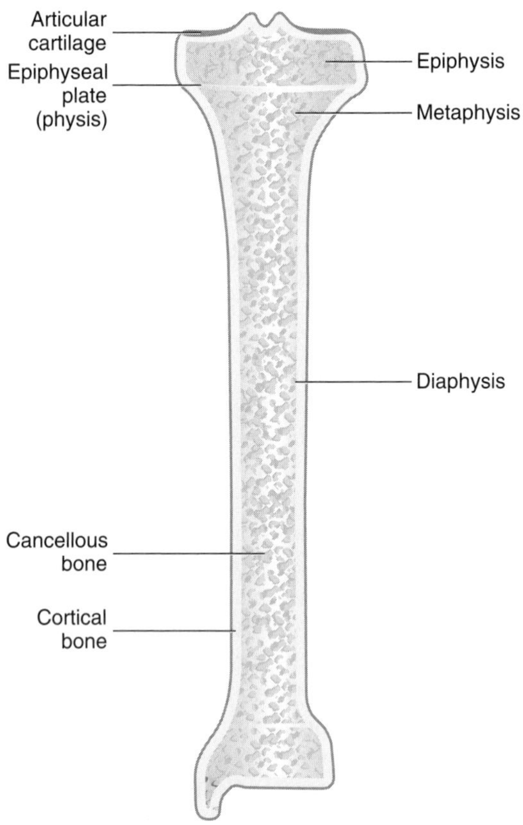

Figure 1–51. The zones of a long bone. (McCarthy E, Frassica F: Pathology of Bone and Joint Disorders, Philadelphia, WB Saunders, 1998.)

D. Osteogenesis (bone development)
1. Cellular players
a. Osteoblasts
(1) Secrete (create) bone. They also play a role in bone remodeling.
(2) Appear as cuboidal cells with a polarized nucleus on the side of the cell opposite from the bony surface.
(3) Synthesize alkaline phosphatase. Note: alkaline phosphatase is also produced in the kidney and liver. Increased serum alkaline phosphatase is often indicative of bone disease.
b. Osteocytes—are osteoblasts that become trapped in bone (i.e., develop from osteoblasts).
c. Osteoclasts
(1) Resorb (destroy) bone.
(2) Appear as multinucleated, giant cells.
(3) Derived from the fusion of blood-borne monocytes.
(4) Bone resorption creates depressions called *Howship's lacunae*.
2. Osteogenesis—two processes:
a. Endochondral ossification
(1) Associated with the growth of long bones.
(2) Increases the length of bones via interstitial growth at the epiphyseal plates.
(3) Includes most skeletal bones (i.e., tibia, fibia, femur) and a few bones in the skull (ethmoid, sphenoid, temporal, occipital bones, and the base of the skull).
(4) Process of bone development (Figure 1–52):
(a) Chondrocytes differentiate from mesenchymal cells present in connective tissue.
(b) Chondrocytes secrete a cartilage (hyaline) matrix, which is covered by perichondrium. The matrix then calcifies.
(c) Chondrocytes die, leaving spaces that become filled with vascular tissue.
(d) Osteoblasts differentiate from mesenchymal cells in adjacent tissues and secrete bone onto the preformed cartilage scaffold.

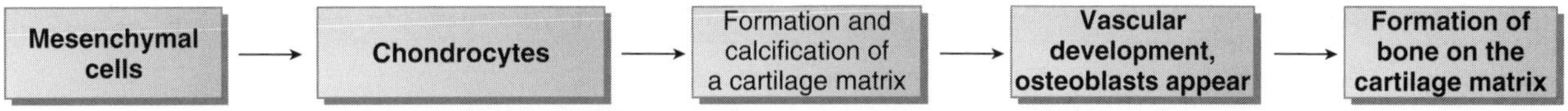

Figure 1–52. Summary of endochondral ossification.

b. Intramembraneous ossification (appositional growth)
   (1) Associated with increasing the diameter or width of flat bones (i.e., bones grow "out.")
   (2) Includes flat bones of the skull, part of the mandible, and a portion of the clavicle.
   (3) Process of bone development (Figure 1–53):
      (a) Osteoblasts differentiate from mesenchymal cells present in connective tissue.
      (b) Osteoblasts secrete bone directly into connective tissues, forming trabeculae (long strands of bone) matrix. This initial type of bony matrix is known as *woven bone*.
      (c) Osteoblasts that become trapped in the matrix, in spaces known as *lacunae*, are called *osteocytes*. They continue to lay down bone, forming compact bone. The bone mineralizes.

c. Bone remodeling—bone is constantly being remodeled. This process includes both osteoclasts removing bone and osteoblasts reforming bone in the resorbed area.

2.3.2 Cartilage

A. Cartilage is a tissue that consists of:
   1. Water.
   2. Type II collagen.
   3. Sulfated proteoglycans, which results in basophilic staining of cartilage.
   4. Chondrocytes.

B. Perichondrium
   1. Fibrous connective tissue that lines the surfaces of cartilage except articulate surfaces (i.e., nonarticulate surfaces).
   2. Is the vascular supply for cartilage.
   3. Cannot be viewed on radiographs due to lack of calcium salts.
   4. Contains chondroblasts.

C. Growth of cartilage
   1. Interstitial growth—growth by cell division of chondrocytes. Note: bones do not grow interstitially (from within), except at the epiphyseal plates. This is one of the ways cartilage growth differs from bone development.
   2. Appositional growth—growth by layering (i.e., deposition of a cartilage matrix by chondroblasts).

D. There are three types of cartilage: hyaline (articular) cartilage, elastic cartilage, and fibrocartilage. Their general characteristics and distribution are summarized in Table 1–30).

2.3.3 Joints

A. Classification of joints
   1. Synarthroses—joints with little or no movement.
      a. Syndesmoses
         (1) Bones joined by dense fibrous tissue. No cartilage is present.
         (2) Example: cranial sutures in children.
         (3) Gomphosis—a type of syndesmoses joint that is described as a cone-shaped process placed in a socket.
         (4) Example: tooth in alveolar bone.
      b. Synchondroses
         (1) Bones joined by cartilage. No synovial cavity is present.

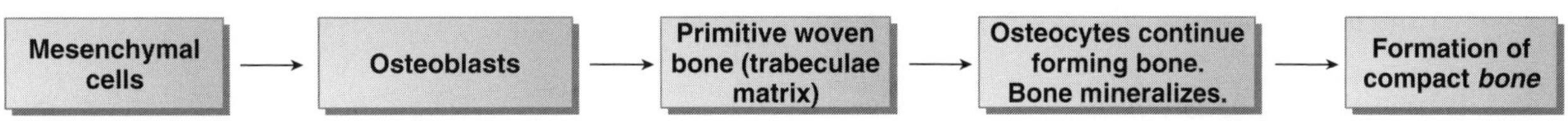

Figure 1–53. Summary of intramembranous ossification.

Table 1–30. Summary of the Three Types of Cartilage

	GENERAL CHARACTERISTICS	DISTRIBUTION
Hyaline (articular) cartilage	Fibrous matrix of type II collagen Slightly elastic Covered by perichondrium	Ends of bones (articular joints) Costal cartilage (ribs) Respiratory cartilage (nasal septum, larynx, trachea, bronchial walls) Auditory cartilage (external auditory meatus, pharyngotympanic tube) Synchondroses Cartilage matrix for endochondrial ossification Embryonic skeleton formation
Elastic cartilage	Like hyaline cartilage with type II collagen, but less dense Elastic Covered by perichondrium	Ear—external ear, pinna, auditory tube Epiglottis
Fibrocartilage	Dense, fibrous matrix of type I collagen Not elastic No perichondrium	Articular discs—TMJ, knee meniscus Intervertebral discs Pubic symphysis Insertions of tendons or ligaments

(2) Example: ribs, sternum.

c. Synostoses
   (1) Bones joined by bone.
   (2) Can, in many circumstances, be considered a pathologic condition (i.e., ankylosis).
   (3) Example: cranial sutures in adults.

d. Symphysis
   (1) Bones joined by fibrocartilage and ligaments.
   (2) May be classified as an amphiarthroses (slightly movable) joint.
   (3) Example: pubic symphysis, intervertebral discs.

2. Synovial (diarthrodial or diarthroses) joints—freely movable joints.
   a. Consists of two bone ends articulating in an enclosed capsule (Figure 1–54).
   b. Articular cartilage
      (1) Consists of hyaline cartilage that covers the ends of the two opposing bones.
      (2) Has no vascular or nerve supply.
      (3) Synovial fluid provides its nourishment.
   c. Articular capsule
      (1) Consists of dense, fibrous connective tissue that encloses the joint space.
      (2) Continuous with the periosteum and synovium.
3. Synovial cavity (joint space)
   a. Synovial fluid
      (1) Fluid that fills the joint space.
      (2) It is responsible for providing lubrication for frictionless movement and nourishment of the articular cartilage.
      (3) Consists of hyaluronic acid, glycoproteins including lubricin, and lysosomal enzymes that are secreted by macrophages.
   b. Synovial membrane (synovium)
      (1) Lines the synovial cavity.
      (2) Secretes synovial fluid.
      (3) Lined with macrophages and fibroblasts.

2.3.4 Blood

In general, circulating blood constitutes 5–7% of our body weight. It is a tissue that consists of

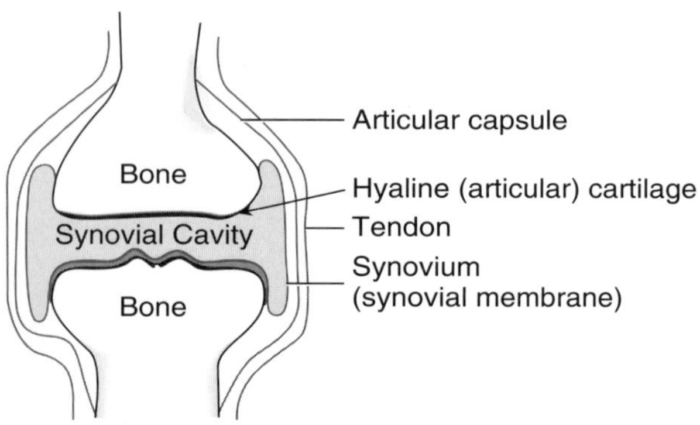

Figure 1–54. Synovial (diarthrodial) joint.

cells and molecules in a fluid medium known as *plasma*.

A. Composition of blood
  1. Plasma—55% of blood volume.
    a. Components:
      (1) Water
      (2) Proteins—three types:
        (a) Carrier proteins—includes albumin and lipoproteins. Albumin makes up two thirds of plasma proteins; it is therefore the major source of colloid osmotic pressure in plasma.
        (b) Immunoproteins—includes immunoglobulins (antibodies) and complement.
        (c) Coagulation proteins—includes fibrinogen, prothrombin, and proteins of the coagulation cascade.
      (3) Other substances, including electrolytes, glucose, hormones, and so forth.
    b. Serum—the supernatant that separates from blood after it has clotted (i.e., plasma without the fibrinogen).
  2. Formed elements (cells)—45% of blood volume.
    a. Erythrocytes (red blood cells [RBCs])
      (1) Shaped as biconcave discs. Do not contain a nucleus or mitochondria.
      (2) Have a life span of 120 days.
      (3) Function to carry oxygen (O_2) and carbon dioxide (CO_2) to or from tissues, respectively.
      (4) Hemoglobin—the protein in RBCs that is responsible for binding O_2 and CO_2.
    b. Platelets (thrombocytes)
      (1) Shaped as disc-shaped fragments. Do not contain a nucleus.
      (2) Play a role, along with coagulation proteins, in blood coagulation.
    c. Leukocytes (white blood cells [WBCs])
      (1) Do contain a nucleus.
      (2) Are capable of locomotion within tissues.
      (3) Play a role in immune defense.
      (4) Cell types include (Figure 1–55):
        (a) Granulocytes—WBCs that are observed with particular nuclear shapes and granules. Includes neutrophils (polymorphonuclear leukocytes), eosinophils, and basophils.
        (b) Lymphocytes (B and T cells)—the smallest leukocyte; they contain a large nucleus with a relatively small amount of cytoplasm.
        (c) Monocytes—contain a kidney-shaped nucleus. They mature into macrophages when they enter tissues.
        (d) Plasma cells.

B. Hematopoiesis (hemopoiesis)
  1. All blood cells develop from a common source of undifferentiated cells (pluripotent hematopoietic stem cells). This process of blood cell differentiation and proliferation is known as *hematopoiesis* (Figure 1–56).
  2. Hematopoiesis occurs in:
    a. Fetus—bone marrow, liver, and spleen.
    b. Adult—bone marrow.
  3. Bone marrow:
    a. Two types:
      (1) Red bone marrow—site of hematopoiesis.
      (2) Yellow bone marrow—consists mainly of fat.
    b. In a growing child, most of the bone marrow is devoted to hematopoiesis (red). As people age, fat (yellow) largely replaces red bone marrow.

2.4 Lymphatic and Circulatory Systems

2.4.1 Circulatory System

A. The heart
  1. The heart and its vessels are enclosed by an outer fibrous sac known as the *pericardium*. It consists of inner (visceral pericardium) and outer (parietal pericardium) sacs that are separated by a layer of pericardial fluid.
  2. The heart wall consists of three layers (listed in order from outer to inner):
    a. Epicardium—the outermost layer of the heart that is equivalent to the visceral pericardium.
    b. Myocardium
      (1) Is the thickest layer of the heart that contains cardiac muscle cells. Cardiac myocytes are incapable of mitosis.

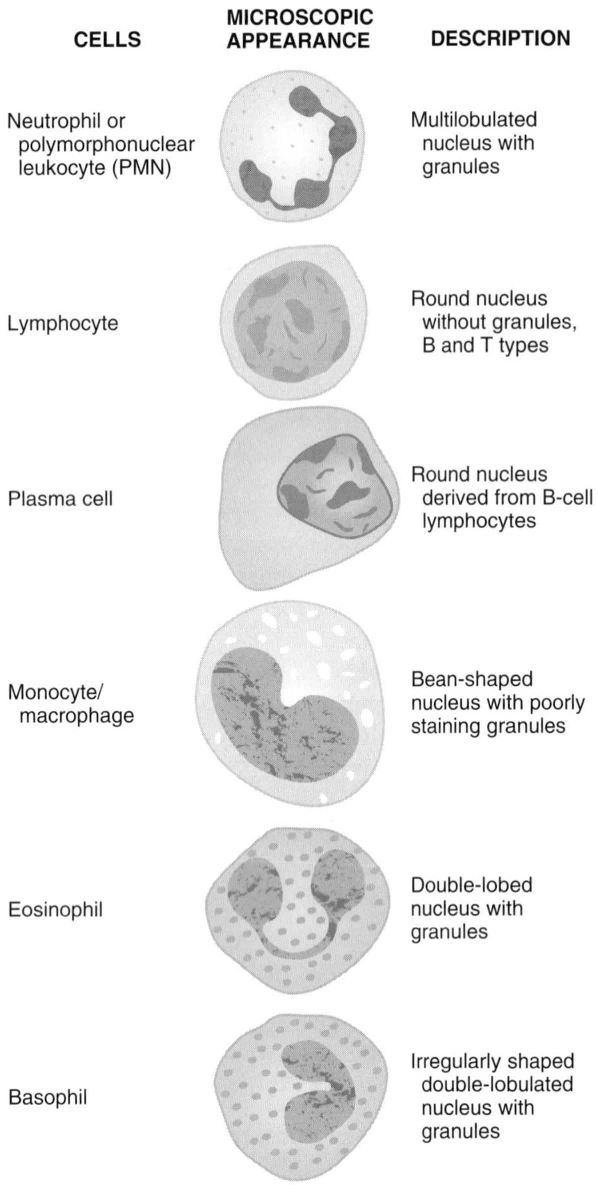

Figure 1–55. Blood cells. (Modified from Bath-Balogh M, Fehrenbach M: Illustrated Dental Embryology, Histology, and Anatomy, ed 2, Philadelphia, WB Saunders, 2006.)

(2) Includes the papillary muscles and chordae tendineae.

c. Endocardium—the innermost layer of the heart that consists of endothelial cells lining the inner chambers and heart valves.

B. Blood vessels

1. Arteries
   a. Arteries transfer blood from the heart to capillary beds throughout the body.
   b. As blood enters the arterial system, it forces arterial walls to expand. The subsequent elastic recoil of these walls aids in the maintenance of blood pressure between ventricular heart beats.
   c. Blood flow to various organs and tissues can be controlled by varying the diameter of small arteries or arterioles (i.e., via vasoconstriction and vasodilatation). This is accomplished by the presence of smooth muscle in the vessel walls, which is primarily controlled by the sympathetic nervous system and hormones from the adrenal medulla.
   d. Three main types of arteries:
      (1) Elastic arteries—the largest arteries that include the aorta, common carotid, subclavian, and pulmonary arteries.
      (2) Muscular arteries—main distribution arterial branches that provide vascular supply to different organs and tissues. These include the radial, femoral, coronary, and cerebral arteries.
      (3) Arterioles—terminal branches of the arterial tree that provide and control the blood supply to the capillary beds.
2. Veins
   a. Veins function under a low pressure system and return blood from the capillary beds back to the heart. More than 70% of total blood volume is in this portion.
   b. Because the pressure in the veins remains low, veins contain valves to help prevent the backflow of blood.
   c. Veins can be categorized as small, medium, or large. Smaller veins are also known as *venules*.
3. The walls of blood vessels are composed of three basic layers:
   a. Tunica intima—the innermost layer that consists of a single layer of endothelial cells and a subendothelial layer of supporting connective tissue.
   b. Tunica media—the middle layer that consists of varying amounts of smooth muscle fibers and elastin. Of the three layers in arterial walls, it is the broadest layer.
   c. Tunica adventitia—the outermost layer that consists of connective tissue containing collagen and elastin. In

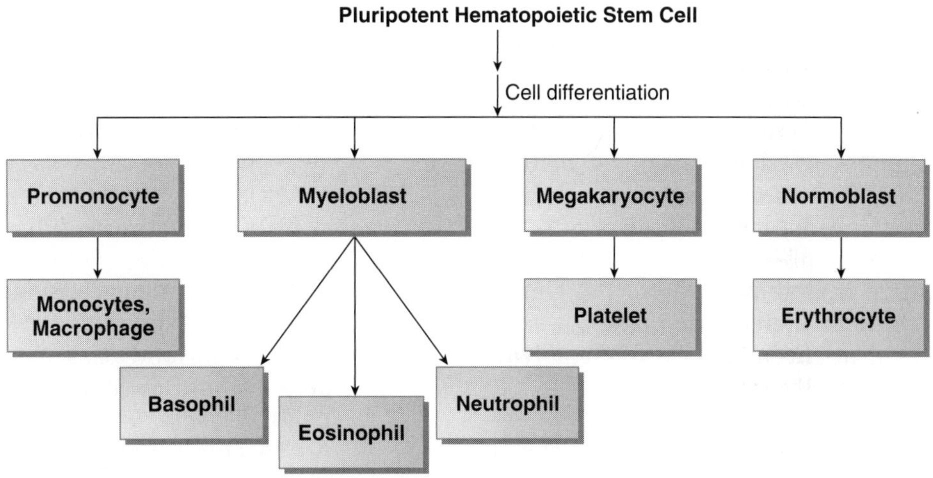

Figure 1–56. Hematopoiesis: lineage of blood cells.

some large vessels, it also contains the vasa vasorum. The vasa vasorum consists of small arteries that provide nutrients to the outer tissues. Of the three layers in the walls of veins, it is the broadest layer. The adventitia frequently contains longitudinal bundles of smooth muscles.

d. Arterial walls—in general, the amount of elastic tissue decreases and the amount of smooth muscle increases as the vessels decrease in size. For example, the tunica media of the aorta is extremely elastic with few smooth muscle fibers. In contrast, the tunica media of arterioles consist mostly of smooth muscle with very few elastic fibers.

e. Venous walls—the walls of veins usually contain little elastin and are thinner than arterial walls. Their tunica media is thin, and the diameter of their lumen is large as compared to that of arteries. In general, the thickness of the tunica adventitia increases as the size of the vein increases.

4. Capillaries
   a. Capillaries consist of a thin layer of endothelial cells with an average diameter of 8 μm (micrometers).
   b. It is in the capillaries that the interchange of gases, fluids, nutrients, and metabolic waste products between the blood and tissues occur.
   c. Blood enters the capillary beds through arterioles. Blood flow is controlled by smooth muscle sphincters, called *precapillary sphincters*, at the arteriole-capillary junctions. Blood from the capillaries drain into venules.
   d. There are three types of capillaries:
      (1) Continuous capillaries—the endothelia contain no pores. They are the most common type of capillary.
      (2) Fenestrated capillaries—the endothelia contain a large number of pores.
      (3) Discontinuous capillaries (sinusoids)—consist of a large lumen and with discontinuous endothelia. They are found in the liver.

2.4.2 Lymphatic System

A. Lymphatic circulation
1. Excess fluid from the circulation (lymph) is drained into the lymphatic circulation. Lymph is first drained into lymphatic capillaries and then transported by a series of progressively larger lymphatic vessels. It is filtered in lymph nodes along the way and will ultimately drain into the venous system via the left or right thoracic duct.
2. Like veins, lymphatic vessels also contain valves, but their lumens are larger and their walls are thinner. They also do not contain any red blood cells.
3. Lymphoid organs
   a. Primary lymphoid organs—site where lymphocyte precursors mature and

are programmed to recognize a specific antigen. Includes the bone marrow (B cell) and thymus (T cell).

b. Secondary lymphoid organs—areas where collected antigens are used to stimulate clonal expansion of mature T and B cells. Examples are lymph nodes, tonsils, and the spleen.

B. Lymph nodes
   1. Lymph is filtered as it enters the lymph node through afferent lymphatics. It exits the gland at the hilum via efferent lymphatic vessel (Figure 1–57).
   2. A secondary lymphoid organ is where antigen-stimulated activation and clonal expansion of T and B cells occur.
   3. Lymph nodes are encapsulated by a layer of dense connective tissue. The capsule is pierced by many afferent lymphatic vessels and has inward trabecular projections that partially compartmentalize the cortex.
   4. Consists of a cortex and medulla.
      a. Cortex
         (1) Outer cortex—consists of B cells, organized in lymphoid follicles. Germinal centers (the central, lighter-staining areas) may be observed in the follicles.
         (2) Paracortex—consists of T cells and is found between the outer cortex and medulla.
      b. Medulla
         (1) Located centrally in the lymph node.
         (2) Is less cellular than the cortex.
         (3) Contain the medullary sinuses.

C. Tonsils
   1. Partially or nonencapsulated masses of lymphoid tissue that are found near the airway and food passages. Unlike lymph nodes, they are not located along lymphatic vessels.
   2. Are located in the lamina propria of oral mucosa. Their epithelial lining consists of stratified squamous epithelium that is continuous with the surrounding oral mucosa.
   3. Palatine tonsils
      a. Located bilaterally at the opening of the pharynx, between the anterior and posterior faucial pillars.
      b. Histologically consists of lymphatic nodules with germinal centers. There are also numerous epithelial invaginations, which form tonsillar crypts (Figure 1–58).

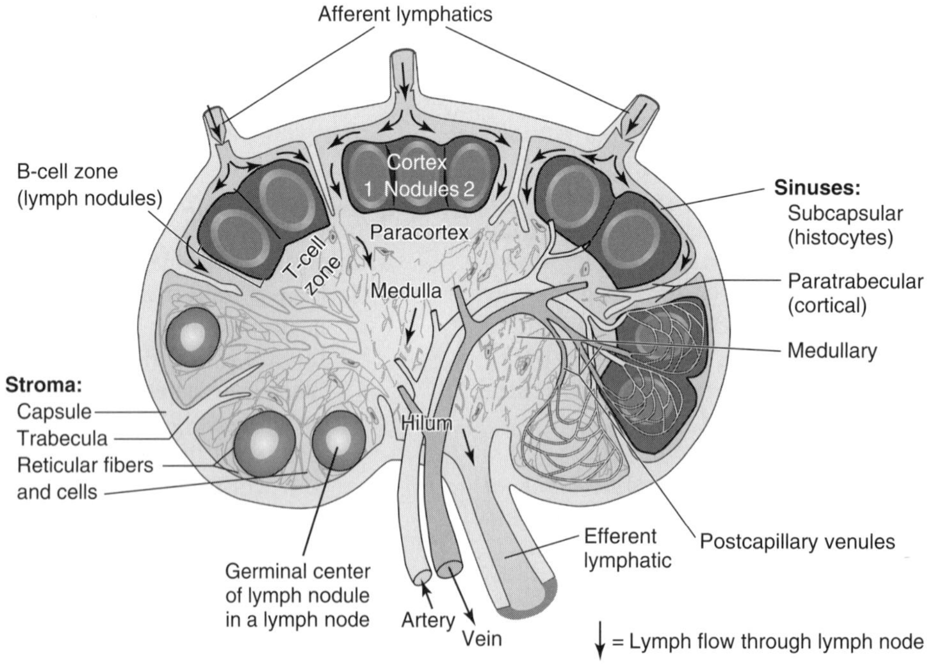

Figure 1–57. Cross-section: lymph node. *Arrows* show the direction of lymph flow through the lymph node. (From Burns ER, Cave MD: Histology and Cell Biology, St. Louis, Mosby, 2002.)

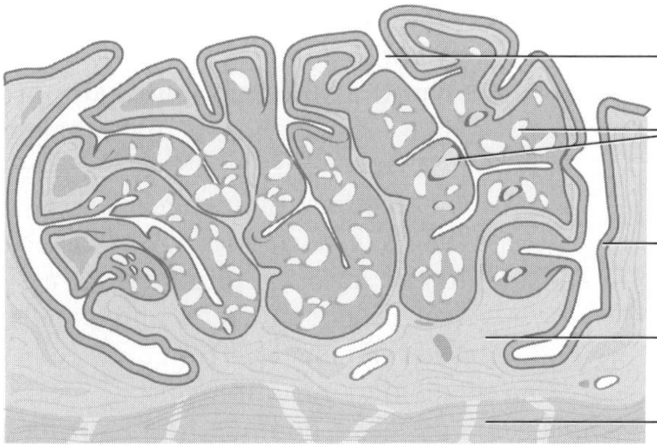

Figure 1–58. Histological features of the palatine tonsil. (Modified from Bath-Balogh M, Fehrenbach M: Illustrated Dental Embryology, Histology, and Anatomy, ed 2, Philadelphia, WB Saunders, 2006.)

4. Pharyngeal tonsil
   a. A single tonsil that lies in the superposterior portion of the pharynx.
   b. It has no crypts, has a thinner capsule, and is composed of mucosa overlying diffuse lymphoid tissue and nodules.
5. Lingual tonsil
   a. Located at the base of the tongue.
   b. Histologically consists of lymphatic nodules with germinal centers and one associated tonsillar crypt.
6. Together, the palatine, lingual, and pharyngeal tonsils form a tonsillar ring, known as *Waldeyer's ring.*

D. Spleen
1. A secondary lymph organ, the functions of which include:
   a. The filtration of blood. This includes removing pathogens and destroying defective or old red blood cells from the circulation.
   b. Antigen-stimulated activation of lymphocytes, which is similar to the function of a lymph node.
   c. In the fetus, it also plays a role in hematopoiesis (forming red blood cells).
2. Can be divided into two parts, the red and white pulps:
   a. White pulp
      (1) Site of activation and clonal expansion lymphocytes.
      (2) T cells congregate around central arteries of the white pulp, forming the periarterial lymphatic sheath. B cells are found in follicles, adjacent to the arterioles.
   b. Marginal zone
      (1) The sinusoidal interface between the red and white pulp.
      (2) Area where antigen-presenting cells interact and activate T-helper cells that, in turn, activate B cells.
   c. Red pulp
      (1) Site of blood filtration.
      (2) Consists of cords (Billroth's cords) containing numerous macrophages that lie between the venous sinusoids.

E. Thymus
1. A primary lymph organ that is the site of T-cell maturation. Since it is not involved in filtering lymph, it contains no afferent lymphatic vessels. It does contain efferent lymphatic vessels.
2. Is located in the anterior mediastinum.
3. Is active at birth and increases in size until puberty, after which it gradually atrophies and is replaced by fatty tissue.
4. Can be divided into two parts separated by connective tissue capsules:
   a. Cortex—outer zone
      (1) The darker-staining, outer zone consists of T cells and epithelial reticular cells.
      (2) Is the site of T-cell maturation, where T cells are programmed to recognize specific antigens.
   b. Medulla—central zone
      (1) The lighter-staining (less dense) central area, where mature T cells leave the medulla.
      (2) Contain Hassall's corpuscles, which consist of epithelial cells with keratohyaline granules.

2.5 Endocrine System

2.5.1 Pituitary Gland (Hypophysis)

The pituitary gland is found in the hypophyseal fossa, protected in the sella turcica of the sphenoid bone. The two components of the pituitary gland are functionally different and are of separate embryological origins: the oral (Rathke's pouch) and neural ectoderm. The two regions of the pituitary gland are divided into an anterior and posterior lobe.

A. Anterior pituitary (adenohypophysis, anterior lobe)
   1. Hormones
      a. Anterior pituitary hormones: growth hormone (GH, somatotropin), prolactin, adrenocorticotropin (ACTH), thyroid-stimulating hormone (TSH), follicle-stimulating hormone (FSH), and luteinizing hormone (LH).
      b. Hypothalamic control:
         (1) The control of hormone secretion from the anterior pituitary is mediated by specific releasing and inhibitory hormones from the hypothalamus (e.g., growth hormone-releasing hormone [GHRH]), with the exception of prolactin, which is under the inhibitory control of dopamine.
         (2) Hypothalamo-hypophyseal portal veins—the axons of hypothalamic neurosecretory cells terminate in the median eminence. The hypothalamic hormones are transferred to the anterior pituitary via a system of portal veins and capillary beds (Figure 1–59).
   2. Can be divided into three parts:
      a. Pars distalis—contains endocrine cells. It serves as the primary source of hormones of the anterior pituitary.
      b. Pars tuberalis—surrounds the infundibulum and carries portal veins of the hypophyseal portal system. Does contain endocrine cells but only plays a minor role.
      c. Pars intermedia
         (1) A thin layer of tissue found between the anterior and posterior lobes.
         (2) Is rudimentary in humans but may play a role in the synthesis and secretion of melanocyte-stimulating hormone (MSH).

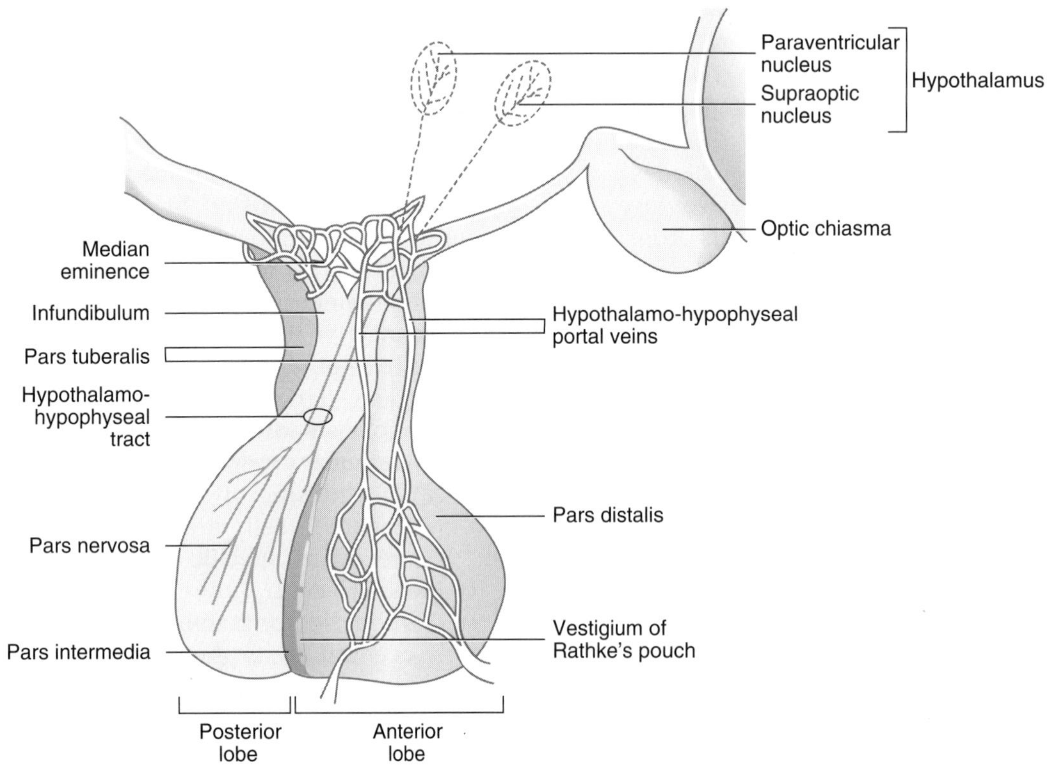

Figure 1–59. Pituitary gland. (Modified from Burkitt HG, Young B, Heath J: Wheater's Functional Histology, ed 3, Churchill Livingstone, 1993.)

(3) A vestigial cleft consisting of cyst-like spaces (Rathke's cysts) may be found between the pars intermedia and anterior lobe. It represents the vestigial lumen of Rathke's pouch (see Figure 1–59).

3. Consists of two groups of cells:
   a. Chromophils—secrete hormones. There are two cell types that are divided according to their histological staining:
      (1) Acidophils—stain a pinkish or orange color and include the following cells:
         (a) Somatotrophs—secrete GH.
         (b) Mammotrophs (lactotrophs)—secrete prolactin.
      (2) Basophils—stain a bluish color and include the following cells:
         (a) Corticotrophs—secrete ACTH.
         (b) Thyrotrophs—secrete TSH.
         (c) Gonadotrophs—secrete FSH and LH.
   b. Chromophobes—have no secretory function. They likely represent degranulated chromophils.

B. Posterior pituitary (neurohypophysis, pars nervosa, posterior lobe)
   1. Hormones
      a. Posterior pituitary hormones: antidiuretic hormone (ADH, vasopressin) and oxytocin.
      b. Hypothalamic control and synthesis:
         (1) The control of hormone secretion from the posterior pituitary is via nerve impulses from the hypothalamus, a regulation process known as *neurosecretion*.
         (2) Hypothalamo-hypophyseal (hypothalamo-pituitary) tract: the hormones are synthesized by neurosecretory cells of the supraoptic nuclei (produce ADH) and paraventricular nuclei (produce oxytocin) of the hypothalamus. The hormones pass down the axons of these cells, called the *hypothalamo-hypophyseal tract*, into the pars nervosa. They are stored in the terminal parts of the axon, known as *Herring bodies*.
   2. The posterior lobe is divided into two parts:
      a. Pars nervosa—consists of:
         (1) The nonmyelinated axons of neurosecretory cells, whose cell bodies remain in the hypothalamus.
         (2) Pituicytes, which are similar neuroglial cells of the CNS and act as supporting cells for the axons of neurosecretory cells.
      b. Infundibulum—connects the pars nervosa to the hypothalamus. It also carries axons of neurosecretory cells.

2.5.2 Thyroid

The thyroid is the largest endocrine gland. It consists of a right and left lobe that are connected by an isthmus. It is located anterior to the trachea, around the level of the cricoid cartilage.

A. Thyroid hormone
   1. There are two forms of thyroid hormone: tri-iodothyronine (T_3) and thyroxine (T_4). T_3 contains three iodine molecules and is the more potent form; T_4 contains four iodine molecules. Although there is more T_4 secreted, T_4 is converted (deiodinated) to T_3 in peripheral tissues.
   2. Synthesis, storage, and secretion of T_3 and T_4. (Note: the numbers below correspond to the numbers shown in Figure 1–60.)
      a. Synthesis and storage: (1) hyroglobulin synthesis from amino acids occurs on rough endoplasmic reticulum within follicular cells; (2) thyroglobulin is released into the colloid in the follicle, where (3) iodination (catalyzed by thyroid peroxidase) of thyroglobulin occurs. This results in the formation of T_3 and T_4 on tyrosine residues of thyroglobulin.
      b. Secretion of hormone: (4) Thyroid-stimulating hormone (TSH) from the anterior pituitary stimulates the release of thyroid hormone. Endocytosis of colloid (containing iodinated thyroglobulin) occurs. A lysosome fuses with the endocytosed vacuole, allowing for lysosomal enzymes to cleave the hormone from thyroglobulin; (5) T_3 and T_4 are secreted into the bloodstream.

B. Thyroid follicles
   1. Site of synthesis, storage, and release of thyroid hormone.
   2. Are spherical structures that make up the thyroid gland. They consist of follicular cells surrounding a lumen filled with colloid (Figure 1–61).
   3. Follicular cells
      a. Derived from the endoderm of the thyroglossal duct.

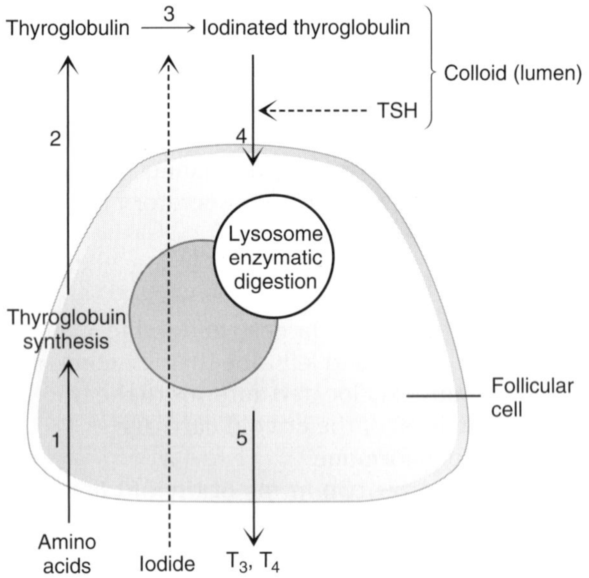

Figure 1–60. Synthesis, storage, and secretion of thyroid hormone. Numbers in the figure correspond to the numbers shown in the text, under the Thyroid Hormone section.

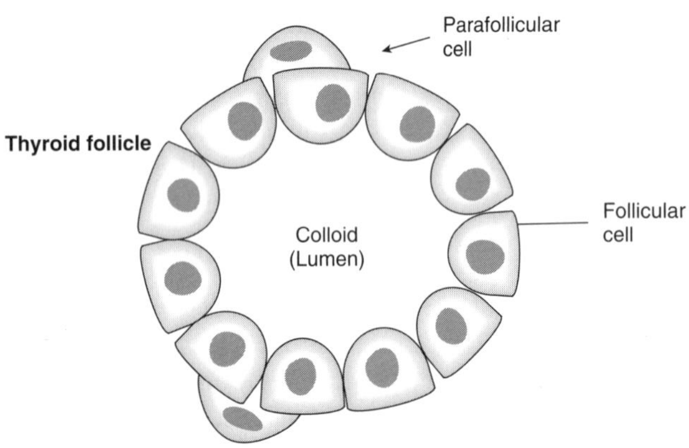

Figure 1–61. Diagram of a cross-section of a thyroid follicle.

b. Histologically, during the synthesis of thyroglobulin, the morphology of the cell appears as low cuboidal cells. During the secretion of thyroid hormone, their morphology changes to resemble taller cuboidal cells.
c. Their apical membranes (facing the colloid) contain thyroid peroxidase, an enzyme that iodinates tyrosine residues of thyroglobulin.

4. Colloid
   a. Fills the lumen of the thyroid follicle.
   b. Consists of a viscous gel that primarily contains iodinated thyroglobulin (i.e., it also serves as a storage reserve for thyroid hormone).

C. Parafollicular cells (clear cells)
1. Derived from the endoderm of the ultimobranchial body, a diverticulum of the fifth pharyngeal pouch.
2. Are located at the periphery of thyroid follicles.
3. Histologically, as compared to follicular cells, their cytoplasm appears paler in color.
4. Secrete calcitonin, a hormone that plays an important role in the regulation of calcium and phosphates. It suppresses bone resorption, by decreasing calcium and phosphate release.

2.5.3 Parathyroid Gland

There are usually four parathyroid glands in humans. The glands are located just posterior to the thyroid gland. Parathyroid hormone (PTH) plays an important role in the metabolism of calcium.

A. Parathyroid hormone
1. Is synthesized and secreted by the parathyroid gland.
2. Is secreted when calcium levels fall.
3. Overall effects of PTH:
   a. Increased serum calcium.
   b. Decreased serum phosphate.
4. Actions of PTH include:
   a. Bone: increased resorption by stimulating osteoblasts to release osteoclast-activating factor.
   b. Kidney: increased calcium resorption (i.e., decreased calcium excretion), decreased phosphate resorption.
   c. Digestive tract: indirectly increases absorption of dietary calcium by stimulating vitamin D activity.
   d. Activation of vitamin D in the kidney.

B. Parathyroid gland
1. Usually there are two pairs of glands.
2. Chief (principal) cells:
   a. Secrete PTH.
   b. Histologically, active cells have dark cytoplasm (basophilic) with numer-

ous granules. Inactive cells have light cytoplasm (acidophilic) with fewer granules.

2.5.4 Adrenal (Suprarenal) Glands

The adrenal glands are located superior and medial to the upper pole of each kidney. The gland consists of two components that function independently and have different embryological origins. The two regions are the adrenal cortex and medulla.

A. Adrenal cortex
   1. Derived from the mesodermal epithelium from the root of the dorsal mesentery.
   2. Divided into three zones (Figure 1–62):
      a. Zona glomerulosa
         (1) Secretes mineralocorticoids (mainly aldosterone), which are important in the regulation of electrolyte and water balance.
         (2) Secretory cells are arranged in irregular, ovoid clumps.
      b. Zona fasciculata
         (1) Secretes glucocorticoids (mainly cortisol), which play a role in the regulation of general metabolism.
         (2) Secretory cells are arranged in narrow cords.
      c. Zona reticularis
         (1) Secretes androgens. The androgens produced are considered weak, but they can be converted in peripheral tissues to testosterone or the estrone estrogen.
         (2) Secretory cells are arranged in an irregular network of anastomosing cords and clumps.

B. Adrenal medulla
   1. Derived from neuroectoderm (neural crest cells).
   2. Consists of chromaffin cells:
      a. Are modified postganglionic sympathetic neurons that synthesize, store, and secrete catecholamines.
      b. There are two types of chromaffin cells: one produces epinephrine (75%) and the other produces norepinephrine (25%).
   3. Secretion of catecholamines is stimulated by the release of acetylcholine from preganglionic-type sympathetic axons that form junctions on chromaffin cells.

2.5.5 Endocrine Pancreas

The pancreas functions as both an exocrine and endocrine gland. The exocrine portion makes up more than 95% of the pancreatic mass and consists of a network of ducts and pancreatic cells, including acinar and centroacinar cells. The endocrine tissue (islets of Langerhans) can be found scattered throughout the exocrine pancreas.

A. Islets of Langerhans
   1. Are most numerous in the tail of the pancreas.
   2. Cell types

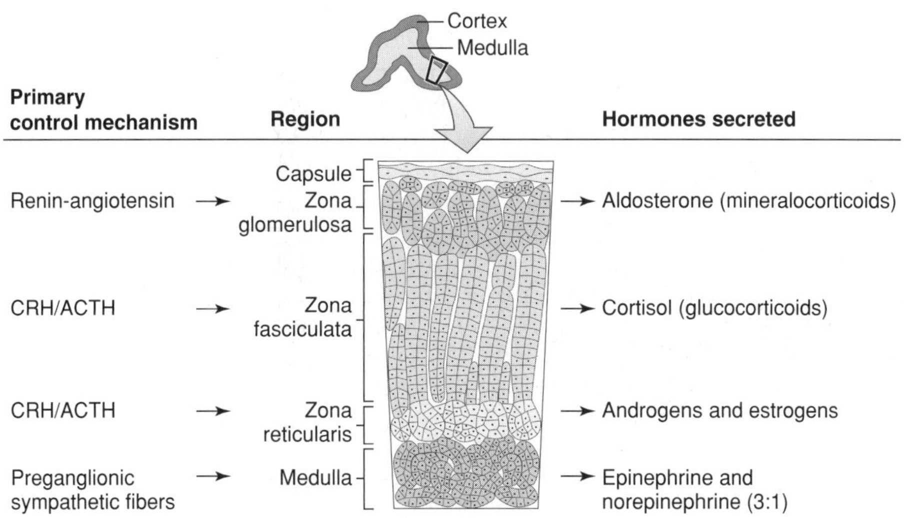

Figure 1–62. Adrenal gland: the three zones of the cortex and the adrenal medulla. (From Burns ER, Cave MD: Histology and Cell Biology, St. Louis, Mosby, 2002.)

a. Alpha (A) cells—secrete glucagon, which, in response to low levels of blood glucose, raises blood glucose levels.
b. Beta (B) cells—secrete insulin, which, in response to high levels of blood glucose, lowers blood glucose levels.
c. Delta (D) cells—secrete somatostatin, an inhibitory hormone that inhibits the release of numerous hormones, including glucagon, insulin, and GH.
d. F cells—secrete pancreatic polypeptide.

2.5.6 Pineal Gland (Epiphysis Cerebri)

A very small gland located along the roof of the third ventricle. It is contained within the pia mater and is largest in early childhood. It secretes the hormone melatonin.

A. Melatonin
 1. Is produced from serotonin.
 2. Circadian fluctuations—blood melatonin levels are three times higher at night than during the day.
 3. Antigonadotropic effect
  a. Has an inhibitory effect on hypothalamic gonadotrophin-releasing hormones.
  b. Since the pineal gland involutes rapidly toward puberty, it plays a role in the onset of puberty (i.e., early destruction of the pineal gland causes precocious puberty).
  c. Administration of melatonin to a child delays the onset of puberty.

B. Cell types
 1. Pinealocytes—produce serotonin and melatonin.
 2. Neuroglial cells—act as support cells to the pinealocytes.

2.6 Respiratory System

The respiratory system consists of progressively smaller passageways that lead to the alveoli where exchange of gases occurs. The system is characterized by respiratory epithelium throughout the conducting portion and the respiratory portion itself.

A. Respiratory epithelium—composed of pseudostratified ciliated columnar epithelium, which lines all or part of the larger conducting areas.
 1. Cell types located in respiratory epithelium
  a. Goblet cells—contain mucin granules. The mucus they secrete traps inhaled particles such as bacteria and dust.
  b. Ciliated columnar cells—move mucus upward toward the oropharynx to remove particles so they may be swallowed or expectorated.
  c. Nonciliated columnar cells—have microvilli on their apical surface; however, they do not possess cilia.
  d. Basal cells—stem cells that will differentiate into goblet cells or columnar cells.
  e. Small granule cells—synthesize and release catecholamines.
 2. Lamina propria deep to respiratory epithelium—is formed of loose areolar connective tissue. It contains seromucous and mucous glands and diffuse lymphatic tissue, including plasma cells, lymphocytes, and macrophages.

B. Conducting portion

Air is warmed, moistened, and cleaned as it passes through the conducting portion. The order of passage is from the nasal cavity to nasopharynx and oropharynx, larynx, trachea, bronchi, bronchioles, and terminal bronchioles.

 1. Nasal cavity and nasopharynx
  a. Oral epithelium composed of a nonkeratinized stratified squamous epithelium that covers some of the areas of the nasopharynx inspired air first crosses.
  b. Blood vessels in the lamina propria help warm air, and watery secretions moisten it.
  c. Olfactory mucosa extending from the third cranial nerve is present in the superior aspect of the nasal cavity.
 2. Larynx—hyaline and elastic cartilage helps support the walls of the larynx.
  a. Epiglottis—the anterior superior extension of the larynx. It protects the airway during swallowing.
   (1) Elastic cartilage surrounded by lamina propria is at the core of the epiglottis.
   (2) The digestive part of the epiglottis is covered by oral epithelium.
   (3) The respiratory part of the epiglottis is covered by respiratory epithelium.

3. Vocal apparatus—consists of two pairs of folds of the laryngeal mucosa that span the laryngeal space.
   a. False vocal cords are the superior pair of folds. They are covered by respiratory epithelium and contain seromucous glands in the lamina propria.
   b. True vocal cords are the inferior pair of folds. They produce sound when air passes over them. They are covered by oral epithelium and do not have seromucous glands in the lamina propria.
4. Trachea
   a. The mucosa of the trachea is covered with respiratory epithelium.
   b. The submucosa is separated from the mucosa by elastic fibers. The submucosa contains seromucous glands.
   c. Hyaline cartilage rings lie deep to the submucosa.
      (1) The cartilage is covered by a perichondrium, surrounded by an adventitia of loose connective tissue that is shared with the esophagus.
      (2) The hyaline cartilage is shaped like a C; the open end of the ring faces toward the posterior.
      (3) Smooth muscle extends across the open end of each cartilage.
   d. Extrapulmonary bronchi arise by division of the trachea outside the lungs and are histologically similar to trachea.
5. Intrapulmonary bronchi—divide many times within the lungs.
   a. Hyaline cartilage provides structure. The pieces are variably shaped and break up into small blocks in the walls of intrapulmonary bronchi.
   b. The layers of the wall become thinner as the bronchi penetrate farther into the lung.
6. Conducting bronchioles—are characterized by an absence of cartilage and smooth muscle in the walls.
   a. The diameter of the bronchioles is controlled by contraction of smooth muscle under sympathetic control of the autonomic nervous system. Epinephrine causes relaxation of these muscles.
   b. The epithelium changes from respiratory to ciliated columnar, ciliated cuboidal, and nonciliated cuboidal as the bronchioles become smaller in diameter.
   c. In contrast to the trachea, there are no seromucous glands in the conducting bronchioles.
   d. Goblet cells are found only in the larger bronchioles.
7. Terminal bronchioles
   a. The most distal part of the conducting tree.
   b. No goblet cells, so no mucus produced.
   c. Contains ciliated cuboidal cells.

C. Respiratory portion
1. Pulmonary lobules—the lung is composed of lobules, distal to terminal bronchioles.
   a. Each lobule contains a central respiratory bronchiole, leading to alveolar ducts.
   b. The alveolar ducts terminate in alveolar sacs.
   c. Pulmonary veins drain oxygenated blood from the periphery of each lobule.
2. Alveoli—the sites of gaseous exchange in the lungs.
   a. Adjacent alveoli are separated by connective tissue partitions called *interalveolar septa*, which contain pulmonary capillaries.
   b. Alveoli share air through pores of Kohn in interalveolar septa.
   c. Alveolar walls are lined by an epithelium with two kinds of pneumocytes.
      (1) Type I pneumocytes—cover most of the alveolar surface. They are connected by tight junctions, and the basal lamina of these cells may be fused with the basal lamina of nearby capillary endothelial cells.
      (2) Type II pneumocytes—may also be called *greater alveolar cells*. They bulge into the alveolar lumen and function as cells that repair the alveoli by dividing and replacing type I pneumocytes, which do not divide.
   d. Pulmonary surfactant is a phospholipid-protein mixture secreted by type II pneumocytes that spreads over alveolar walls.
      (1) The surfactant reduces surface tension in the alveoli, allowing them to expand easily during inspiration and contract without collapsing during expiration.

3. Gaseous exchange
   a. Oxygen diffuses from the alveolar airspace into red blood cells, where it binds to heme groups in hemoglobin. Carbon dioxide diffuses back to the alveolar airspace.
   b. The respiratory membrane is about 0.2 μm thick.
   c. The respiratory membrane contains the following elements, in order from lung surface: surfactant, type I pneumocyte, basal lamina of type I pneumocyte, basal lamina of capillary endothelial cell, endothelial cell, blood plasma, plasmalemma of red blood cell.
4. Alveolar macrophages—called *dust cells* are derived from monocytes. They migrate from capillaries in the interalveolar septa and ingest bacteria and other inhaled substances on the alveolar surface.

E. Visceral and parietal pleurae
1. Serous membranes—the pleural cavity contains serous membranes composed of surface mesothelium and an underlying lamina propria.
   a. Visceral pleura invests the lungs, and parietal pleura lines the thoracic cavity.
   b. Visceral and parietal pleura slide over one another to permit movement of the lungs within the thoracic cavity.

2.7 Gastrointestinal System

The gastrointestinal system consists of a hollow tube, also known as the *alimentary canal*, extending from the lips to the anus. The digestive system also includes several extramural glands, including the salivary glands, liver, and gallbladder. The secretions of these glands are delivered to the gastrointestinal system.

A. Major layers—the wall of the gastrointestinal system consists of four major layers.
1. Mucosa—lines the lumen of the gastrointestinal tract. It has three distinct sublayers.
   a. A nonkeratinized stratified, squamous epithelium with secretory, absorptive, and protective functions.
   b. A lamina propria of loose areolar connective tissue deep to the epithelium. The lamina propria contains glands and gut-associated lymphatic tissue.
   c. A muscularis mucosae with one to three layers of fine smooth muscle.
2. Submucosa—is composed of dense, irregular connective tissue.
   a. The submucosa contains (Meissner's) autonomic plexuses or ganglia.
3. Muscularis externa—contains an inner circular and an outer longitudinal layer of smooth muscle.
   a. The muscularis externa contains (Auerbach's) myenteric autonomic plexus or ganglia between the layers of muscle.
4. Serosa or fibrosa (adventitia)
   a. The serosa consists of a mesothelial lining and a layer of submesothelial connective tissue.
      (1) It forms the visceral peritoneum, a reflection of the parietal peritoneum that forms the serosal lining of the abdominal wall.
      (2) It covers the intraperitoneal portions of the alimentary canal, surface of the gallbladder exposed to the peritoneal cavity, and surface of the colon facing the peritoneal cavity.
   b. Fibrosa—consists of dense, irregular connective tissue containing adipose.
      (1) It blends with connective tissue around adjacent organs.
      (2) It covers retroperitoneal portions of the alimentary canal, surface of gallbladder embedded in the liver, and surface of the colon facing the posterior body wall.

B. Innervation

Peristalsis of the gastrointestinal tract is dependent upon innervation to the smooth muscle.
1. Postganglionic sympathetic fibers from the sympathetic chain pass through the gut wall to glands and smooth muscle.
2. Preganglionic parasympathetic fibers arrive on cell bodies of parasympathetic postganglionic neurons in ganglia in the gut wall.
3. Postganglionic parasympathetic fibers pass to glands and smooth muscle.

C. Gut-associated lymphoid tissue (GALT)

Lining epithelium is coated with secretory Immunoglobulin A (IgA) produced by Peyer's patches and other GALT.
1. Lymph follicles
   a. Specialized squamous epithelial cells called *M cells*, located in the luminal epithelium, acquire antigens from the lumen and transport them to lymph follicles in the underlying lamina propria.

   b. Antigen-stimulating B cells within follicles differentiate into IgA-secreting plasma cells.
2. Diffuse lymphatic tissue of the lamina propria, including lymphocytes, macrophages, and IgA-secreting plasma cells.
3. Aggregated lymph follicles
   a. Waldeyer's ring of tonsillar tissue in the oropharynx.
   b. Peyer's patches in the submucosa of the ileum.

D. Oral cavity—extends from the lips to the pharynx.
1. Lips
   a. The lips have a core of skeletal muscle, the orbicularis oris.
   b. The anterior surface is covered with dermis and epidermis.
   c. The posterior surface is covered by a nonkeratinized, stratified squamous epithelium (oral epithelium) and a lamina propria.
2. Teeth
   a. Cementum covers the external surface of the tooth root. It is similar to bone in composition. Sharpey's fibers extend from the surface of the cementum into the bony tooth socket.
   b. Enamel covers the external surface of the tooth crown. It is highly mineralized, contains 98% hydroxyapatite by weight, and is the hardest substance in the body.
   c. Dentin is found around the pulp in both the crown and root of the tooth. It forms the bulk of the tooth.
   d. Pulp contains fibroblasts, odontoblasts, nerves, and blood vessels.
3. Tongue—a strong, muscular organ with specialized mucosa for taste.
   a. The skeletal muscle fibers of the tongue run in three different directions.
   b. The mucosa of the tongue lacks a muscularis mucosa on the dorsal surface and an underlying submucosa on the dorsal surface.
      (1) The ventral surface is covered by oral epithelium, a nonkeratinized, stratified squamous epithelium.
      (2) The dorsal surface is covered by a parakeratinized, stratified squamous epithelium.
   c. Lingual papillae project from the dorsal surface of the anterior two thirds of the tongue.
      (1) Filiform papillae do not have taste buds.
      (2) Fungiform and circumvallate papillae have taste buds.
      (3) Glands of von Ebner rinse out the trenches surrounding circumvallate papillae with a serous secretion.
4. Hard palate
   a. The mucosa of the hard palate is firmly attached to the bone.
   b. Nasal mucosa is lined with a pseudostratified, ciliated, columnar epithelium, called *respiratory epithelium*, containing seromucous glands.
   c. Lingual mucosa is lined with parakeratinized, stratified, squamous epithelium containing mucous glands.
5. Soft palate
   a. The mucosa is similar to the lingual mucosa of the hard palate.
   b. The uvula is surfaced by oral epithelium.
6. Pharynx—is continuous with both the nasal and oral cavities and with the lumen of the esophagus.
   a. Pharyngeal mucosa contains respiratory epithelium where air transits, and oral epithelium where food passes.
   b. Pharyngeal constrictor muscles are found beneath the mucosa.

E. Alimentary canal
1. Esophagus
   a. Mucosa—has surface mucosal folds when food is not present.
      (1) The mucosa is surfaced by oral epithelium, a nonkeratinized, stratified, squamous epithelium.
   b. Muscularis externa
      (1) The upper third of the esophagus contains skeletal muscle.
      (2) The middle third of the esophagus contains both skeletal and smooth muscle.
      (3) The lower third of the esophagus contains smooth muscle.
   c. Mucous glands
      (1) The submucosa contains esophageal glands.
      (2) The lamina propria contains esophageal cardiac glands.
2. Stomach
   a. The gastric mucosa is surfaced by a simple epithelium of mucous columnar cells.

b. The muscularis externa has a third layer, an inner oblique layer of smooth muscle.
c. Gastric glands are simple, branched tubular glands. These glands consist of an isthmus opening into the bottom of a gastric pit, a neck, and a base or fundus that traverses the lamina propria (Figure 1–63).
   (1) Mucous neck cells secrete mucus.
   (2) Stem cells proliferate and differentiate to replace the other cells of the gland, pit, and surface epithelium.
   (3) Chief cells secrete pepsinogen.
   (4) Parietal cells located primarily in the body and fundus of the stomach secrete intrinsic factor needed for absorption of vitamin B_{12} and manufacture HCl.
   (5) Enteroendocrine cells secrete hormones toward capillaries in the lamina propria.

3. Small intestine—has a number of specializations that increase the surface area for absorption, including microvilli, villi, and plicae circulares.
   a. Glands with secretions that enter the intestinal lumen.
      (1) Brunner's glands are submucosal glands in the duodenum that secrete an alkaline mucus.
      (2) Goblet cells within the epithelium of the lumen.
      (3) Crypts of Lieberkühn open between adjacent villi and extend to muscularis mucosae.
   b. Cells of the intestinal lining
      (1) Enterocytes are the primary cell type of surface epithelium.
         (a) They are tall, columnar cells containing closely packed microvilli forming a brush border.
      (2) Goblet cells containing mucigen granules.
      (3) Enteroendocrine cells producing hormones.
      (4) Paneth's cells containing eosinophilic granules. These cells secrete digestive enzymes and lysosome, and phagocytize some micro-organisms.
      (5) Stem cells replace cells of the intestinal lining.

4. Large intestine—The primary function of the large intestine is to absorb water and electrolytes and lubricate feces with mucus.
   a. From caecum to the anal canal, enterocytes decrease.
   b. Goblet cells increase in number.
   c. The outer longitudinal layer of muscularis externa forms three strong, flat strips.

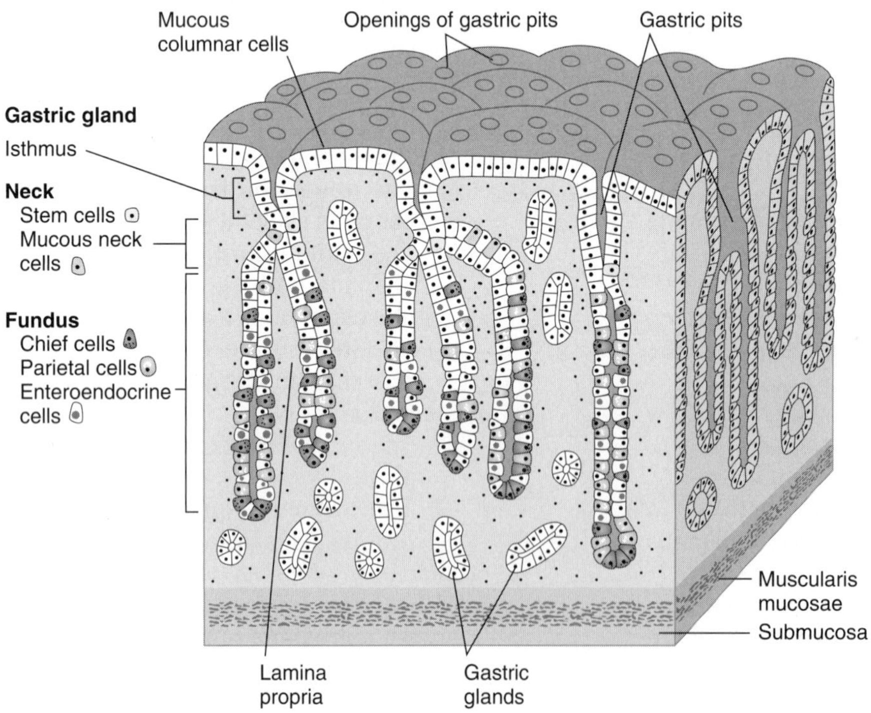

Figure 1–63. Lining of the stomach showing the relation of gastric glands to gastric pits and the underlying muscularis mucosae. (From Burns ER, Cave MD: Histology and Cell Biology, St. Louis, Mosby, 2002.)

d. Myenteric (Auerbach's) ganglia are located between taeniae coli and the subjacent circular layer of smooth muscle.

5. Anal canal
   a. The upper portion is continuous with the rectum.
   b. The lower portion is surfaced by nonkeratinized, stratified, squamous epithelium.

F. Extramural glands of the digestive system—exocrine secretions enter the oral cavity from the salivary glands, and the small intestine from the liver, gallbladder, and pancreas.

1. Major salivary glands
   a. Components of saliva
      (1) Water and salivary glycoproteins clean and lubricate the oral cavity.
      (2) IgA, lysozyme, and lactoferrin defend against pathogens.
      (3) Amylase begins the digestion of carbohydrates.
   b. Liver
      (1) Hepatic sinusoids arise near the periphery of the lobule and course between cords of hepatocytes to drain toward the central vein. The sinusoids are lined by sinusoidal endothelial cells and Kupffer's cells, which are phagocytic.
      (2) The space of Disse between sinusoid endothelium and adjacent hepatocytes contains reticular fibers, which are lipocytes (Ito cells) that store vitamin A, and blood plasma minus formed elements.
      (3) Hepatocytes exchange material with contents of spaces of Disse.
         (a) Microvilli are present on surfaces facing spaces of Disse.
         (b) Bile canaliculi occur as tiny grooves between abutting surfaces of adjacent hepatocytes.
         (c) Basophilic cytoplasmic regions contain rough endoplasmic reticulum and free polysomes.
         (d) Acidophilic cytoplasmic regions contain mitochondria and peroxisomes.
         (e) Unstained cytoplasmic regions contain multiple Golgi bodies, glycogen inclusions, and droplets of lipid.
   c. Gallbladder—releases bile in response to the presence of fat in the duodenum. Cholecystokinin released by enteroendocrine cells in the duodenum stimulates release of bile.
      (1) The mucosa is composed of simple, columnar epithelium with microvilli and junctional complexes and a richly vascularized lamina propria.
      (2) The muscularis externa is thin, with three indistinct layers.
      (3) The external surface has serosa facing the peritoneal cavity and fibrosa facing the liver.
   d. Exocrine pancreas
      (1) Pancreatic acinar cells contain basally located nuclei and rough endoplasmic reticulum, prominent Golgi apparatus, and apically located secretory granules.
      (2) Centroacinar cells within the acini form the beginning of the duct system.

2.8 Genitourinary System

2.8.1 Male Reproductive System

A. Structure

1. The testes produce male gametes (spermatozoa).
   a. The tunica albuginea is a connective tissue capsule surrounding each testis.
      (1) The thickened, posterior region of each capsule contains incomplete connective tissue septa. The septa divide each testis into numerous lobules.
      (2) Each lobule contains two to four highly convoluted seminiferous tubules.
         (a) Seminiferous epithelium lining the tubules is a specialized, gland-like epithelium where spermatogenesis occurs.
      (3) Intratesticular ducts conveying spermatozoa to the surface of the testis include tubuli recti and rete testis.
         (a) Tubuli recti are straight, terminal portions of the seminiferous tubules lined by simple columnar epithelium. They drain into the rete testis.
         (b) Rete testis are an anastomosing network of channels located at the mediastinum and lined by simple cuboidal epithelium.

2. Extratesticular ducts conduct spermatozoa outside the body.
3. Specialized glands produce and release secretions that provide nutritive and lubricative elements to semen.
   a. Seminal vescicles.
   b. Prostate gland.
   c. Bulbourethral (Cowper's) glands.
4. Glandular function of the testes.
   a. Exocrine function
      (1) Production of a holocrine cytogenic secretion containing spermatozoa occurs within the seminiferous epithelium.
   b. Endocrine function
      (1) Synthesis and secretion of hormones is carried out by Leydig cells within the interstitium and by Sertoli cells within the seminiferous epithelium.

B. Spermatogenesis
1. Composition of seminiferous epithelium.
   a. Spermatogenic cells
      (1) Present in a gradient from undifferentiated cells to differentiated spermatids that are ready to be released into the lumen.
   b. Sertoli cells
      (1) Tall, columnar cells extending from the basement membrane to the lumen.
      (2) Support and protect germ cells within the seminiferous epithelium.
      (3) Secrete inhibin and androgen-binding protein.
      (4) Are nondividing cells and remain in the senescent gonad after degeneration of germ cells.

C. Hormonal control of male reproductive system
1. Pituitary hormones—release of pituitary hormones that promote testicular hormone production is stimulated by gonadotropin-releasing hormone from the hypothalamus.
   a. Luteinizing hormone stimulates Leydig cells to release testosterone.
   b. Follicle-stimulating hormone stimulates Sertoli cells to secrete inhibin and androgen-binding protein.
2. Effects of testicular hormones
   a. Testosterone
      (1) Promotes development of secondary sex characteristics.
      (2) Stimulates spermatogenesis.
      (3) Maintains the function of ducts and accessory glands.
      (4) Acts on the hypothalamus to reduce release of gonadotropin-releasing hormone (GnRH), exhibiting negative feedback on LH and FSH secretion.
   b. Androgen-binding protein
      (1) Binds testosterone and helps transport it across seminiferous epithelium to tubular lumen.
      (2) Helps maintain high local concentration of testosterone.
      (3) Inhibin acts on the anterior pituitary to decrease FSH secretion.

2.8.2 Female Reproductive System

A. Structure—organs of the female reproductive system.
1. Ovaries
   a. Features
      (1) A simple, squamous to cuboidal epithelium covers the surface.
      (2) The tunica albuginea of fibrous connective tissue lies under the surface epithelium.
      (3) The cortex contains ovarian follicles in various stages of maturation.
      (4) The medulla is not well-defined.
2. Oviducts
   a. Regions
      (1) The infundibulum is a funnel-shaped free end with fingerlike projections called *fimbria*.
      (2) The ampulla is a dilated region proximal to the infundibulum where fertilization usually occurs.
      (3) The isthmus is a nondilated region proximal to the ampulla.
      (4) Pars intramuralis is the part passing through the uterine wall.
   b. Oviduct wall
      (1) The mucosa is a simple, columnar epithelium containing ciliated cells and secretory cells.
      (2) The lamina propria is edematous during the premenstrual phase.
      (3) Contractions of the muscularis stimulates movement of the zygote toward the uterus.
3. Uterus
   a. Uterine wall
      (1) The perimetrium is an external uterine covering that is serosa or adventitia, depending upon the peritoneal reflection.

(2) The myometrium is the vascularized smooth muscle tunic of the uterus.
(3) The endometrium is the mucosal lining of the uterus. It is composed of a simple, columnar epithelium, highly vascular lamina propria, and endometrial glands.

4. Breasts
   a. Lobes
      (1) Each gland has 15 to 25 lobes that are separated by a dense connective tissue septa.
      (2) Each lobe has compound tubuloalveolar glands that drain into intralobular ducts, interlobular ducts, lactiferous sinus, lactiferous duct, and finally the nipple.
   b. Lactiferous ducts
      (1) Stratified cuboidal and columnar epithelium lines the largest ducts, and simple cuboidal lines the smallest.
      (2) The epithelium is surrounded by loose areolar connective tissue, outside of which is dense irregular connective tissue with adipose cells.
   c. Alveoli
      (1) Dilated ends of intralobular ducts are lined by simple cuboidal epithelium and surrounded by a discontinuous layer of stellate myoepithelial cells.

B. Oogenesis
1. Formation of primordial follicles
   a. Primordial germ cells migrate from yolk-sac endoderm into the ovaries early in the embryonic period.
   b. Oogonia proliferate until 20 to 28 weeks of gestation, yielding 3 million oogonia per ovary.
      (1) After ceasing mitosis, oogonia are arrested in prophase I of meiosis.
      (2) Additional oocytes are not formed later in life.
   c. The primordial follicle consists of one primary oocyte surrounded by a single layer of squamous epithelial cells and a basal lamina.
      (1) The number of primordial follicles is reduced to approximately 200,000 per ovary at menarche.
2. Maturation of ovarian follicles—characterized by progressive morphologic changes in the oocyte, surrounding follicular cells, and adjacent stroma.
   a. Unilaminar primary follicle
      (1) Simple, squamous epithelium changes to a single layer of cuboidal follicular cells.
      (2) Differentiation of primary oocyte begins, marked by increases in size and number of mitochondria, Golgi apparatus, rough endoplasmic reticulum, and polysomes, which augment the synthetic capacity of the oocyte.
      (3) Zona pellucida, synthesized by both the oocyte and follicular cells, begins to form around the oocyte.
   b. Multilaminar primary follicle
      (1) Stratification of cuboidal follicular cells occurs, forming a granulosa layer.
      (2) Stromal cells begin to form the thecal layer around the follicle.
   c. Secondary (antral) follicle
      (1) Spaces filled with fluid appear between granulosa cells. They eventually coalesce into a single large antrum.
      (2) A mound of granular cells called the *cumulus oophorus* attaches the oocyte to the follicular wall.
      (3) The theca interna secretes a 17-ketosteroid, which is known as *androstenedione*.
         (a) Androstenedione is enzymantically converted to testosterone.
         (b) FSH stimulates enzymatic conversion of these androgens to estrogen in granulosa cells.
   d. Graafian follicle
      (1) The primary oocyte completes its first meiotic division within the mature follicle shortly before ovulation, forming a large secondary oocyte and small polar body.
      (2) The secondary oocyte enters the second meiotic division but is halted in metaphase II at the time of ovulation.
3. Ovulation and the fate of secondary oocyte
   a. A surge of LH, induced by a rising level of estrogen, triggers the release of a secondary oocyte surrounded by its corona radiata from a graafian follicle.
   b. The ovulated secondary oocyte normally is caught in the fimbria of the oviduct.

2.8.3 Urinary System

The urinary system consists of the paired kidneys and ureters and the unpaired bladder and urethra.

A. Structure
  1. The uriniferous tubule is a continuous tubular structure with regional specializations that constitute the functional unit of the kidney.
     a. Each uriniferous tubule consists of a nephron and the collecting tubules into which it drains.
        (1) The nephron includes a renal corpuscle, a proximal convoluted tubule (PCT), the loop of Henle, and a distal convoluted tubule (DCT).
        (2) Collecting tubules extend from arched collecting tubules to the papillary duct.

B. Uriniferous tubules and urine production (Figure 1–64).
  1. Renal (malpighian) corpuscle—consists of the glomerulus and Bowman's capsule.
     a. Glomerulus
        (1) Blood flows from the afferent arteriole through the glomerular capillary network to the efferent arteriole.
        (2) Mesangial cells are located around glomerular capillaries. These cells are phagocytic and help support capillary loops.

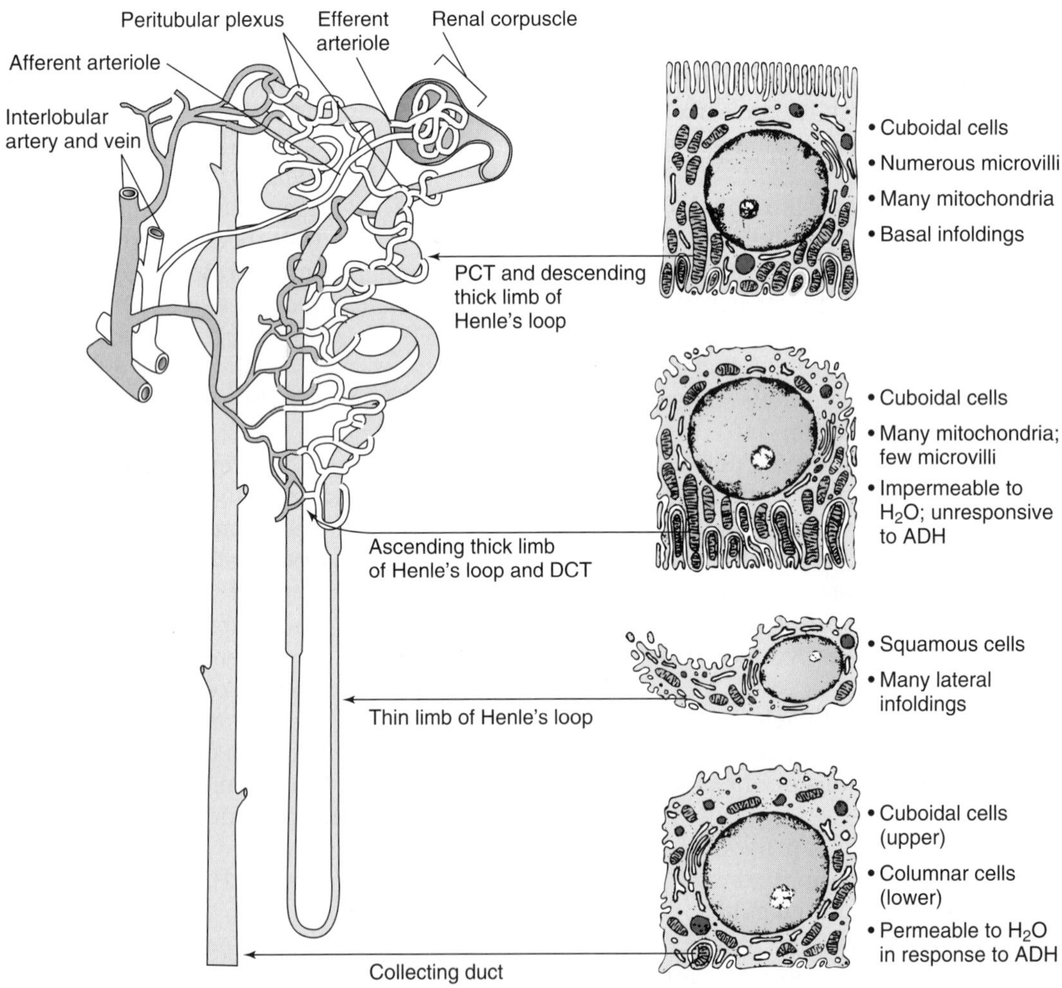

Figure 1–64. Schematic depiction of the uriniferous tubule and associated blood vessels. Microscopic appearance of the epithelial cells at various points reveals their characteristic ultrastructure. The long, thin limb of Henle's loop in juxtamedullary nephrons is surrounded by small vessels (vasa recta), which are not shown.

b. Bowman's capsule
   (1) The visceral layer is formed of podocytes, which are responsible for synthesis of the glomerular basement membrane.
   (2) Bowman's urinary space is the narrow cavity between the visceral and parietal layers into which the glomerular filtrate drains.
   (3) The parietal layer is composed of simple, squamous epithelium and forms the outer wall of Bowman's capsule.

2. Renal tubule
   a. Proximal convoluted tubule
      (1) The wall is composed of large, cuboidal epithelial cells and a number of structures.
         (a) Abundant microvilli called a *brush border.*
         (b) Apical tubular invaginations called *canaculi*, *vesicles*, and *granules*.
         (c) Infoldings of basal plasmalemma.
         (d) Numerous mitochondria.
   b. Thin segment of the loop of Henle.
      (1) The wall is composed of squamous epithelial cells.
      (2) Apical surfaces possess sparse microvilli.
   c. Thick ascending segment of the loop of Henle.
      (1) The wall is composed of cuboidal epithelial cells.
   d. Distal convoluted tubule
      (1) The wall is similar to the thick ascending segment of the loop of Henle; it also is impermeable to water.
   e. Collecting tubules and ducts
      (1) The arched collecting tubule is lined by simple cuboidal epithelium, which connects the distal convoluted tubule of a nephron and the collecting tubule into which it drains.
      (2) The collecting duct is a straight tubule formed by the convergence of arched tubules from multiple nephrons.
         (a) The upper, cortical portion has cuboidal epithelium and lies within a medullary ray.
         (b) The lower, medullary portion has columnar epithelium and lies within a medullary pyramid.
      (3) Papillary ducts of Bellini are large collecting tubules with simple columnar epithelium.

C. Juxtaglomerular apparatus—functions in the regulation of blood pressure.
   1. Components
      a. Macula densa are specialized cells of the distal convoluted tubule where it contacts the afferent arteriole.
      b. Juxtaglomerular cells are myoepithelial cells derived from smooth muscle in the tunica media of the afferent arteriole.
   2. Renin-angiotensin-aldosterone system (RAAS)
      a. Renin is secreted by juxtaglomerular cells in response to a decrease in blood pressure.
      b. Renin converts angiotensin I to angiotensin II in circulation.
      c. Angiotensin-converting enzyme (ACE) is located in endothelial cells of blood vessels and hydrolyzes angiotensin I to angiotensin II.
      d. Angiotensin II increases blood pressure:
         (1) Directly by stimulating vasoconstriction.
         (2) Indirectly by stimulating aldosterone secretion.

2.9 Integument

The integument consists of the skin and its appendages, such as hair follicles, nails, sweat glands, and sebaceous glands.

A. Components
   1. Epidermis—a superficial layer of stratified, squamous, keratinized epithelium.
   2. Dermis—a dense, fibrous, irregular connective tissue layer beneath the epidermis.
   3. Hypodermis—a layer of loose connective tissue underlying the dermis.
      a. The hypodermis binds skin to adjacent tissue.

B. Epidermis
   1. Keratinocytes—form a stratified, squamous, keratinized epithelium containing five strata.
      a. Stratum basale—the deepest layer of epidermis; it is a single layer of cuboidal to columnar keratinocytes.
         (1) These keratinocytes are mitotically active.

(2) The keratinocytes are attached to the basement membrane by hemidesmosomes.
(3) The keratinocytes produce low-molecular-weight keratins.
(4) Basal cells give rise to additional nondifferentiating stem cells, which remain in this layer, as well as to differentiating keratinocytes, which migrate into the stratum spinosum.

b. Stratum spinosum—contains several layers of polyhedral-shaped keratinocytes (prickle cells) that proliferate and differentiate.
(1) High-molecular-weight keratins are produced and assembled into intermediate filaments (tonofibrils) that terminate in numerous desmosomes.
(2) Lamellar bodies containing lipid, carbohydrate, and hydrolytic enzymes become evident.
(3) The stratum germinativum consists of the stratum basale and stratum spinosum.

c. Stratum granulosum—consists of three to five layers of flattened keratinocytes.
(1) Disulfide bonds begin to cross-link keratin filaments.
(2) Glycolipid and sterols secreted from lamellar bodies into the intercellular space form an impermeable, waterproof barrier.
(3) Lysosomal activity degrades organelles as cells move superficially.

d. Stratum lucidum—a clear and homogenous layer composed of flat keratinocytes lacking nuclei and organelles.
(1) The cytoplasm consists almost entirely of keratin filaments.
(2) The layer is well-defined only in thick skin.

e. Stratum corneum—the most superficial layer, composed of 5 to 50 layers of flattened, keratinized dead cells.
(1) The cells, called *squames*, are filled with cross-linked keratin filaments.
(2) Squames are continuously shed from the surface and are replaced with differentiating cells from the basal layer.

2. Nonkeratinocytes include melanocytes, Langerhans cells, and Merkel cells.

a. Melanocytes—synthesize melanin, which absorbs ultraviolet (UV) radiation and protects cells in the skin from UV-induced damage.
(1) Melanocytes are located in the stratum basale, the papillary layer of the dermis, and hair follicles.
(2) Synthesis of melanin occurs in melanosomes, granules containing tyrosinase and other enzymes that participate in the metabolic pathway whereby tyrosine is converted to melanin.
(3) Chromatophores are cells in the dermis that take up melanin by phagocytosis.

b. Langerhans' cells
(1) Langerhans' cells are located primarily in the stratum spinosum.
(2) They are derived from precursor cells in bone marrow.

c. Merkel cells
(1) Contain small granules filled with catecholamines.
(2) May act as sensory mechanoreceptors or as diffuse neuroendocrine cells.

C. Dermis—composed of dense, fibrous, irregular connective tissue.

1. Layers—both the papillary and reticular layers of dermis contain an elastic fiber network continuous throughout the bundles of collagen.

a. Papillary layer
(1) The papillary layer is composed of moderately dense connective tissue arranged in fine, interlacing bands of thin, collagenous bundles.

b. Reticular layer
(1) The reticular layer is composed of dense connective tissue arranged in thick, interlacing collagenous bands.

D. Appendages

Hair follicles and glands extend into the dermis and occasionally the hypodermis.

1. Hair and hair follicles

a. Structure: the hair shaft is located in a multilayered follicle.
(1) Ducts of sebaceous glands and apocrine sweat glands empty into hair follicles.
(2) A dermal sheath surrounds each follicle and extends a protrusion

through the follicular layers into the base of the shaft.

(3) The arrector pili muscle originates on the dermal sheath of the hair follicle and inserts into the papillary layer of the dermis.

2. Glands in the skin (Table 1–31)
   a. Glands in the skin include sebaceous, eccrine sweat, and apocrine sweat glands.
3. Nails
   a. The proximal root is embedded in epidermis.
      (1) The eponychium (cuticle) is the stratum corneum of the nail fold that overlies the proximal root.
      (2) The nail matrix is the area of epidermal cells covered by eponychium where nail synthesis takes place.
      (3) The lunula is an extension of the nail matrix beyond the eponychium. It is visible as a white crescent.
   b. The distal free edge is underlaid by hyponychium, a thickened stratum corneum.

E. Vasculature of the skin—the epidermis does not have a blood supply; the deeper layers and all skin appendages have a network of small vessels.
   1. Arterial plexuses
      a. Rete cutaneum at the border of the dermis and hypodermis.
      b. Rete subpapillare at the border of papillary and reticular layers of the dermis.
         (1) Arterioles from this plexus give rise to a single capillary loop around each dermal papilla.
   2. Venous plexuses
      a. Located in the middle of the dermis, between papillary and reticular layers of the dermis, and at the border of the dermis and hypodermis.
   3. Arteriovenous anastomoses
      a. Direct connections between arterioles and venules (AV shunts). They occur in deeper skin and are important in thermoregulation.
      b. Blood flow through AV shunts is regulated by autonomic nerve fibers and certain hormones.

F. Nerves of the skin
   1. Motor nerves are postganglionic fibers from sympathetic ganglia of the paravertebral chain.
      a. Autonomic nerve supply functions primarily in thermoregulation.
   2. Sensory nerve endings
      a. Free nerve endings are located at epidermal openings, and the root sheaths of hair follicles function as mechanoreceptors.
      b. Encapsulated sensory receptors, located in the skin and associated mucous membranes, include the Pacinian corpuscle, the Meissner corpuscle, and the Krause end bulb.

TABLE 1–31. GLANDS OF THE SKIN

	TYPE OF GLAND		
PROPERTY	**SEBACEOUS**	**ECCRINE SWEAT**	**APOCRINE SWEAT**
Location within skin	Dermis	Dermis	Dermis and hypodermis
Body distribution	Throughout body except for palms and soles	Throughout body	Axilla, mons pubis, areola of nipple, perianal region
General structure	Branched acinar gland with short duct	Simple, tubular gland	Large, complex gland
Myoepithelial cells	Absent	Present	Present
Type of secretion	Thick, lipid-containing substance (sebum)	Clear, watery secretion	Viscous substance rich in protein and cellular debris
Secretion mechanism	Holocrine	Merocrine	Mixed
Duct opening	Hair follicle (usually)	Surface of skin (sweat pore)	Hair follicle
Period of activity	Inactive until puberty	Active throughout life	Inactive until puberty
Other features	Excess androgen-mediated secretion can plug hair follicles, predisposing to acne	Secretion stimulated by high temperature and stress	Activity is linked to menstrual cycle in girls and women

From Burns ER, Cave MD: Histology and Cell Biology, Mosby, St. Louis, 2002.

3.0 ORAL HISTOLOGY

3.1 Tooth and Supporting Structures

A. Enamel
1. Composition
   a. Inorganic (96%)—calcium hydroxyapatite crystals.
   b. Organic (4%)—water and proteins, including amelogenins and enamelins.
2. Structural characteristics and microscopic features
   a. Enamel rods or prisms
      (1) Basic structural unit of enamel.
      (2) Consists of tightly packed hydroxyapatite crystals. Hydroxyapatite crystals in enamel are four times larger and more tightly packed than hydroxyapatite found in other calcified tissues (i.e., it is harder than bone).
      (3) Each rod extends the entire thickness of enamel and is perpendicular to the dentinoenamel junction (DEJ).
   b. Aprismatic enamel
      (1) The thin outer layer of enamel found on the surface of newly erupted teeth.
      (2) Consists of enamel crystals that are aligned perpendicular to the surface.
      (3) It is aprismatic (i.e., prismless) and is more mineralized than the enamel beneath it.
      (4) It results from the absence of Tomes' processes on the ameloblasts during the final stages of enamel deposition.
   c. Lines of Retzius (enamel striae)
      (1) Microscopic features
         (a) In longitudinal sections, they are observed as brown lines that extend from the DEJ to the tooth surface.
         (b) In transverse sections, they appear as dark, concentric rings similar to growth rings in a tree.
      (2) The lines appear weekly during the formation of enamel.
      (3) Although the cause of striae formation is unknown, the lines may represent appositional or incremental growth of enamel. They may also result from metabolic disturbances of ameloblasts.
      (4) Neonatal line
         (a) An accentuated, dark line of Retzius that results from the effect of physiological changes on ameloblasts at birth.
         (b) Found in all primary teeth and some cusps of permanent first molars.
   d. Perikymata
      (1) Lines of Retzius terminate on the tooth surface in shallow grooves known a *perikymata*.
      (2) These grooves are usually lost through wear but may be observed on the surfaces of developing teeth or nonmasticatory surfaces of formed teeth.
   e. Hunter-Schreger bands
      (1) Enamel rods run in different directions. In longitudinal sections, these changes in direction result in a banding pattern known as *Hunter-Schreger bands*.
      (2) These bands represent an optical phenomenon of enamel and consist of a series of alternating dark and light lines when the section is viewed with reflected or polarized light.
   f. Enamel tufts
      (1) Consist of hypomineralized groups of enamel rods.
      (2) They are observed as short, dark projections found near or at the DEJ.
      (3) They have no known clinical significance.
   g. Enamel lamellae
      (1) Small, sheet-like cracks found on the surface of enamel that extend its entire thickness.
      (2) Consist of hypocalcified enamel.
      (3) The open crack may be filled with organic material from leftover enamel organ components, connective tissues of the developing tooth, or debris from the oral cavity.
      (4) Both enamel tufts and lamellae may be likened to geological faults in mature enamel.
   h. Enamel spindle
      (1) Remnants of odontoblastic processes that become trapped after crossing the DEJ during the differentiation of ameloblasts.

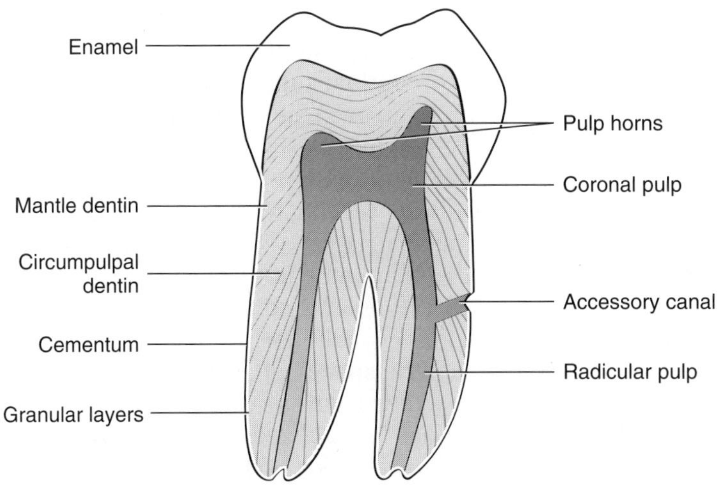

Figure 1–65. Lateral cross-section of a tooth: dental tissues. (Modified from Bath-Balogh M, Fehrenbach M: Illustrated Dental Embryology, Histology, and Anatomy, ed 2, Philadelphia, WB Saunders, 2006.)

(2) Spindles are more pronounced beneath the cusps or incisal edges of teeth (i.e., areas where occlusal stresses are the greatest).

i. Note: to microscopically evaluate enamel, slides cannot be decalcified due to the low content of organic matrix in enamel. Only ground sections can be used.

B. Dentin

1. Composition
   a. Inorganic (70%)—calcium hydroxyapatite crystals.
   b. Organic (30%)—water and type I collagen.
2. Types of dentin
   a. Primary dentin
      (1) Dentin formed during tooth development, before completion of root formation. It constitutes the majority of dentin found in a tooth.
      (2) It consists of a normal organization of dentinal tubules.
      (3) Circumpulpal dentin
         (a) The layer of primary dentin that surrounds the pulp chamber (Figure 1–65). It is formed after the mantle dentin.
         (b) Its collagen fibers are parallel to the DEJ.
   b. Secondary dentin
      (1) Dentin formed after root formation is complete.
      (2) Is deposited unevenly around the pulp chamber, forming along the layer of dentin closest to the pulp. It therefore contributes to the decrease in the size of the pulp chamber as one ages.
      (3) It consists of a normal, or slightly less regular, organization of dentinal tubules. However, as compared to primary dentin, it is deposited at a slower rate.
      (4) Although the dentinal tubules in secondary dentin can be continuous with those in primary dentin, there is usually a tubular angle change between the two layers.
   c. Tertiary (reparative, reactive) dentin
      (1) Dentin that is formed in localized areas in response to trauma or other stimuli such as caries, tooth wear, or dental work.
      (2) Its consistency and organization vary. It has no defined dentinal tubule pattern (Figure 1–66).

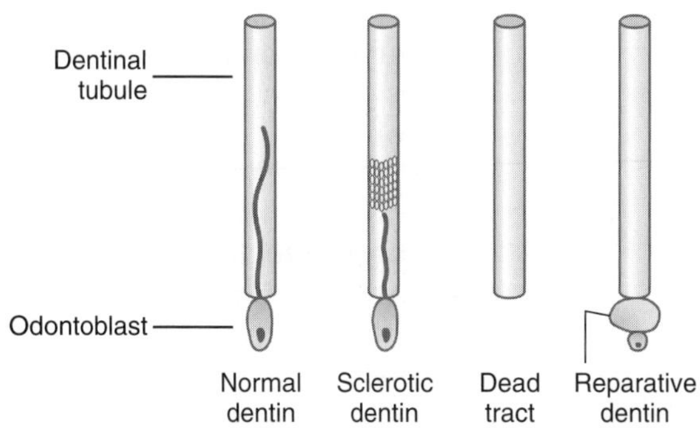

Figure 1–66. Diagram of sclerotic and reparative dentin, and dead tract. The odontoblast-like layer and the tubules in reparative dentin lack a defined organization.

d. Mantle dentin
   (1) The outermost layer of dentin (see Figure 1–65).
   (2) Is the first layer of dentin laid down by odontoblasts adjacent to the DEJ.
   (3) Is slightly less mineralized than primary dentin.
   (4) Has collagen fibers that are perpendicular to the DEJ.
   (5) Dentinal tubules branch abundantly in this area.

e. Sclerotic (transparent) dentin
   (1) Describes dentinal tubules that have become occluded with calcified material (see Figure 1–66).
   (2) Occurs when the odontoblastic processes retreat, filling the dentinal tubule with calcium phosphate crystals.
   (3) Occurs with aging.

f. Dead tracts
   (1) When odontoblasts die, they leave behind empty dentinal tubules, or dead tracts (see Figure 1–66).
   (2) Occurs with aging or trauma.
   (3) Empty tubules are potential paths for bacterial invasion.

3. Structural characteristics and microscopic features:
   a. Dentinal tubules
      (1) Tubules extend from the DEJ to the pulp chamber.
      (2) The tubules taper peripherally (i.e., their diameters are wider as they get closer to the pulp). Since the tubules are distanced farther apart at the periphery, the density of tubules is greater closer to the pulp.
      (3) Each tubule contains an odontoblastic process or Tomes' fiber. Odontoblastic processes are characterized by the presence of a network of microtubules, with occasional mitochondria and vesicles present. Note: the odontoblast's cell body remains in the pulp chamber.
      (4) Coronal tubules follow an S-shaped path, which may result from the crowding of odontoblasts as they migrate toward the pulp during dentin formation.

   b. Peritubular dentin (intratubular dentin)
      (1) Is deposited on the walls of the dentinal tubule, which affects (i.e., narrows)the diameter of the tubule (Figure 1–67).
      (2) It differs from intertubular dentin by lacking a collagenous fibrous matrix. It is also more mineralized than intertubular dentin.

   c. Intertubular dentin
      (1) The main part of dentin, which fills the space between dentinal tubules (see Figure 1–67).
      (2) Is mineralized and contains a collagenous matrix.

   d. Interglobular dentin
      (1) Areas of hypomineralized or unmineralized dentin caused by the failure of globules or calcospherites to fuse uniformly with mature dentin.
      (2) Dentinal tubules are left undisturbed as they pass through interglobular dentin; however, no peritubular dentin is present.
      (3) Interglobular dentin is found in the:
         (a) Crown—just beneath the mantle dentin.
         (b) Root—beneath the dentinocemental junction, giving the root the appearance of a granular layer (of Tomes).

   e. Incremental lines
      (1) Dentin is deposited at a daily rate of approximately 4 microns.
      (2) As dentin is laid down, small differences in collagen fiber orientation result in the formation of incremental lines.

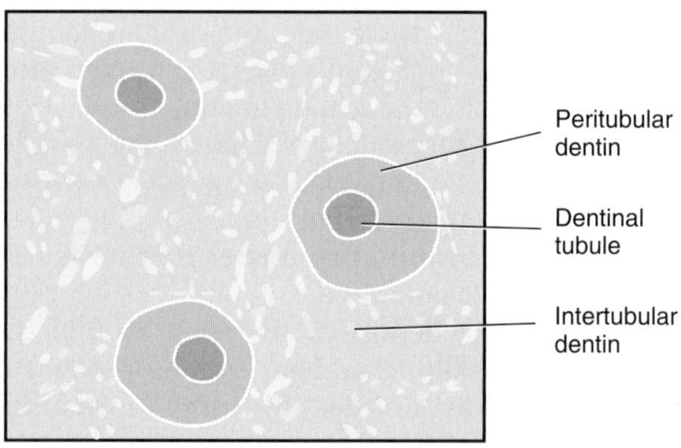

Figure 1–67. Transverse section of dentin.

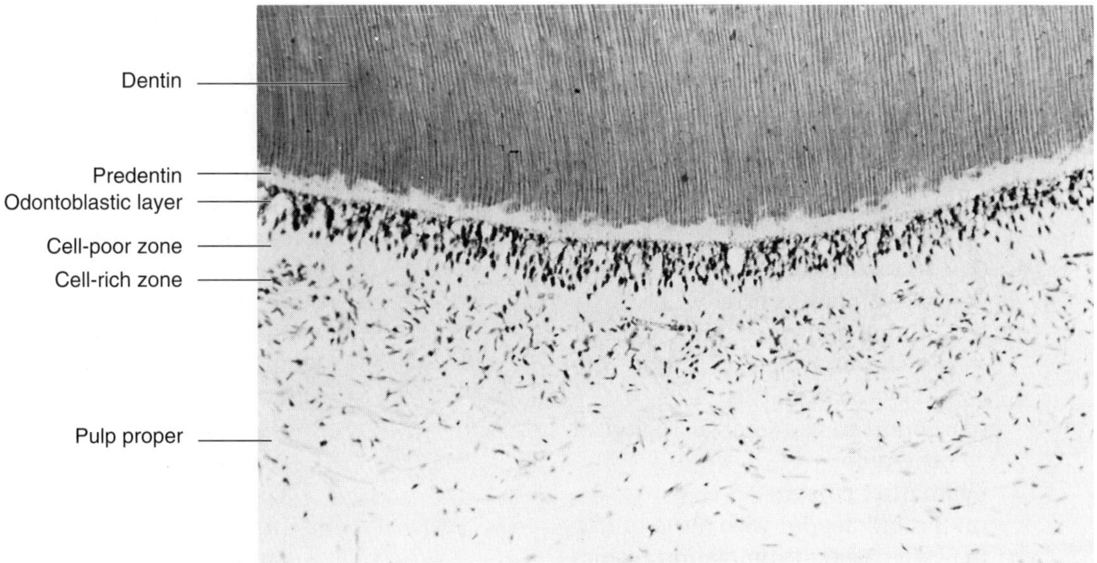

Figure 1–68. Morphologic zones of the dental pulp. (Modified from Cohen S, Hargreaves K: Pathways of the Pulp, ed 9, St. Louis, 2006.)

(3) Called *imbrication lines of von Ebner.*

(a) Every 5 days, or about every 20 μm, the changes in collagen fiber orientation appear more accentuated. This results in a darker staining line, known as the *imbrication line of von Ebner.*

(b) These lines are similar to the lines of Retzius seen in enamel.

f. Contour lines of Owen

(1) An optical phenomenon that occurs when the secondary curvatures of adjacent dentinal tubules coincide, resulting in the appearance of lines known as *contour lines of Owen.*

(2) Contour lines of Owen may also refer to lines that appear similar to those just described; however, these lines result from disturbances in mineralization.

g. Granular layer of Tomes

(1) A granular or spotty-appearing band that can be observed on the root surface adjacent to the dentinocemental junction, just beneath the cementum.

(2) The cause is unknown.

C. Pulp

1. Four zones—listed from dentin inward (Figure 1–68):

a. Odontoblastic layer

(1) Contains the cell bodies of odontoblasts. Note: their processes remain in dentinal tubules.

(2) Capillaries, nerve fibers, and dendritic cells may also be present.

b. Cell-free or cell-poor zone (zone of Weil)

(1) Contains capillaries and unmyelinated nerve fibers.

c. Cell-rich zone

(1) Consists mainly of fibroblasts. Macrophages, lymphocytes, and dendritic cells may also be present.

d. The pulp (pulp proper, central zone)

(1) The central mass of the pulp.

(2) Consists of loose connective tissue, larger vessels, and nerves. Also contains fibroblasts and pulpal cells.

2. Pulpal innervation

a. When pulpal nerves are stimulated, they can only transmit one signal—pain.

b. There are no proprioceptors in the pulp.

c. Types of nerves:

(1) A-delta fibers

(a) Myelinated sensory nerve fibers.
(b) Stimulation results in the sensation of fast, sharp pain.
(c) Found in the coronal (odontoblastic) area of the pulp.

(2) C-fibers
(a) Unmyelinated sensory nerve fibers.
(b) Transmits information of noxious stimuli centrally.
(c) Stimulation results in pain that is slower, duller, and more diffuse in nature.
(d) Found in the central region of the pulp.

(3) Sympathetic fibers
(a) Found deeper within the pulp.
(b) Sympathetic stimulation results in vasoconstriction of vessels.

3.1.1 Periodontium

The periodontium consists of tissues supporting and investing the tooth and includes cementum, the periodontal ligament (PDL), and alveolar bone. Parts of the gingiva adjacent to the tooth also give minor support, although the gingiva is not considered to be part of the periodontium in many texts. For our purposes here, the groups of gingival fibers related to tooth investment are discussed in this section.

A. Cementum
1. Composition
a. Inorganic (50%)—calcium hydroxyapatite crystals.
b. Organic (50%)—water, proteins, and type I collagen.
c. Note: Compared to the other dental tissues, the composition of cementum is most similar to bone; however, unlike bone, cementum is avascular (i.e., no Haversian systems or other vessels are present).
2. Main function of cementum is to attach PDL fibers to the root surface.
3. Cementum is generally thickest at the root apex and in interradicular areas of multirooted teeth. It is thinnest in the cervical area.
4. Types of cementum
a. Acellular (primary) cementum
(1) A thin layer of cementum that surrounds the root, adjacent to the dentin.
(2) May be covered by a layer of cellular cementum, which most often occurs in the middle and apical root.
(3) It does not contain any cells.
b. Cellular (secondary) cementum
(1) A thicker, less-mineralized layer of cementum that is most prevalent along the apical root and in interradicular (furcal) areas of multirooted teeth.
(2) Contains cementocytes.
(3) Lacunae and canaliculi:
(a) Cementocytes (cementoblasts that become trapped in the extracellular matrix during cementogenesis) are observed in their entrapped spaces, known as *lacunae*.
(b) The processes of cementocytes extend through narrow channels called *canaliculi*.
(4) Microscopically, the best way to differentiate between acellular and cellular cementum is the presence of lacunae in cellular cementum.
c. A summary of the differences between acellular and cellular cementum is listed in Table 1–32.

B. Periodontal ligament
1. Composition
a. Consists mostly of collagenous (alveolodental) fibers. Note: the portions of the fibers embedded in cementum and the alveolar bone proper are known as *Sharpey's fibers*.
b. Oxytalan fibers (a type of elastic fiber) are also present. Although their function is unknown, they may play a role in the regulation of vascular flow.

TABLE 1–32. SUMMARY OF DIFFERENCES BETWEEN ACELLULAR AND CELLULR CEMENTUM

	ACELLULAR CEMENTUM	CELLULAR CEMENTUM
Presence of cells	None	Cementocytes
Dentin border	Not clearly demarcated	Clearly demarcated
Rate of development	Slow	Fast
Incremental lines	Close together	Relatively wide apart
Precementum layer	Largely absent	Present
Function	Anchorage	Adaptation and repair

c. Contains mostly type I collagen, although smaller amounts of type III and XII collagen are also present.
d. Has a rich vascular and nerve supply. Both sensory and autonomic nerves are present.
   (1) The sensory nerves in the PDL differ from pulpal nerves in that PDL nerve endings can detect both proprioception (via mechanoreceptors) and pain (via nociceptors).
   (2) The autonomic nerve fibers are associated with the regulation of periodontal vascular flow.
   (3) Nerve fibers may be myelinated (sensory) or unmyelinated (sensory or autonomic).

2. Cells
   a. Cells present in the PDL include fibroblasts; epithelial cells; cementoblasts and cementoclasts; osteoblasts and osteoclasts; and immune cells such as macrophages, mast cells, or eosinophils.
   b. These cells play a role in forming or destroying cementum, alveolar bone, or PDL.
   c. Epithelial cells often appear in clusters, known as *rests of Malassez*.
3. Types of alveolodental fibers (Figure 1–69)
   a. Alveolar crest fibers—radiate downward from cementum, just below the cementoenamel junction (CEJ), to the crest of alveolar bone.
   b. Horizontal fibers—radiate perpendicular to the tooth surface from cementum to alveolar bone, just below the alveolar crest.
   c. Oblique fibers
      (1) Radiate downward from the alveolar bone to cementum.
      (2) The most numerous type of PDL fiber.
      (3) Resist occlusal forces that occur along the long axis of the tooth.
   d. Apical fibers
      (1) Radiate from the cementum at the apex of the tooth into the alveolar bone.
      (2) Resist forces that pull the tooth in an occlusal direction (i.e., forces that try to pull the tooth from its socket).
   e. Interradicular fibers
      (1) Only found in the furcal area of multi-rooted teeth.
      (2) Resist forces that pull the tooth in an occlusal direction.

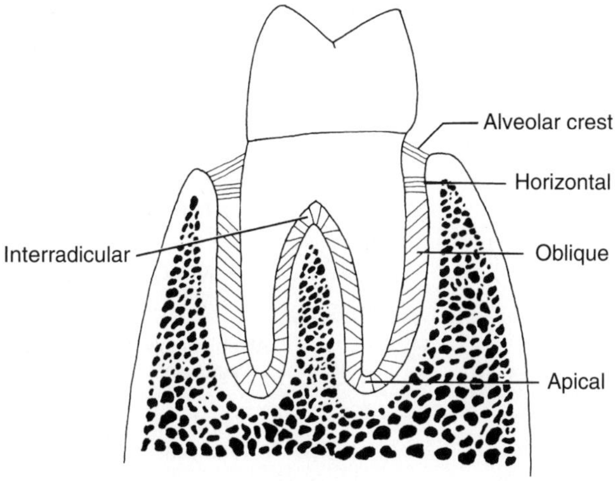

Figure 1–69. PDL (alveolodental) fibers: five groups. (From Brand R, Isselhard D: Anatomy of Orofacial Structures, St. Louis, Mosby, 2003.)

4. Gingival fibers
   a. The fibers of the gingival ligament are not strictly part of the PDL, but they play a role in the maintainence of the periodontium.
   b. Gingival fibers are packed in groups and are found in the lamina propria of gingiva (Figure 1–70).
   c. Gingival fiber groups:
      (1) Transseptal (interdental) fibers
         (a) Extend from the cementum of one tooth (just apical to the junctional epithelium), over the alveolar crest, to the corresponding area of the cementum of the adjacent tooth.
         (b) Collectively, these fibers form the interdental ligament (Figure 1–71), which functions to resist rotational forces and retain adjacent teeth in interproximal contact.
         (c) These fibers have been implicated as a major cause of postretention relapse of teeth that have undergone orthodontic treatment.
      (2) Circular (circumferential) fibers
         (a) Extend around tooth near the CEJ.
         (b) Function in binding free gingiva to the tooth and resisting rotational forces.
      (3) Alveologingival fibers—extend from the alveolar crest to lamina propria of free and attached gingiva.

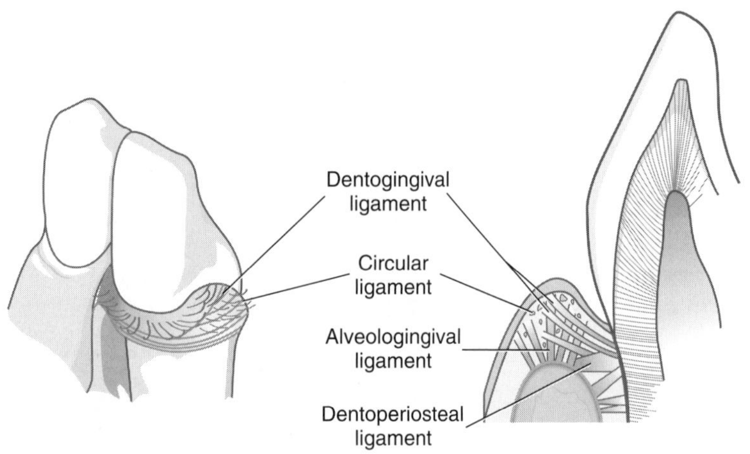

Figure 1–70. Arrangement of gingival fiber groups in the lamina propria of gingiva. (Modified from Bath-Balogh M, Fehrenbach M: Illustrated Dental Embryology, Histology, and Anatomy, ed 2, Philadelphia, WB Saunders, 2006.)

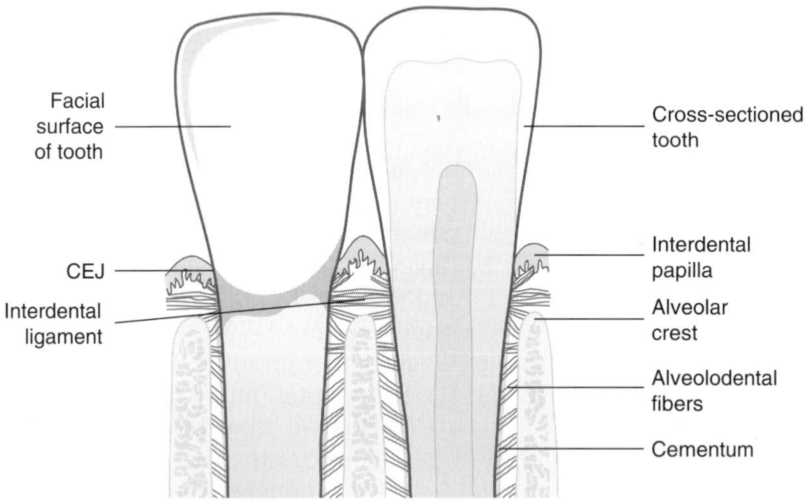

Figure 1–71. Interdental ligament. (Modified from Bath-Balogh M, Fehrenbach M: Illustrated Dental Embryology, Histology, and Anatomy, ed 2, Philadelphia, WB Saunders, 2006.)

(4) Dentogingival fibers—extend from cervical cementum to the lamina propria of free and attached gingiva.
(5) Dentoperiosteal fibers—extend from cervical cementum, over the alveolar crest, to the periosteum of the alveolar bone.

C. Alveolar bone (process)
1. The bone in the jaws that contains the teeth alveoli (sockets).
2. Three types of bone (Figure 1–72):
a. Cribriform plate (alveolar bone proper)
(1) Directly lines and forms the tooth socket. It is compact bone that contains many holes, allowing for the passage of blood vessels. It has no periosteum.
(2) Serves as the attachment site for PDL (Sharpey's) fibers.
(3) The tooth socket is constantly being remodeled in response to occlusal forces. The bone laid down on the cribriform plate, which also provides attachment for PDL fibers, is known as *bundle bone*.
(4) It is radiographically known as the *lamina dura*.
b. Cortical (compact) bone
(1) Lines the buccal and lingual surfaces of the mandible and maxilla.
(2) Is typical compact bone with a periosteum and contains Haversian systems.
(3) Is generally thinner in the maxilla and thicker in the mandible, especially around the buccal area of the mandibular premolar and molar.

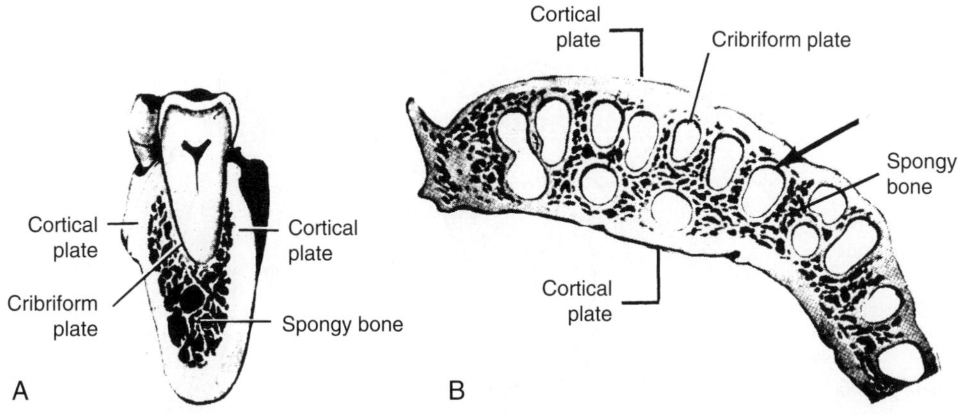

Figure 1–72. Alveolar bone. A, Cross-section view through a mandible. **B.** A longitudinal horizontal section through a mandible. Notice the thickened lamina dura *(arrow)*. (From Brand R, Isselhard D: Anatomy of Orofacial Structures, St. Louis, Mosby, 2003.)

c. Trabecular (cancellous, spongy) bone
   (1) Is typical cancellous bone containing Haversian systems.
   (2) Is absent in the maxillary anterior teeth region.

3. Alveolar crest (septa)
   a. The height of the alveolar crest is usually 1.5 to 2 mm below the CEJ junction.
   b. The width is determined by the shape of adjacent teeth.
      (1) Narrow crests—found between teeth with relatively flat surfaces.
      (2) Widened crests—found between teeth with convex surfaces or teeth spaced apart.

3.2 Soft Oral Tissues

3.2.1 Oral Mucosa

The oral mucosa consists mainly of two types of tissues: the oral epithelium, which consists of stratified, squamous epithelium, and the underlying connective tissue layer, known as the *lamina propria* (Figure 1–73). There are three variations of oral mucosa.

A. Oral epithelium
   1. Consists of stratified, squamous epithelium.
   2. Four layers (Note: Cells mature as they progress from the deepest [basal] layer to the most superficial [cornified] layer)
      a. Basal layer (stratum germinativum or basale)
         (1) A single layer of cuboidal or columnar cells overlying the lamina propria.
         (2) Contains progenitor cells and thus provides cells to the epithelial layers above.
         (3) Site of cell division (mitosis).
      b. Prickle cell layer (stratum spinosum)
         (1) Consists of several layers of larger, ovoid-shaped cells.
      c. Granular layer (stratum granulosum)
         (1) Cells appear larger and flattened.
         (2) Granules (known as *keratohyaline granules*) are present in the cells.
         (3) This layer is absent in nonkeratinized epithelium.
      d. Cornified layer (stratum corneum, keratin, or horny layer)
         (1) In keratinized epithelium:
            (a) Orthokeratinized epithelium—the squamous cells on the surface appear flat and contain keratin. They have no nuclei present.
            (b) Parakeratinized epithelium—the squamous cells appear flat and contain keratin; nuclei are present within the cells.
         (2) In parakeratinized epithelium, both squamous cells without nuclei and cells with shriveled (pyknotic) nuclei are present.
         (3) In nonkeratinized epithelium, the cells appear slightly flattened and contain nuclei.

B. Lamina propria
   1. Consists of type I and III collagen, elastic fibers, and ground substance. It also contains many cell types, including fibroblasts, endothelial cells, immune cells, and a rich vascular and nerve supply.
   2. Two layers:
      a. Superficial, papillary layer

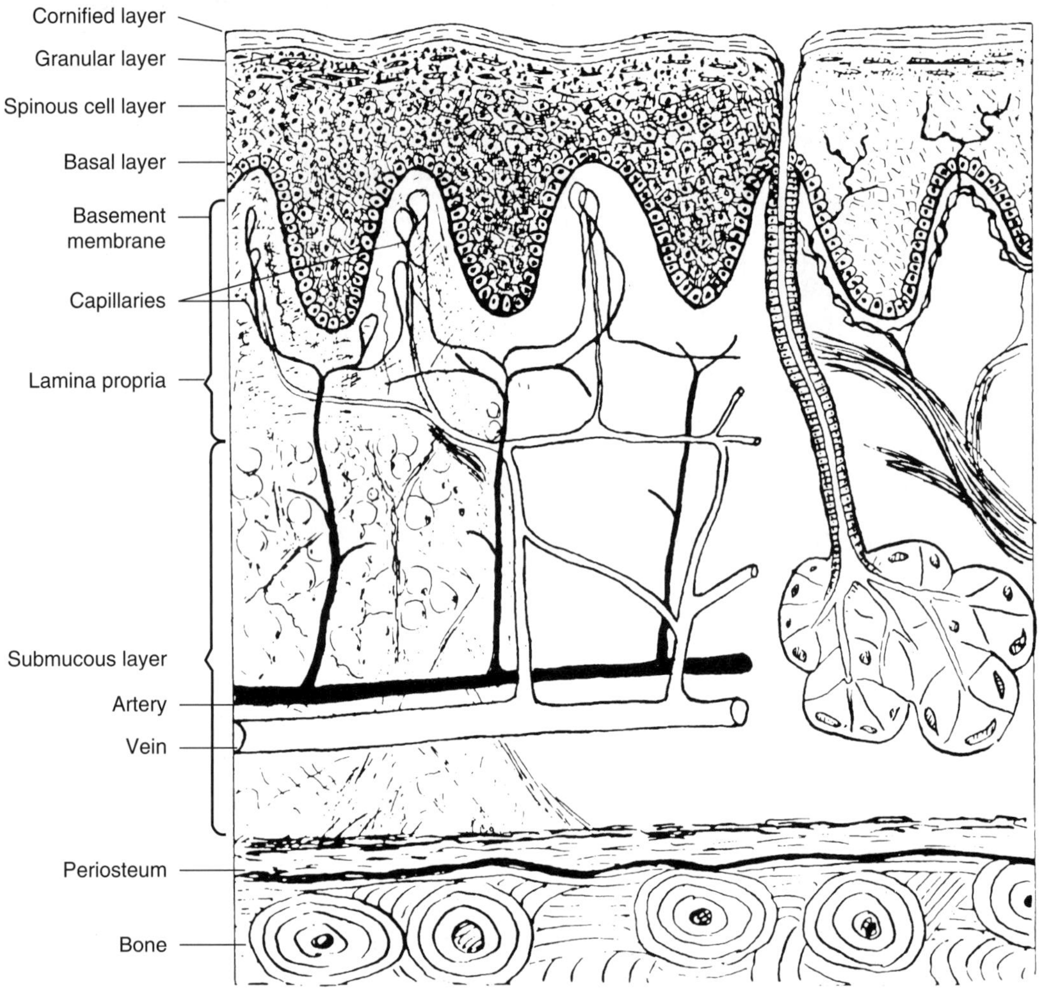

Figure 1–73. Oral mucosa: epithelium and lamina propria. Also shown are submucosal layer and bone. (From Brand R, Isselhard D: Anatomy of Orofacial Structures, St. Louis, Mosby, 2003.)

(1) Located around and between the epithelial ridges.
(2) Collagen fibers are thin and loosely arranged.

b. Reticular layer
   (1) Located beneath the papillary layer.
   (2) Collagen fibers are organized in thick, parallel bundles.

C. Types of oral mucosa (summarized in Table 1–33).
1. Masticatory mucosa
   a. Found in areas that have to withstand compressive and shear forces.
   b. Clinically, it has a rubbery, firm texture.
   c. Regions: gingiva, hard palate.
2. Lining mucosa
   a. Found in areas that are exposed to high levels of friction, but must also be mobile and distensible.

TABLE 1–33. THREE TYPES OF ORAL MUCOSA

	MUCOSA	REGIONS
Masticatory mucosa	Thick epithelium Keratinized Numerous rete ridges Long papilla	Gingiva (free, attached) Hard palate
Lining mucosa	Thin epithelium* Nonkeratinized Few rete ridges Short papilla	Alveolar mucosa Labial and buccal mucosa Lips Floor of mouth Ventral side of tongue Soft palate
Specialized mucosa	Nonkeratinized Forms lingual papillae	Dorsum of tongue

*An exception is the epithelium of labial and buccal mucosa—it is thick.

b. Clinically, it has a softer, more elastic texture.
c. Regions: alveolar mucosa, buccal mucosa, lips, floor of the mouth, ventral side of the tongue, and soft palate.

3. Specialized mucosa
   a. Similar to masticatory mucosa, specialized mucosa is able to tolerate high compressive and shear forces; however, it is unique in that it forms lingual papillae.
   b. Region: dorsum of the tongue.

D. Submucosa
1. The connective tissue found beneath the mucosa (see Figure 1–73). It contains blood vessels and nerves and may also contain fatty tissue and minor salivary glands.
2. Submucosa is not present in all regions of the oral cavity, such as attached gingiva, the tongue, and hard palate. Its presence tends to increase the mobility of the tissue overlying it.

E. Gingiva
1. The portion of oral mucosa that attaches to the teeth and alveolar bone.
2. There are two types of gingiva: attached and free gingiva. The boundary at which they meet is known as the *free gingival groove* (Figure 1–74).
   a. Attached gingiva
      (1) Directly binds to the alveolar bone and tooth.
      (2) It extends from the free gingival groove to the mucogingival junction.
   b. Free gingiva
      (1) Coronal to the attached gingiva, it is not bound to any hard tissue.

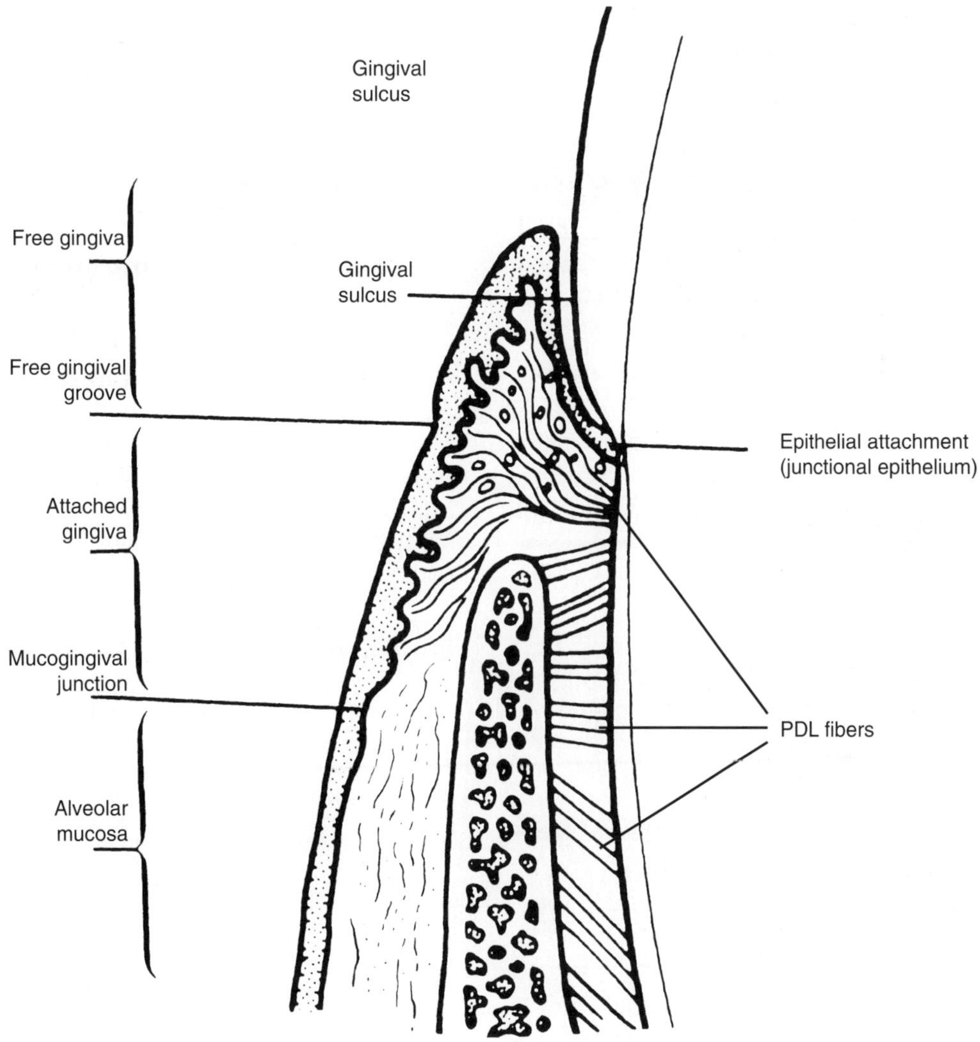

Figure 1–74. The gingival sulcus and tissues that form it. (From Brand R, Isselhard D: Anatomy of Orofacial Structures, St. Louis, Mosby, 2003.)

(2) It extends from the gingival margin to the free gingival groove.

c. Together, the free and attached gingiva form the interdental papilla (described below).

F. Alveolar mucosa
1. The tissue just apical to the attached gingiva.
2. The alveolar mucosa and attached gingiva meet at the mucogingival junction (Figure 1–74).
3. Histological differences in mucosal structure between gingiva and alveolar mucosa are summarized in Table 1–34.

G. Junctional epithelium
1. Area where the oral mucosa attaches to the tooth, forming the principal seal between the oral cavity and underlying tissues.
2. Is unique in that it consists of two basal lamina, an internal and external (Figure 1–75). The internal basal lamina, along with hemidesmosomes, comprises the attachment apparatus (the epithelial attachment). This serves to attach the epithelium directly to the tooth.
3. Histologically, it remains as immature, poorly differentiated tissue. This allows it to maintain its ability to develop hemidesmosomal attachments.
4. Has the highest rate of cell turnover of any oral mucosal tissue.

H. Interdental papilla (interdental gingiva)
1. Occupies the interproximal space between two teeth. It is formed by free and attached gingiva.
2. Functions to prevent food from entering the (interproximal) area beneath the contact point of two adjacent teeth. It therefore plays an important role in maintaining the health of the gingiva.
3. Col
   a. If the interdental papilla is cross-sectioned in a buccolingual plane, it would show two peaks (buccal and lingual) with a dip between them, known as the *col* or *interdental col*. This depression occurs around the contact point of the two adjacent teeth.
   b. Histologically, col epithelium is the same as junctional epithelium.

Table 1–34. Gingiva and Alveolar Mucosa: Differences in Mucosal Structure

	GINGIVA	ALVEOLAR MUCOSA
Oral mucosa type	Lining mucosa	Masticatory mucosa
Epithelium	Thick, keratinized stratified squamous	Thin, nonkeratinized stratified squamous
Lamina propria	Long papillae Very vascular	Short, poorly developed papillae Less vascular
Submucosa	No distinct layer	Extensive layer

3.3 Temporomandibular Joint

A. Description
1. The TMJ features two types of movements: rotary and translatory (gliding). It is therefore described as a synovial sliding-ginglymoid joint. It may also be referred to as a *hinge* and *sliding joint.*
2. The TMJ is unlike other diarthrodial joints in that its articulating surfaces are

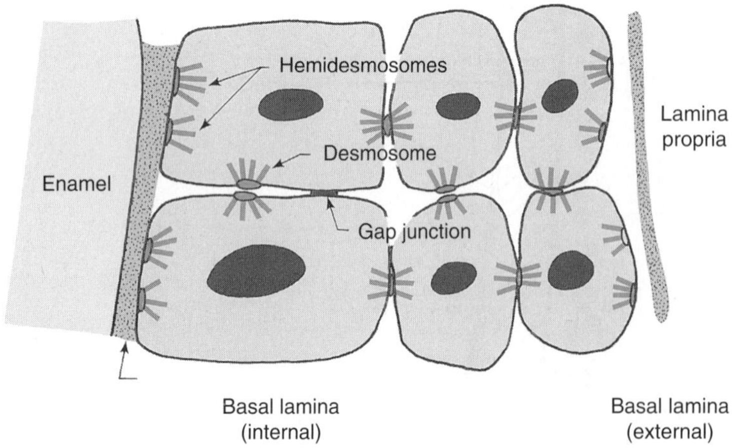

Figure 1–75. Diagram of junctional epithelium. (From Berkovitz BK, Holland G, Moxham B: Oral Anatomy, Histology, and Embryology, St. Louis, Mosby, 2002.)

covered with fibrocartilage rather than hyaline cartilage.

3. The TMJ is unlike compound (complex) joints, which consist of three bones. The TMJ consists of two bones and a disc.

B. Structure and anatomy
   1. Bones
      a. The TMJ is formed from two bones: the temporal bone (mandibular fossa) and the mandible (condyle).
      b. Mandibular (articular) fossa
         (1) Part of the squamous portion of the temporal bone (see Figure 1–19).
         (2) Anterior to the mandibular fossa is the articular eminence. Posterior to it lies the postglenoid process.
      c. The articulating surfaces of the TMJ are covered with fibrocartilage, directly overlying periosteum. The nonarticulating surfaces are covered with periosteum.
   2. Articular (joint) capsule
      a. The thick, fibrous capsule that encloses the joint space (Figure 1–76).
      b. Attachments:
         (1) Superiorly, the capsule attaches to the margin of the articular eminence (anteriorly) and fossa and extends posteriorly to the squamotympanic fissure of the temporal bone.
         (2) Inferiorly, it attaches to the neck of the condyle.
      c. Consists of two layers:
         (1) Outer layer—thick, fibrous tissue that is supported laterally by the temporomandibular ligament.
         (2) Inner layer—consists of synovial membrane, which secretes synovial fluid to help lubricate and nourish the joint.
      d. Note: the superior head of the lateral pterygoid muscle attaches to the anterior portion of the articular capsule (see Figure 1–76). When chewing food, the contraction of the superior head helps to stabilize the TMJ on the nonchewing side.
   3. Articular disc (meniscus)
      a. Consists of dense, fibrous tissue.
      b. Divides the TMJ into two compartments: the upper and lower synovial cavities. These two cavities are involved in translational and rotational TMJ movements, respectively (refer to TMJ movements, later).

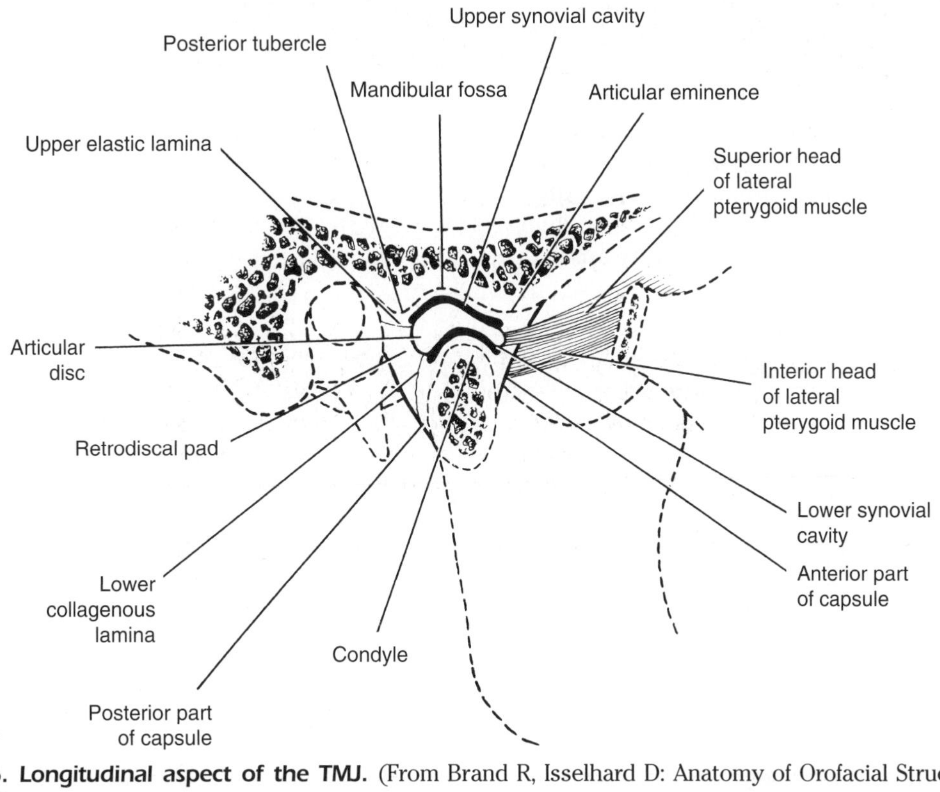

Figure 1–76. Longitudinal aspect of the TMJ. (From Brand R, Isselhard D: Anatomy of Orofacial Structures, St. Louis, Mosby, 2003.)

c. Disc thickness:
   (1) Lateral aspect (from widest to narrowest): posterior → anterior → middle.
   (2) Coronal aspect: medial side is wider than the lateral side (Figure 1–77).

d. Attachments:
   (1) The anterior end of the disc fuses with the articular capsule.
   (2) The posterior end is divided into two sections: the upper portion attaches to the postglenoid process of the temporal bone; the lower portion attaches to the neck of the condyle.
   (3) Fibers of the superior head of the lateral pterygoid muscle attach to the anterior end of the disc. This helps to balance and stabilize the disc during closure.

e. The central part of the disc is void of any blood vessels or nerves. The posterior portion of the disc (specifically, the retrodiscal space between the upper and lower posterior portions) contains vascular and nerve tissue.

4. Upper elastic lamina (superior retrodiscal lamina)
   a. Attachments: extends from the tympanic plate of the temporal bone to the upper portion of the posterior disc (see Figure 1–76).
   b. Contains elastic fibers.
   c. Produces a posterior pull on the disc.
      (1) During mouth opening, the condyles will rotate forward. The disc, attached to the poles of the condyle, has a tendency to move forward with it. The elastic lamina, however, pulls the disc back, allowing the disc and condyle to rotate on one another.
      (2) During retrusion (i.e., as the mandible returns to centric relation), the superior head of the lateral pterygoid will relax. This relaxation will balance the posterior pull of the elastic lamina.

5. Lower collagenous lamina
   a. Attachments: extends from the posterior condylar neck to the lower portion of the posterior disc.
   b. Prevents anterior displacement of the disc and upper elastic lamina.

6. Functional ligaments
   a. Collateral (discal) ligaments
      (1) Attach to the medial and lateral sides of the disc (Figure 1–77).
      (2) The lateral side is shorter than the medial side.
      (3) These ligaments help to restrict medial and lateral rotation of the disc.
   b. Capsular ligament
      (1) Wraps around the entire ligament.
      (2) Helps to keep the disc together.
   c. Temporomandibular (lateral) ligament
      (1) Prevents posterior, inferior, and some lateral displacement of the mandible.
      (2) Provides lateral reinforcement to the articular capsule.
      (3) Consists of two ligaments (running in different directions), which function as a single unit (Figure 1–78):
         (a) Oblique—outer ligament
            (i) Extends from the articular eminence posteriorly and

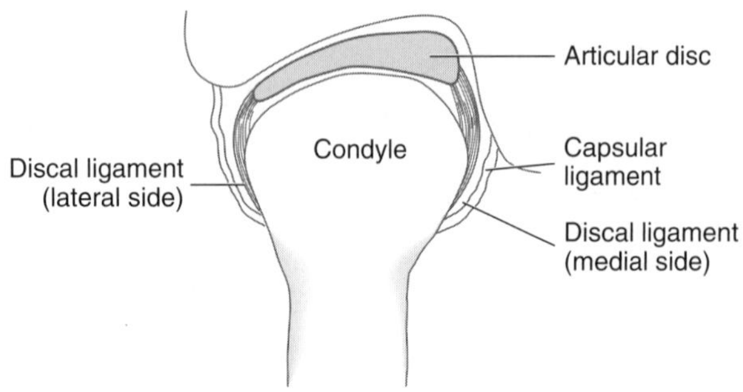

Figure 1–77. Coronal aspect of right TMJ: functional ligaments.

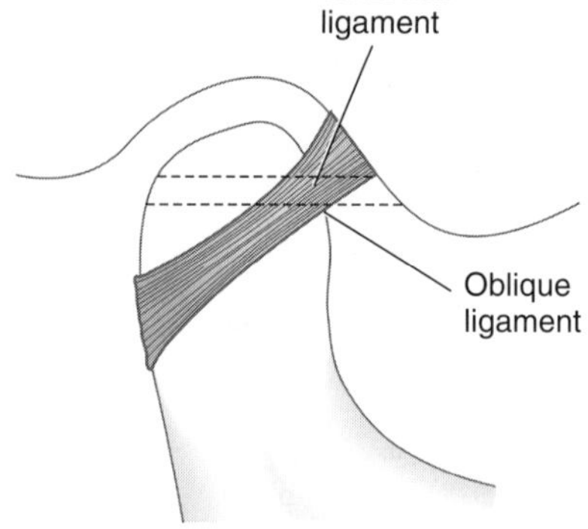

Figure 1–78. Lateral aspect: temporomandibular ligament.

inferiorly to the outer surface of the neck of the condyle.

(ii) Prevents lateral and inferior displacement of the mandible.

(b) Horizontal—inner ligament

(i) Extends from the articular eminence posteriorly to the lateral pole of the condyle.

(ii) Prevents posterior displacement of the mandible.

7. Accessory ligaments

a. Sphenomandibular ligament

(1) Extends from the spine of the sphenoid bone to the lingula of the mandibular foramen.

(2) Local anesthesia considerations—the inferior alveolar nerve (IAN) courses between the sphenomandibular ligament and the ramus of the mandible before entering the mandibular foramen. The sphenomandibular ligament may thus be damaged during the administration of an IAN block.

b. Stylomandibular ligament

(1) Extends from the styloid process of the temporal bone to the angle of the mandible.

(2) Restricts anterior (protrusive) movement of the mandible.

C. Nerve and vascular supply

1. Innervation—provided by branches of the trigeminal nerve, mandibular division (V_3), including:

a. Auriculotemporal nerve.

b. Sensory fibers from the masseteric and posterior temporal nerve.

2. Blood supply—provided by branches of the external carotid artery, including:

a. Superficial temporal artery.

b. Branches from the deep auricular, anterior tympanic, ascending pharyngeal, and maxillary arteries may also be involved.

D. TMJ movement

1. Two motions:

a. Rotational

(1) A hinge-like motion, which occurs around a horizontal axis.

(2) Isolated rotation is possible only when the mandible is retruded, in the centric relation position.

(3) Involves the disc and condyle in the lower synovial cavity (i.e., during rotation, the shape of the lower synovial cavity will be more affected).

(4) Terminal hinge movement—rotation that occurs when the discs are positioned superiorly in the articular fossa, with the condyles directly underneath them.

b. Translational, sliding motion

(1) Translation occurs as the disc slides along the slope of the articular eminence.

(2) Isolated translation occurs during protrusion (i.e., when the jaw moves forward).

(3) Involves the disc and anterior eminence in the upper synovial cavity.

2. Mouth opening—when the mouth opens, both rotational and translational movements occur. The condyles initially rotate and then translate forward (Note: rotational movement continues during translation) (Figure 1–79).

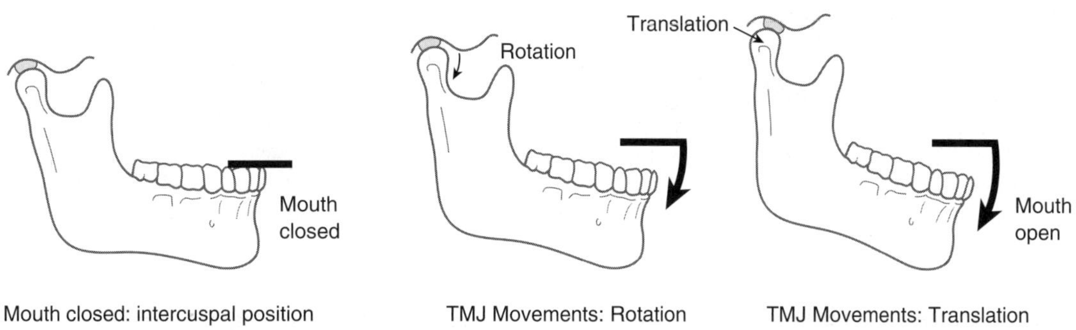

Figure 1–79. TMJ movements: rotation and translation.

4.0 DEVELOPMENTAL BIOLOGY

4.1 Osteogenesis

A. Intramembranous ossification

The process of intramembranous ossification involves differentiation of mesenchyme directly into bone without formation of an intervening cartilage. Flat bones of the skull and subperiosteal lamellar bone are formed by intramembranous ossification.

1. Steps in intramembranous ossification
   a. Stellate mesenchymal cells differentiate into osteoblasts and form spicules of aggregated cells.
   b. Osteoblasts commence producing osteoid
      (1) Osteiod traps some of the osteoblasts, which will form osteocytes in the interior of spicules.
   c. Mineralization of the developing spicule occurs gradually.
      (1) The basophilic core is composed of mineralized, older osteoid.
      (2) The thin, eosinophilic peripheral zone is composed of nonmineralized, younger osteoid.
   d. Spicules anastomose with one another to produce immature woven bone.
      (1) Woven bone does not contain lamellae.
      (2) It has loosely packed, randomly arranged collagen fibers.
      (3) It has a greater cell density than mature bone.
   e. Anastomosing spicules eventually enclose mesenchymal areas, which contain blood vessels and nerves.
   f. Deposition of osteoid is greatest on the side of the spicule nearest the vessels
2. Remodeling of immature bone creates mature compact bone.

B. Endochondral ossification

This process of bone formation begins with differentiation of mesenchyme into a hyaline cartilage model. It is then reworked into adult compact bone. Long bones of the limbs, vertebral column, shoulder and pelvic girdles, and ribs are formed by endochondral ossification.

1. Formation of diaphyseal (primary) center of ossification
   a. Based upon the hyaline cartilage model.
      (1) Structure is formed from fetal mesenchyme containing chondroblasts and chondrocytes. It is surrounded by perichondrium except at the ends.
      (2) Interstitial growth increases the length of the model.
      (3) Appositional growth increases the width.
   b. Vascularization of the perichondrium induces differentiation of osteoblasts from regional mesenchyme.
      (1) The outer layer is transformed into periosteum.
   c. The periosteal collar of bone is produced by intramembranous ossification of the periosteum.
   d. Hypertrophy and death of chondrocytes at the center of the cartilage leaves spicules of calcified cartilage and lacunae.
      (1) These will form the primitive marrow cavity.
      (2) Enlargement of the cavity will occur by addition of bone on the outside of the diaphyseal collar and removal of bone from its endosteal surface.
   e. The periosteal bud, containing blood vessels, osteoprogenitor cells, and mesenchymal cells, extends from the diaphyseal periosteum into the center of the degenerating cartilage.
   f. Osteoprogenitor cells of the periosteal bud attach to spicules of calcified cartilage and become osteoblasts.
      (1) This establishes the primary center of ossification.
   g. Osteoblasts begin elaborating matrix, which will become mineralized to form a spicule.
      (1) Spicules have calcified cartilage in the center surrounded by mineralized bone matrix.
      (2) The mineralized bone matrix is surrounded by mineralized bone matrix, surfaced by a thin zone of unmineralized matrix under the layer of osteoblasts.
   h. The formation of bone proceeds toward both epiphyseal ends.
   i. The marrow cavity is enlarged by osteoclastic removal of the oldest spicules of endochondral ossification.
2. Formation of epiphyseal centers of ossification
   a. Following birth, a center of ossification develops in each epiphysis.

(1) This occurs by the same process used in formation of the diaphyseal center.

b. Epiphyseal and diaphyseal centers of ossification are separated by epiphyseal plates composed of hyaline cartilage.
c. Addition of new hyaline cartilage at the epiphyseal ends of long bones, and its replacement by bone at the diaphyseal ends, cause migration of the epiphyseal plates outward, leading to lengthening of long bones.
d. Cartilage is enlarged by interstitial growth of hyaline cartilage in the articular region and its ossification.
e. Epiphyseal surfaces remain covered by hyaline cartilage and have no periosteum.

C. Epiphyseal plates

Bone formation at the epiphyseal plates is stimulated by pituitary growth hormone.

1. Zones in epiphyseal plates can be distinguished histologically.
2. The zones occur in this order from epiphyseal to diaphyseal side:
   a. Zone of resting cartilage composed of small, randomly arranged chondrocytes.
   b. Zone of proliferation composed of rows of isogenous cell groups due to interstitial growth of chondrocytes.
   c. Zone of hypertrophy composed of enlarged chondrocytes that release alkaline phosphatase.
   d. Zone of calcified cartilage containing dead or dying chondrocytes and calcified cartilage spicules.
   e. Zone of ossification with a continuous secretion of osteoid by osteoblasts attached to spicules of calcified cartilage and subsequent mineralization of older osteoid.
3. Closure of epiphyses occurs within epiphyseal plates and makes them nonfunctional.
   a. Closure occurs in young adults at 20 to 30 years of age.
   b. Epiphyseal closure marks the end of growth in length of long bones.

D. Remodeling of bone

1. Bone remodeling results from combined activity of osteoclasts and osteoblasts.
2. Adult bone turns over completely in about 7 to 10 years.

4.2 Tooth Development, Eruption, and Movement

A. Tooth development

1. Dental lamina
   a. Neural crest cells migrate down the sides of the head and induce oral epithelial cells to form the dental lamina.
   b. The first sign of a dental structure is a narrow band of thickened oral epithelium.
   c. The lamina will form the oral epithelium that will subsequently develop into the inner enamel epithelium and, in turn, will induce the formation of dentin from mesenchymal cells.
   d. After forming, the lamina then wraps around the perimeter of the jaws, and 20 tooth buds appear.
   e. The buds may be called the *enamel organ*.
   f. The enamel organ consists of knobs of tissue that periodically arise from the dental lamina.
   g. The lamina then develops 32 permanent tooth buds lingual to the primary buds.
      (1) If the permanent tooth follows a primary tooth, it develops from successional lamina.
      (2) If there was no primary tooth, it develops as did the primary teeth from general lamina.

B. Stages of tooth development

1. Bud
   a. A localized growth of epithelial cells that develops from the dental lamina to create an enamel organ.
2. Cap
   a. The cells acquire a concave lower surface.
   b. The epithelial cells now become the enamel organ and remain attached to the lamina.
   c. Mesenchymal cells form the dental papilla, which becomes the pulp.
   d. The tissue surrounding these structures is the dental follicle.
3. Bell
   a. The enamel organ has developed into an outer and inner enamel epithelium.
   b. The inner enamel epithelium differentiates into ameloblasts that will create enamel.
   c. The ameloblasts induce cells in the dental papillae to differentiate into

odontoblasts that start to lay down dentin before the ameloblasts start laying down enamel.

d. Between the inner and outer enamel epithelium are stellate reticulum cells.

e. Another layer adjacent to the inner enamel epithelium in the enamel organ is called the *stratum intermedium*.

C. Dental papilla

1. Densely packed fibroblasts are seen in the dental papilla.
2. These cells are thought to be significant in furthering the formation of the enamel organ in the bud and cap stages.
3. Blood vessels and nerves may also be seen, initially in the central region.

D. Dentinogenesis

1. Odontoblasts move toward the pulp, forming increments of dentin.
2. First, the dentin matrix is a matrix of collagen fibers, but it becomes calcified within 24 hours.
3. Dentinogenesis takes place in two phases:
   a. The initial collagen matrix formation.
   b. Deposition of calcium phosphate crystals (hydroxyapatite).
      (1) The crystals grow, spread, and coalesce until the matrix is mineralized.

E. Amelogenesis

1. Ameloblasts begin to deposit enamel shortly after dentin deposition has begun.
2. The enamel matrix is formed within the cell and migrates in vesicles to the apical end of the cell, where it is deposited.

F. Root sheath

1. Inner and outer enamel epithelial cells lengthen after crown completion.
2. The double layer of cells is called the *epithelial root sheath (Hertwig's sheath)*.
   a. At the apex it bends inward at a 45-degree angle (epithelial diaphragm).
3. The inner cell layer induces odontoblasts to form root dentin.
4. The outer cell layer deposits a cuticular membrane (enameloid) on the root surface.
5. Mesenchymal cells appear in the pulp in what is known as the *pulp proliferative zone*.
6. These cells create new odontoblasts for dentin and fibroblasts for pulp.
7. The dentin tapers to the apical foramen.

G. Single root formation

1. Following deposition of enameloid, the root sheath breaks up, creating epithelial rests (rests of Malassez).
2. Mesenchymal cells move in to contact the root surface and become cementoblasts.
3. Cementoblasts secrete cementoid, which mineralizes to form cementum.
4. Near the CEJ, cementum is thinner and acellular.
5. Cementum nearer the apex is thicker and cellular.
6. It contains cementocytes and is formed following tooth eruption.

H. Multiple root formation

1. The shape of roots depends on the interaction of the inner and outer enamel epithelial cells and adjacent pulp mesenchymal cells.
2. Extensions of the epithelial diaphragm grow at an increased rate until they fuse.
3. Each extension forms the same as a single rooted tooth.

I. Supporting structures

1. The periodontal ligament connects cementum and alveolar bone.
2. The periodontal ligament and alveolar bone form from mesenchymal cells in the dental follicle.
3. Fibroblasts develop from mesenchyme and appear on cementum in the cervical area of the tooth.
4. Fibroblasts produce the collagen that forms connective tissue.
5. The alveolar process develops as a bony trench around the teeth.
6. Septa appear between teeth to create crypts.
7. The collagen formed by fibroblasts attaches to cementum on one end and alveolar bone on the other to create the periodontal ligament.

J. Prefunctional eruptive phase

1. The prefunctional eruptive phase continues until the clinical crown contacts the opposing crown.
2. Macrophages appear in soft tissue and release enzymes along the eruptive path, causing bone resorption.
3. For permanent teeth replacing primary teeth, the resorptive process is similar to bony resorption in primary teeth.
4. Monocytes form osteoclasts that resorb bone and primary roots.
5. The alveolus grows in size as the tooth root grows.
6. Occasionally, trauma may cause primary or permanent teeth to fuse to bone (ankylosis).

7. Compensating alveolar process development continues while teeth are in function.
8. It may take 2 or 3 years for completion of root formation after teeth are in function.
9. Teeth may erupt slightly even later in life to compensate for wear.

K. Physiological tooth movement
1. The arches grow in a vertical, facial, and buccal direction.
2. The alveolar process must compensate for growth of the roots of permanent incisors and changes in position.
3. Children pass through a mixed dentition stage as teeth erupt.
4. Anterior force on teeth causes them to drift forward toward the midline (mesial drift).
5. The teeth are also wearing occlusally and proximally.
6. Mesial drift may create anterior crowding that is accentuated as a person ages.
7. Crowding may create oral hygiene difficulties and periodontal problems.

L. Orthodontic movement of teeth
1. Bone is more easily remodeled than cementum.
2. Remodeled bone will show arrest and reversal lines.
3. It is easier to tilt teeth rather than move them bodily, and extrude rather than intrude teeth.

4.3 Facial and Branchial Arch Development

A. Development of the oropharynx

The face begins forming in the fourth week; at that time the body is about $^1/_{16}$ inch long.
1. The neural plate bends ventrally, pushing the heart ventrally.
   a. An oral pocket develops between the forebrain and the heart that will eventually become the oral cavity.

B. Branchial arches
1. Externally, they appear as swellings; internally, they form pharyngeal pouches.
   a. Resemble gill slits.
2. Externally, they will disappear by the end of the fifth week as the second grows down to contact the fifth branchial arch.
   a. There are five or six branchial arches.
   b. They are separated by branchial clefts or grooves.

C. Branchial grooves and pharyngeal pouches
1. The clefts seen between the arches.
   a. The first branchial groove deepens to become the external auditory canal leading to the middle ear.
   b. The membrane at the depth of the first branchial groove becomes the tympanic membrane.
   c. The middle ear and eustachian tube develop from the corresponding first pharyngeal pouch.
   d. The second pharyngeal pouch becomes the palatine tonsils.
      (1) Tonsils function in the development of lymphocytes.
   e. The third pharyngeal pouch becomes the inferior parathyroids and thymus.
   f. The fourth pharyngeal pouch becomes the superior parathyroid.
   g. The fifth pharyngeal pouch becomes the ultimobranchial body.
      (1) Ultimobranchial function is unknown.

D. Vascular development

Each of the branchial arches has a right and left aortic arch vessel that leads from the heart through the arches to the face, brain, and posterior of the body.
1. The first and second branchial arches begin to develop in the fourth week and disappear in the fifth week.
2. The third arch vessels then become prominent, taking over the facial area from the first two.
3. As the fourth and fifth arch vessels arise, the fourth becomes prominent and the fifth disappears.
4. Finally, the sixth arch vessels arise and become dominant, along with the third and fourth.
5. The third arch vessels become the common carotid arteries, which supply the neck, face, and brain.
6. The fourth arch vessels become the dorsal aorta, which supplies the rest of the body.
7. The sixth arch vessels supply the lungs.

E. Muscular and neural development

Muscle cells become apparent in the first arch in the fifth week.
1. They spread within the mandibular arch into each muscle's site of origin in the sixth and seventh weeks.

2. The muscles of the first arch become the muscles of mastication.
3. By the tenth week, the muscles of the second arch have formed a thin sheet extending over the face and posterior to the ear.
4. The muscles of the fourth arch form the pharyngeal constrictor muscles.
5. By the end of the seventh week, cranial nerve (CN) V (first arch) and CN VII (second arch) have interdigitated with their respective muscle groups.
6. The CN IX interdigitates with the third arch.
7. The CN X interdigitates with the fourth arch.

F. Cartilagenous skeletal development
1. Meckel's cartilages appear bilaterally in the first arch.
    a. These structures will later be absorbed into the forming jaw.
    b. Their posterior hinge will become the malleus of the ear.
2. Reichert's cartilage appears in the second arch.
    a. The stapes, styloid process, lesser horn, and upper body of the hyoid arise from this arch.
3. The third arch forms the greater horn and lower part of the hyoid.
4. The fourth arch forms hyoid cartilage.
5. The fifth arch has no adult cartilage derivative.
6. The sixth arch forms the laryngeal cartilage.

G. Cartilages of the face

The cartilaginous nasal capsule (ethmoid), the sphenoid, the auditory capsules, and the basioccipital cartilages are the first skeletal structures seen in the craniofacial area.
1. They are called the *cranial base*.
2. Later, these will separate to form individual bones by endochondral bone formation.

H. Bones of the face
1. The protective bones of the face do not form from cartilage.
    a. These include the frontal, parietal, and squamous portions of the temporal and interoccipital bones.
2. Facial bones also do not form from cartilage.
    a. They include the premaxillary, maxillary, zygomatic, and petrous portions of the temporal bone.
3. Maxillary bones also grow medially into the palate to support the palatine shelf tissue.
4. Mandibular bones grow laterally to the first arch cartilage and posteriorly to meet the bony body of the cartilaginous condyle.
5. Together these will replace Meckel's cartilage.
6. The mandible forms from several units:
    a. Condylar
        (1) Forms the articulation.
    b. Body
        (1) Center of all growth.
    c. Angular process
        (1) Responds to lateral pterygoid and masseter muscles.
    d. Coronoid process
        (1) Responds to temporalis muscle development.
    e. Alveolar process
        (1) Responds to development of the teeth.

I. Sutures of the face

Sutures are fibrous joints (articulations) in which opposing surfaces are closely joined.
1. Sutures are named for the bones they join.
    a. The articulations may consist of a band of connective tissue.
2. External face
    a. All sutures have a central zone or proliferating connective tissue cells along peripheral bony fronts.
    b. All are surrounded by fibrous connective tissue.
    c. There are three types of sutures of the face:
        (1) Simple.
        (2) Serrated.
            (a) Interdigitating type of suture.
        (3) Squamosal.
            (a) Beveled or overlapping.
3. Internal face
    a. A synchondrosis—all have an interposing band of cartilage.
    b. Grow by forming new cartilage in the center of the suture.

J. Structures derived from branchial arches
1. Branchial arch I—Mandibular
    a. Most of maxilla.
    b. Mandible lateral to left and right Meckel's cartilage.
    c. One-half of the external ear.
        (1) Three hillocks here and three from the second branchial arch.
    d. Incus and malleus.
    e. Muscles of mastication.
    f. Trigeminal nerve (V).

g. Maxillary and mandibular branches supply structures of branchial arch I.
2. Branchial arch II—Hyoid
a. Stapes.
b. Styloid process.
c. The other three hillocks forming the external ear.
d. Hyoid bone (most).
e. Muscles of facial expression.
f. Facial nerve (VII)
(1) Supplies structures of the second branchial arch.
(2) Taste to anterior two thirds of the tongue.
3. Branchial arch III
a. Forms part of the hyoid bone.
b. Glossopharyngeal nerve (IX)
(1) Supplies structures of the third branchial arch.
(2) Taste to posterior one third of the tongue.
4. Branchial arches IV, V, and VI
a. Larynx.
b. Pharyngeal constrictor muscles.
c. Vagus nerve (X)
(1) Supplies structures of the fourth, fifth, and sixth branchial arches.

K. Formation of structures
1. Week by week
a. Between the fourth and eighth weeks, all structures are formed and are recognizable. From that point on, they add mass.
2. Week 4
a. By the end of the third week, branchial arch I (called the *mandibular arch*) has divided into left and right maxillary and mandibular processes.
b. By the beginning of the fourth week, the primitive mouth (stomodeum) has formed.
c. The buccopharyngeal membrane separates the stomodeum and foregut and is located in the area of the palatine tonsils.
3. Week 5
a. The embryo is $\frac{1}{4}$ inch long.
b. Depressions called *nasal pits* appear in the frontal process.
c. Nasal pits divide the frontal process into the:
(1) Medial nasal processes.
(2) Lateral nasal processes.
d. Oropharyngeal membrane ruptures.
e. Eyes form on side of the head.
4. Week 6
a. Globular processes appear on the medial nasal process.
(1) Will form the philtrum of the lip.
b. The primary palate forms, later known as the *premaxilla*.
c. The globular processes then begin to fuse with the lateral nasal processes and the maxillary processes.
(1) Takes about 2 weeks.
5. Week 7
a. The face has a more human appearance.
b. Lateral growth of the brain moves eyes to the front of the face.
c. Upper lip has fused, creating the medially located philtrum.
d. The hillocks have fused to form the ears.

L. Development of vascular blood supply to the face
1. Aortic arch formation and changes.
2. A dorsal aortic arch forms corresponding to each branchial arch.
a. The first and second aortic arch shrivel.
b. The third aortic arch becomes the common carotid.
c. The fourth aortic arch becomes the dorsal aorta.
d. The dorsal aorta becomes the internal carotid, which develops a stapedial artery.
e. The sixth aortic arch forms the pulmonary circulation.
f. The ventral aorta becomes the ventral pharyngeal artery.
3. Shift from internal to external carotid artery
a. The stapedial artery dwindles, and vessels arising from it become attached to the external carotid artery, which will supply the face.
b. The internal carotid subsequently supplies the brain.

M. Medial and lateral palatal processes

The palate develops from an anterior, wedge-shaped medial part and two lateral palatine processes.
1. Medial palate
a. Also called the *primary palate*.
b. Develops from the globular processes near the end of the sixth week.
c. Is a floor to the nasal pits.
2. Lateral palatine processes
a. Appear at the eighth week.

b. Arise as left and right (L/R) palatine processes coming off the L/R maxillary processes.
c. Will form the posterior portion of the hard palate and the soft palate.

N. Palatal elevation
1. Occurs rapidly as the palatine processes flip up over the descending tongue.
2. Fusion of the hard palate begins in the ninth week, following palatal elevation.
3. Contact between segments is initially made behind the medial palatine segment.
a. Continues in an anterior and posterior direction until the entire palate is complete by the end of the twelfth week.

4.3.1 Internal Facial Development

A. Muscle development
1. Muscle cells become apparent during the fifth week and spread during the sixth and seventh weeks.
a. They grow over the face and attach to developing bones.

B. Neural development
1. The CNS begins forming during the third week.
2. Cranial nerves grow from the area of the developing brain to innervate the muscles of the head.
a. CN V—innervates the muscles of mastication.
b. CN VII—innervates stylohyoid and stapedius muscles and the posterior belly of the digastric muscle.
c. CN IX—innervates the stylopharyngeal and upper pharyngeal constrictor muscles.
d. CN X—innervates the inferior constrictor and laryngeal muscles.

C. Cartilaginous skeletal development
1. First branchial arch
a. Meckel's cartilage
(1) Originally articulates with the malleus, which will become a hearing bone of the middle ear.
b. Eventually the TMJ becomes functional, and Meckel's cartilage is incorporated into the mandible.
2. Second branchial arch
a. Reichert's cartilage
(1) Will form the stapes, styloid process, and the lesser horn and upper part of the body of the hyoid.
3. Third branchial arch
a. Will form the greater horn and lower part of the hyoid body.
4. Fourth branchial arch
a. Will form the thyroid cartilage.
5. Sixth branchial arch
a. Will form the laryngeal cartilage.

D. Tongue
1. Muscles of the head (including the tongue) arise from blocks of mesoderm (the myotomes).
2. Nerves
a. CN V—sensory nerve to anterior tongue.
b. CN VII—special sensory nerve to anterior two thirds (body) of tongue.
c. CN IX—sensory nerve to posterior third (base) of tongue.
d. CN X—also innervates the base of the tongue.
3. Body
a. The anterior, more movable, part of the tongue develops from the first branchial arch during the fourth week.
b. Extends from the tip to a V-shaped groove called the *terminal sulcus* behind the circumvallate papillae.
4. Root
a. The posterior, less movable, part of the tongue develops from the second and third branchial arches.
5. Development
a. Arises from two mounds of tissue called *lateral lingual swellings* and the *tuberculum impar*.
b. The lateral parts rapidly enlarge and merge.
c. A U-shaped sulcus develops around the anterior part of the tongue.

E. Thyroid gland

At the point of the V-shaped groove (called the *terminal sulcus*) is a depression known as *foramen caecum*.
1. This location is the embryologic beginning point of the thyroid gland.
2. During development, the epithelium in this area begins to migrate into the neck.
3. The path is called the *thyroglossal duct*.
4. The glandular tissue that will form the thyroid is carried into the neck with the epithelium.
5. Eventually, the pathway usually disappears.
6. A remnant can persist, and aberrant thyroid tissue that can cause a cyst may be found anywhere along the path.

F. Facial clefts
1. May be unilateral, bilateral, or medial.
2. May be complete with no joining of tissue.

3. May be incomplete with joining of soft tissue but not bone.
4. Normally, philtrum ridges are the line of fusion.

G. Palatal clefts
1. Most cleft palates occur in combination with cleft lips.
2. They may also occur as isolated defects.
3. Palatal clefts must extend around the medial palatal segment before they reach the midline.

H. Other defects—are involved with defects in fusion and merging.
1. Fusion
   a. Epithelial adhesion followed by reorganization of the deep tissues to mesenchyme.
   b. After the ectoderm has fused, it is replaced by mesenchyme.
   c. Sometimes globules of ectoderm persist and become epithelial rests, which may become cysts.
2. Merging
   a. Filling in of a cleft
   b. If failure occurs at the junction of the lateral nasal and maxillary processes, it causes an oblique facial cleft.
   c. If failure occurs at the globular processes, it causes a midsagittal cleft in the upper lip.

4.4 General Embryology

The study of embryology allows us to see how a single cell can develop to form an entire person. The journey begins with fertilization of the egg. After fertilization, the egg (now called a *zygote*) begins a trip along the fallopian tube toward the uterus. As it travels it starts to divide, first into two cells, then four, then eight, and so on. Eventually it forms a solid ball called a *morula* (for mulberry). The morula continues to grow, and as it does, the interior becomes hollow. At this stage the aggregation of cells is called a *blastocyst*. Along the interior of one side of the blastocyst, a mass of cells begins forming; it arches into the cavity of the blastocyst until there is a second, smaller cavity under the group of cells. The organism itself will form from this small group of cells, with the majority of the blastocyst forming the yolk sac and the yolk that will be consumed by the developing organism.

The small mass of cells is called the *embryonic disk*. At first, it is only one cell layer thick; however, it soon divides into three layers. These primordial layers are significant because each will form distinct structural parts of the body.

The layer facing the smaller cavity is called *ectoderm*. Ectoderm will form nervous tissue, sensory epithelia of the eye, ear, and nose, epidermis, hair, and nails, mammary and cutaneous glands, epithelia of sinuses, oral and nasal cavities, intraoral glands, and tooth enamel.

The middle layer is called *mesoderm*. Mesoderm will form muscles, connective tissue, bone, cartilage, blood, dentin, cementum, pulp, and the periodontal ligament.

The layer facing the larger cavity will form endoderm. Endoderm will form the gastrointestinal tract epithelium.

A. Parts and organelles
1. Cell structure and function
   a. Cells are composed of a nucleus, containing a nucleolus and the surrounding cytoplasm, organelles, inclusions, and a surrounding cell membrane.
      (1) Within each cell is intracellular material.
      (2) Surrounding each cell is intercellular material.
   b. They are connected by cell junctions including desmosomes, tight junctions, and gap junctions.
2. Nucleus and nuclear membrane
   a. A nucleus is found in all cells except mature RBCs and platelets.
      (1) Usually round.
      (2) Usually singular.
   b. Binucleate nucleus in cardiac muscle and parenchymal liver cells.
   c. Multinucleate in osteoclasts and skeletal muscle cells.
3. The nucleus contains DNA in chromosomes, which is the location of the genetic code.
   a. DNA is only visible during cell division; at other times it is dispersed and is called *chromatin*.
4. Nucleolus
   a. Round and dense bodies in the nucleus.
      (1) Up to four may be found.
      (2) Contain the RNA in the nucleus.
      (3) RNA carries instructions from the nucleus to sites of protein synthesis (rough endoplasmic reticulum) in the cytoplasm.
5. Nucleus and nuclear membrane (nuclear envelope)
   a. The nucleus is bound by a nuclear envelope with openings at the nuclear pores.

   b. Its outer thickness is contiguous with the endoplasmic reticulum.
6. Cytoplasm
   a. Contains structures needed for absorption and creation of cell products.
   b. The cytosol acts as a factory, taking in raw material and producing products.
7. Endoplasmic reticulum
   a. A system of parallel membrane-bound cavities in the cytoplasm.
   b. Contains newly acquired and synthesized protein.
   c. A channel for the movement of materials.
   d. May be continuous with the nuclear membrane, plasma membrane, or Golgi apparatus.
   e. There are two types, depending on whether ribosomes are present:
      (1) Rough
         (a) Ribosomes are present.
         (b) The site of protein synthesis.
      (2) Smooth
         (a) Ribosomes are not present.
         (b) The site of lipid manufacture.
8. Ribosomes
   a. Small, granular bodies that are the site of protein synthesis.
   b. May be found free in the cytoplasm.
   c. Produce proteins for cell's own use.
   d. May be found attached to endoplasmic reticulum.
   e. Produce proteins for export.
   f. Three types of RNA are necessary for protein synthesis: mRNA, tRNA, rRNA.
9. Golgi apparatus
   a. Connected to the endoplasmic reticulum.
   b. Composed of cisternae (flat plates) or saccules, small vesicles, and large vacuoles.
   c. Sorts, condenses, packages, and delivers proteins from the endoplasmic reticulum to the cell membrane for export from the cell.
10. Lysosomes
   a. Surrounded by a membrane.
   b. Contain acids and digestive enzymes.
   c. Common in macrophages and leukocytes.
   d. Can digest substances both within and around the cell, including bacteria, parts of injured cells, or an entire cell.
11. Peroxisomes
   a. Similar to lysosomes.
   b. A membrane-surrounded body containing various enzymes.
   c. Contain catalase, which catalyzes hydrogen peroxide to water and oxygen.
12. Mitochondrion
   a. Small, variable-shaped, membrane-bound organelles free in the cytoplasm.
   b. The powerhouse of the cell.
   c. Up to 6000 or 7000 per cell.
   d. Has its own DNA.
   e. Inner layer of their membrane is composed of cristae.
   f. Generate ATP through the Kreb's cycle, producing chemical energy from food.
13. Microtubules
   a. Composed of the protein tubulin.
   b. Appear as singular, doublet, or triplet entities.
   c. Function as structural and force-generating elements.
   d. Centrioles are composed of microtubules.
      (1) Centrioles replicate before mitosis begins.
14. Microfilaments
   a. A thin sheath just below the plasmalemma.
   b. Solid rods of actin protein.
   c. Help cell move through cilia and flagella.
   d. Also give shape to the cell.
   e. Associated with endocytosis, exocytosis.
15. Vacuole
   a. Space inside the cell.
   b. Purpose is not known.
16. Vesicles
   a. Sacs containing various substances within the cell.
   b. Transport vesicles.
      (1) Move proteins from endoplasmic reticulum to Golgi apparatus.
   c. Secretory vesicles
      (1) Neurotransmitters.
      (2) Mucus.
      (3) Inorganic substances.
      (4) Other substances.
17. Cell membrane
   a. The external boundary of a cell.
   b. Also called the *plasma membrane* or *plasmalemma*.
   c. Composed primarily of lipid and protein, with some carbohydrate.
   d. Lipid bilayer is oriented with hydrophilic ends outward and hydrophobic ends inward.

(1) Functions as a selective barrier and site of transport.
(2) Has specialized areas of interconnection with other cells for attachment and communication.

e. Desmosomes—between cells.
f. Hemidesmosomes—into the basement membrane.

B. Cell division
1. Both somatic and sex cells divide.
a. In somatic cells, division (mitosis) ensures that the resulting cells contain all of the same genetic material as the original cell.
b. In sex cells, division (meiosis) ensures that the resulting cells contain half of the genetic material that the original mother and father cells contained.
(1) Meiosis is also known as *reduction division*.

2. Mitosis

Mitosis has four phases, plus interphase (a resting phase).

a. Prophase
(1) Chromatin in the nucleus thickens to become visible chromosomes.

b. Metaphase
(1) The chromosomes line up on the equatorial plate.
(2) The two chromatids comprising a chromosome split at their centromere.

c. Anaphase
(1) Each chromatid migrates toward the centriole at the poles of the newly forming cells.

d. Telophase
(1) Cytokinesis divides the cell into two, each containing all the genetic information.

3. Meiosis
a. Occurs in two stages, the second of which mirrors mitosis.
(1) When the chromosomes line up at the equatorial plate for the first division, one whole chromosome of each pair migrates to opposite poles rather than splitting at the centromere.
(2) This has the effect of reducing the chromosome count in resulting cells from 46 to 23.
(3) Four daughter cells are created from one parent cell.

C. Definition of basic terms
1. Embryology
a. The study of the development of the individual during the first 8 weeks following conception.
(1) Formation of the organs occurs in this period.

b. Histology
(1) Microscopic anatomy.
(2) That portion of anatomy dealing with the minute structure, composition, and function of tissues.

c. Cytology
(1) The study of individual cells and their parts.

D. Embryo
1. Periods of prenatal development:
a. 0 to 2 weeks—proliferative.
(1) Includes fertilization, implantation, and formation of the embryonic disc.

b. 2 to 8 weeks—embryonic.
(1) Tissues develop to create organ systems.

c. 8 weeks to 9 months—fetal.
(1) Increase in body weight and size.

2. Fertilization—the egg is fertilized in the distal portion of the uterine tube, which is called the *ampulla of the oviduct*.
a. The fertilized egg is first called a *zygote*.
b. As it travels toward the uterus the number of cells begins to increase, but the size does not increase at first.
(1) At this point, the many-celled ball is called a *morula*.

c. After 5 to 6 days, it has 16 to 32 cells and reaches the uterus, where the endometrium has developed to receive it.
(1) The morula becomes a blastocyst as it increases in size and becomes hollow.

3. Implantation—usually occurs 6 to 10 days after conception.
a. Soon after entering the uterine cavity, the blastocyst sticks to the uterine lining.
b. The lining deteriorates at the site of adhesion, and the blastocyst becomes embedded in the wall of the endometrium.

4. Blastocyst—a hollow mass of cells that forms as cells pull away from the center of the morula.

a. The peripheral cells are called the *trophoblast*, with the blastocele being the cavity.
b. This hollow ball of cells develops an inner cell mass against one wall.
c. The small mass enlarges to form an area separating two small cavities.
   (1) This layer is called the *embryonic disc*.
d. Cells facing the smaller cavity form the primordial ectodermal layer, and cells facing the larger one form the primordial endodermal layer.

5. Yolk sac—implantation of the blastocyst causes breakdown of endometrial tissue.
   a. This provides food and materials for the embryo for a few weeks.
   b. The embryo sends out branches of umbilical arteries and veins.
   c. The yolk supplies nutrition to the embryo through the vitelline arteries.
   d. At the same time, the placenta and its blood supply are forming.
   e. When the yolk sac becomes depleted, the placenta takes over supplying nutrients and removing waste.
   f. Five weeks after implantation, the umbilical and placental system is in place.
   g. Nutrients and wastes cross, but maternal and fetal blood do not mix.
6. Extraembryonic coelem—at 9 or 10 days, the trophoblast portion of the blastocyst produces mesoblasts, which begin to fill the blastocyst cavity.
   a. The blastocyst grows faster than these cells can fill the space, so they end up lining the cavity around the actual embryo.
   b. These cells will form the amnion, vitelline sac, and chorion.

E. Primordial layers
   1. Ectoderm
      a. Forms:
         (1) Nervous system.
         (2) Sensory epithelium of eye, ear, nose.
         (3) Epidermis, hair, nails.
         (4) Mammary and cutaneous glands.
         (5) Epithelium of sinuses, oral and nasal cavities, intraoral glands.
         (6) Tooth enamel.
   2. Mesoderm—arises between the ectodermal and endodermal layers of the embryonic disc.
      a. Forms:
         (1) Muscles.
         (2) Connective tissue derivatives: bone, cartilage, blood, dentin, pulp, cementum, periodontal ligament.
   3. Endoderm
      a. Forms:
         (1) Gastrointestinal (GI) tract epithelium and associated glands.

F. Development of human tissues
   1. Epithelial structures and derivatives
      a. Mesoderm
         (1) Forms the dermis of the epithelium and the visceral mesoderm that covers the yolk sac and subsequently becomes the GI tract.
      b. Ectoderm
         (1) Initially, the embryo is covered by a single layer of ectodermal cells.
         (2) By 11 to 12 weeks, this thickens into four layers.
         (3) Later melanocytes invade and pigment the skin.
   2. Nervous system
      a. Folds arise in the neural plate in the third week.
         (1) The fold facing the smaller cavity will show three areas that will form the forebrain, midbrain, and hindbrain.
      b. The forebrain curls down toward the chest as the cranial nerves develop.
   3. Connective tissue
      a. Develops from somites as fibroblasts migrating from either side of the neural tube.
   4. Cartilage and bone—cartilage cells arise from the sclerotome and migrate to surround the notochord and spinal cord.
      a. The skeleton forms in a segmental pattern.
      b. Cartilage grows both by apposition and interstitial growth.
      c. Bone replaces cartilage through a process called *endochondral bone development* or by intramembranous bone formation.
   5. Muscle

      By the tenth prenatal week, myoblasts migrate from the myotome.
   6. Cardiovascular system—originates from angioblasts, which arise from mesoderm in the walls of the yolk sac.
      a. For the first few weeks, nutrition is provided through the vitelline vascular system.
      b. The heart starts pumping in the fourth week.

Sample Questions

1. ***The lateral pterygoid muscle attaches to which of the following?***
   A. Lateral surface of the lateral pterygoid plate.
   B. Medial surface of the lateral pterygoid plate.
   C. Lateral surface of the medial pterygoid plate.
   D. Medial surface of the medial pterygoid plate.
   E. Pyramidal process of palatine bone.
2. ***Which of the following muscles is responsible for the formation of the posterior tonsillar pillar?***
   A. Stylopharyngeus.
   B. Tensor veli palatine.
   C. Palatoglossus.
   D. Palatopharyngeus.
   E. Levator veli palatine.
3. ***The superior and inferior ophthalmic veins drain into the ______.***
   A. Internal jugular vein
   B. Pterygoid plexus
   C. Frontal vein
   D. Infraorbital vein
   E. Facial vein
4. ***The masseter originates from the ______.***
   A. Condyle of the mandible
   B. Infratemporal crest of the sphenoid bone
   C. Inferior border of the zygomatic arch
   D. Pyramidal process of the palatine bone
   E. Mastoid process of temporal bone
5. ***Which of the following muscles adducts the vocal cords?***
   A. Lateral cricoarytenoid.
   B. Posterior cricoarytenoid.
   C. Cricothyroid.
   D. Vocalis.
   E. Tensor veli palatine.
6. ***Which of the following strata of oral epithelium is engaged in mitosis?***
   A. Basale.
   B. Granulosum.
   C. Corneum.
   D. Spinosum.
7. ***The auriculotemporal nerve encircles which of the following vessels?***
   A. Maxillary artery.
   B. Superficial temporal artery.
   C. Deep auricular artery.
   D. Middle meningeal artery.
   E. Anterior tympanic artery.
8. ***The muscle that is found in the walls of the heart is characterized by ______.***
   A. A peripherally placed nucleus
   B. Multiple nuclei
   C. Intercalated discs
   D. Fibers with spindle-shaped cells
9. ***All of the following are found in the posterior triangle of the neck* except *one. Which one is the* exception?**
   A. External jugular vein.
   B. Subclavian vein.
   C. Hypoglossal nerve.
   D. Phrenic nerve.
   E. Brachial plexus.
10. ***Deoxygenated blood from the transverse sinus drains into the ______.***
    A. Inferior sagittal sinus
    B. Confluence of sinuses
    C. Sigmoid sinus
    D. Straight sinus
    E. Internal jugular vein
11. ***The vestigial cleft of Rathke's pouch in the hypophysis is located between the ______.***
    A. Anterior and posterior lobes
    B. Anterior lobe and hypothalamus
    C. Posterior lobe and hypothalamus
    D. Median eminence and the optic chiasm
12. ***Involution of the thymus would occur following which year in a healthy individual?***
    A. 0 years (at birth).
    B. 12th year.
    C. 20th year.
    D. 60th year.
13. ***Blood from the internal carotid artery reaches the posterior cerebral artery by the ______.***
    A. Anterior cerebral artery
    B. Anterior communicating artery
    C. Posterior communicating artery
    D. Posterior superior cerebellar artery
    E. Basilar artery
14. ***The infraorbital nerve is a branch of the ______.***
    A. Optic nerve
    B. Oculomotor nerve
    C. Ophthalmic nerve
    D. Maxillary nerve
    E. Mandibular nerve
15. ***Which of the following cells are capable of mitosis?***
    A. Smooth muscle.
    B. Skeletal muscle.
    C. Cardiac muscle.
    D. Type I pneumocytes.
    E. Neurons.
16. ***Which of the following types of epithelium lines acinar units of salivary glands?***
    A. Simple squamous.
    B. Stratified squamous.
    C. Simple cuboidal.
    D. Simple columnar.
    E. Pseudostratified columnar.

17. ***To which of the following bones is the tensor tympani attached?***
    A. Incus.
    B. Malleus.
    C. Stapes.
    D. Hyoid.
    E. Mandible.
18. ***In mature dentin, the ratio of inorganic to organic matter is approximately _____.***
    A. 94:6
    B. 50:50
    C. 70:30
    D. 80:20
    E. 60:40
19. ***Which of the following cells forms the myelin sheath around myelinated nerves in the central nervous system?***
    A. Schwann cells.
    B. Astrocytes.
    C. Microglia.
    D. Oligodendrocytes.
    E. Amphicytes.
20. ***Which of the following nerves supplies taste sensation to the anterior two-thirds of the tongue?***
    A. Hypoglossal.
    B. Glossopharyngeal.
    C. Lingual.
    D. Facial.
    E. Mental.

Test items 21–26 refer to the following testlet.

A 24-year-old man presents to your office for an emergency visit, after being hit on the left side of his face with a soccer ball. He complains that his "tooth got knocked out" and that his jaw feels "out of place." He has no other medical conditions.

21. ***During intraoral examination, you find that the patient's lower second premolar is missing. Which type of alveolodental fibers was* least *involved in resisting the force that pulled this patient's tooth out of its socket?***
    A. Apical.
    B. Oblique.
    C. Alveolar crest.
    D. Interradicular.
22. ***You also notice that a cusp of his mandibular second molar has fractured off and that dentin is exposed. If this patient were to drink something cold, what will he sense?***
    A. Pain.
    B. Pressure.
    C. Vibration.
    D. Temperature.
23. ***You decide to take a radiograph of the fractured tooth. On the first film you miss the apex of the tooth, so you decide to take another radiograph. Relaxation of which of the patient's muscles would help you in taking the second film?***
    A. Geniohyoid.
    B. Stylohyoid.
    C. Mylohyoid.
    D. Levator veli palatine.
    E. Palatopharyngeus.
24. ***On further examination, you determine that the articular disc of the patient's temporomandibular joint has been displaced. If the patient contracts his lateral pterygoid muscle, the disc will move _______.***
    A. Posteriorly and medially
    B. Anteriorly and medially
    C. Posteriorly and laterally
    D. Anteriorly and laterally
25. ***During the examination, the patient observes that he cannot feel it when you touch part of his cheek and his upper lip. Which of the following nerves was probably damaged during the accident?***
    A. Lingual.
    B. Maxillary.
    C. Long buccal.
    D. Superior alveolar.
    E. Inferior alveolar.
26. ***You decide to restore the missing cusp on the patient's molar. During the administration of the inferior alveolar nerve block, which of the following ligaments is* most *likely damaged?***
    A. Sphenomandibular.
    B. Stylomandibular.
    C. Temporomandibular.
    D. Interdental.

27. ***The lateral thoracic wall of the axilla is covered by which of the following muscles?***
    A. Pectoralis major.
    B. Pectoralis minor.
    C. Serratus anterior.
    D. Subscapularis.
    E. Latissimus dorsi.
28. ***The trochlea of the humerus bone articulates with the _______.***
    A. Ulna of the forearm
    B. Radius of the forearm
    C. Coronoid process of the ulna of the forearm
    D. Olecranon of the ulna of the forearm
    E. Medial epicondyle
29. ***Which of the following muscles of the back is supplied by the CN XI?***
    A. Levator scapulae.
    B. Latissimus dorsi.
    C. Trapezius.
    D. Major rhomboid.
    E. Minor rhomboid.

30. There are _____ pairs of true ribs.
A. Four
B. Five
C. Seven
D. Eleven
E. Twelve

31. ______ vertebrae are characterized by a heart-shaped body.
A. Cervical
B. Thoracic
C. Lumbar
D. Sacral
E. Coccygeal

32. The sternal angle between the manubrium and the sternum marks the position of the _____ rib.
A. First
B. Second
C. Third
D. Fourth
E. Fifth

33. Which muscle of the anterolateral abdominal wall is described as being belt- or strap-like?
A. External oblique muscle.
B. Internal oblique muscle.
C. Transversus abdominis muscle.
D. Rectus abdominis muscle.
E. Quadratus lumborum muscle.

34. In addition to the esophagus itself, which of the following structures also passes through the diaphragm through the esophageal opening?
A. The aorta.
B. The inferior vena cava.
C. The azygos vein.
D. The posterior and anterior vagal trunks.
E. The splanchnic nerves.

35. The inferior aspect of the diaphragm is supplied with blood by which of the following arteries?
A. Median sacral artery.
B. Lumbar arteries.
C. Inferior phrenic arteries.
D. Celiac trunk.
E. Superior mesenteric artery.

36. Oral epithelium is composed of ______ epithelium.
A. Keratinized simple squamous
B. Keratinized stratified squamous
C. Nonkeratinized simple squamous
D. Nonkeratinized stratified squamous
E. Nonkeratinized stratified columnar

37. Which of the following statements is true of the histology of the trachea?
A. The mucosa is covered with oral epithelium.
B. Elastic cartilage rings lie deep to the submucosa.
C. The cartilage is ring-shaped; the open end of the ring faces anterior.
D. The cartilage is covered by a perichondrium.
E. Skeletal muscle extends across the open end of each cartilage.

38. Terminal bronchioles are characterized by _____ cells.
A. Goblet
B. Ciliated cuboidal
C. Nonciliated cuboidal
D. Ciliated squamous
E. Nonciliated squamous

39. The most superficial layer of the epidermis is the stratum _____.
A. Spinosum
B. Basale
C. Granulosum
D. Lucidum
E. Corneum

40. Langerhans cells are located primarily in stratum _____.
A. Corneum
B. Lucidum
C. Granulosum
D. Spinosum
E. Basale

41. Arteriovenous anastomoses in deeper skin are important in _____.
A. Immunity
B. Thermoregulation
C. Controlling the arrector (erector) pili muscle
D. Pigmentation
E. Pain sensation

42. Which of the following bones is formed by intramembranous ossification?
A. Humerus.
B. Lumbar vertebrae.
C. Frontal bone of the skull.
D. Ribs.
E. Clavicle.

43. Osteocytes are found in _____ in mature bone.
A. Trabeculae
B. Lacunae
C. The central canal
D. Canaliculi
E. Spicules

44. _____ marks the end of growth in length of long bones.
A. Diaphyseal closure
B. Epiphyseal closure
C. Ossification
D. Formation of periosteum
E. Cessation of bone remodeling

45. The branchial arches disappear when the _____ branchial arch grows down to contact the _____.
A. second; third branchial arch
B. second; fifth branchial arch
C. third; fifth branchial arch
D. first; first branchial groove
E. first; sixth branchial groove

46. Facial nerves are derived from the ____ branchial arch.
A. First
B. Second
C. Third
D. Fourth
E. Fifth and sixth

47. ***Cytochrome P450 enzymes may be found in which of the following cellular organelles?***
A. Mitochondria.
B. Golgi apparatus.
C. Lysosome.
D. Ribosome.
E. Endoplasmic reticulum.

48. ***What type of collagen is found in cementum?***
A. Type I collagen.
B. Type II collagen.
C. Type III collagen.
D. Type IV collagen.
E. Type V collagen.

49. ***Calcium binds to which of the following for contraction in smooth muscle?***
A. Troponin C.
B. Calmodulin.
C. Myosin.
D. Actin.
E. Desmosomes.

50. ***Lymph from the mandibular incisors drain chiefly into _____.***
A. Submandibular nodes
B. Submental nodes
C. Superficial parotid nodes
D. Deep cervical nodes
E. Occipital nodes

51. ***Which of the following muscle attaches to the anterior end of the articular disc of the temporomandibular joint?***
A. Superficial head of the medial pterygoid muscle.
B. Deep head of the medial pterygoid muscle.
C. Superior head of the lateral pterygoid muscle.
D. Inferior head of the lateral pterygoid muscle.

52. ***All of the following arteries are branches of the mandibular division of the maxillary artery*** **except** ***one. Which one is the*** **exception?**
A. Incisive artery.
B. Submental artery.
C. Middle meningeal artery.
D. Mylohyoid artery.
E. Deep auricular artery.

53. ***The maxillary nerve passes through which of the following?***
A. Superior orbital fissure.
B. Internal acoustic meatus.
C. Foramen ovale.
D. Foramen rotundum.
E. Foramen spinosum.

54. ***Injury to which of the following nerves would affect abduction of the eyeball?***
A. Optic nerve.
B. Oculomotor.
C. Trochlear.
D. Trigeminal.
E. Abducens.

55. ***Nucleus ambiguus contains the cell bodies of which of the following cranial nerves?***
A. III, IV, and V.
B. VII, IX ,and X.
C. VII, IX, and XI.
D. IX, X, and XI.
E. IX, X, and XII.

56. ***The articulating surfaces of the temporomandibular joint are covered with _____.***
A. Fibrocartilage
B. Hyaline cartilage
C. Articular cartilage
D. Elastic cartilage
E. Perichondrium

57. ***The primary sensory neurons' nucleus of termination involved in the jaw jerk reflex is the _____.***
A. Facial nucleus
B. Trochlear nucleus
C. Mesencephalic nucleus
D. Spinal trigeminal nucleus
E. Nucleus of solitary tract

58. ***Red pulp in the spleen consists of _____.***
A. Fibroblasts
B. T lymphocytes
C. B lymphocytes
D. Macrophages
E. Chromaffin cells

59. ***The vertebral artery meets with the basilar artery at the lower border of the _____.***
A. Midbrain
B. Pons
C. Medulla
D. Temporal lobe
E. C1

60. ***Where are the cells that produce calcitonin located?***
A. Red marrow.
B. Adrenal gland.
C. Parathyroid gland.
D. Thyroid gland.
E. Spleen.

61. ***Chromosomes line up at a cell's equator during which phase of mitosis?***
A. Telophase.
B. Metaphase.
C. Interphase.
D. Anaphase.
E. Prophase.

62. ***Which of the following types of epithelium lines the oropharynx?***
A. Simple squamous.
B. Stratified squamous.
C. Simple cuboidal.
D. Simple columnar.
E. Pseudostratified columnar.

63. ***Which of the following organelles is surrounded by a double membrane?***
    A. Ribosome.
    B. Golgi apparatus.
    C. Lysosome.
    D. Cytoplasmic inclusion.
    E. Mitochondria.
64. ***Hassall's corpuscles are found in the medulla of which of the following glands?***
    A. Thymus.
    B. Thyroid.
    C. Parathyroid.
    D. Pineal.
    E. Suprarenal.
65. ***Which of the following are the* most *abundant in the fovea centralis of the eyeball?***
    A. Rod cells.
    B. Cone cells.
    C. Rod and cone cells.
    D. Amacrine cells.
    E. Ganglion cells.
66. ***Which of the following bones is part of the superior wall (roof) of the orbit?***
    A. Zygomatic.
    B. Lacrimal.
    C. Sphenoid.
    D. Maxilla.
    E. Ethmoid.

Test items 67–70 refer to the following testlet.

A 30-year-old woman comes to your office for a dental examination. She has not been to the dentist in 2 years. The patient has type I diabetes, which requires her to take insulin. She is otherwise in good health. On intraoral examination, you notice that the dorsum of her tongue has a thick, matted appearance and diagnose her with hairy tongue. You also find that the patient has deep caries in her upper second maxillary molar.

67. ***Which type of papillae is affected that causes the hair-like appearance of her tongue?***
    A. Foliate.
    B. Circumvallate.
    C. Fungiform.
    D. Filiform.
68. ***On the patient's radiograph, you notice that the pulp chamber in the carious molar appears smaller than the surrounding teeth. This is* most *likely due to the deposition of which type of dentin?***
    A. Secondary.
    B. Tertiary.
    C. Mantle.
    D. Sclerotic.
69. ***You decide to remove the caries and prepare the patient for anesthesia. Which nerve must you anesthetize to ensure adequate anesthesia for the patient?***
    A. Nasopalatine nerve.
    B. Greater palatine nerve.
    C. Anterior superior alveolar nerve.
    D. Middle superior alveolar nerve.
    E. Posterior superior alveolar nerve.
70. ***After administering the anesthetic, the patient complains that her "heart feels like it's racing." You explain to her that it may be from the epinephrine in the anesthesia. Which of the following glands could* most *likely cause the same symptoms in the patient?***
    A. Hypophysis.
    B. Thyroid.
    C. Pineal.
    D. Suprarenal.

71. ***All of the following are rotator cuff muscles* except:**
    A. Supraspinatous muscle
    B. Infraspinatous muscle
    C. Teres minor muscle
    D. Teres major muscle
    E. Subscapularis muscle
72. ***The brachial plexus of nerves arises from which of the following roots of the anterior primary rami of spinal nerves?***
    A. All cervical roots (C1–C8).
    B. All thoracic roots (T1–T12).
    C. C 8 and T1.
    D. C5 through C8 and T1.
    E. C5 through C8 and T1 through T4.
73. ***The right subclavian artery arises from the _____ and the left subclavian artery arises from the _____.***
    A. Axillary artery; aortic arch
    B. Brachiocephalic artery; aortic arch
    C. Aortic arch; brachiocephalic artery
    D. Brachiocephalic artery; axillary artery
    E. Axillary artery; brachial artery
74. ***The pulmonary vein of the lung carries:***
    A. Unoxygenated blood from the lungs to the heart
    B. Oxygenated blood from the lungs to the heart
    C. Unoxygenated blood to the lungs from the heart
    D. Oxygenated blood to the lungs from the heart
    E. Oxygenated blood from the heart to the lungs
75. ***The _____ of the heart is also known as the mitral valve.***
    A. Right atrioventricular valve
    B. Left atrioventricular valve
    C. Pulmonary valve
    D. Aortic valve
    E. Tricuspid valve

76. The cricopharyngeus muscle of the esophagus _____.

A. Is a parasympathetic stimulator of peristalsis
B. Is a sympathetic inhibitor of peristalsis
C. Prevents swallowing air at the pharyngeal end
D. Prevents regurgitation of stomach contents at the abdominal end
E. Controls the gag reflex

77. The pancreas is enveloped at its head by the _____.

A. First part of the duodenum
B. Second part of the duodenum
C. Third part of the duodenum
D. Fourth part of the duodenum
E. First part of the jejunum

78. The gallbladder arises from the _____.

A. Common hepatic duct
B. Common bile duct
C. Left hepatic duct
D. Cystic duct
E. Bile canaliculi

79. The apex of a medullary pyramid in the kidney is called the _____.

A. Cortex
B. Medulla
C. Renal papilla
D. Major calyx
E. Minor calyx

80. Ureters travel inferiorly just _____ the parietal peritoneum of the posterior body wall. They pass _____ to the common iliac arteries as they enter the pelvis.

A. Above; posterior
B. Above; anterior
C. Below; posterior
D. Below; anterior
E. Above; superior

81. The lumen of the gastrointestinal tract is lined with _____.

A. Mucosa
B. Submucosa
C. Muscularis externa
D. Fibrosa
E. Adventitia

82. Gut-associated lymphoid tissue (GALT) produces secretory _____.

A. IgA
B. IgD
C. IgE
D. IgG
E. IgM

83. The muscularis externa has a third layer in the _____.

A. Esophagus
B. Stomach
C. Liver
D. Small intestine
E. Large intestine

84. Which portion of uriniferous tubules contains squamous epithelial cells?

A. Proximal convoluted tubule.
B. Thick descending limb of Henle's loop.
C. Thin segment of Henle's loop.
D. Thick ascending segment of Henle's loop.
E. Distal convoluted tubule.

85. The _____ is a component of the juxtaglomerular apparatus which functions in regulation of blood pressure.

A. Proximal convoluted tubule
B. Distal convoluted tubule
C. Bowman's capsule
D. Glomerulus
E. Macula densa

86. Urinary filtrate is most hypotonic in the _____.

A. Proximal convoluted tubule
B. Descending limb of Henle's loop
C. Thin segment of Henle's loop
D. Thick ascending segment of Henle's loop
E. Distal convoluted tubule

87. The _____ differentiates into ameloblasts.

A. Stellate reticulum
B. Inner enamel epithelium in the cap stage
C. Inner enamel epithelium in the bell stage
D. Outer enamel epithelium in the cap stage
E. Outer enamel epithelium in the bell stage

88. The dental lamina arises from _____.

A. Somites
B. Neural crest cells
C. The first branchial arch
D. The second branchial arch
E. The buccopharyngeal membrane

89. The correct order of tooth formation is _____.

A. Ameloblasts form, odontoblasts form, ameloblasts start to form enamel, odontoblasts start to form dentin
B. Ameloblasts form, odontoblasts form, odontoblasts start to form dentin, ameloblasts start to form enamel
C. Odontoblasts form, odontoblasts start to form dentin, ameloblasts form, ameloblasts start to form enamel
D. Ameloblasts form, ameloblasts start to form enamel, odontoblasts form, odontoblasts start to form dentin
E. Odontoblasts form, ameloblasts form, odontoblasts start to form dentin, ameloblasts start to form enamel

90. The auricular hillocks are derived from the _____.

A. First branchial arch
B. Second branchial arch
C. First and second branchial arch
D. Lateral nasal process
E. Medial nasal process

91. Reduction division occurs during the _____.
A. First stage of mitosis
B. Second stage of mitosis
C. First stage of meiosis
D. Second stage of meiosis
E. Third stage of meiosis

92. The embryo develops specifically from the _____.
A. The entire blastocyst
B. The entire trophoblast
C. The embryonic disc
D. The extraembryonic coelem
E. The morula

93. Tooth enamel is derived from _____.
A. Endoderm
B. Mesoderm
C. Ectoderm
D. Endoderm and mesoderm
E. Ectoderm and mesoderm

94. The olecranon fossa is located on the _____ surface of the _____.
A. Superior; radius
B. Anterior; humerus
C. Posterior; humerus
D. Anterior; radius

95. The latissimus dorsi muscle is supplied by the _____ nerve.
A. Medial pectoral
B. Cranial nerve XI
C. Dorsal scapular
D. Thoracodorsal

96. The middle trunk of the brachial plexus of nerves arises from:
A. C5
B. C6
C. C7
D. C8

97. Which of the following ribs cannot be palpated?
A. First
B. Second
C. Third
D. A and B

98. An infection in a mandibular incisor with an apex below the mylohyoid muscle drains into which of the following spaces?
A. Sublingual space
B. Submental space
C. Submandibular space
D. Parapharyngeal space

99. The spread of an odontogenic infection to which of the following spaces would MOST likely be considered life-threatening?
A. Submandibular space
B. Sublingual space
C. Parapharyngeal space
D. Retropharyngeal space
E. Pterygomandibular space

100. The median pharyngeal raphe serves as the attachment site for which of the following muscles?
A. Lateral pterygoid muscle
B. Palatopharyngeus muscle
C. Levator veli palatine muscle
D. Salpingopharyngeus
E. Superior constrictor muscle

2

Biochemistry and Physiology

KENNETH R. ETZEL

OUTLINE

1.0 BIOLOGICAL COMPOUNDS

Biological systems depend upon molecules that serve various functions. They may serve as structural components, regulatory agents, energy sources, enzymatic agents, osmotic regulators, transport agents, and agents of hereditary information. Each of these compounds has unique characteristics that enable them to perform their function in both the intracellular and extracellular environments. This section will focus on these biochemical agents and relate their function to biological systems in which they participate.

1.1 Sugars and Carbohydrates

A. Carbohydrate terminology
   1. Empirical formula $(CH_2O)_n$.
   2. Classified based on the number of carbons.
      a. Trioses (3)
      b. Tetroses (4)
      c. Pentoses (5)
      d. Hexoses (6)
   3. Aldoses—contain an aldehyde as their most oxidized functional group. Can contain any number of carbons.
      a. Glyceraldehydes (aldotriose)
      b. Glucose (aldohexose)
   4. Ketoses—contain a keto group as their most oxidized functional group. Fructose is a ketohexose.
   5. Isomers—the chemical formula is the same, but the structure is different.
   6. Epimers—configuration around one carbon differs.
   7. Glycosidic bonds—bonds formed between two sugars or a sugar and another non-carbohydrate molecule.

B. Carbohydrate classification—carbohydrates are classified based on the number of simple sugar units they contain. Examples are given in Figure 2-1.
   1. Monosaccharides (glyceraldehydes, ribose, xylose, glucose, mannose, galactose, fructose).
   2. Disaccharides (lactose, maltose, sucrose).
   3. Oligosaccharides (often found in glycoprotein).
   4. Polysaccharides.
      a. Amylose—unbranched glucose chain of $\alpha(1,4)$ glycosidic bonds).

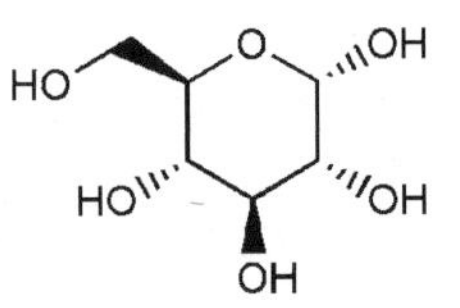

Glucose

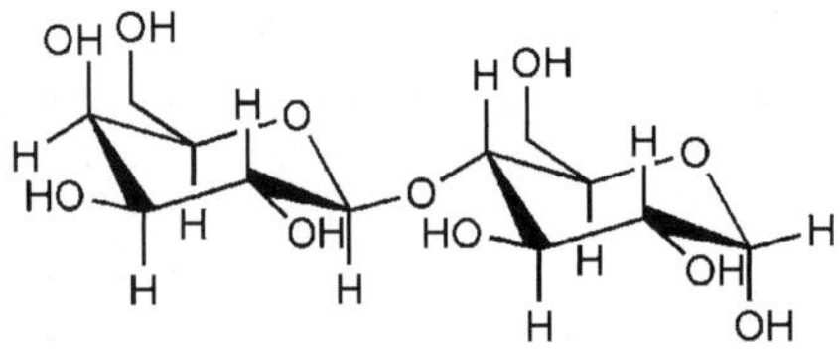

Lactose

Figure 2-1. Chemical structures of glucose and lactose.

b. Amylopectin—α(1–4) glucose chains with branches of α(1,6) glycosidic bonds).
c. Glycogen—α(1–4) glucose chains with highly branched α(1,6) glycosidic bonds, which is the principal carbohydrate storage molecule in vertebrates.
d. Cellulose—polymer of glucopyranose linked by β(1,4) glycosidic bonds. Major structural polysaccharide in plants.
e. Mucopolysaccharidoses are hereditary disorders (deficiency of lysosomal hydrolases, which degrade heparin sulfate or dermatan sulfate), which result in the accumulation of glycosaminoglycans in tissues.

C. Function of carbohydrates
1. Important source of energy.
2. Component of RNA and DNA.
3. Structural component of plants and animals.

D. Nutritional implications of carbohydrates
1. Monosaccharides are absorbed by a secondary active transport system (Na^+ and sugar cotransported) or facilitated diffusion.
2. Disaccharides are absorbed by secondary active transport followed by digestion by brush border enzymes (lactase, maltase, sucrase).
3. Polysaccharides are digested by amylase secreted by the salivary glands and pancreas.
4. Refer to the metabolism section for discussion of regulation of blood glucose and glycogen metabolism.

1.2 Amino Acids and Proteins

A. Protein terminology
1. Amino acids—building blocks of proteins consisting of a carboxyl group, an amino group, and a distinctive side chain attached to the α carbon. Depending on the side chain, each amino acid has specific characteristics (Figure 2-2).

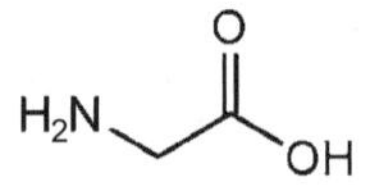

Glycine

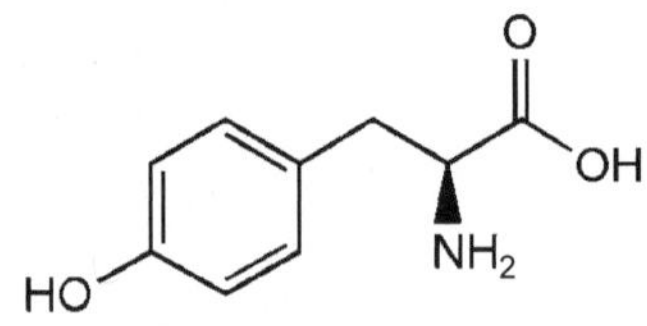

Tyrosine

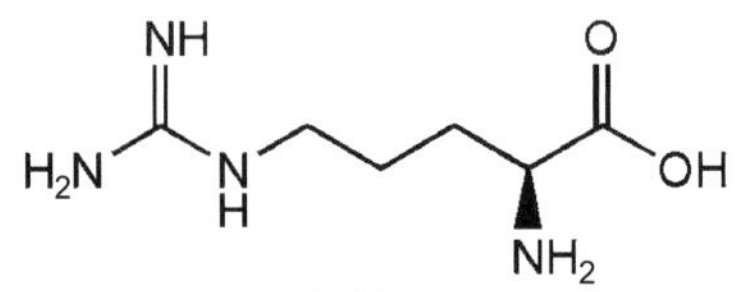

Arginine

Figure 2-2. Chemical structures of three amino acids.

a. Nonpolar side chains (glycine, alanine, valine, leucine, isoleucine, phenylalanine, tryptophan, methionine, and proline). These promote hydrophobic interactions.
b. Uncharged polar side chains (asparagine, cysteine, glutamine, tyrosine, threonine, serine). These have no charge at neutral pH but may participate in hydrogen bond formation with other compounds.
c. Acidic side chains (aspartic acid, glutamic acid). These have negative charges at neutral pH due to the charge on the carboxyl group.
d. Basic side chains (arginine, lysine, and histidine). Have positive charges at neutral pH due to the ability to accept protons.
e. Peptide bond—a covalent linkage that is formed between the free amino end of the peptide or amino acid and the free carboxyl end of the peptide or amino acid. It is responsible for the formation of the primary structure of a protein.

2. Characteristics of weak acids and weak bases. The Henderson-Hasselbalch equation describes the relationship between pK and pH. Can be used to determine the dissociation of ionizable groups at a given pH.

a. pH = –log [H^+].
b. pK of an acid is defined as the pH at which the acid is half-dissociated. pK = –log K.
c. Hydrogen bond—responsible for the secondary structure of proteins. Formed through interactions of the carbonyl oxygens and amide hydrogens that are a part of the peptide.
   (1) α helix—coiled polypeptide core with amino acid side chains extending outward to avoid steric interference. Keratins and myoglobin are examples.
   (2) β sheets—characterized by hydrogen bonds between two or more polypeptide chains.
d. Tertiary structure—the three-dimensional structure of a protein due to side chain interactions of the peptide. May be due to hydrophobic or hydrophilic interactions, hydrogen binding, disulfide bonds, or ionic interactions.
e. Hydrophilic groups—amino acids that are found on the surface of the molecule. Responsible for tertiary structure of proteins.
f. Hydrophobic groups—amino acids that are found in the interior of the molecule. Responsible for tertiary structure of proteins.
g. Disulfide bonds—a covalent link between cysteine groups, which results in a folding of the primary structure. Also responsible for the tertiary structure of protein.
h. Protein misfolding is associated with a number of diseases (amyloidoses), including Alzheimer disease and bovine spongiform encephalopathy (mad cow disease).
i. Hemoglobinopathies are disorders produced by abnormal hemoglobin molecules or insufficient amounts of the globular protein. Examples include sickle cell anemia (abnormal β chain of the globulin molecule) and thalassemia (imbalance of α and β chains).

1.3 Lipids

A. Lipid terminology
1. Fatty acids are straight-chained compounds containing an even number of hydrocarbons. They possess a terminal carboxyl group that provides polarity to the molecule. Because of this characteristic, fatty acids are amphipathic (contain both hydrophilic and hydrophobic moieties).
   a. Saturated fatty acid—contains no double bonds.
   b. Unsaturated fatty acid—contains double bonds that are identified with δ or ω terminology. May be either monounsaturated or polyunsaturated.
   c. Triacylglycerols (triglycerides)—esters of glycerol and three fatty acids. These are hydrophobic since the carboxyl group is covalently linked to glycerol.
2. Essential fatty acids cannot be synthesized in the body.
   a. Linoleic acid.
   b. Linolenic acid.
   c. Arachidonic acid (if linoleic acid is missing from the diet).
3. Lipoproteins—a complex consisting of a hydrophobic core surrounded by a hydrophilic shell. Serves as a vehicle for transporting triacylglcerol and cholesterol in plasma. Based on density (protein content), they are classified into several categories (see Lipoproteins, B.3. below).
4. Cholesterol—characterized by a four-ring sterol ring, hydrocarbon (hydrophobic) tail, and hydroxyl (polar) site on the steroid nucleus.

B. Classification of lipids
1. Phospholipids—composed of glycerol or sphingosine, two fatty acids, and phosphoric acid. They are an important component of membranes since they have hydrophobic (fatty acid) and hydrophilic (phosphoric acid) domains. In an aqueous environment, they form bimolecular layers, which are the biological basis of membranes.
   a. Phosphoglycerides—composed of glycerol, fatty acids, and phosphate.
      (1) Phosphatidic acid (PA) is a common precursor of other phosphoglycerides.
      (2) PA and serine = phosphatidylserine (important component of membranes).
      (3) PA and ethanolamine = phosphatidylethanolamine or cephalin (important for mitochondrial activity).
      (4) PA and choline = phosphatidylcholine or lecithin (major constituent of surfactant).

(5) Respiratory distress syndrome is caused by the inability to synthesize surfactant (dipalmitoyllecithin).
(6) PA and inositol = phosphatidylinositol (precursor of second messengers diacylglycerol and inositol trisphosphate) (Figure 2-3).
(7) PA and glycerol = phosphatidylglycerol.

b. Sphingophospholipids—composed of sphingosine, fatty acid, phosphoric acid, and choline. Sphingomyelin, a member of this group, is an important constituent of myelin.

2. Glycolipids (glycosphingolipids)—composed of carbohydrate, sphingosine, and fatty acid. These compounds are often found on plasma membrane surfaces, especially in nervous tissue. Gangliosides are members of this group and appear to have a role in receptor function.
3. Lipoproteins (found in plasma)
   a. Chylomicron—composed primarily of dietary triacylglycerol.
   b. Very-low-density lipoprotein (VLDL)—transports endogenous triacylglycerol from liver to cells.
   c. Intermediate-density lipoprotein (IDL)—returns endogenous cholesterol to liver.
   d. Low-density lipoprotein (LDL)—transports cholesterol from liver to cells.
   e. High-density lipoprotein (HDL)—transports cholesterol from cells to IDL and LDL and back to the liver.
4. Apoproteins
   a. Apo A required for cholesterol transport from peripheral tissue to the liver.

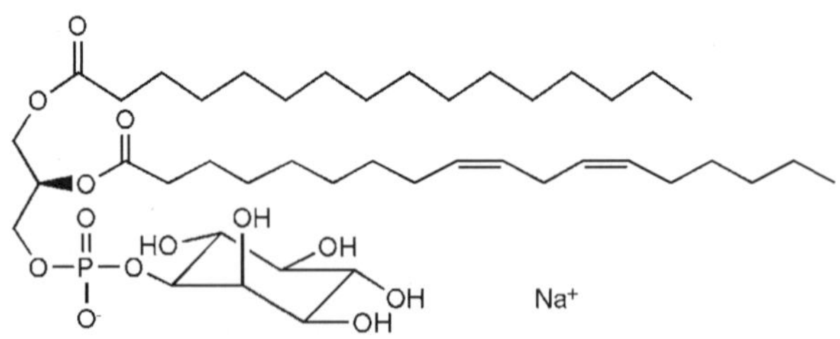

Phosphatidylinositol

Figure 2–3. Structure of phosphatidylinositol, showing the inositol bound to the phosphate group, which is attached to the glycerol backbone. Two fatty acids, palmitic and linoleic (unsaturated), are shown in ester linkage to glycerol.

   b. Apo B is required for binding of LDL to cell surface receptors.
   c. Apo C regulates the activity of lipoprotein lipase.
   d. Apo E is required for the removal of chylomicrons and IDL from plasma.

C. Function of lipids
   1. Component of biological membranes (phospholipids and sphingolipids).
   2. Facilitate the interactions between membrane proteins and hydrophobic environments in the membrane (a function, for instance, of covalent modification of the protein with myristic and palmitic acids).
   3. Source of energy (triacylglycerol).
   4. Provides insulation and protection (triacyglycerol).
   5. Precursor of hormones and intracellular messengers (fatty acids).
   6. Precursor of steroid hormones, bile acids and salts, membranes (cholesterol).

D. Nutritional implication of lipids
   1. Essential fatty acids—cannot be synthesized by mammals and therefore must be obtained from the diet (linoleic and linolenic). Arachidonic acid is synthesized from linoleic acid. Arachidonic acid is a precursor of the eicosanoids, which function as hormone-like molecules in most tissues (Figure 2-4). Prostaglandins, thromboxanes, and leukotrienes are examples of these molecules. If linoleic acid is missing from the diet, arachidonic acid becomes essential.
   2. Nonessential fatty acids—can be synthesized by enzyme systems in the body.
   3. In general, the more saturated the fat, the more solid it is at room temperature.
   4. Triacyglycerols release 9.3 kcal/g and therefore are an important source of energy.

1.4 Nucleic Acids and Metabolism

A. Nucleic acid terminology (Figure 2-5):
   1. Nucleic acids—complex molecules that combine with several different classes of smaller molecules to form either deoxyribonucleic acid or ribonucleic acid.
   2. Bases of nucleic acids
      a. Purines (adenine and guanine).
      b. Pyrimidines (cytosine, thymine, and uracil).

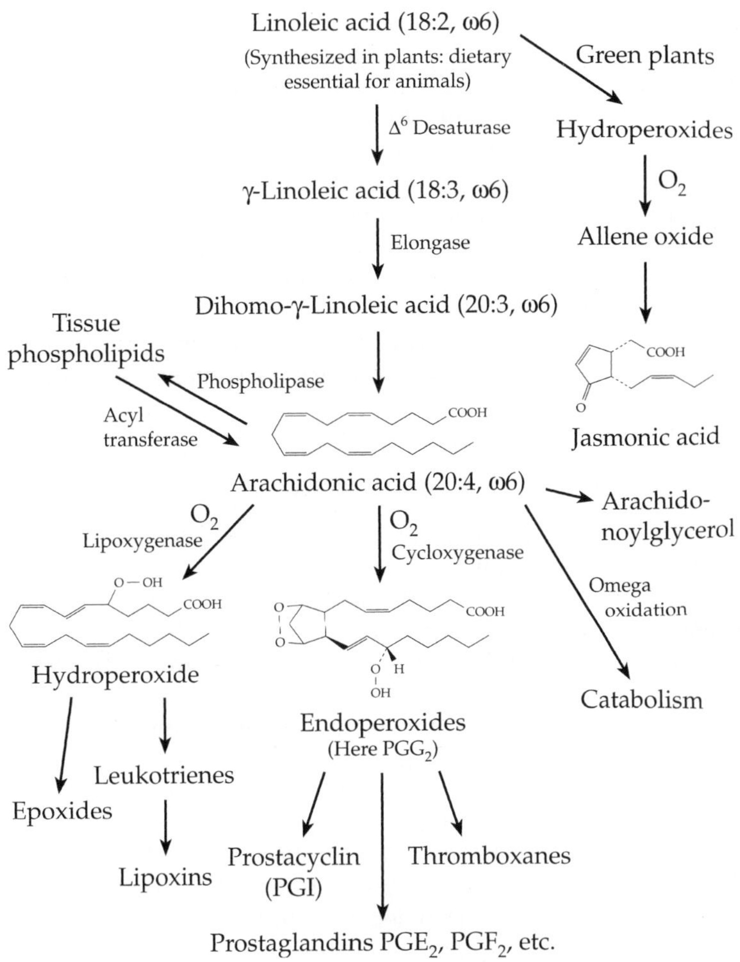

Figure 2–4. Arachidonic acid is a precursor of the eicosanoids, which function as hormone-like molecules in most tissues. (From Metzler DE: Biochemistry, ed 2, Academic Press, San Diego, 2003.)

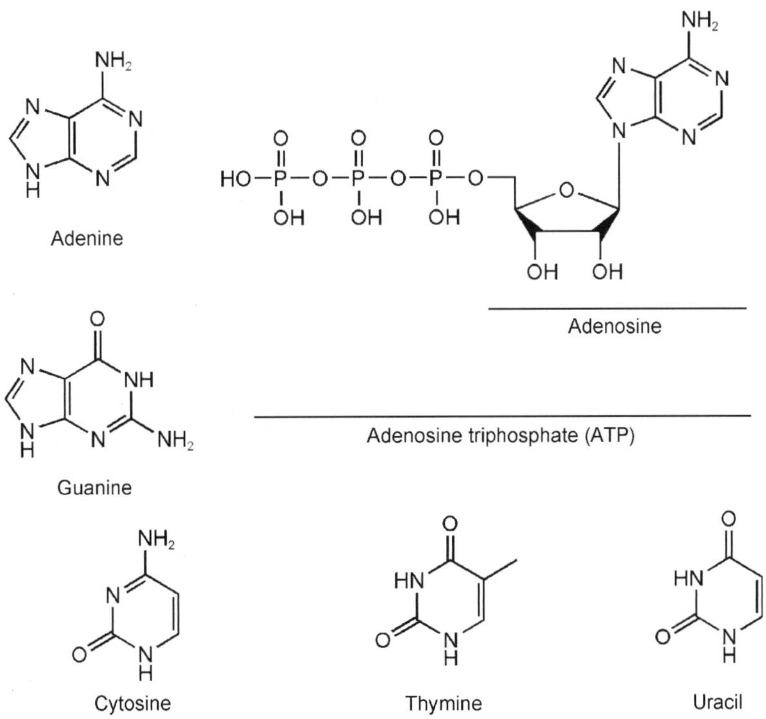

Figure 2–5. Chemical structures of the purines, adenine, and guanine and pyrimidines, cytosine, thymine, and uracil. The structures of the nucleoside, adenosine, and the nucleotide, adenosine triphosphate, are also shown.

3. Nucleosides—compounds formed when either a purine or pyrimidine base is linked to a sugar molecule. Examples:
   a. Adenine + ribose = adenosine.
   b. Cytosine + deoxyribose = deoxycytidine.
4. Nucleotides—the molecule formed by linking phosphate groups to nucleosides. Examples:
   a. Adenine + ribose + phosphate = adenosine monophosphate.
   b. Cytosine + deoxyribose + phosphate = deoxycytidine monophosphate.
5. Adenonosine triphosphate (ATP)—high-energy nucleotide used as an energy source in numerous biological systems.
6. Polynucleotides—by removing a molecule of water between the phosphate group of one nucleotide and the sugar group of the other (phosphate–ester bond), a polynucleotide chain is formed. The chains formed are either polyribonucleotides (RNA) or polydeoxyribonucleotides (DNA).
7. Transcription—making RNA from DNA.
8. Translation—the production of a polypeptide using an mRNA template.

B. Classification of nucleic acids
1. DNA
   a. Composed of four bases linked to deoxyribose and phosphate.
      (1) Adenine
      (2) Guanine
      (3) Cytosine
      (4) Thymine
   b. Consists of two strands of nucleotides in the form of a double helix.
   c. The double helix is held together by hydrogen bonds.
   d. Only adenine and thymine and guanine and cytosine are paired. Thus, the two strands are said to be complementary.
2. RNA
   a. Composed of four bases linked to ribose and phosphate.
      (1) Adenine
      (2) Guanine
      (3) Cytosine
      (4) Uracil
   b. Types of RNA
      (1) Ribosomal RNA (rRNA)—integral component of ribosomes, the site of protein synthesis.
      (2) Messenger RNA (mRNA)—carries the genetic information of DNA to the site of protein synthesis.
      (3) Transfer RNA (tRNA)—transfers amino acids to the site of protein synthesis.

C. Function of nucleic acids
1. DNA is responsible for transmitting genetic information from generation to generation.
2. RNA transmits the genetic information stored in DNA for the synthesis of proteins.

1.5 Nutrients and Minerals

A Vitamins—traditionally divided into fat and water-soluble vitamins. Vitamins A, D, K, and E are fat-soluble, and the remaining nine are water-soluble. Due to the ability of the fat-soluble vitamins to be retained in lipid throughout the body, the potential for toxicity is, in general, greater than that of the water-soluble vitamins.

1. Thiamin (B_1)
   a. Coenzyme form: thiamine pyrophosphate.
   b. Involved in two key cell reactions: decarboxylation and transketolation.
   c. Deficiency results in the impairment of carbohydrate metabolism and lipid biosynthesis. Beriberi is a disease of the peripheral nerves caused by thiamin deficiency.
2. Riboflavin (B_2)
   a. Coenzyme form: flavin mononucleotide (FMN) and flavin adenine dinucleotide (FAD).
   b. Catalyzes important reactions in the respiratory chain of cellular energy metabolism.
   c. Deficiency results in oral symptoms, including angular cheilosis and glossitis.
3. Nicotinamide (niacin)
   a. Coenzyme form: nicotinamide adenine dinucleotide (NAD) and nicotinamide adenine dinucleotide phosphate (NADP).
   b. Participates in reversible oxidation-reduction reactions that are necessary for the utilization of all major nutrients.
   c. Deficiency results in pellagra (dermatitis, diarrhea, and dementia). Oral symptoms are also possible.
4. Pantothenic acid
   a. Coenzyme form: coenzyme A.

   b. Involved in many reversible acetylation reactions in carbohydrate, fat, and amino acid metabolism.
5. Pyridoxine (B_6)
   a. Coenzyme form: pyridoxal phosphate.
   b. Involved in a number of enzyme systems essential for normal amino acid metabolism.
   c. Deficiency results in seborrheic dermatitis, cheilosis, glossitis, and stomatitis.
6. Biotin
   a. Functions as a coenzyme involved in the process of carboxylation.
   b. Works with acetyl CoA in reactions that transfer carbon dioxide from one compound to another.
7. Folic acid
   a. Coenzyme form: tetrahydrofolate.
   b. Plays a major role as an intermediate carrier of one-carbon units to appropriate metabolites in the synthesis of nucleic acids and porphyrin compounds.
   c. Since folic acid is essential for normal cell division and replication, a deficiency will manifest itself in the most rapidly growing tissues such as in bone marrow and the gastrointestinal tract. Megaloblastic anemia is symptomatic of folic acid deficiency. Maternal deficiency is also associated with neural tube defects in pregnancy.
8. Cyanocobalamine (B_{12})
   a. Coenzyme form: adenosyl cobalamine.
   b. Plays a role in the transfer of single carbon intermediates (primarily methyl groups) from one compound to another.
   c. Deficiency is often found in individuals who lack the normal intrinsic factor for the proper absorption of vitamin B_{12}. This results in pernicious anemia characterized by a megaloblastic macrocytic anemia and progressive neurological degeneration.
9. Ascorbic acid (C)
   a. Plays a role in the metabolism of amino acids, in particular the final oxidation of phenylalanine and tyrosine. Also essential for the normal elaboration of the intercellular substance of collagenous and fibrous tissue in animals. As a cofactor in the enzymatic hydroxylation of proline to 4-hydroxyproline, it is required for the formation and maintenance of bone matrix, cartilage, dentin, collagen, and connective tissue in general.
   b. Deficiency results in scurvy, which exhibits symptoms related to connective tissue weakening.
10. Vitamin A
    a. Vitamin A plays a role in maintaining the normal structure and function of biological membranes both as components of intracellular organelles or peripheral cell membranes. Epithelial cells also depend upon vitamin A for optimal growth and integrity. The vitamin is also essential for osteoblast and osteoclast activity.
    b. Deficiency is associated with night blindness since retinol is limited and the amount of rhodopsin is decreased.
    c. Can be synthesized from carotenoids in the diet. Preformed vitamin A is potentially very toxic.
11. Vitamin E
    a. A generic name for a group of compounds with vitamin E activity, of which α-tocopheral is the most significant.
    b. Plays a major role in protecting cellular and subcellular membranes from deterioration. As an antioxidant, vitamin E protects the polyunsaturated fatty acids in lipid membranes from oxidation.
12. Vitamin K
    a. The major function of vitamin K is to catalyze the posttranslational modification of blood-clotting factors in the liver. These include four factors:
       (1) Factor II, prothrombin.
       (2) Factor VII, serum prothrombin conversion factor.
       (3) Factor IX, plasma thromboplastin component.
       (4) Factor X, Stuart factor.
    b. Warfarin, a vitamin K analog, interferes with vitamin K activity.
13. Vitamin D
    a. Cholesterol serves as the precursor for the synthesis of vitamin D_3 (cholecalciferol). This step requires UV light.
    b. Enzymes in the liver (25-hydroxylase) and kidney (1-hydroxylase) are required for the synthesis of the active 1,25 dihydroxycholecalciferol.
    c. Vitamin D increases Ca^{2+} and P_i intestinal absorption and mobilization from bone.

   d. Deficiency results in rickets (children) and osteomalacia (adults).

B. Minerals—in biological systems, minerals are often associated with enzymes, and they function as cofactors. The following are examples of cofactors (minerals) and the enzymes with which they are associated:
   1. Fe^{2+} or Fe^{3+}—cytochrome oxidase, catalase, peroxidase.
   2. Cu^{2+}—cytochrome oxidase.
   3. Zn^{2+}—DNA polymerase, carbonic anhydrase, alcohol dehydrogenase.
   4. Mg^{2+}—hexokinase, glucose-6-phosphatase.
   5. Mn^{2+}—arginase.
   6. K^{+}—pyruvate kinase.
   7. Ni^{2+}—urease.
   8. Mo—nitrate reductase.
   9. Se—glutathione peroxidase.

2.0 METABOLISM

2.1 Bioenergetics

The study of the energy transductions that occur in living cells and the chemical processes underlying these transductions.

A. Terminology
   1. Entropy (δS)—degree of randomness in a system.
   2. Enthalpy (δH)—heat change during a chemical reaction due to differences in bond energy.
   3. Exergonic—the free energy of the products is lower than the free energy of the reactants ($\delta G < 0$). (Net energy is released as a result of the reaction.)
   4. Endergonic—the free energy of the products is higher than the free energy of the reactants ($\delta G > 0$). (Net energy is consumed as a result of the reaction.)
   5. Equilibrium constant (K_{eq})—the ratio of the concentration of products to reactants when the reaction reaches equilibrium. The larger the K_{eq}, the more favorable the reaction.
   6. Free energy (δG)—the energy that can drive a chemical reaction.
      a. Negative δG—the reaction proceeds in the direction written.
      b. Positive δG—the reaction goes in the opposite direction.
      c. δG is 0—the reaction is at equilibrium.
   7. Free energy of activation—energy required to reach the transition state.
   8. Transition state—highest energy arrangement of the atoms that occurs between the reactants and the products.
   9. Thermodynamics—the energy state of a system and the direction in which the reaction will proceed.
   10. Kinetics—the rate of the reaction and the factors that affect the rate. The rate of the reaction can be increased in two ways:
      a. Increase the temperature to activate more molecules to reach the transition state.
      b. Lower the activation of energy of the transition state by using a catalyst.

2.2 Enzymology

Enzymes are biological compounds that catalyze chemical reactions. Enzymes can alter the rates of reactions but cannot alter the equilibrium of the reaction. Most enzymes are highly specific since they associate with substrates through specific sites in the catalytic center of the enzyme.

A. Classification of enzymes
   1. Oxidoreductases—one substrate is oxidized, while at the same time, the other is reduced.
   2. Transferases—transfer functional groups between two substrates.
   3. Hydrolases—catalyze the hydrolysis of proteins, carbohydrates, and so forth.
   4. Lyases—remove two groups from a substrate, leaving a double bond.
   5. Isomerases—interconvert isomers.
   6. Ligases—catalyze the formation of covalent bonds, utilizing the hydrolysis of ATP or some other high-energy compound.

B. Michaelis-Menten equation—examines the kinetics of enzyme catalyzed reactions.

C. Enzyme kinetics plot (velocity versus substrate) (Figure 2-6):
   1. V_{max} = maximum velocity of the reaction.
   2. K_m = the substrate concentration at which the velocity is 50% of the maximum velocity.

D. Enzyme inhibition—numerous substances (including drugs and metabolites) can interfere with enzyme activity. This inhibition may be reversible or irreversible. Three types of reversible inhibitory mechanisms can be identified by enzyme kinetic plots.

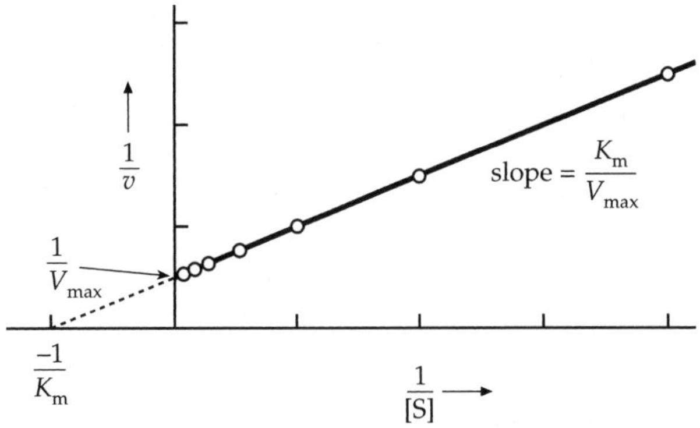

Figure 2–6. Double-reciprocal or Lineweaver-Burk plot of 1/v versus 1/[S]. The intercept on the vertical axis gives $1/V_{max}$ and the slope gives K_m/V_{max}. The intercept on the horizontal axis equals $-1/K_m$. (From Metzler DE: Biochemistry, ed 2, Academic Press, San Diego, 2003.)

1. Competitive inhibition
   a. Substances are similar to the substrate and therefore compete for binding at the active site.
   b. K_m is increased but there is no change in V_{max}.
2. Uncompetitive inhibition
   a. The inhibitor binds only to the substrate–enzyme complex.
   b. Both the V_{max} and K_m are reduced.
3. Noncompetitive inhibition
   a. The inhibitor can bind to the substrate-enzyme complex or free enzyme.
   b. V_{max} is decreased, but K_m is unaffected.

E. Enzyme regulation can occur by the following mechanisms:
1. Increased synthesis of the enzyme.
2. Activation or inactivation by proteolytic enzymes.
3. Activation or inactivation by covalent modification (phosphorylation).
4. Allosteric modification.
5. Degradation of enzymes by proteases.

F. Measurement of enzymes is useful in the diagnosis of disease. For example, alanine aminotransferase (liver damage), creatine kinase, troponin T, and lactate dehydrogenase (myocardial infarction).

2.3 Catabolism

The degradation of large complex molecules into smaller, simple products

A. Carbohydrate catabolism
1. Glycolysis (Figure 2-7)—a series of reactions that convert glucose to pyruvate or lactate. Also produce intermediate for other pathways of metabolism.
   a. The process is located in the cytosol.
   b. Under aerobic conditions, pyruvate, NADH, and ATP are produced.
   c. Under anaerobic conditions, lactate and ATP are produced by utilizing NADH.
   d. Important enzymes:
      (1) Hexokinase (most cells)—irreversible reaction trapping glucose in cell.
      (2) Glucokinase—found in liver; has high K_m and V_{max}.
      (3) Phosphofructokinase—irreversible reaction forming fructose-1,6-bisphosphate. The rate-limiting step in the pathway.
      (4) Pyruvate kinase—catalyzes the formation of ATP and production of pyruvate.
   e. Regulators
      (1) Hexokinase—inhibited by glucose 6-phosphate.
      (2) Glucokinase—via glucokinase regulatory protein.
         (a) Inhibited by fructose 6-phosphate.
         (b) Stimulated by glucose.
      (3) Phosphofructokinase—inhibited by ATP and citrate, stimulated by AMP and fructose-2, 6-bisphosphate.
      (4) Pyruvate kinase—in muscle activated by fructose-1, 6-bisphosphate and inhibited by ATP. In the liver, inhibited by ATP and alanine.
      (5) Lactic acidosis occurs when pyruvate metabolism is blocked.
   f. Endocrine regulation of glycolysis
      (1) Insulin stimulates.
      (2) Glucagon inhibits.
      (3) Epinephrine stimulates in muscle, inhibits in liver.
2. Pentose phosphate pathway
   a. Source of pentoses for nucleotide synthesis.
   b. Major source of NADPH for synthesis of fatty acids, cholesterol, steroids, and so forth.
   c. Overall reaction (glucose-6-P + 2 NADP $\rightarrow$ ribulose—5 P +CO_2 and 2 NADPH).
   d. Transketolase and transaldolase catalyze reversible reactions in the pathway.

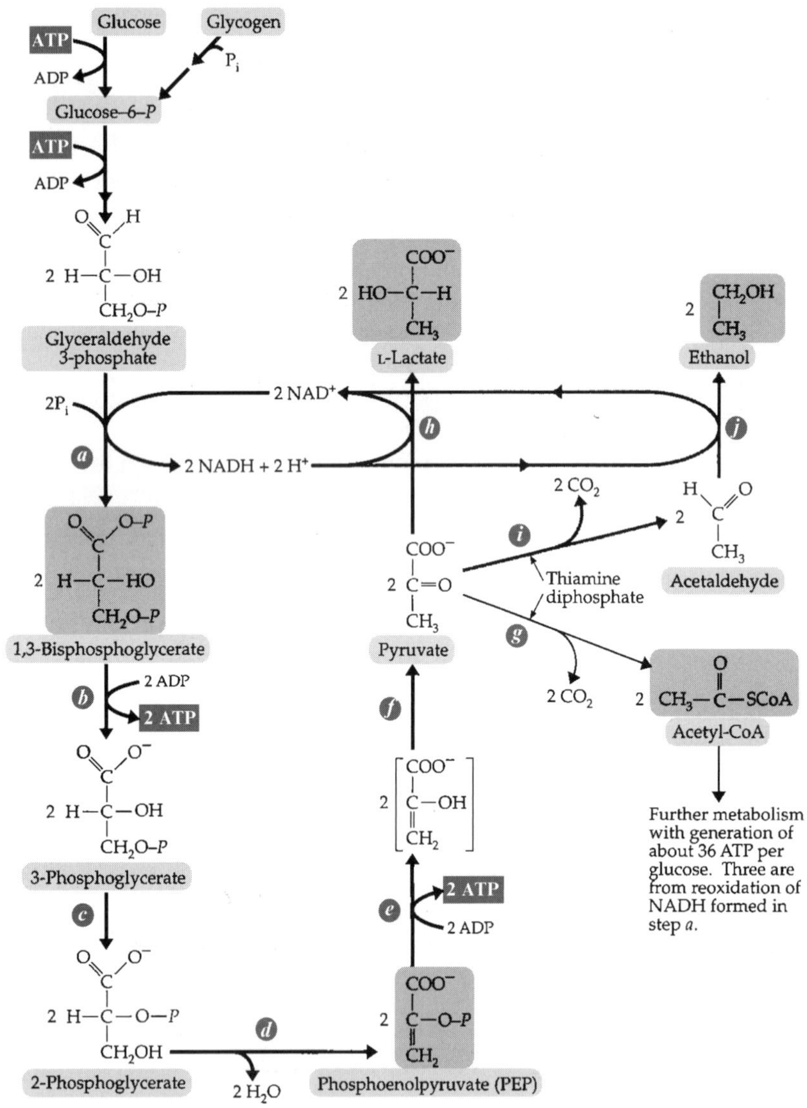

Figure 2–7. Coupling of the reactions of glycolysis with formation of lactic acid and ethanol in fermentations. Steps *a* through *g* describe the Embden-Meyerhof-Parnas pathway. Generation of 2 ATP in step *b* can provide all of the cell's energy. (From Metzler DE: Biochemistry, ed 2, Academic Press, San Diego, 2003.)

3. Tricarboxylic acid (TCA) cycle (Krebs cycle, citric acid cycle) (Figure 2-8):
   a. Metabolizes acetyl CoA to form ATP (12 molecules) and CO_2.
   b. Process located in mitochondria.
   c. Consists of eight reactions that require the following five coenzymes:
      (1) FAD
      (2) Thiamine pyrophosphate
      (3) Lipoic acid
      (4) Coenzyme A
      (5) NAD^+
   d. Provides substrates for biosynthetic processes.
      (1) Citrate used for fatty acid synthesis.
      (2) Succinyl CoA for heme synthesis.
      (3) Oxaloacetate for glucose synthesis.
      (4) Alpha ketoglutarate for nonessential amino acid synthesis.
   e. Important irreversible regulatory enzymes
      (1) Alpha ketoglutarate dehydrogenase—inhibited by NADH.
      (2) Citrate synthase—inhibited by NADH.
      (3) Isocitrate dehydrogenase—inhibited by ATP and stimulated by ADP. This also is the rate-limiting step in the cycle.
   f. Overall reaction (each acetyl CoA = 12 ATP)
      (1) Acetyl CoA + 3 NAD + FAD + GTP + P_i = 2 CO_2 + 3 NADH + $FADH_2$ + GTP.

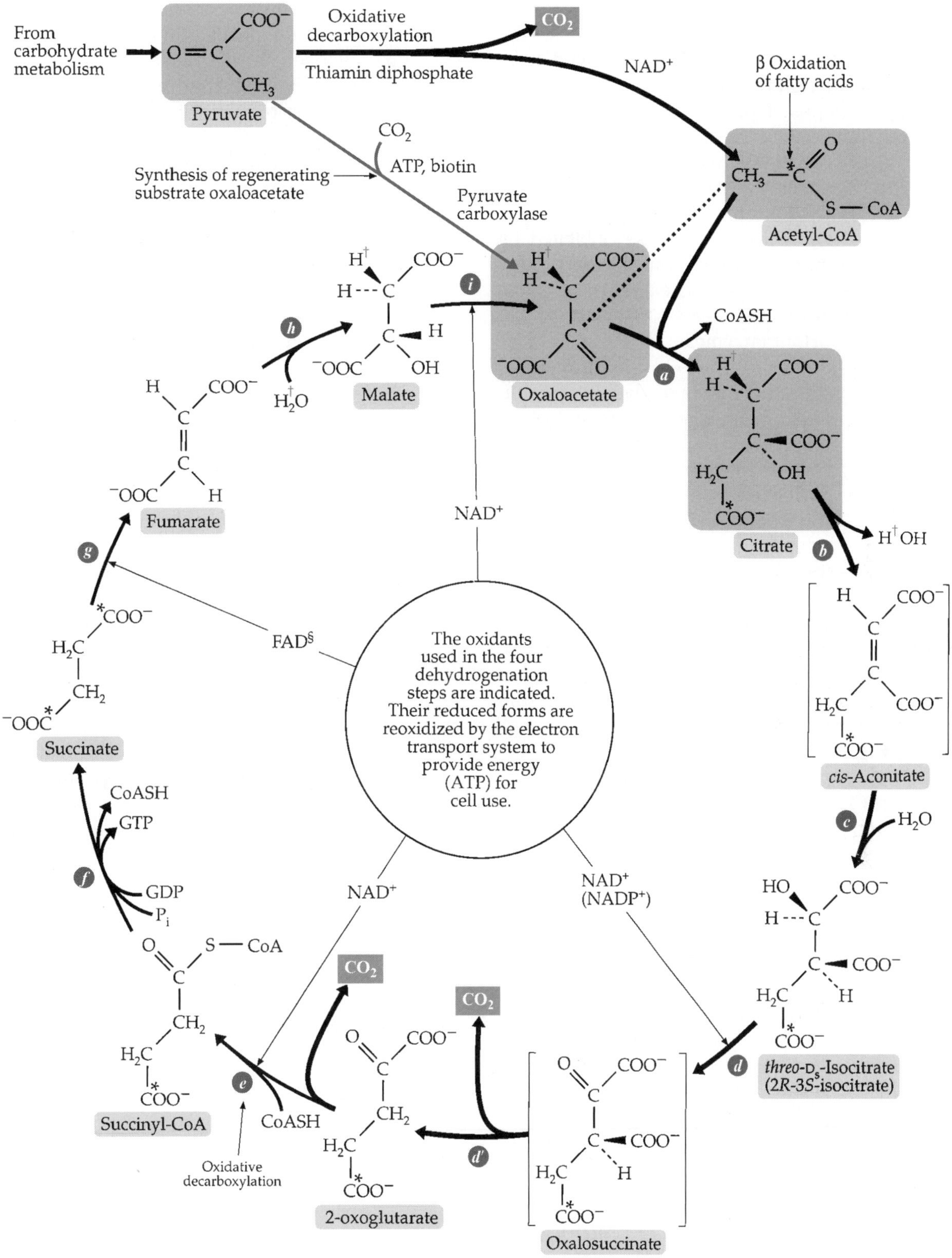

Figure 2–8. Reactions of the citric acid cycle (Krebs tricarboxylic acids cycle). Asterisks designate positions of labeled carboxyl groups from acetate introduced into the cycle. Note that it is *not* the two-carbon atoms from acetyl CoA that are immediately removed as CO_2, but two atoms from oxaloacetate. Only after several turns of the cycle are the carbon atoms of the acetyl CoA completely converted to CO_2. Nevertheless, the cycle can properly be regarded as a mechanism of oxidation of acetyl groups to CO_2. Daggers (†) designate the position of ^2H introduced into malate as $^2H^+$ from the medium. FAD§ designates covalently bound 8-histidyl-FAD. 2-oxyglutarate = α-ketoglutarate. (From Metzler DE: Biochemistry, ed 2, Academic Press, San Diego, 2003.)

4. Electron transport chain (Figure 2-9):
   a. Located in the mitochondria where NADH and $FADH_2$ are produced from oxidation reactions.
   b. Composed of four protein complexes (all contain iron):
      (1) NADH-CoQ reductase.
      (2) Succinyl-CoQ reductase.
      (3) Cytochrome c reductase.
      (4) Cytochrome c oxidase (inhibited by cyanide, carbon monoxide, and azide).
5. Glycogenolysis—the breakdown of glycogen to form glucose.
   a. Important enzymes
      (1) Phosphorylase—phosphorylates the α 1, 4 bonds of glycogen, resulting in the release of glucose 1-phosphate.
      (2) Debranching enzyme and α 1, 6 glucosidase—responsible for cleaving α 1, 6 bonds in a two-step process to release glucose-1-phosphate and free glucose.
   b. Regulation
      (1) Glucagons and epinephrine through cAMP activate protein kinases, which phosphorylate the phosphorylase enzyme, converting it to the active form of the enzyme.
      (2) Insulin dephosphorylates the phosphorylase enzyme, inactivating it.
      (3) Allosteric inhibitors of phosphorylase include ATP, creatine phosphate, and glucose-6-phosphate.
      (4) Allosteric stimulators include AMP and glucose (in liver).
6. Glycogen storage disease refers to a number of diseases that result from defects in enzymes required for glycogen synthesis or glycogen degradation (Von Gierke disease results from deficiencies of glucose-6-phosphatase).

B. Lipid catabolism (Figure 2-10):
1. β oxidation—the process by which fatty acids are broken down to acetyl CoA and ultimately utilized as a source of energy in the TCA cycle.
2. The process is located in the mitochondria.
3. Fatty acids are delivered to the mitochondria from cytoplasm by the carnitine shuttle.
   a. Two enzymes are involved in transporting large fatty acids into mitochondria:
      (1) Carnitine acyltransferase-1—associates carnitine with the fatty acid to form acyl carnitine (releases CoA).
      (2) Carnitine acyltransferase-2—reassociates the fatty acid with CoA. This enzyme is inhibited by malonyl CoA.
4. Important enzymes for β oxidation
   a. Fatty acyl CoA dehydrogenases—specific for fatty acids of different chain lengths. Ultimately this produces a β ketoacyl CoA and NADH.
   b. Thiolase—adds a CoA, which results in the release of acetyl CoA.

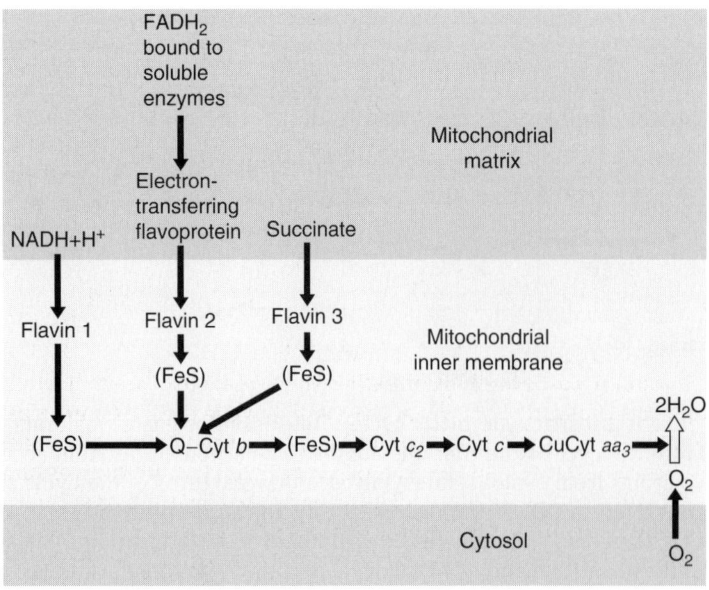

Figure 2–9. An abbreviated version of the electron transport chain of mitochondria. Four electrons reduce O_2 to $2H_2O$. (From Metzler DE: Biochemistry, ed 2, Academic Press, San Diego, 2003.)

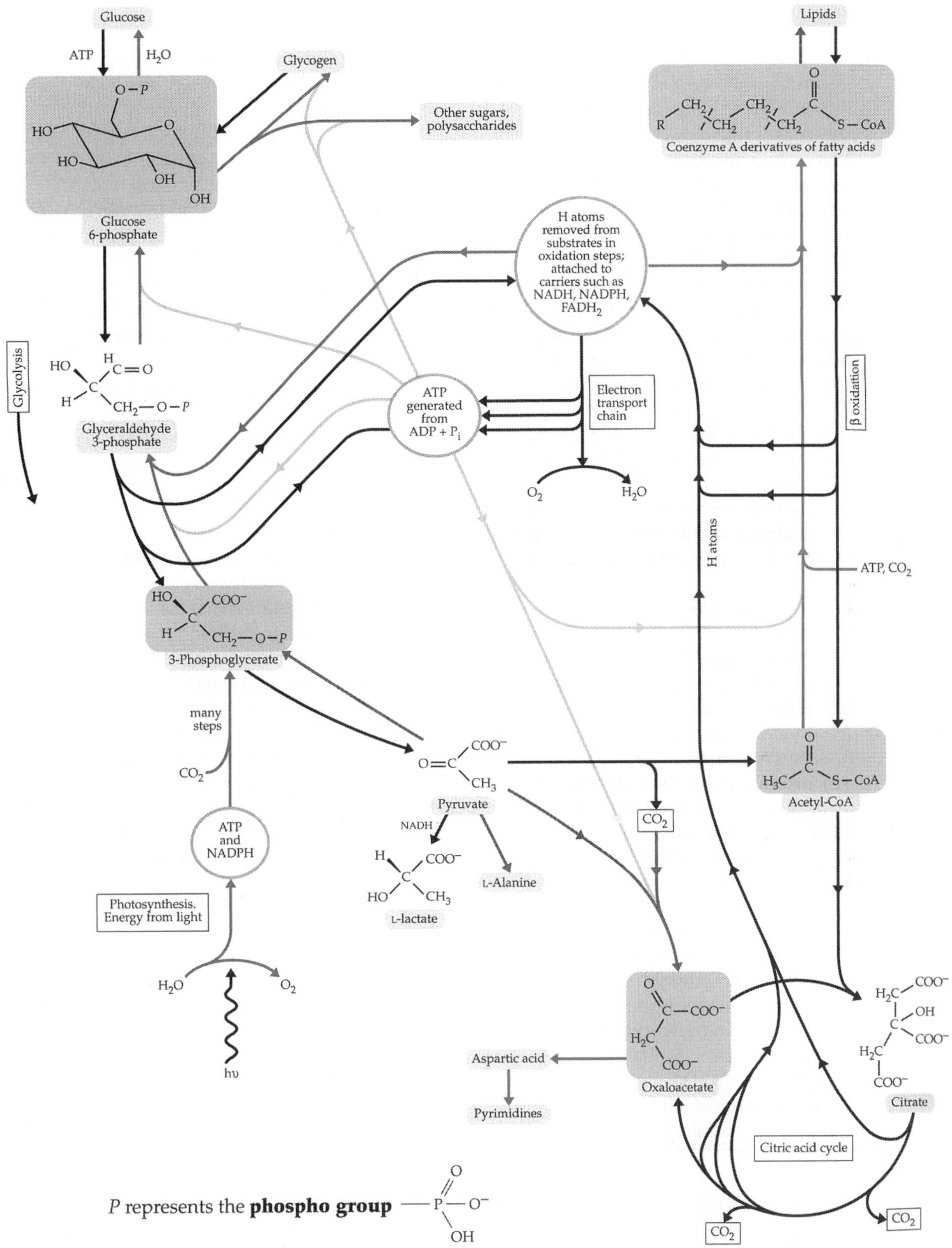

Figure 2–10. An overall view of some metabolic sequences. Several major pathways of catabolism are indicated by heavy lines. The glycolysis pathway, leading to pyruvate and lactate, starts at the top left, while the β oxidation pathway of fatty acids is on the right. Biosynthetic routes are shown in thin, dark lines. A few of the points of synthesis and utilization of ATP are indicated by light lines. Some of the oxidation–reduction reactions that produce or utilize the reduced hydrogen carriers NADH, NADPH, and $FADH_2$ are also indicated. The citric acid cycle, a major supplier of these molecules, is shown at the bottom right, while photosynthesis, the source of reduced hydrogen, carries in green plants, and the source of nearly all energy for life, is shown at the bottom left. (From Metzler DE: Biochemistry, ed 2, Academic Press, San Diego, 2003.)

5. Regulators
   a. Regulation of lipid catabolism is primarily through activation of hormone-sensitive lipase, which degrades triglycerides into fatty acids and glycerol. Free fatty acids readily enter the cell and become fatty acid acyl CoA by fatty acyl CoA synthetase.
      (1) Glucagons, epinephrine, and ACTH stimulate lipase.
      (2) Insulin inhibits lipase.
6. Ketone metabolism—under conditions of reduced intake of carbohydrate and increased β oxidation of fatty acids, ketone bodies are formed. Since most of the oxaloacetate is being utilized for gluconeogenesis, acetyl CoA resulting from β oxidation cannot be condensed and further metabolized in the TCA cycle. Acetyl CoA is then conserved by converting it to acetoacetate and β-hydroxybutyrate in the liver.
   a. Ketone bodies may serve as a source of energy for extrahepatic tissues.
      (1) Heart
      (2) Skeletal muscle
      (3) Kidney
      (4) Brain
   b. Accumulation of ketone bodies results in ketoacidosis.
   c. Ketoacidosis is associated with excessive fatty acid oxidation associated with a lack of insulin.
   d. Hyperlipidemia results from defects in lipoprotein metabolism.
      (1) Type I results from the accumulation of triglycerides.
      (2) Type II results from the accumulation of cholesterol.
      (3) Type III results from the accumulation of both triglyceride and cholesterol.

C. Cholesterol catabolism (Figure 2-11):
   1. Most cholesterol is eliminated from the body via the feces after conversion to bile salt in the liver.
      a. Cholic acid and chenodeoxycholic acid are the major bile acids.
      b. Bile salts are produced by the addition of an amino acid to the bile acid.
         (1) Glycocholate (cholic acid and glycine).
         (2) Glycochenodeoxycholic (chenodeoxycholic acid and glycine).
         (3) Taurine may also be added to bile acids to produce comparable bile salts.
   2. Enterohepatic circulation accounts for the resorption of most of the bile acids secreted from the liver.

D. Protein catabolism
   1. Two major enzyme systems are responsible for protein degradation:
      a. Ubiquitin-proteosome mechanism—proteins tagged with molecules of ubiquitin are recognized by the proteolytic molecule proteasome, which degrades the protein to amino acids.
      b. Lysosomes—primarily responsible for digesting extracellular enzymes.
   2. Pyridoxal phosphate (vitamin B_6) is an important coenzyme in transamination reactions using a class of enzymes known as *aminotransferases*. This is important since the products of this reaction (α keto acids and glutamate) can be used as amino group donors for the synthesis of essential amino acids (glutamate) or enter metabolic pathways for energy metabolism (α keto acids).
   3. The liver is the main site for amino acid catabolism where amino groups are removed, converted to urea, and excreted.
   4. Every amino acid has a corresponding α keto acid that can be metabolized for energy.
      a. α ketoglutarate (glutamate).
      b. Oxaloacetate (aspartate).
      c. Pyruvate (alanine).
   5. The carbon groups are further metabolized to pyruvate, acetyl CoA, acetoacetyl CoA, α ketoglutarate, succinyl CoA, fumarate, or oxaloacetate.
   6. Peripheral amino acids can be transported to the liver as part of alanine (alanine aminotransferase), glutamate (glutamate aminotransferase), or glutamine.
   7. Phenylketonuria, caused by a deficiency of phenylalanine hydroxylase, results in the inability to metabolize phenylalanine. Aspartame, since it contains phenylalanine, is also contraindicated in individuals with this deficiency.
   8. Maple syrup urine disease is caused by a deficiency in branched-chain α ketoacid dehydrogenase.
   9. Albinism is caused by a defect in tyrosine metabolism and subsequent inability to produce melanin.
   10. Since these enzymes are normally intracellular enzymes, elevated plasma levels of aminotransferases indicate damage to tissues containing cells rich in these enzymes (i.e., the liver).

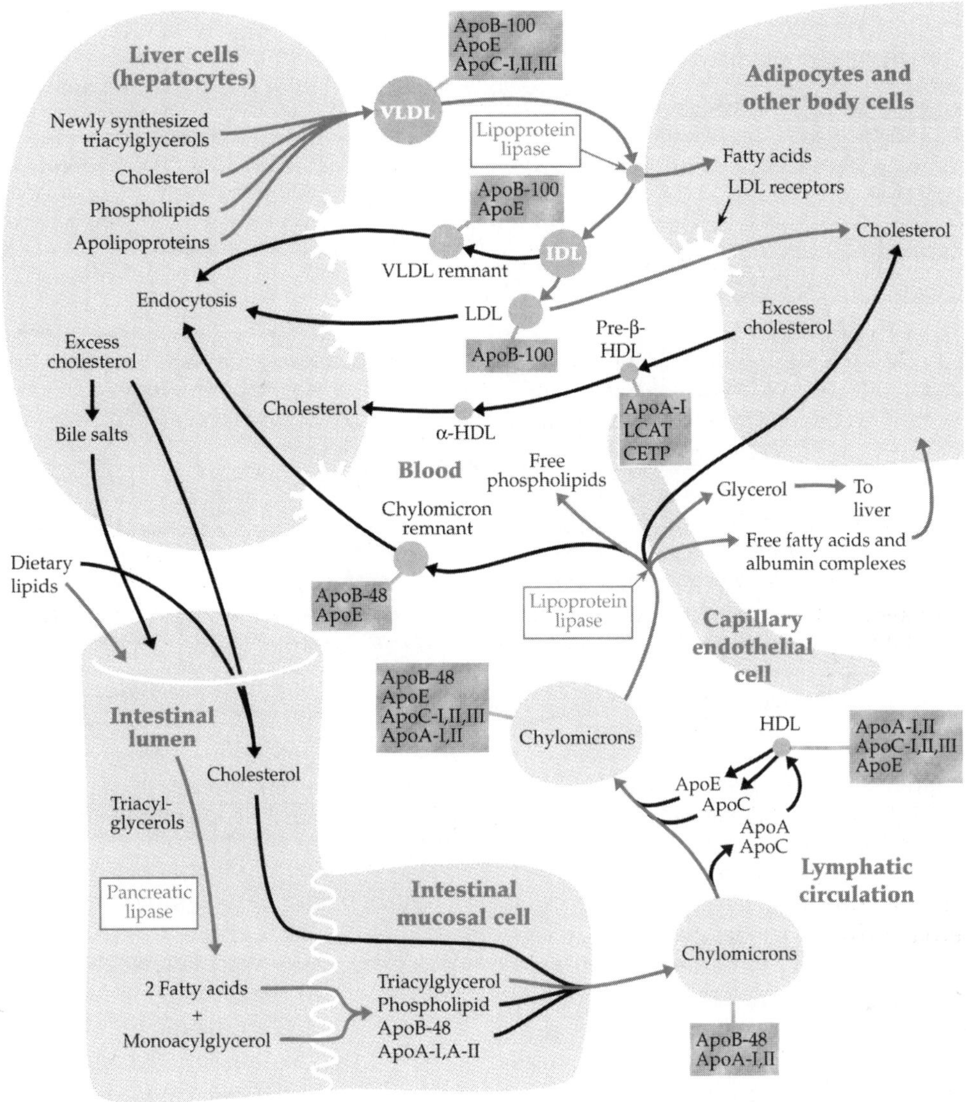

Figure 2–11. Movement of triacylglycerols from liver and intestine to body cells and lipid carriers of blood. *VLDL*, very-low-density lipoprotein that contains triacylglycerols, phospholipids, cholesterol, and apolipoproteins B and C; *IDL*, intermediate-density lipoproteins found in human plasma; *LDL*, low-density lipoproteins that have lost most of their triacylglycerols. (From Metzler DE: Biochemistry, ed 2, Academic Press, San Diego, 2003.)

11. Only the liver can make urea since it is the only tissue that has arginase. Four ATPs are needed for each cycle.
12. Urea cycle (Figure 2-12):

E. Nucleotide catabolism
   1. Purine nucleotides—degraded to uric acid through a series of reactions catalyzed by the following enzymes:
      a. Adenosine deaminase—removes the amino group.
      b. 5′ nucleotidase—converts the nucleotide to nucleoside.
      c. Purine nucleoside phosphorylase—releases the bases (guanine and hypoxanthine).
      d. Guanine is deaminated and hypoxanthine oxidized to xanthine.
      e. Xanthine is oxidized to uric acid.
      f. Gout—caused by the overproduction or under-excretion of uric acid.
   2. Pyrimidine nucleotides—pyrimidine ring is opened and degraded to β alanine and β aminoisobutyrate, which can be further metabolized in the citric acid cycle.

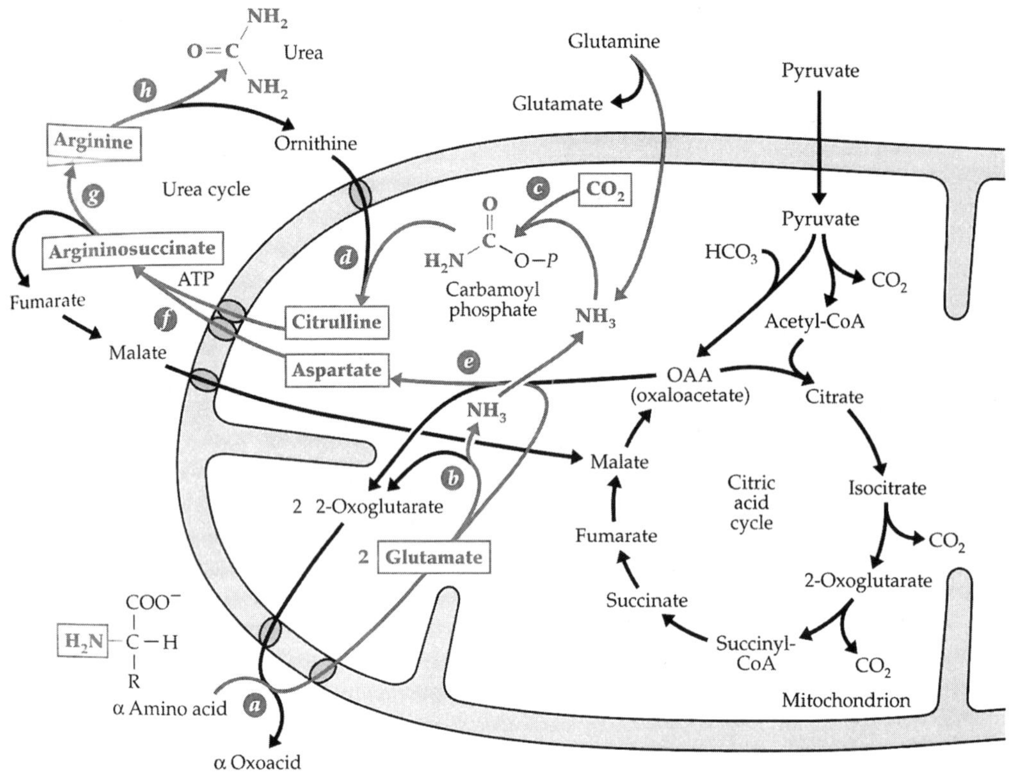

Figure 2–12. Integration of the urea cycle with mitochondrial metabolism. Thinner lines trace the flow of nitrogen into urea upon deamination of amino acids or upon removal of nitrogen from the side chain of glutamine. (From Metzler DE: Biochemistry, ed 2, Academic Press, San Diego, 2003.)

2.4 Anabolism

The process by which small simple compounds are used to synthesize more complex molecules, including carbohydrates, lipids, proteins, and nucleic acids.

A. Carbohydrate anabolism
   1. Glycogenesis—the process by which glucose is stored as a polymer consisting of α 1, 4 and α 1, 6 glycosidic bonds.
   2. Process occurs in the liver and muscle.
   3. Important enzymes for glycogen synthesis:
      a. Glycogen is synthesized from a series of reactions that utilize glucose-6-phosphate trapped within the cell by either glucokinase (liver) or hexokinase (muscle).
      b. Glucose-6-phosphate is converted to glucose-1-phosphate, which reacts with UTP, producing UDP-glucose (irreversible step).
      c. UDP-glucose is then added to a glycogen primer catalyzed by glycogen synthase (UDP-glycosyl transferase).
      d. Once the chain contains 6 to 11 residues, a branching enzyme transfers the oligosaccharide to an interior site of the glycogen molecule, creating an α 1, 6 glycosidic bond.
   4. Regulation of glycogen synthesis is by insulin that activates protein phosphatase 1, which, by removing phosphate groups from glycogen synthase, activates the enzyme.

B. Lipid anabolism—occurs when energy sources (acetyl CoA, citrate) are high.
   1. Synthesis of fatty acids occurs in the cytoplasm by sequential addition of two carbon units (acetyl CoA) to the carboxyl end.
   2. Acetyl CoA carboxylase (biotin serving as a coenzyme) catalyzes the rate-limiting step in the production of malonyl CoA, which is the committed step in the synthesis of fatty acids. The enzyme is regulated by two mechanisms:
      a. Allosteric control
         (1) Citrate activates.
         (2) Malonyl CoA, AMP inhibit.
      b. Covalent modulation (phosphorylation/dephosphorylation)

(1) Insulin activates.
(2) Epinephrine and glucagons inactivate.
3. Fatty acid synthase—a multienzyme complex that synthesizes palmitic acid.
   a. Utilizes NADPH as reducing source.
   b. Located in cytosol.
   c. Net reaction: 8 acetyl CoA + 7 ATP + 14 NADPH + H^+ → palmitate + 14 NADP + + 8 CoA + 6 H_2O + 7 ADP + 7 P_i.
4. Synthesis of triacylglycerides (triglycerides)
   a. Glycerol phosphate serves as the initial acceptor of the fatty acid. Glycerol phosphate can be synthesized by glycolysis in liver and adipose cells or from glycerol in liver.
   b. The fatty acids are activated by thiokinases (CoA attachment).
   c. Final synthetic pathway involves the addition of the fatty acids and phosphate removal.

C. Cholesterol anabolism
1. Synthesized through a series of reactions from carbon atoms provided by acetyl CoA.
2. Rate-limiting step and control of synthesis is exerted through the regulation of HMG CoA reductase.
   a. Inhibitors of HMG CoA reductase—cholesterol, glucagons, glucocorticoids, bile acids, and medications (statin drugs).
   b. Stimulators of HMG CoA reductase—insulin, thyroxin, and fat ingestion.
3. Familial hypercholesterolemia is caused by a defect in the LDL receptor.

D. Protein anabolism
1. Protein synthesis involves transcription and translation of DNA and RNA (see Molecular Biology on following page).
2. Essential amino acids must be obtained in the diet, because humans cannot synthesize them in sufficient quantities (isoleucine, leucine, lysine, methionine, phenylalanine, valine, tryptophan, threonine).
3. Nonessential amino acids—can be synthesized in humans.
   a. Alanine—transamination from pyruvate.
   b. Aspartate—transamination from oxaloacetate.
   c. Asparginine—addition of ammonia to aspartate.
   d. Cysteine—skeleton from serine and sulfur from methionine.
   e. Glutamate—transamination from α-ketoglutarate.
   f. Glutamine—addition of ammonia to glutamate.
   g. Glycine—removal of hydroxymethyl from serine, de novo synthesis by action of glycine synthetase or oxidation of choline.
   h. Proline—from α ketoglutarate.
   i. Serine—from 3-phosphoglycerate and transamination.
   j. Tyrosine—from phenylalanine.
4. Products/utilization of individual amino acids
   a. Precursor of gamma-aminobutyric acid (GABA), important intermediate in transamination reactions.
   b. Alanine—important in gluconeogenesis.
   c. Glycine—precursor for purine and porphyrin synthesis.
   d. Aspartate—involved in purine synthesis, urea structure, and gluconeogenesis.
   e. Serine—source of one-carbon fragments for folic acid coenzymes.
   f. Proline—major collagen amino acid. Converted to hydroxyproline.
   g. Glutamine—major role in NH_4^+ metabolism and transfer of amino groups to sugars, pyrimidines, and purines.
   h. Histidine—precursor of histamine.
   i. Tyrosine—precursor of thyroxin, melanin, and catecholamines.
   j. Arginine—precursor of urea and creatine.
   k. Phenylalanine—precursor of tyrosine.
   l. Tryptophan—precursor of serotonin.
   m. Cysteine—precursor of taurine and source of sulfur.
   n. Methionine—precursor of cysteine, adenosylmethionine (transmethylation reactions), and source of sulfur.
   o. Nitric oxide (NO)—mediator of numerous physiological activities, including smooth muscle relaxation, macrophage stimulation, and inhibition of platelet aggregation. Its synthesis requires NO synthase. In the reaction arginine, O_2, and NADPH are converted to NO and citrulline.

E. Nucleotide anabolism
1. Purine biosynthesis
   a. Addition of amino group from glutamine to phosphoribosyl-1-pyrophosphate.

(amido-phoshoribosyl transferase catalyzes this committed step). This addition is inhibited by purines.
   b. Closure of rings by addition of single carbons utilizing tetrahydrofolate, biotin, and cobalamine.
   c. Purines can also be synthesized from intact bases obtained from dietary sources or nucleotide degradation.
2. Pyrimidine biosynthesis
   a. Orotate is synthesized from carbamyl phosphate in cytosol.
   b. Ribose phosphate is added followed by subsequent reductase reactions to form UMP, UTP, and CTP.

3.0 MOLECULAR AND CELLULAR BIOLOGY

3.1 DNA/RNA and Protein Synthesis

A. DNA
1. Structure and terminology (Figure 2-13):
   a. D-2-deoxyribose (2′ position lacks the hydroxyl group).
   b. Bases:
      (1) Purine bases (adenine and guanine).
      (2) Pyrimidine bases (thymine and cytosine).
   c. Deoxynucleosides—deoxyribose with a base covalently attached (glycosidic bond) to the 1′ hydroxyl group.
   d. Deoxynucleotides—a deoxynucleoside phosphorylated at the 5′ position. The number of phosphate groups may be one (mono), two (di) or three (tri) and will be named accordingly.
   e. Single-stranded DNA
      (1) Polymer of deoxynucleotides bound together by phosphodiester linkages.
      (2) By convention, the sequence of the polymer is always 5′ to 3′ based on the ribose hydroxyl groups.
   f. Double-stranded DNA (helix)
      (1) Bases in one strand are hydrogen-bonded to bases on complementary strand.
      (2) Base pairing—due to conformational restraints, bases must be paired.
         (a) Thymine pairs with adenine.
         (b) Guanine pairs with cytosine.

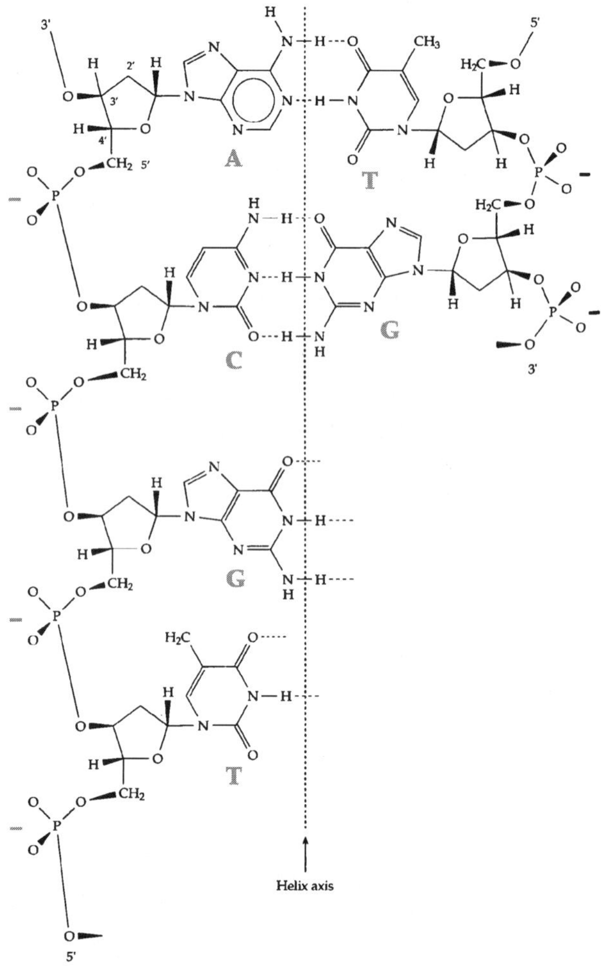

Figure 2–13. A distorted (flattened) view of the Watson-Crick structure of DNA showing the hydrogen-bonded base pairs. (From Metzler DE: Biochemistry, ed 2, Academic Press, San Diego, 2003.)

   g. Chromosomes—very long molecules of DNA-containing genes.
2. DNA replication
   a. DNA double helix is unwound by helicases, exposing single strands to serve as templates for reproduction.
   b. DNA polymerase III adds nucleoside triphosphates (5′ to 3′) under the direction of the template sequence. This is referred to as *chain elongation.*
   c. DNA polymerase I fills in regions of RNA primers, which are used to simultaneously replicate the complementary strand.
   d. Primase synthesizes RNA primers of the lagging (complementary) strand of DNA.

e. DNA ligase forms phosphodiester bonds between 5′ P and 3′ OH group of newly synthesized DNA fragments (Okazaki fragments).

B. RNA
1. Structure and terminology
a. Ribose.
b. Uracil replaces thymine as one of the pyrimidine bases.
c. Adenine pairs with uracil, and guanine pairs with cytosine.
d. Three types of RNA:
(1) Ribosomal (rRNA)—component of ribosomes that has catalytic function.
(2) Transfer RNA (tRNA)—delivers amino acids to ribosome. Cloverleaf structure contains an anticodon triplet of bases to base pair with mRNA.
(3) Messenger RNA (mRNA)—directs protein synthesis.
e. Codon—a triplet of mRNA bases that specifies an amino acid.
2. RNA synthesis
a. DNA serves as a template for replication (transcription).
b. Nucleoside triphosphates are polymerized into a chain catalyzed by RNA polymerase.
c. DNA template is read 3′ to 5′.
d. RNA is synthesized 5′ to 3′.
e. Transcription is terminated by Rho protein.

C. Protein synthesis (translation)—consists of three phases:
1. Initiation
a. Initiation factors GTP and mRNA associate with ribosome.
b. Met-tRNA anticodon binds to fMet codon (fMet = formyl methionine).
c. GTP is hydrolyzed, and the initiation complex is stabilized.
2. Elongation
a. Elongation factor GTP and a second amino acid tRNA bind to the neighboring site.
b. Once mRNA codon and tRNA codon are matched, GTP is hydrolyzed, forming a peptide bond between the amino acids.
c. Ribosome moves on the mRNA to the next site, and tRNA dissociates.
d. Elongation continues to termination.
3. Termination
a. Stop codon release factors bind to the ribosome.
b. Protein is released, and ribosome complex dissociates into subunits.
c. mRNA is released, terminating translation.

3.2 Genetic Engineering

A. Restriction endonucleases
1. Bacterial enzymes that hydrolyze double-stranded DNA at specific sites.
2. The resultant DNA fragments are able to be incorporated into a different DNA molecule utilizing DNA ligase.

B. Complementary DNA libraries
1. Complementary DNA (cDNA) is synthesized using reverse transcriptase, which uses mRNA as a template.
2. Multiple copies of cDNA can be made using DNA polymerase (polymerase chain reaction).
3. All the cell's expressed genes can be cloned once this library is made.

C. Polymerase chain reaction (PCR)
1. A sample of DNA is added to a mixture of RNA primer, dNTPs (deoxynucleotide triphosphates), and a thermophilic DNA polymerase.
2. The mixture is heated to separate the strands of DNA, which permits the primers to bind.
3. The mixture is cooled, and polymerase synthesizes complementary DNA.
4. The mixture is again heated, and strands separate, permitting primers to bind to DNA.
5. The mixture is cooled, permitting another synthesis of complementary DNA.
6. The process continues through many cycles, resulting in many copies.

D. Genetic transfer (genetic engineering)
1. Cloned cDNA is incorporated into a vector (bacterial plasmids, bacterial virus), which introduces the cDNA into a host DNA.
2. The host DNA is then able to express the cDNA product.

E. Terminology
1. Southern blots analyze DNA.
2. Northern blots analyze RNA.
3. Western blots analyze protein.
4. ELISA assays analyze protein.

3.3 Cell cycle for growth and division (Figure 2-14):

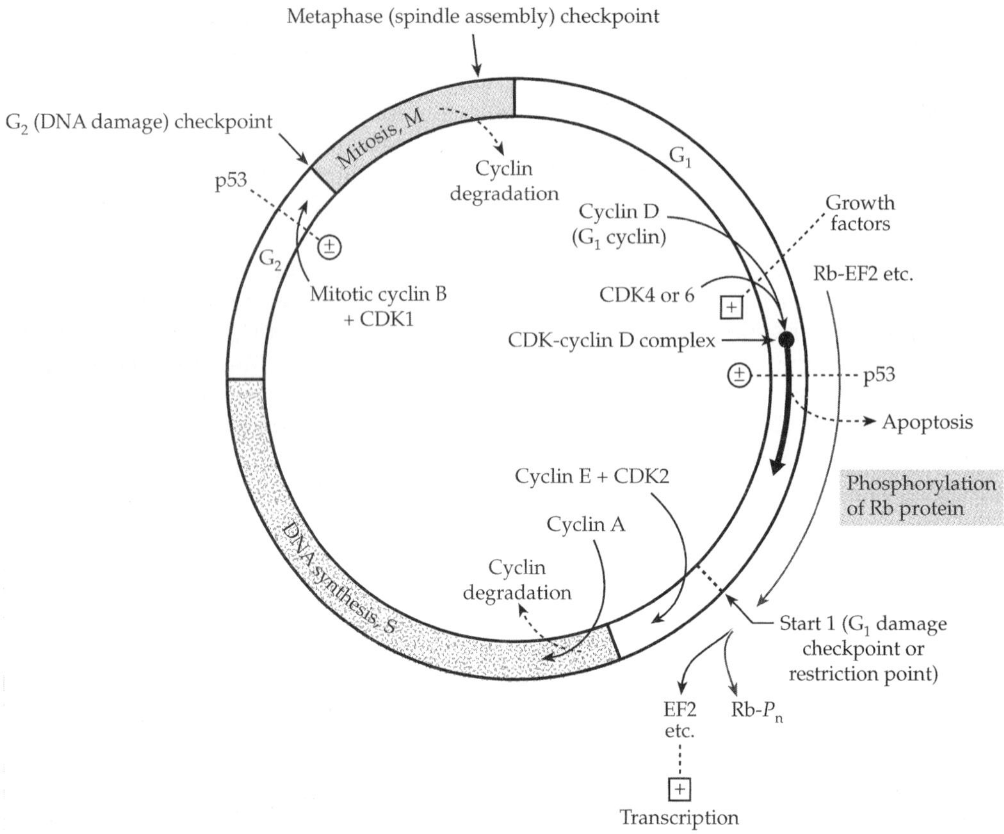

Figure 2–14. The cell cycle, which depicts the relative lengths of time for each stage of cell growth and division. After mitosis (*M*), the cell grows during the G_1 (gap) period. At the G_1 checkpoint, the cell prepares to divide, with DNA synthesis occurring during the S-phase. After a second gap (G_2), mitosis takes place to complete the cycle. (From Metzler DE: Biochemistry, ed 2, Academic Press, San Diego, 2003.)

4.0 CONNECTIVE TISSUE AND BONE

A. Collagen
1. Most abundant protein in humans, characterized by its high rigidity and tensile strength.
2. Approximately one-third of collagen is glycine (every third position), and 10% is proline.
3. Hydroxyproline and hydroxylysine are formed from proline and lysine, respectively, after translation (posttranslational modification). This requires ascorbate, Fe^{2+}, and O_2.
4. The tertiary structure is a triple helix (tropocollagen) formed by hydrogen bonds and modified by glycosylation of hydroxylysine.
5. Tropocollagen spontaneously aggregates, and crosslinks form between lysine and hydroxylysine.
6. Several types of collagen exist:
   a. Type I—skin, tendon, bone, dentine.
   b. Type II—cartilage.
   c. Type III—aorta, fetal skin.
   d. Type IV—basement membrane.
   e. Type V—placenta, skin.
7. Collagen is degraded by mammalian enzymes, which cleave tropocollagen. Cleavage of tropocollagen permits further digestion by proteases.
8. Osteogenesis imperfecta is an inherited disease that is due to an amino acid substitution in collagen that interferes with the normal folding of the protein into a triple helix conformation.

B. Elastin
1. Rich in proline and other nonpolar side chains. Approximately one-third of elastin amino acids are glycines.
2. Does not have a stable tertiary structure, but crosslinks are derived from lysine condensation.
3. Due to its elastic properties, it is found in arterial walls, lung pleura, and parenchyma.
4. Elastin is degraded by elastases synthesized by inflammatory cells or cells involved in tissue remodeling.

C. Keratin
1. Fibrous, insoluble proteins derived from epidermis.
2. Forms a helical structure stabilized by hydrogen bonds.
3. Overall properties depend on the degree of disulfide crosslinking.
   a. Low level of crosslinking—more flexibility (e.g., hair, skin).
   b. High level of crosslinking—less flexibility (e.g., nails).

D. Hydroxyapatite
1. $Ca_{10} (PO_4)_6 (OH)_2$.
2. Hydroxyapatite can vary in ion content. Most substituted ions increase the solubility of the crystal. Fluoride *lowers* the solubility.
   a. Ca^{+2} may be substituted by Mg^{2+}, Sr^{2+}, and Pb^{2+}.
   b. $PO_4^{\ 3-}$ may be substituted by HPO_4^- and citrate.
   c. OH^- may be substituted by Cl^-, F^-, and HCO_3^-.
3. Mineralization
   a. Supersaturated solutions of calcium and P_i (1.5 mM of each) may exist without hydroxyapatite formation (crystals of hydroxyapatite will promote precipitation).
   b. Increasing the concentration of calcium and P_i >3 mM of each results in the formation of amorphous calcium phosphate $CaHPO_4$-$2H_2O$ (brushite).
   c. Mineralization process
      (1) Initiation—ions become aligned on the surface of the initiator protein (phosphoryns).
         (a) Contain phosphorylated side chains for binding Ca^{2+}.
         (b) Cationic side chains attract PO_4^{3-} and OH^-.

Table 2–1. Composition of Calcified Tissue

TISSUE	% INORGANIC	% ORGANIC	% H_2O
Enamel	95	1	4
Dentin	70	20	10
Bone	60	25	15
Calculus	84	10	6

      (2) Crystal growth
         (a) Osteoblasts (and odontoblasts) secrete phosphoryns between collagen matrix.
         (b) Growth of crystals facilitated by concentrating Ca and P_i in matrix vesicles.
            (i) Phospholipid membrane vesicles produced by budding from osteoblasts.
            (ii) Calcium pump driven by ATP hydrolysis.
         (c) Composition of mineralized tissues (Table 2-1).

5.0 MEMBRANES

5.1 Structure

A. Lipid composition
1. Phospholipids—amphipathic compounds having a hydrophobic end (internally located) and a hydrophilic end (interfaces with internal and external aqueous environment). These compounds permit the formation of bilayer structures, which contain the following phospholipids:
   a. Phosphatidylcholine
   b. Phosphatidylinositol
   c. Phosphatidylserine
   d. Phosphatidylethanolamine
2. Cholesterol—stabilizes the membrane, maintains fluidity.
3. Glycolipids—have several functions:
   a. Surface markers to regulate tissue growth.
   b. Important for cell recognition.

B. Protein composition (Fig. 2-15)
1. Intrinsic or integral proteins.
   a. Mostly composed of hydrophobic amino acids.
   b. Difficult to remove from the membrane.
   c. Often extend through the entire thickness of the membrane.
   d. Examples include the following:

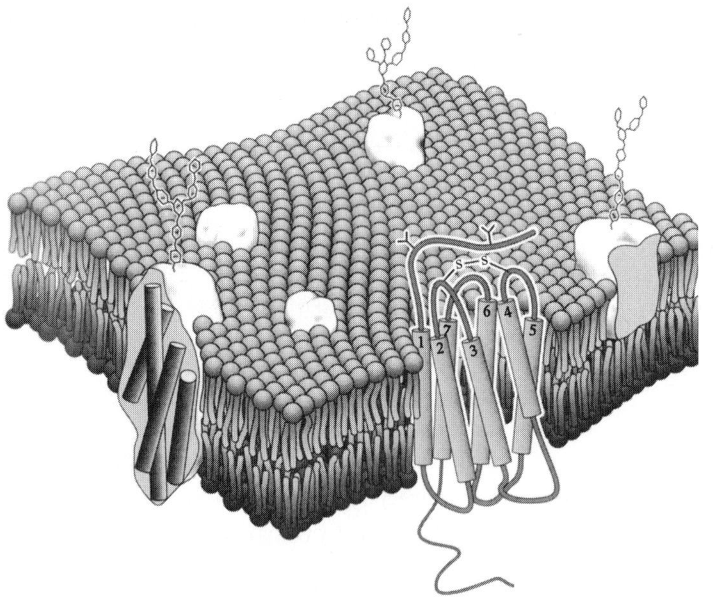

Figure 2–15. The fluid mosaic model of Singer and Nicholson. Some integral membrane proteins, which are shown as irregular solids, are dissolved in the bilayer. Transmembrane proteins protrude from both sides. One of these is pictured as a seven-helix protein, a common type of receptor for hormones and for light absorption by visual pigments. Other proteins adhere to either the outer or the inner surface. Many membrane proteins carry complex oligosaccharide groups, which protrude from the outer surface. A few of these are indicated here as chains of sugar rings. (From Metzler DE: Biochemistry, ed 2, Academic Press, San Diego, 2003.)

(1) Regulated channels that selectively permit ions to move across the membrane.
(2) Carrier molecules unique to certain tissues.
(3) Receptor proteins—specific surface molecules that initiate membrane and cellular events (may require second messenger systems).

2. Extrinsic or peripheral proteins
   a. Composed of both hydrophobic and hydrophilic amino acids.
   b. Found near the surface of the membrane.
   c. Function as enzymes or in a structural capacity.

5.2 Function

A. Membranes function in several capacities
   1. Provide a means for selective movement of molecules into and out of the cell or organelle. In doing so, they serve as selective permeability barriers.
   2. Establish membrane potentials by separating ionic charges.
   3. Facilitate cell adhesions and specialized cell junctions.

B. Membrane transport
   1. Passive transport (diffusion)—movement across a membrane without utilizing energy. Movement continues until gradient is eliminated. May be either simple diffusion or facilitated diffusion.
      a. Simple diffusion—down a concentration gradient without the need for carrier proteins. Osmosis and bulk flow are associated with simple diffusion. Since the membrane is primarily lipid in nature, hydrophobic molecules and very small molecules (such as O_2 and CO_2) diffuse across the lipid bilayer. Charged molecules (ions) utilize transmembrane protein channels.
      b. Facilitated diffusion—utilizes intrinsic proteins to transport large, lipid-insoluble molecules (amino acids, glucose). Also moves down a concentration gradient. Intrinsic proteins undergo conformational changes to facilitate diffusion (saturable and specific). Does not require energy. Shows Michaelis-Menten kinetics (glucose transport).
      c. Osmosis—diffusion of water from lower solute concentration to higher solute concentration. Extracellular fluid and intracellular fluid have the same osmolarity (~300 mOsm).
         (1) Isotonic extracellular solution—no cell volume change.
         (2) Hypertonic extracellular solution—cells will shrink.
         (3) Hypotonic extracellular solution—cells will swell.
   2. Active transport—movement across a membrane from an area of low concentra-

tion to high concentration. Since carriers are involved, it demonstrates Michaelis-Menten kinetics. It is a unidirectional transport that requires energy (ATP).

a. Endocytosis—vacuole formation utilizing plasma membrane and released inside the cell. May result in degradation. If vacuole is fused with lysozymes, results in degradation.
   (1) Pinocytosis—internalization of interstitial fluid.
   (2) Phagocytosis—internalization of material and subsequent lysosomal digestion.
   (3) Receptor mediated endocytosis—selective internalization of receptor/ligand complex. Receptor complex may return to surface.
b. Exocytosis—secretory vesicle membrane from within the cell fuses with the plasma membrane, and the contents of the vesicle are released outside the cell.
c. Primary active transport—energy derived from ATP. Specific carriers are utilized, which are saturable.
   (1) Ca^{2+}-ATPase pumps are important active transports in sarcoplasmic reticulum membranes.
   (2) Na^+K^+-ATPase pump is present in all plasma membranes.
      (a) Establishes and maintains a Na^+ and K^+ gradient by transporting Na^+ out and K^+ into the cell.
      (b) The Na^+ concentration gradient is the force for secondary active transport mechanisms.
d. Secondary active transport—ATP establishes an ionic gradient, which is the driving force (secondary transport).
   (1) Na^+ gradient established by membrane pumps drive this system.
   (2) Protein carriers bind both the substance transported and Na^+.
   (3) Cotransport systems—Na^+ and substance transported move in the same direction. Examples include:
      (a) Glucose and galactose across GI mucosa and resorption in renal tubule.
      (b) Amino acid transport in GI mucosa and renal tubules.
   (4) Countertransport—Na^+ and transported substance move in opposite directions. Examples include:
      (a) Na^+/H^+ exchange (H^+ out and Na^+ into cells).
      (b) Na^+/Ca^{2+} exchange (Ca^{2+} out and Na^+ into cells).

3. Transport protein terminology
   a. Uniport proteins—transport a single molecule.
   b. Coupled or cotransport proteins—transport two different compounds simultaneously. Both must be bound for transport to occur.
      (1) Symport—coupled transport in the same direction.
      (2) Antiport or exchange—coupled transport in opposite directions.

C. Membrane potentials—the measured potential difference measured across a cell membrane in millivolts (measured charge is inside the cell). This results from concentration differences of permeable ions.
   1. The separation of charges (ions) results in a slight excess of negative charges inside and more positive charges outside.
   2. An electrochemical gradient is established due to the ion and chemical concentration differences. The electrochemical gradient determines the diffusion of ions.
   3. Resting membrane potential is determined by the diffusion potentials of the ions and membrane.
      a. At rest, K^+ is far more permeable than Na^+.
      b. Table 2-2 shows the composition of ECF and ICF.

TABLE 2–2. APPROXIMATE COMPOSITIONS OF EXTRACELLULAR AND INTRACELLULAR FLUIDS

SUBSTANCE AND UNITS	EXTRACELLULAR FLUID	INTRACELLULAR FLUID*
Na^+ (mEq/L)	140	14
K^+ (mEq/L)	4	120
Ca^{2+}, ionized (mEq/L)	2.5†	1×10^{-4}
Cl^- (mEq/L)	105	10
HCO_3^- (mEq/L)	24	10
pH‡	7.4	7.1
Osmolarity (mOsm/L)	290	290

*The major anions of intracellular fluid are proteins and organic phosphates.
†The corresponding total [Ca^{2+}] in extracellular fluid is 5 mEq/L or 10 mg/dL.
‡pH is $-\log_{10}$ of the [H^+]; pH 7.4 corresponds to [H^+] of 40×10^{-9} Eq/L.
From Costanzo LS: Physiology, ed 3, WB Saunders, Philadelphia, 2004.

c. Due to the diffusion of K^+ out of the cell, the resting membrane potential is negative and near the equilibrium potential of K^+.

d. The resting membrane potential is maintained by the Na^+-K^+-ATPase pump (−40 to −90 mV).

e. Hyperkalemia reduces the concentration gradient for potassium out of the cell, thus making the inside less negative.

D. Graded membrane potentials—local changes in membrane potentials that result in gradations of membrane potentials and sensitivity to stimulation. Examples include:

1. Postsynaptic potentials in synapses.
2. Sensory receptor potentials.
3. Skeletal muscle end-plate potential.
4. Pacemaker potential in cardiac and smooth muscle.

E. Action potentials—changes in membrane potentials.

1. Terminology

a. Depolarization—process of making the membrane potential less negative. Usually due to the opening of voltage-sensitive sodium channels opening and sodium diffusing into the cell (inward current).

b. Hyperpolarization—process of making the membrane potential more negative due to the outward flow of positive ions (outward current).

c. Threshold potential—the membrane potential which, when reached, results in an action potential.

d. Action potential—an all-or-none response producing a fast depolarization followed by repolarization back to the resting membrane potential. The action potential propagates from one site to adjacent sites.

e. Refractory period—the period during which another normal action potential cannot be elicited.

(1) Relative refractory period—action potential can be elicited only if a greater than usual depolarization is applied.

(2) Absolute refractory period—another action potential cannot be elicited.

2. Ionic basis for action potentials (Figure 2-16):

3. Propagation of action potential—occurs by local currents depolarizing adjacent areas of membrane. Propagation velocity

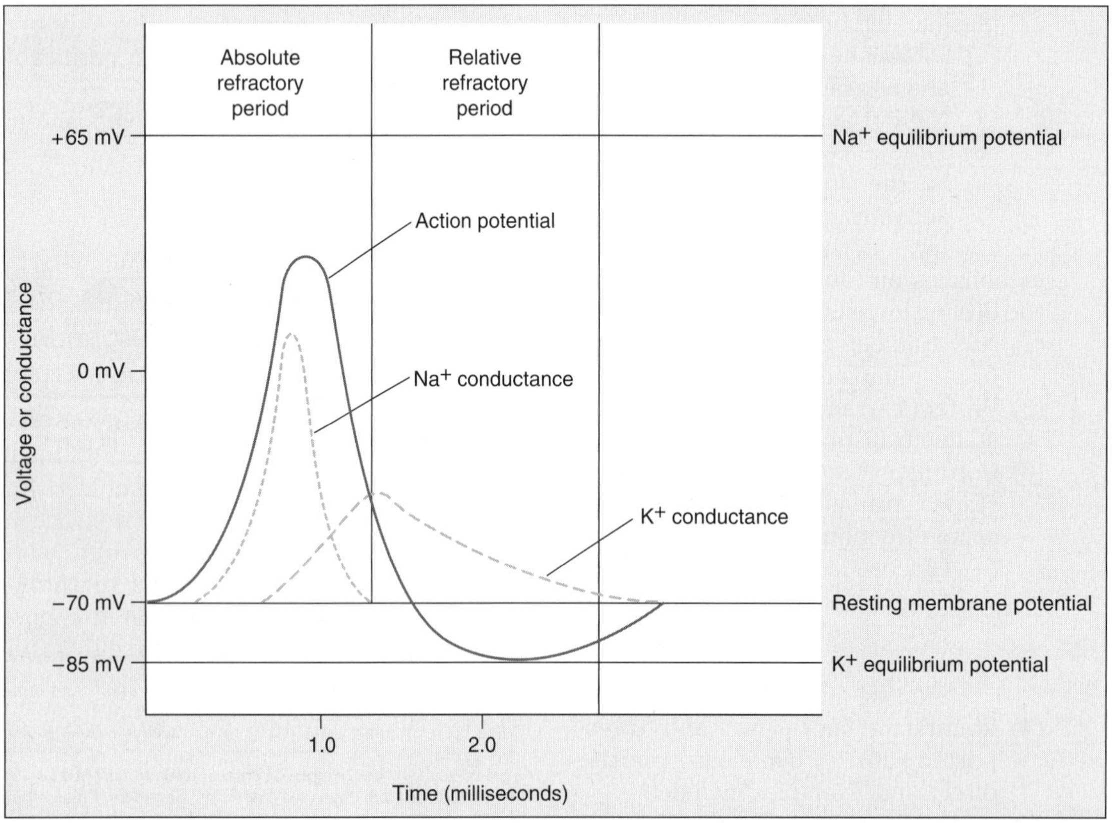

Figure 2–16. Relationship of action potential and refractory periods to sodium and potassium conductance.

can be increased by the following factors:
a. Increasing fiber size.
b. Increasing stimulation intensity.
c. Myelination, which results in action potentials jumping from node to node (saltatory conduction).

6.0 NERVOUS SYSTEM

6.1 General Properties

A. The central nervous system (CNS) consists of highly integrated neurons (spinal cord and brain) surrounded by cerebral spinal fluid (CSF).
B. The peripheral nervous system is an interface between the CNS and the environment.
   1. Autonomic neurons
      a. Parasympathetic.
      b. Sympathetic.
      c. Enteric.
   2. Sensory receptors and afferent neurons (vision, hearing, chemical, touch).
   3. Somatic motor neurons (muscle, endocrine, and exocrine gland secretion).

6.2 Central Nervous System

A. Spinal cord—contains sensory (afferent/ascending pathways) and motor (efferent/descending pathways) nerves.
B. Brainstem
   1. Medulla—responsible for regulating and/or coordination of:
      a. Blood pressure.
      b. Breathing.
      c. Swallowing.
      d. Coughing.
      e. Vomiting.
   2. Pons—participates in respiratory regulation and the relay of information from cerebral hemispheres to the cerebellum.
   3. Midbrain—participates in coordination of visual and auditory systems.
C. Cerebellum—responsible for posture and coordination of movement.
D. Thalamus—processes sensory information going to and motor information coming from the cerebral cortex.
E. Hypothalamus—essentially an endocrine gland that is involved with the regulation of body temperature, water balance, and food intake (see Endocrine section).
F. Cerebral cortex—receives and processes sensory information and integrates motor function in response to peripheral input.
G. Basal ganglia—involved with movement control. Modulates information from the thalamus to the motor cortex in the execution of movement. GABA (γ aminobutyric acid) is an important neurotransmitter for many inhibitory synaptic connections.
H. Hippocampus and amygdala—involved with emotions and the autonomic responses mediated through the hypothalamus (pupil size, heart rate, hypothalamic hormone secretion).

6.3 Autonomic Nervous System

Involuntary regulation of visceral organs. Highly integrated in the hypothalamus but reflexes often involve only the medulla or spinal cord. Most tissues are tonically innervated by both sympathetic and parasympathetic systems, resulting in dual control (inhibitory/stimulatory). An exception is the salivary gland, where both systems are stimulatory.

A. Parasympathetic system (Figure 2-17)
   1. Preganglionic neurons have cell bodies in brainstem or sacral region of spinal cord (S1–S4) (long fibers).
   2. Postganglionic cell bodies are found in ganglia located near target tissues (short fibers).
   3. Both preganglionic and postganglionic neurons are cholinergic (acetylcholine is synthesized, stored, and used as a neurotransmitter in nerve terminal).
   4. Two types of cholinergic receptors (cholinoreceptors) exist (Table 2-3)
      a. Nicotinic receptors
         (1) Found in autonomic ganglion, neuromuscular junction of skeletal muscle, and chromaffin cells of the adrenal medulla.
         (2) Agonists include acetylcholine, nicotine, and carbachol.
         (3) Antagonists include curare (skeletal neuromuscular junction-selective) and hexamethonium (ganglion-selective).
         (4) Activation of the receptor by the agonist results in the opening of Na^+/K^+ ion channels, resulting in excitation.
      b. Muscarinic receptors
         (1) Found in all effector organs of the parasympathetic nervous system (smooth muscle, cardiac muscle, and most glands) and in sweat

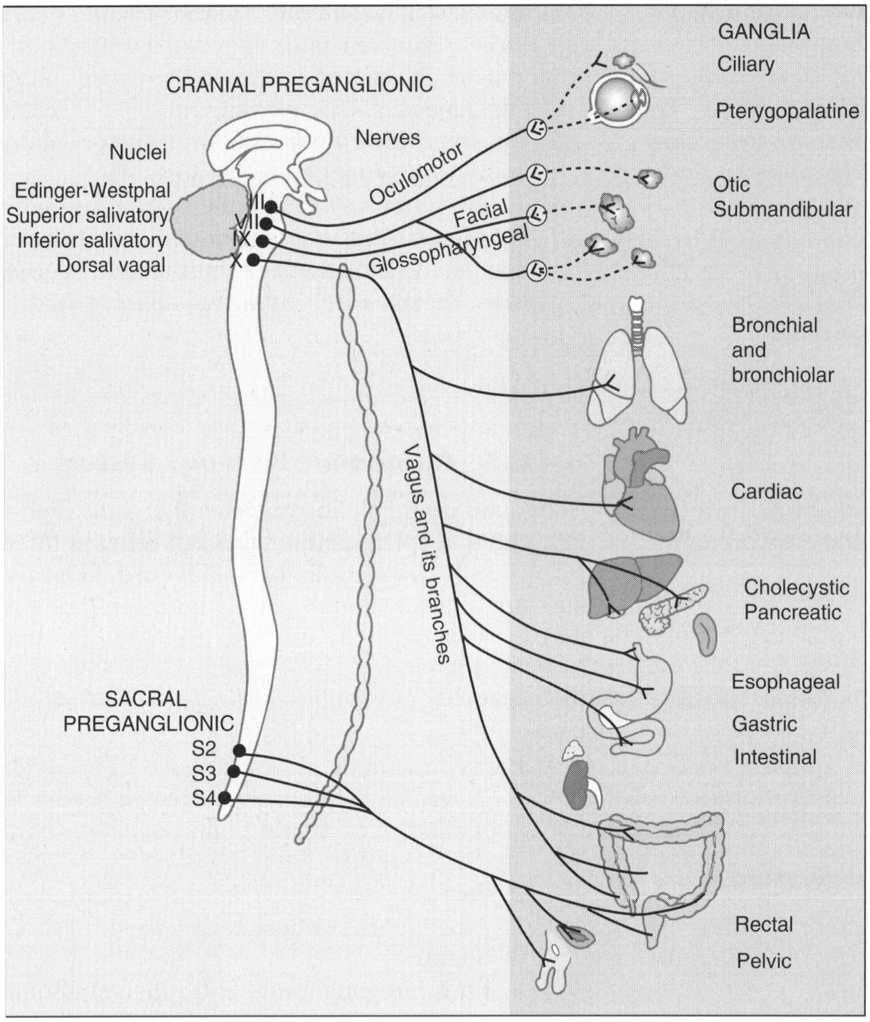

Figure 2–17. Parasympathetic nervous system. (From Berne RM, Levy MN: Principles of Physiology, ed 4, St. Louis, Mosby, 2006.)

glands (innervated by the sympathetic nervous system).

(2) Activation results in G protein-mediated activation of phospholipase C, generation of IP_3 and diacylglycerol with subsequent release of Ca^{2+} to produce tissue-specific physiological actions (similar to α_1 adrenoreceptors).

(3) Other muscarinic receptors utilize G proteins to directly act upon ion channels (e.g., K^+ channels in cardiac tissue).

5. Acetylcholine activity is terminated through the activity of acetyl cholinesterase, which degrades acetylcholine.

B. Sympathetic system (Figure 2-18)

1. Preganglionic neurons have cell bodies in the thoracolumbar spinal cord segments (T1–L3).
2. Postganglionic cell bodies are located in the vertebral ganglia or paravertebral ganglia (e.g., mesenteric or celiac).
3. Preganglionic neurons are cholinergic; release acetylcholine to interact with nicotinic receptors.
4. Postganglionic neurons are adrenergic; synthesize, store, and release norepinephrine to interact with adrenoceptors. (Postganglionic neurons to sweat glands are cholinergic.)
5. The adrenal medulla is a specialized endocrine organ, which, upon stimulation from sympathetic neurons, secretes catecholamines (80% epinephrine and 20% norepinephrine).
6. Several classes of adrenergic receptors exist (Table 2-3).
7. Norepinephrine is removed from the terminal by neuronal reuptake and then reutilized or metabolized by monoamine oxidase (MAO).

C. Enteric system—the intrinsic neuronal system of the gastrointestinal tract. Neurons and neuromodulators are contained totally in the tissues but are influenced by input

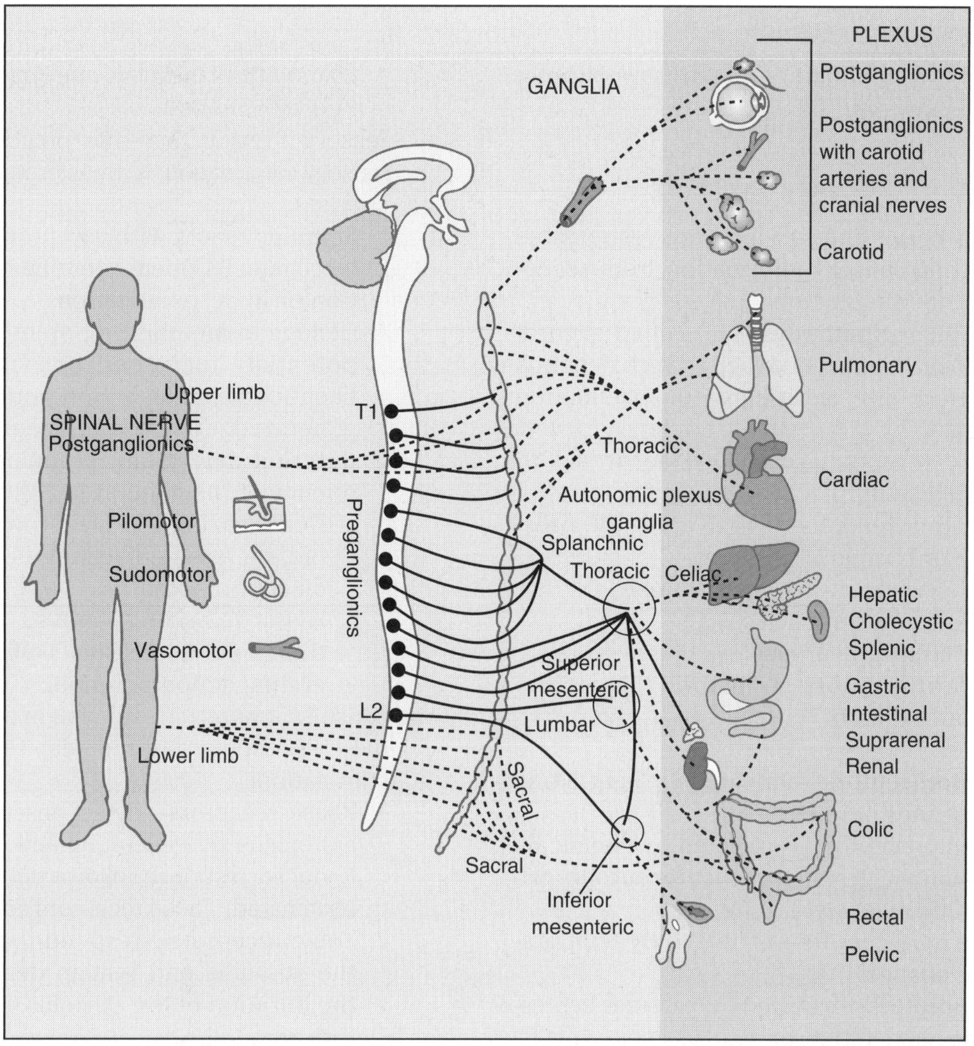

Figure 2–18. Sympathetic nervous system. (From Berne RM, Levy MN: Principles of Physiology, ed 4, St. Louis, Mosby, 2006.)

TABLE 2–3. LOCATION AND MECHANISM OF ACTION OF AUTONOMIC RECEPTORS

RECEPTOR	TARGET TISSUE	SIGNALING MECHANISM
Adrenoceptors		
α_1	Vascular smooth muscle, skin, renal, and splanchnic Gastrointestinal tract, sphincters Bladder, sphincter Radial muscle, iris	IP_3, ↑ intracellular (Ca^{2+})
α_2	Gastrointestinal tract, wall Presynaptic adrenergic neurons	Inhibition of adenylyl cyclase, ↓ cAMP
β_1	Heart Salivary glands Adipose tissue Kidney	Stimulation of adenylyl cyclase, ↑ cAMP
β_2	Vascular smooth muscle of skeletal muscle Gastrointestinal tract, wall Bladder, wall Bronchioles	Stimulation of adenylyl cyclase, ↑ cAMP
Cholinergic receptors		
Nicotinic	Skeletal muscle, motor end plate Postganglionic neurons, SNS and PNS Adrenal medulla	Opening Na^+ and K^+ channels → depolarization
Muscarinic	All effector organs, PNS Sweat glands, SNS	IP_3, ↑ intracellular (Ca^{2+})

cAMP, Cyclic adenosine monophosphate; *PNS*, parasympathetic nervous system; *SNS*, sympathetic nervous system.
From Costanzo LS: Physiology, ed 3, WB Saunders, Philadelphia, 2004.

from the sympathetic and parasympathetic nervous system.

6.4 Sensory Systems

Consist of nerve fibers, which are responsible for transmitting sensory information from receptors to the CNS (afferent input).

A. Nerve fibers (pathways)—classified according to their conduction velocity, which depends upon their size and degree of myelination (Table 2-4).
B. Sensory receptors—classified according to their specificity.
   1. Mechanoreceptors—activated by pressure or change in pressure.
      a. Hair cells in the organ of Corti.
      b. Pacinian corpuscles.
      c. Meissner's corpuscles.
      d. Baroreceptors in carotid sinus and carotid arch.
      e. Golgi tendo organs.
   2. Photoreceptors—activated by light (rods and cones in retina).
   3. Chemoreceptors—activated by chemicals (olfactory, gestation, osmoreceptors, pH, O_2, CO_2 receptors).
   4. Thermoreceptors—activated by temperature change.
   5. Nociceptors—activated by extremes in pressure, temperature, or noxious chemicals.
   6. Receptors for pain are free nerve endings. Fast pain is carried by group Aδ fibers, slow pain by C fibers. Among the neurotransmitters is substance P (release inhibited by opioids).
C. Sensory transduction—the process by which sensory information is transformed into nerve impulses.
   1. Stimulus reacts with receptor.
   2. Ion channels open, producing depolarization or hyperpolarization.
   3. Change in membrane potential (receptor potential) increases or decreases the likelihood that an action potential will be generated. The type, magnitude, and duration determine the number and frequency of the generated action potential.
      a. Depolarizing—moves toward threshold, increasing likelihood of generating an action potential.
      b. Hyperpolarizing—moves away from threshold, decreasing likelihood of generating action potential.
D. Sensory adaptation—the fall in action potential frequency with time despite continuous stimulation.
   1. Phasic receptors—detect onset and offset of a stimulus by generating action potentials. Reduced response follows until stimulus is terminated. These receptors adapt rapidly.
   2. Tonic receptors—respond to the onset of the stimulus and remain depolarized for the duration of the stimulus. These receptors adapt slowly.
E. Somatosensory pathways
   1. Dorsal column system—responsible for transmitting information about discrimi-

TABLE 2–4. CLASSIFICATION OF NERVE FIBERS

CLASSIFICATION	TYPE OF NERVE FIBER	EXAMPLE	RELATIVE DIAMETER	RELATIVE CONDUCTION VELOCITY	MYELINATION
Sensory and motor	A alpha (Aα)	α Motoneurons	Largest	Fastest	Yes
	A beta (Aβ)	Touch, pressure	Medium	Medium	Yes
	A gamma (Aγ)	γ Motoneurons to muscle spindles (intrafusal fibers)	Medium	Medium	Yes
	A delta (Aδ)	Touch, pressure, temperature, pain	Small	Medium	Yes
	B	Preganglionic autonomic nerves	Small	Medium	Yes
	C	Slow pain; postganglionic autonomic nerves; olfaction	Smallest	Slowest	No
Sensory only	Ia (Aα)	Muscle spindle afferents	Largest	Fastest	Yes
	Ib (Aα)	Golgi tendon organ afferents	Largest	Fastest	Yes
	II (Aβ)	Secondary afferents of muscle spindles; touch, pressure	Medium	Medium	Yes
	III (Aδ)	Touch, pressure, fast pain, temperature	Small	Medium	Yes
	IV (C)	Pain, temperature; olfaction	Smallest	Slowest	No

From Costanzo LS: Physiology, ed 3, WB Saunders, Philadelphia, 2004.
The numerical system is an alternative way to classify sensory nerves.

native touch, pressure, vibration, and proprioception.

2. Anterolateral system—responsible for transmitting information about pain, temperature, and light touch.
3. General patterns of transmission:
   a. First-order neuron (primary afferent neuron)—signal transmitted to the CNS by the primary afferent neuron. The nerve cell body is located in the dorsal root.
   b. Second-order neuron—signal is transmitted from first-order neurons, and the information is then transmitted to the thalamus. Located in spinal cord or brainstem.
   c. Third-order neuron—located in the somatosensory nuclei of thalamus. Projects information to cerebral cortex.
   d. Fourth-order neuron—located in the somatosensory cortex. Responsible for conscious perception of the stimulus.

6.5 Neurotransmission

A. Synaptic transmission—the transfer of information from one cell to another.
   1. Electrical synapse—current moves from one cell to another through areas of low resistance (gap junctions). Examples include muscle in cardiac, uterine, and bladder tissue.
   2. Chemical synapse—information transferred through the synaptic cleft by the release of neurotransmitters (e.g., acetylcholine, norepinephrine, dopamine).
      a. Presynaptic neuron
         (1) Action potential causes Ca^{2+} channels to open, which causes neurotransmitters stored in vesicles to be released.
         (2) Neurotransmitters diffuse across cleft to interact with postsynaptic receptors.
      b. Postsynaptic neuron
         (1) Neurotransmitter interacts with receptor to open ion channels, which can either be excitatory (cause depolarization by opening sodium ion channels) or inhibitory (cause hyperpolarization by opening chloride ion channels).
         (2) Postsynaptic neurons receive input from many presynaptic terminals which, when integrated, result in overall stimulation (excitatory postsynaptic potential or EPSP) or overall inhibition (inhibitory postsynaptic potential or IPSP). These potentials are graded so the magnitude determines the frequency of the action potential transmitted down the postsynaptic neuron.
            (a) Spatial summation—occurs when multiple neurons arrive at the postsynaptic neuron simultaneously.
            (b) Temporal summation—occurs when multiple presynaptic inputs arrive in rapid succession, permitting the inputs to overlap in time.

B. Neurotransmitters
   1. Acetylcholine
      a. Neuromuscular transmission.
      b. Neurotransmitter in all parasympathetic preganglionic and postganglionic neurons.
      c. Neurotransmitter from all sympathetic preganglionic neurons and from most sympathetic postganglionic neurons to sweat glands.
      d. The activity is terminated through the action of acetycholinesterase.
      e. Myasthenia gravis is an autoimmune disease that interferes with the acetylcholine receptors on the motor end-plates.
   2. Catecholamines (epinephrine, norepinephrine, and dopamine)
      a. Synthesized from tyrosine.
      b. Activity is terminated by catechol-*O*-methyl transferase (COMT) (in tissues) or MAO (in nerve).
   3. Serotonin—synthesized from tryptophan.
   4. Histamine—synthesized from histidine.
   5. Glutamate—excitatory neurotransmitter in CNS.
   6. Glycine
      a. Inhibitory neurotransmitter in CNS.
      b. Causes hyperpolarization by increasing chloride ion conductance.
   7. GABA
      a. Synthesized from glutamic acid.
      b. Causes hyperpolarization by increasing chloride conductance ($GABA_A$) or potassium conductance ($GABA_B$) in postsynaptic cell.
      c. $GABA_A$ is the receptor site for the action of benzodiazepines and barbiturates.

6.6 Somatic Nervous System (Motor Neurons)

A. Motor unit—the single neuron and the muscle fibers it innervates
   1. Fine movements—single motor neurons innervating a small number of muscle fibers.
   2. Forceful movements—single motor neurons innervating many fibers.

B. Muscle reflexes—an automatic response produced through the stimulation of receptors (sensors) in muscle
   1. Knee-jerk reflex—due to stretching of muscle spindles (intrafusal fibers arranged in parallel with the larger, force-generating extrafusal fibers).
      a. Mechanical stretch of muscle spindle increases afferent fiber firing.
      b. Afferent fibers synapse (monosynaptic reflex) with α motor neuron in spinal cord.
      c. Alpha motor neuron stimulates muscle contraction, returning muscle length to normal.
      d. Muscle spindles are responsible for maintenance of posture and resting muscle length.
      e. Knee-jerk reflex is used to test function of CNS.
   2. Withdrawal reflex—response to noxious stimulus (polysynaptic reflex).
   3. Golgi tendon reflex—responds to too much tension and results in inhibition of alpha motor neurons.

7.0 MUSCLE

7.1 Skeletal Muscle

A. Skeletal muscle—general considerations
   1. Location—attached to bone, skin-deep fascia.
   2. Appearance—striated, many nuclei in each fiber, unbranched.
   3. Nervous control—voluntary. Controlled by somatic nerves.
   4. Function
      a. Movement of skeletal system.
      b. Maintain posture.
      c. Movement of diaphragm to change intrathoracic volume.

B. Skeletal muscle—structural considerations

Functional unit—each muscle fiber is innervated by a motor neuron and contains bundles of myofibrils (bundles of muscle fibers/cells) arranged in repeating structures called *sarcomeres*. Sarcomeres (covered by sarcolemmal membranes) contain repeating units of contractile filaments.
   1. Thick filaments—composed primarily of myosin.
      a. Present in the A band.
      b. Contain two myosin heads that bind ATP and are responsible for cross-bridging to actin.
   2. Thin filaments—composed of actin, tropomyosin, and troponin.
      a. Actin is a globular (spherical) protein that contains binding sites for myosin, tropomyosin, and troponin.
      b. Tropomyosin—elongated protein that covers the cross-bridge binding sites when the muscle is resting.
      c. Troponin—regulator protein that permits cross-bridging when it binds calcium.
      d. Transverse tubules (T-tubules)—sarcolemmal membrane that invaginates into the muscle fiber.

C. Skeletal muscle—excitation-contraction coupling (Figure 2-19)
   1. Action potential—depolarization initiated at the neuromuscular junction due to the release of acetylcholine and graded end-plate potential (see Neuromuscular junction/Somatic nervous system).
   2. Depolarization of the T-tubules—produces a conformational change in the sarcoplasmic reticulum to release Ca^{2+}.
   3. Ca^{2+} binds to troponin C, producing a conformational change on the thin filament, which causes tropomyosin to be moved out of the way so cross-bridging can begin.
   4. Cross-bridges form between actin and myosin. Without ATP, this remains tightly bound, resulting in rigor.
   5. ATP binding to myosin produces a conformational change, decreasing its affinity for actin and causing a displacement of myosin.
   6. ATP is hydrolyzed to ADP and P_i, permitting myosin to bind to a new site on actin, thus constituting the force-generating power stroke.
   7. The cross-bridging continues as long as Ca^{2+} is bound to troponin. When Ca^{2+} is sequestered again by the sarcoplasmic reticulum, calcium is released from troponin, and tropomyosin returns to its resting position, blocking the myosin-binding site on actin (Figure 2-19).

Position of Actin and Myosin During Cross-Bridge Cycling	Events	ATP/ADP
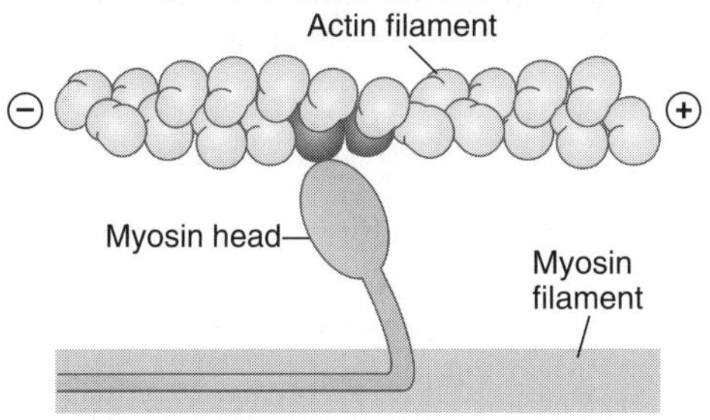	Rigor	No nucleotides bound
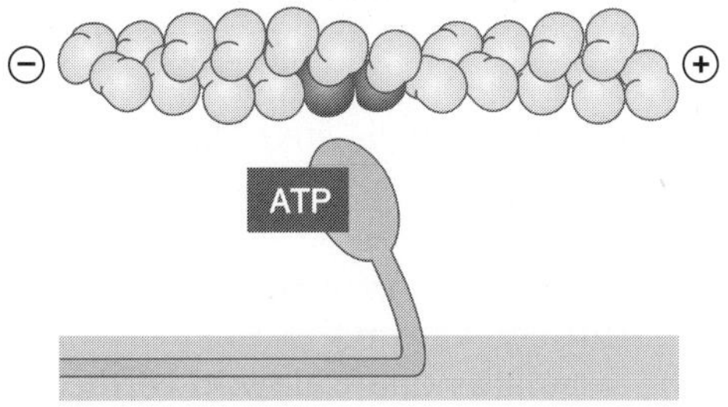	ATP binds to cleft on myosin head Conformational change in myosin Decreased affinity of myosin for actin Myosin released	ATP bound
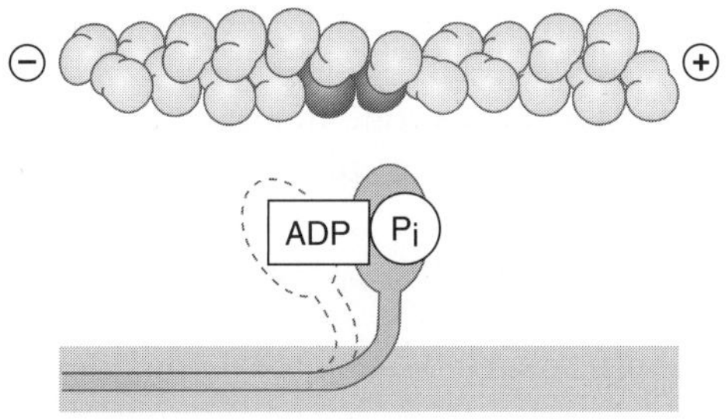	Cleft closes around ATP Conformational change Myosin head displaced toward ⊕ end of actin ATP hydrolysis	ATP → ADP + P_i ADP + P_i bound
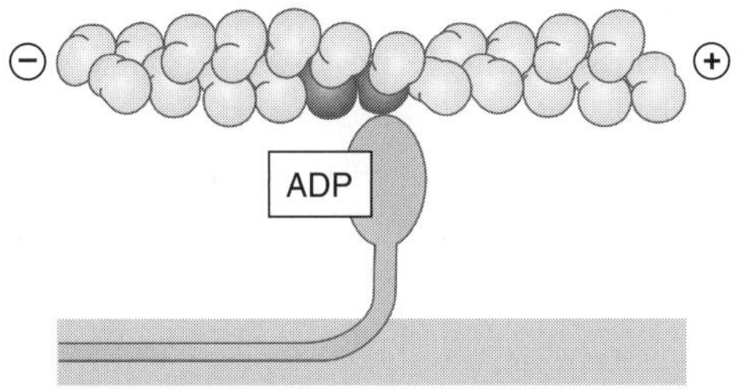	Myosin head binds new site on actin Power stroke = force	ADP bound
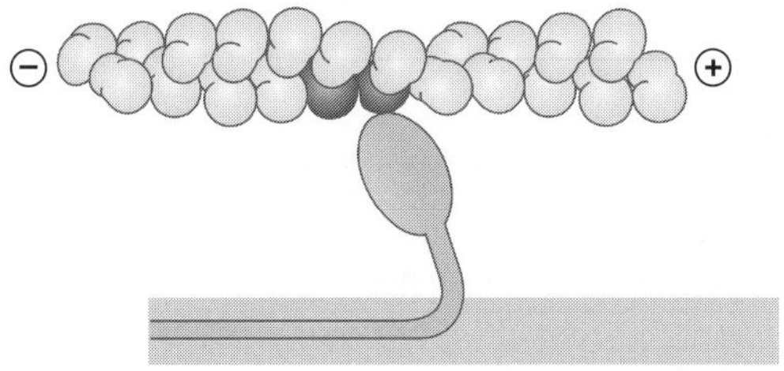	ADP released Rigor	No nucleotides bound

Figure 2–19. Cross-bridge cycle in skeletal muscle.

D. Skeletal muscle mechanics
   1. Spatial summation—more motor units (fibers) recruited, resulting in greater tension and stronger contraction.
   2. Temporal summation—increased frequency of stimulation to each motor unit, resulting in a summation of twitches.
   3. Tetanus—maximum, sustained muscle contraction with rapid stimulation.

E. Length–tension relationship
   1. Isometric—tension developed but muscle does not shorten. Load is too great to permit shortening.
   2. Isotonic—muscle tension remains constant, and the muscle shortens.

F. Energy sources for muscle contraction
   ATP is necessary for muscle contraction but limited amounts available. ATP can be generated by different metabolic pathways.
   1. Creatine phosphate—serves as a storage pool of high-energy phosphate. Important supply for short bursts of high-intensity activity.
   2. Glycolysis
      a. Aerobic—supply ATP at very high rates (two ATP produced when pyruvate is formed from glucose).
      b. Anaerobic—in the absence of oxygen, ATP is produced, and lactic acid is formed from pyruvate.
   3. Oxidative phosphorylation—a slow process that uses O_2 and substrates to generate ATP.

G. Fiber types—based on ATP production and consumption rates
   1. Type I—(oxidative metabolism) slow speed, weak contractions, resistant to fatigue.
   2. Type IIB—(glycolytic metabolism) fast speed, strong contraction, fatigable.
   3. Type IIA—(oxidative metabolism) fast speed, intermediate strength of contraction, resistant to fatigue.

7.2 Smooth Muscle

A. Smooth muscle—general considerations
   1. Location
      a. Walls of hollow organs.
      b. Blood vessels.
      c. Iris and ciliary muscles of eye.
      d. Erector pili (hair).
   2. Appearance—no striations, single nucleus, spindle-shaped fibers.
   3. Nervous control—involuntary control of the autonomic nervous system.
   4. Function
      a. Mixes and propels luminal contents through GI tract.
      b. Regulates blood flow in cardiovascular system.
      c. Contracts urinary bladder, gallbladder, and spleen.
      d. Modulates tone in sphincter muscles.
      e. Regulates pupil diameter and lens shape.
      f. Causes hair to stand up (erector pili muscles).

B. Smooth muscle—structural considerations
   1. Multiunit—little or no coupling between cells. Must be directly stimulated for contraction (examples are iris and vas deferens).
   2. Unitary (single unit)—have gap junctions that permit fast spread of electrical activity and coordinated contraction

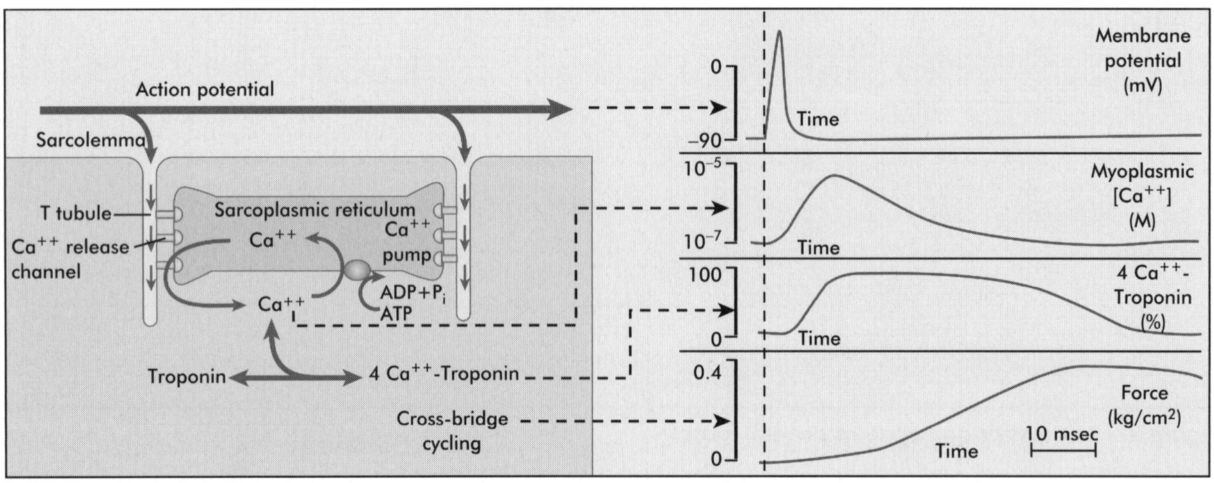

Figure 2–20. Excitation-contraction coupling in skeletal muscle. (From Berne RM, Levy MN: Principles of Physiology, ed 4, St. Louis, Mosby, 2006.)

(examples are gastrointestinal tract, bladder, uterus, and ureter). Characterized as having pacemaker (slow wave) activity.

C. Smooth muscle—excitation-contraction coupling (see Fig. 2-20)
   1. Action potential—depolarization opens voltage-gated Ca^{2+} channels in the sarcolemmal membrane, producing an increase in intracellular Ca^{2+} concentration.
   2. Hormones and neurotransmitters—may produce an additional increase in intracellular Ca^{2+} via ligand-gated Ca^{2+} channels or IP_3-gated Ca^{2+} release channels.
   3. Calmodulin binding—the increased Ca^{2+} binds to calmodulin, which activates myosin-light-chain kinase.
   4. Myosin phosphorylation—produced by myosin phosphorylase, which permits it to bind actin to form cross-bridges and produce a contraction. ATP is consumed in the process.
   5. Myosin dephosphorylation—due to reduced intracellular Ca^{2+}, which activates myosin-light-chain phosphatase. Myosin and actin remain attached but not by cross-bridges.
   6. Relaxation—occurs when intercellular Ca^{2+} levels fall below the level necessary to form Ca^{2+}-calmodulin complexes.

7.3 Cardiac Muscle

A. Cardiac muscle—general considerations
   1. Location—heart.
   2. Appearance—striated, single nucleus, branched, fibers with intercalated discs.
   3. Nervous control—involuntary, controlled by the autonomic nervous system.
   4. Function—propel blood through the cardiovascular system.

B. Cardiac muscle—structural considerations
   1. Structure of cardiac muscle is similar to that of striated muscle.
   2. Contraction of cardiac muscle is similar to that of skeletal muscle.

C. Cardiac muscle—excitation-contraction coupling (Figure 2-21)

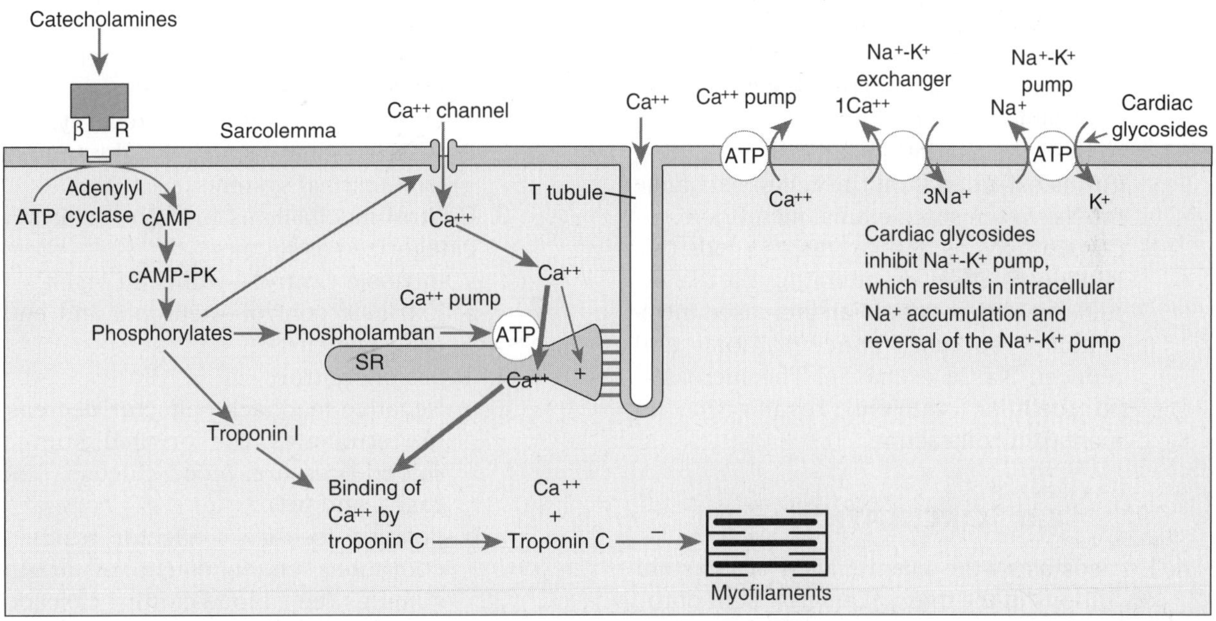

Figure 2–21. Excitation-contraction coupling in skeletal muscle. The action potential depolarizing the sarcolemma via T-tubular membranes spreads into the interior of the cells. The T-tubules are anatomically coupled to Ca^{2+}-release channels in the sarcoplasmic reticulum that open momentarily with the fall in voltage. Ca^{2+} is the intracellular messenger, coupling electrical events at the cell membranes to activation of the contractile apparatus. Ca^{2+} rapidly diffuses down its concentration gradient from the sarcoplasmic reticulum store to the myoplasm, where it binds to sites on troponin, a thin filament protein. Ca^{2+} binding to troponin induces a conformational change in the thin filament that allows cross-bridge attachment and cycling with force development and shortening. Increases in the myoplasmic Ca^{2+} also activate Ca^{2+} pumps in the sarcoplasmic reticulum membrane, and Ca^{2+} is returned to the sarcoplasmic reticulum. The fall in myoplasmic Ca^{2+} causes bound Ca^{2+} to dissociate from troponin, and the thin filaments return to the "off" conformation with cessation of cross-bridge attachment and relaxation. (From Berne RM, Levy MN: Principles of Physiology, ed 4, St. Louis, Mosby, 2006.)

1. Action potential—initiated in the myocardial cell membrane and spreads to the interior of the cell by way of the T-tubules. This causes an influx of Ca^{2+} from the extracellular fluid to the intracellular fluid. This increase in Ca^{2+} triggers more release of Ca^{2+} from the sarcoplasmic reticulum.
2. Intercellular Ca^{2+} binds to troponin C, producing a conformational change on the thin filament, which causes tropomyosin to be moved out of the way so cross-bridging can begin.
3. Cross-bridges form between actin and myosin. Without ATP, this remains tightly bound, resulting in rigor.
4. ATP binding to myosin produces a conformational change, decreasing its affinity for actin and causing a displacement of myosin.
5. ATP is hydrolyzed to ADP and P_i, permitting myosin to bind to a new site on actin, thus constituting the force-generating power stroke.
6. The cross-bridging continues as long as Ca^{2+} is bound to troponin.
7. The magnitude of tension developed by myocardial cells is proportional to the intracellular Ca^{2+} concentration.
8. When Ca^{2+} is sequestered by the sarcoplasmic reticulum by the action of Ca^{2+} ATPase, relaxation occurs. In addition, Ca^{2+} is extruded from the cell in exchange for Na^+ in the sarcolemmal membrane.
9. Cardiac glycosides produce a positive inotrophic effect by inhibiting the Na^+/K^+ ATPase. This results in an increased intracellular sodium concentration and reduced Na/Ca exchange. The increased intracellular calcium results in an increased contraction.

8.0 CIRCULATION

A. Homeostasis—the maintenance of constant conditions in the internal environment of the body. This is accomplished through the coordinated efforts of organ systems in the body, which are integrated through neuronal and endocrine communication.
   1. Internal environment (of a 70-kg adult human)—maintained by organ systems.
      a. Extracellular fluid (20% of total body weight, 14 L), which includes the following:
         (1) Interstitial fluid (11 L)
            (a) High in sodium and chloride.
            (b) Low in potassium, magnesium, and phosphate.
         (2) Plasma (3 L)
            (a) Similar ionic composition to interstitial fluid.
            (b) Higher concentration of protein compared to interstitial fluid.
      b. Intracellular fluid (28 L), separated from the extracellular fluid by the cell membrane, which is highly permeable to water but not to many of the electrolytes and proteins.
         (1) High in phosphate and potassium.
         (2) Low in calcium ions.
   2. Factors that must be maintained within very narrow limits, and the organs responsible for regulating the concentrations of each include the following:
      a. Electrolytes—gastrointestinal and renal systems.
      b. Water—gastrointestinal, circulatory, and renal systems.
      c. pH—renal and respiratory systems.
      d. Temperature—cardiovascular, respiratory, musculatory, and integumentary systems.
      e. Nutrients—cardiovascular, renal, gastrointestinal systems.
      f. O_2, CO_2—respiratory and renal systems.
      g. Wastes—circulatory, renal, and gastrointestinal systems.
   3. Control mechanisms for homeostasis are categorized as follows:
      a. Intrinsic control—within an organ.
      b. Extrinsic control—neuronal and endocrine systems.
   4. Types of control
      a. Negative feedback—effector decreases or terminates the original stimulus (blood pressure, blood glucose, blood gases, and pH).
      b. Positive feedback—effector results in continued enhancement of original stimulus (e.g., blood-clotting cascade).

B. Anatomical considerations
   1. Arteries
      a. Large vessels containing numerous layers of elastin (stretch) and collagen (tensile strength).
      b. Due to their large radius, offer little resistance to flow.
      c. Capable of elastic recoil; therefore, serve as a pressure reservoir.
   2. Arterioles
      a. Less elastic and more muscular.

b. Provide the greatest resistance to blood flow.

3. Capillaries
   a. Heavily branched, thin-walled vessels (one cell thick).
   b. Location of the exchange of fluid and substances between blood and interstitial fluid.
   c. Precapillary sphincter muscles regulate local blood flow.
4. Veins
   a. Have large radii, low resistance to flow.
   b. Valves ensure one-way flow.
   c. Serve as a blood reservoir.
5. Lymphatics
   a. One-way vessels that return interstitial fluid and contents to venous circulation.
   b. One-way valves and skeletal muscle contraction ensure proper flow.

C. Pressure, resistance, and flow
1. Relationship of pressure, flow, and resistance.
   a. Pressure gradient (δP)—the difference in pressure between the beginning and end of a vessel. This is the driving force for blood flow. Blood flows from high to low pressure.
   b. Resistance (R)—impediment to blood flow.
   c. Flow rate (Q)—the volume of blood through a vessel per unit of time.
   d. Ohm's Law $Q = \delta P/R$.
2. Blood flow is characterized as two types:
   a. Laminar flow
      (1) Velocity is greatest in the center of the vessel.
      (2) Fluid passes more readily through a large vessel than through a small vessel because a given volume of blood comes into contact with more surface area in the small vessel.
   b. Turbulent flow
      (1) Blood flows crosswise.
      (2) Caused by obstructions to flow and rough surfaces in the vessel.
3. Resistance
   a. Caused by friction between the moving blood and the vessel wall.
   b. As the blood flows through the vessel, the pressure decreases due to frictional losses.
      (1) As resistance increases, flow decreases.
      (2) In order to maintain the same flow with increased resistance, pressure must increase.
   c. Resistance to blood flow depends upon three factors:
      (1) Viscosity of blood.
      (2) Vessel length (usually remains the same).
      (3) Vessel radius (most important factor since this can change).
   d. Poiseuille's Law—the effect of vessel diameter (or radius, r) on resistance and flow.
      (1) Flow is proportional to r^4, or resistance is inversely proportional to r^4. Fluid passes more readily through a large vessel because a given volume of blood comes into contact with more surface area in a small vessel.
      (2) Resistance is proportional to $1/r^4$ and, since radius can be regulated, this is the most important factor in controlling overall resistance to blood flow.
   e. Viscosity and blood flow
      (1) Viscosity increases as hematocrit (percent of cells in blood) increases.
      (2) The greater the hematocrit, the less the flow due to increased resistance.

D. Blood pressure and vascular compliance
1. Blood pressure—depends on the volume of blood contained within the vessel and the compliance or distensibility of the vessel wall.
   a. Systolic pressure—the pressure at the height of each pulse. Measured when the ventricle ejects the stroke volume (normal average = 120 mmHg).
   b. Diastolic pressure—the lowest point pressure (normal average = 80 mmHg).
   c. Pulse pressure (systolic pressure minus the diastolic pressure). This depends upon two factors:
      (1) Stroke volume output.
      (2) Compliance (total dispensability) of arterial tree.
   d. Mean arterial pressure—the average of all pressures measured at any time point.

E. Arteriole resistance—very important to the understanding of blood pressure.
1. The radii of the arterioles are responsible for regulation of blood pressure and the distribution of cardiac output.
2. Vascular tone—the normal state of partial vascular constriction due to inherent contractile activity and ongoing sympathetic stimulation.

3. Arteriole smooth muscle is responsible for adjustments in arteriole resistance. This may result in either vasoconstriction or vasodilation. Factors that produce these changes are both intrinsic (local) or extrinsic (neuronal or hormonal).
   a. Local factors producing vasodilation:
      (1) Increased CO_2.
      (2) Decreased O_2.
      (3) Histamine.
      (4) Heat.
      (5) Decreased myogenic activity in response to:
         (a) Increased metabolism (reactive hyperemia).
         (b) Reduced blood flow (pressure autoregulation).
      (6) Decreased pH (carbonic and lactic acids).
      (7) Increased K^+.
      (8) Increased osmolarity.
      (9) Adenosine (cardiac vessels).
      (10) Prostaglandins (PGE and PGI_2).
      (11) Nitric oxide.
   b. Local factors producing vasoconstriction:
      (1) Decreased CO_2.
      (2) Increased O_2.
      (3) Cold.
      (4) Increased myogenic activity in response to decreased metabolism or increased blood flow and pressure.
   c. Extrinsic factors producing vasodilation are primarily via decreased sympathetic activity.
   d. Extrinsic factors producing vasoconstriction:
      (1) Epinephrine and norepinephrine from adrenal medulla.
      (2) Vasopressin.
      (3) Angiotensin II.
   e. Regulatory factors in special tissues
      (1) Coronary circulation—hypoxia and adenosine.
      (2) Cerebral circulation—CO_2 or H^+.
      (3) Pulmonary circulation—CO_2 causes vasoconstriction.
      (4) Renal circulation—autoregulation.
      (5) Skeletal muscle—sympathetic innervation at rest, local metabolites (lactate, adenosine, and K^+) during exercise.
      (6) Skin—sympathetic innervation and vasoactive substances (histamine).

F. Capillary exchange
   1. Types of exchange
      a. Passive diffusion—the key factor in the exchange of gases, substrates, and waste products between capillaries and tissue cells. This exchange occurs readily due to the following reasons:
         (1) Distance is small.
         (2) Capillary walls are composed of single cells with pores.
            (a) Responsible for passage of water-soluble substances (e.g., ions, amino acids).
            (b) Pore size varies (liver has large pores, brain has no pores).
            (c) Pore size is increased by histamine.
         (3) There are a large number of capillaries.
         (4) Flow in capillaries is slow.
         (5) Lipid-soluble substances and gases pass directly through the capillary membrane.
         (6) Proteins not exchanged by vesicular transport are retained in the capillary.
      b. Bulk flow—the volume of protein-free plasma that passes in and out of the capillary. This determines the distribution of extracellular fluid (ECF) volume between the vascular and interstitial fluid compartment. It is responsible for maintaining the distribution of fluids in the interstitial space and plasma, which, in turn, affects blood volume and blood pressure. Four primary forces determine fluid movement through the capillary membrane:
         (1) Capillary blood pressure (P_c).
            (a) Arteriolar end (30 to 37 mmHg).
            (b) Venous end (10 to 17 mmHg).
            (c) Tends to force fluid out into the interstitial space.
         (2) Interstitial fluid pressure (P_{if}).
            (a) Approximately –3 to 1 mmHg.
            (b) If positive, tends to force fluid into the capillaries.
            (c) Due to the lymphatic drainage, excess fluid is removed.
         (3) Plasma colloid osmotic pressure (π_p).
            (a) Approximately 25 to 28 mmHg.
            (b) Causes osmotic flow of fluid from interstitial space to the plasma.

(c) Due to plasma proteins trapped in the capillary.

(4) Interstitial fluid colloid osmotic pressure (π_{if}).

(a) Usually 0 mmHg.

(b) If raised, tends to cause fluid to move into the interstitial space.

(c) Caused by protein in interstitial space.

c. Overall fluid movement

(1) Ultrafiltration

(a) Bulk movement of fluid from the capillaries to the interstitial areas.

(b) Forces primarily responsible for this are:

(i) Capillary blood pressure.

(ii) Interstitial fluid colloid osmotic pressure.

(2) Resorption

(a) Bulk movement of fluid from interstitial space into capillaries.

(b) Forces primarily responsible for this are:

(i) Plasma colloid osmotic pressure.

(ii) Interstitial fluid pressure.

(3) Net exchange

(a) Net exchange pressure = $(P_c) + (\pi_{if}) - (\pi_p + P_{if})$.

(b) Positive net exchange (outward exceeds inward) = ultrafiltration.

(c) Negative net exchange (inward exceeds outward) = resorption.

d. Edema—the accumulation of excess fluid in the interstitial areas. This may be caused by the following:

(1) Reduced concentration of plasma proteins.

(a) Loss of plasma proteins (burns).

(b) Protein deficiency.

(c) Reduced protein synthesis by liver (liver disease).

(d) Loss of protein in the urine (kidney disease).

(2) Increased permeability of capillary walls.

(a) Histamine and other mediators of allergic reactions and inflammation.

(b) Leakage of plasma proteins into interstitial space due to tissue trauma.

(3) Increased venous pressure.

(a) Congestive heart failure.

(b) Localized edema (pregnancy).

(4) Lymphatic blockage.

(a) Parasitic infection (elephantiasis).

(b) Surgical removal of lymph nodes.

G. Veins

1. Serve as a blood reservoir due to their distensibility (less smooth muscle and elastin compared to arteries).
2. Increased pooling of blood results in reduced cardiac output.
3. Venous return

a. Volume of blood entering each atrium per minute.

b. Factors affecting venous return:

(1) Pressure produced by cardiac contraction.

(2) Sympathetically induced constriction of veins.

(3) Skeletal muscle activity.

(4) One-way venous valves.

H. Cardiodynamics and electrophysiology

1. Anatomical considerations

a. Atria—weak and elastic chambers that receive blood from the veins.

b. Ventricles—heavily muscled chambers.

c. Endocardium—cells that line the chambers of the heart.

d. Myocardium—short, branched, interconnected muscle cells joined together by gap junctions. These cells are electrically joined and behave as a single functional unit (syncytium). The heart muscle will therefore contract with an all-or-none contraction.

e. Epicardium—thin external membrane covering the heart.

f. Fibrous connective tissue—separates atria from the ventricles.

g. Valves

(1) Atrioventricular (AV)—open passively when the pressure in the ventricle falls below the atrial pressure. This permits blood to enter the ventricle. Closing of these valves is associated with the first heart sound.

(a) Tricuspid valve—separates the right atrium and ventricle.

(b) Bicuspid (mitral) valve—separates the left atrium and ventricle.

(2) Semilunar—open when the pressure in the ventricle exceeds the pressure in the aorta or pulmonary artery. This permits blood to be pumped out of the ventricles. Closing of these valves is associated with the second heart sound.
(a) Aortic valve.
(b) Pulmonic valve.

2. Electrical activity
   a. Pacemaker—region demonstrating spontaneous electrical activity.
      (1) Sinoatrial (SA) node—a cluster of specialized cells with inherent contractile rhythm faster than any other cells in the heart.
      (2) Ectopic pacemaker—a pacemaker other than the SA node.
      (3) Pacemaker potential—a spontaneous depolarization produced by the slow depolarization current through the membranes. Both fast and slow channels exist. Repolarization is caused by the outward diffusion of potassium ions.
   b. Conducting tissues of the heart
      (1) Atrioventricular (AV) node—located on the inferior portion of the interatrial septum. These cells conduct more slowly than the atrial cells. Due to fibrous tissue surrounding this node, it is the only normal pathway between the SA node and the ventricles. The reduced rate of conduction through this node is responsible for the atria contracting before the ventricles.
      (2) Atrioventricular bundle (bundle of His)—specialized muscle fibers that conduct impulses through the interventricular septum. Conduction rate is greatly increased compared to ventricular muscle. Responsible for the simultaneous contraction of the ventricles.
      (3) Purkinje fibers—specialized cardiac muscle fibers that carry impulses to ventricular musculature.
3. Action potential in myocardial cells—the heart has an extremely long refractory period (due to calcium channels opening and maintaining a prolonged positive membrane potential), which is almost as long as the contraction. Because of this long refractory period, the heart cannot be tetanized.
4. Cardiac innervation
   a. Parasympathetic stimulation (vagus nerve) is inhibitory since it decreases the rate of spontaneous depolarization in autorhythmic cells. Heart rate is reduced (negative chronotropic effect).
   b. Sympathetic stimulation is stimulatory since it increases the rate of spontaneous depolarization, which results in an increased heart rate (positive chronotropic effect). Sympathetics also produce an increased contractility, which results in a more forceful contraction (positive inotropic effect).
5. Electrocardiogram (ECG)—a standardized measurement of potential difference between two points on body surfaces caused by the electrical activity of the heart.
   a. A typical tracing produces a P-Q-R-S-T wave (Figure 2-22).
      (1) P wave is caused by depolarization of the atria.
      (2) QRS complex represents ventricular depolarization.
      (3) T wave is produced by repolarization of the ventricles.
   b. ECG can be used to monitor abnormal heart rate and rhythm.
      (1) Tachycardia—shorter distances between QRS complexes (>100 bpm).
      (2) Bradycardia—longer distances between QRS complexes (<50 bpm).

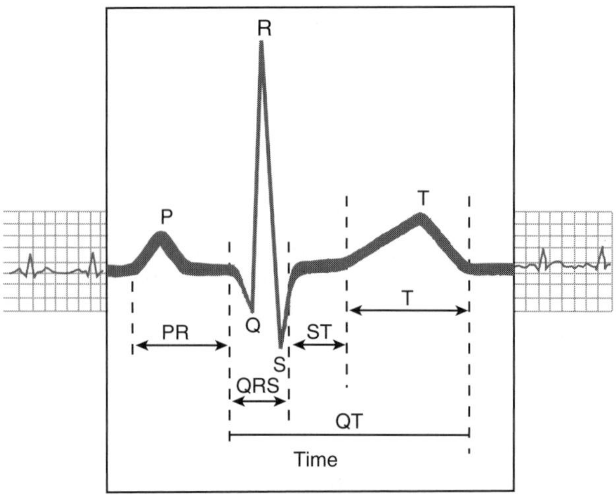

Figure 2–22. The important deflections and intervals of a typical electrocardiogram. (From Berne RM, Levy MN: Principles of Physiology, ed 4, St. Louis, Mosby, 2006.)

(3) Extrasystoles—beats from an ectopic source.
(4) Atrial flutter—very rapid atrial depolarization.
(5) Atrial fibrillation—rapid, irregular uncoordinated atrial depolarization.
(6) Ventricular fibrillation—rapid, uncoordinated ventricular contractions.
(7) Heart block—interruptions of impulses between atria and ventricles.

6. Mechanical events of the cardiac cycle (Figure 2-23)
   a. Early diastole (diastole = periods of relaxation and filling)
      (1) Semilunar valves are closed.
      (2) Due to venous return, atrial pressure is greater than ventricular pressure.
      (3) AV valves are open.
      (4) Ventricular volume increases (rapidly initially, then slowly).
   b. Late diastole
      (1) SA node fires, spreads over the atria (P wave), and atria contract.
      (2) Atrial contraction causes an increase in both atrial and ventricular pressure.
   c. Early systole
      (1) Ventricle has reached the end-diastolic volume (EDV). This is also referred to as the *preload.*
      (2) Impulses pass through the AV node.
      (3) QRS complex represents ventricular depolarization and contraction.
      (4) Ventricular pressure increases.
      (5) AV valves close once pressure in ventricle is greater than pressure in atrium.
   d. Peak systole
      (1) Ventricular pressure continues to rise.
      (2) Both valves are closed so pressure increases with a constant volume (isovolumetric contraction).
      (3) Aortic valve opens when ventricular pressure is greater than aortic or pulmonary pressure.
      (4) Blood is ejected into systemic and pulmonary branches, resulting in increased pressure in these vessels. The *stroke volume,* which is the amount of blood pumped out with each contraction.
      (5) Ventricular volume decreases to the lowest level in the cycle. This is the end systolic volume (ESV), also known as the *afterload.*

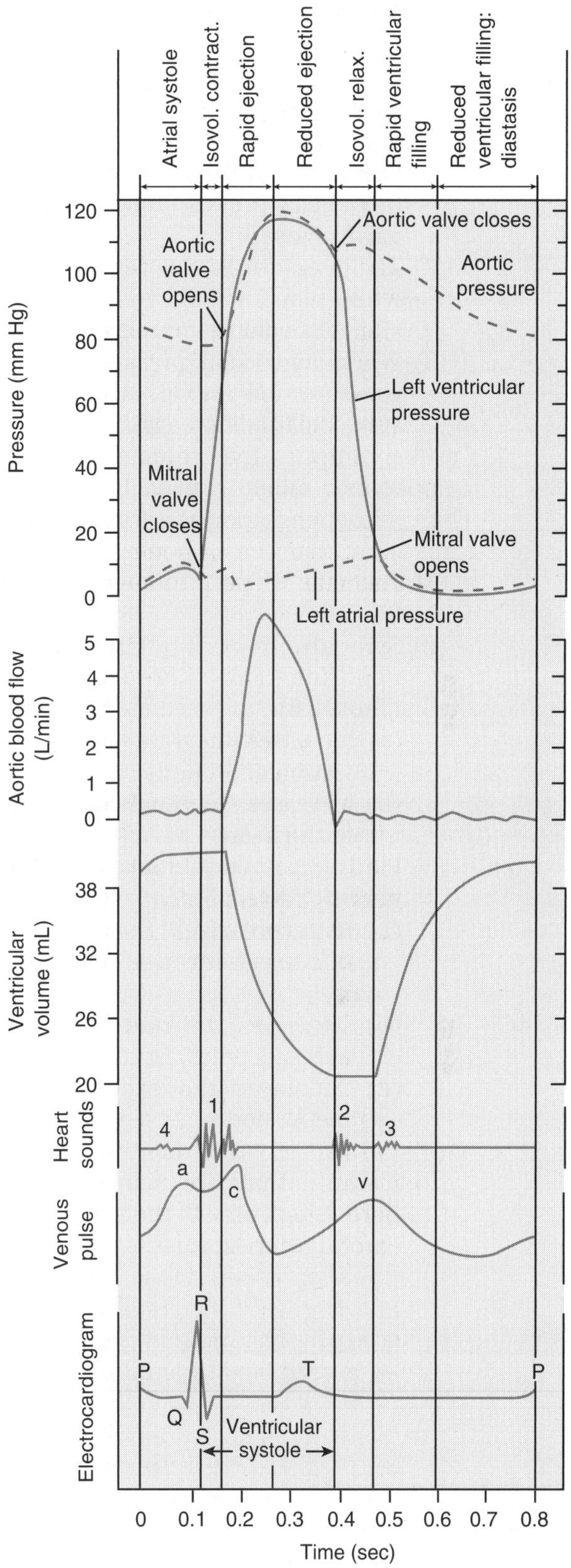

Figure 2-23. Left atrial, aortic, and left ventricular pressure pulses correlated in time with aortic flow, ventricular volume, heart sounds, venous pulse, and the electrocardiogram for a complete cardiac cycle. (From Berne RM, Levy MN: Principles of Physiology, ed 4, St. Louis, Mosby, 2006.)

(6) T wave that represents ventricular repolarization occurs at the end of ventricular systole.

e. Late systole
   (1) Ventricles start to relax and, when the ventricle pressure < aortic or pulmonary pressure, the semilunar valves close.
   (2) The pressure in the ventricle falls while blood volume remains constant (isovolumetric relaxation).
   (3) When ventricular pressure < atrial pressure, the AV valves open, and ventricular filling begins.

7. Cardiac output—the volume of blood pumped per minute by each ventricle. This will depend upon the following factors:
   a. Cardiac rate, which is influenced by:
      (1) SA node.
      (2) Sympathetic stimulation (epinephrine and norepinephrine) (Table 2-5).
         (a) Increases the rate of depolarization of SA node.
         (b) Increases electrical conduction in the heart.
      (3) Parasympathetic stimulation (vagus nerve) (Table 2-5).
         (a) Hyperpolarizes the SA node due to enhanced K^+ permeability.
         (b) Decreases the rate of spontaneous depolarization.
         (c) Decreases the excitability of the AV node.
      (4) Cardiac control centers in the medulla that are influenced by baroreceptors in the aorta and carotid arteries.
   b. Stroke volume, which is influenced by:
      (1) End-diastolic volume (EDV)—the volume of blood in the ventricles at the end of diastole. Stroke volume is directly proportional to EDV.
      (2) Total peripheral resistance (TPR)—the frictional resistance to blood flow in the arteries. Stroke volume is inversely proportional to TPR.
      (3) Contractility—the strength of ventricular contraction. Stroke volume is directly proportional to contractility.
   c. Stroke volume is also regulated by both intrinsic and extrinsic means.
      (1) Intrinsic control—the inherent ability of the heart to vary stroke volume. This is referred to as the *Frank–Starling Law of the Heart.*
         (a) The strength of ventricular contraction varies directly with EDV.
         (b) Increased stretching of cardiac muscle allows for more advantageous overlapping of actin and myosin, resulting in a more forceful contraction.
      (2) Extrinsic control—factors originating outside the heart that affect stroke volume.
         (a) Contraction strength—increasing sympathetic stimulation and epinephrine from the adrenal medulla increases the amount of calcium available for the sarcomeres. This results in an increased stroke volume.
         (b) Increased venous return.
            (i) Increased sympathetic activity stimulates smooth

TABLE 2–5. EFFECTS OF AUTONOMIC NERVOUS SYSTEM ON THE HEART AND BLOOD VESSELS

	SYMPATHETIC		PARASYMPATHETIC	
	ACTION	**RECEPTOR**	**ACTION**	**RECEPTOR**
Heart rate	↑	β_1	↓	M_2
Contractility	↑	β_1	↓ (atria only)	M_2
Conduction velocity (AV node)	↑	β_1	↓	M_2
Vascular smooth muscle (skin, renal, and splanchnic)	Constriction	α_1	Dilation (releases EDRF)	M_3
Vascular smooth muscle (skeletal muscle)	Dilation	β_2	Dilation (releases EDRF)	M_3
	Constriction	α_1		

From Costanzo LS: Physiology, ed 3, WB Saunders, Philadelphia, 2004.
AV, Atrioventricular; *EDRF,* endothelial-derived relaxing factor or nitric oxide; *M,* muscarinic.

muscle contractions in venous walls, increasing venous return.

(ii) Skeletal muscle pump.

(iii) Pressure difference between the thoracic and abdominal muscles.

8. Blood pressure determinants and regulation
   a. Mean arterial pressure = cardiac output multiplied by the total peripheral resistance (MAP = CO × TPR).
   b. Regulatory mechanisms of the autonomic nervous center (vasomotor center). All are located in the medulla.
      (1) Cardioinhibitory center—parasympathetic innervations to SA and AV nodes of the heart.
      (2) Cardiostimulatory center—sympathetic stimulation to SA and AV nodes of the heart and ventricle.
      (3) Vasoconstrictor system—innervates vasoconstrictor fibers to provide vascular tone (sympathetic system acts on alpha adrenergic receptors) (Table 2-5).
   c. Arterial pressure is regulated (adjusted) by both short-term and long-term adjustments.
      (1) Short-term adjustments
         (a) Baroreceptors—respond to increased blood pressure.
            (i) Located in aortic arch and carotid sinus.
            (ii) Afferent nerves carry signals to vasomotor center via glossopharyngeal and vagus nerves.
            (iii) Efferent pathways in autonomic nervous system (ANS) result in decreased sympathetic tone and increased parasympathetic activity.
            (iv) Ultimately produces decreased cardiac output and total peripheral resistance.
         (b) Bainbridge reflex—produces an increased heart rate due to stretching of the right atrium.
         (c) Carotid and aortic chemoreceptors.
            (i) Sensitive to decreased O_2, increased CO_2, and decreased pH.
            (ii) Input acts via CNS vasomotor center.
            (iii) Reductions in blood pressure (resulting in reduced flow through these chemoreceptor areas) result in an increase in blood pressure.
         (d) CNS ischemic response.
            (i) Reduced blood flow in CNS produces increased CO_2.
            (ii) Vasomotor center is stimulated to produce an increased blood pressure.
      (2) Long-term adjustments—adjustments in body fluid by the kidney.
         (a) Renal function curve.
            (i) Increased blood pressure results in increased renal fluid excretion.
            (ii) Increased fluid loss produces the following:
               1. Less extracellular fluid and blood volume.
               2. Less venous return and cardiac output.
               3. Reduced blood pressure.
         (b) Vasopressin (ADH)
            (i) Secreted from the pituitary in response to increased osmolarity.
            (ii) Stimulates the kidney to retain water.
            (iii) Ultimately increases blood volume and increases blood pressure.
         (c) Renin-angiotensin system.
            (i) Reduced renal perfusion pressure leads to renin release (Figure 2-24).
            (ii) Aldosterone
               1. Secreted by the adrenal medulla in response to reduced circulating fluid volume (may be due to chronic sodium depletion) and increased plasma potassium.
               2. Stimulates the resorption of sodium and secretion of potassium in the kidney.
               3. Water is resorbed passively, resulting in increased blood volume and blood pressure.
9. Coagulation (Figure 2-25)

Figure 2–24. The renin-angiotensin II-aldosterone system. P_a, Arterial pressure; TPR, total peripheral resistance.

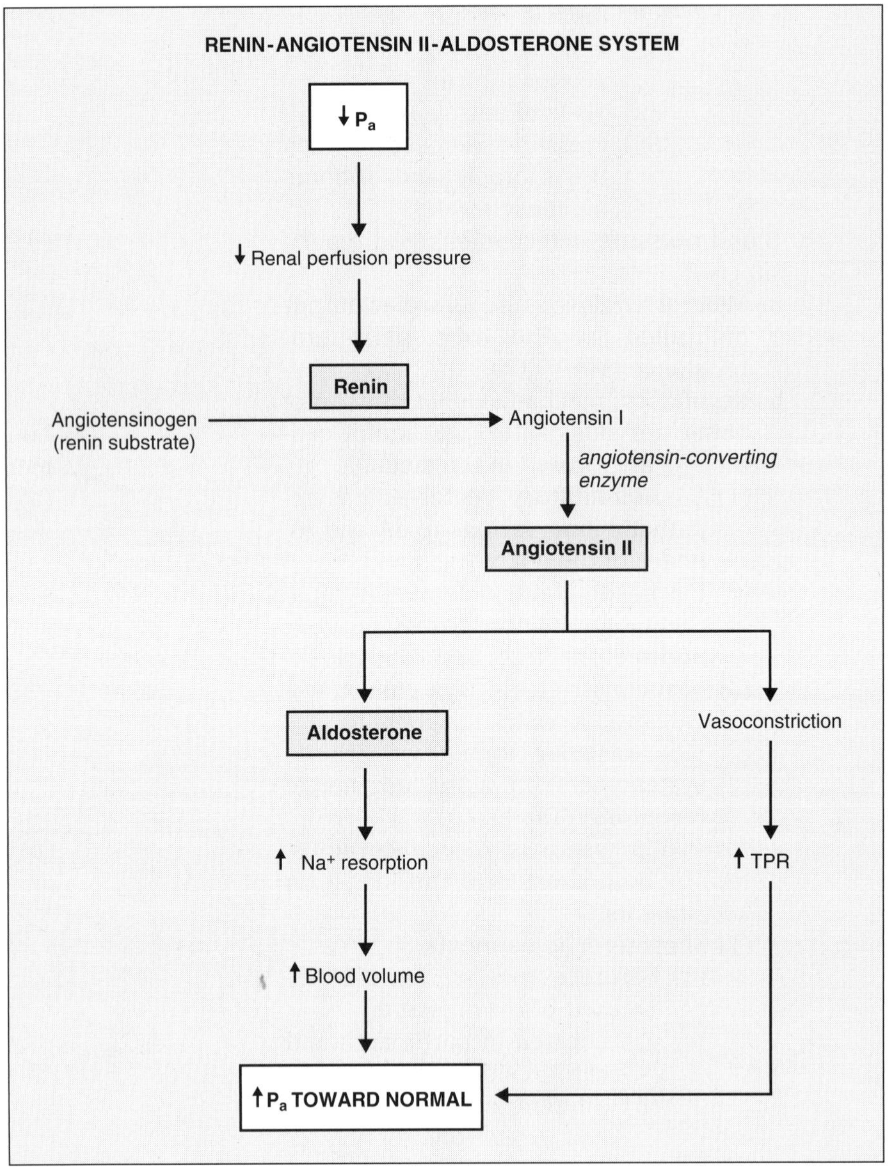

9.0 RESPIRATION

9.1 Mechanical Aspects

A. Conducting zone—responsible for bringing air into and out of the respiratory zone. These structures include the nasal passages, pharynx, trachea, bronchi, bronchioles, and terminal bronchioles.
   1. Lined with mucus and ciliated cells.
   2. Contain smooth muscle, which is innervated by the autonomic nervous system.
      a. Sympathetics—β_2-adrenergic receptors, which produce relaxation and dilation of airways.
      b. Parasympathetics—muscarinic receptors, which produce contraction and constriction of the airways.

B. Respiratory zone—responsible for gas exchange. These structures include the respiratory bronchioles, alveolar ducts, and alveolar sacs.
   1. Respiratory bronchioles have cilia and innervated smooth muscle.
   2. Alveoli exchange O_2 and CO_2 and are composed of three cell types:
      a. Type I—epithelial cells for diffusion (predominant type).
      b. Type II—synthesize surfactant.
      c. Alveolar macrophages—remove foreign material from alveoli.

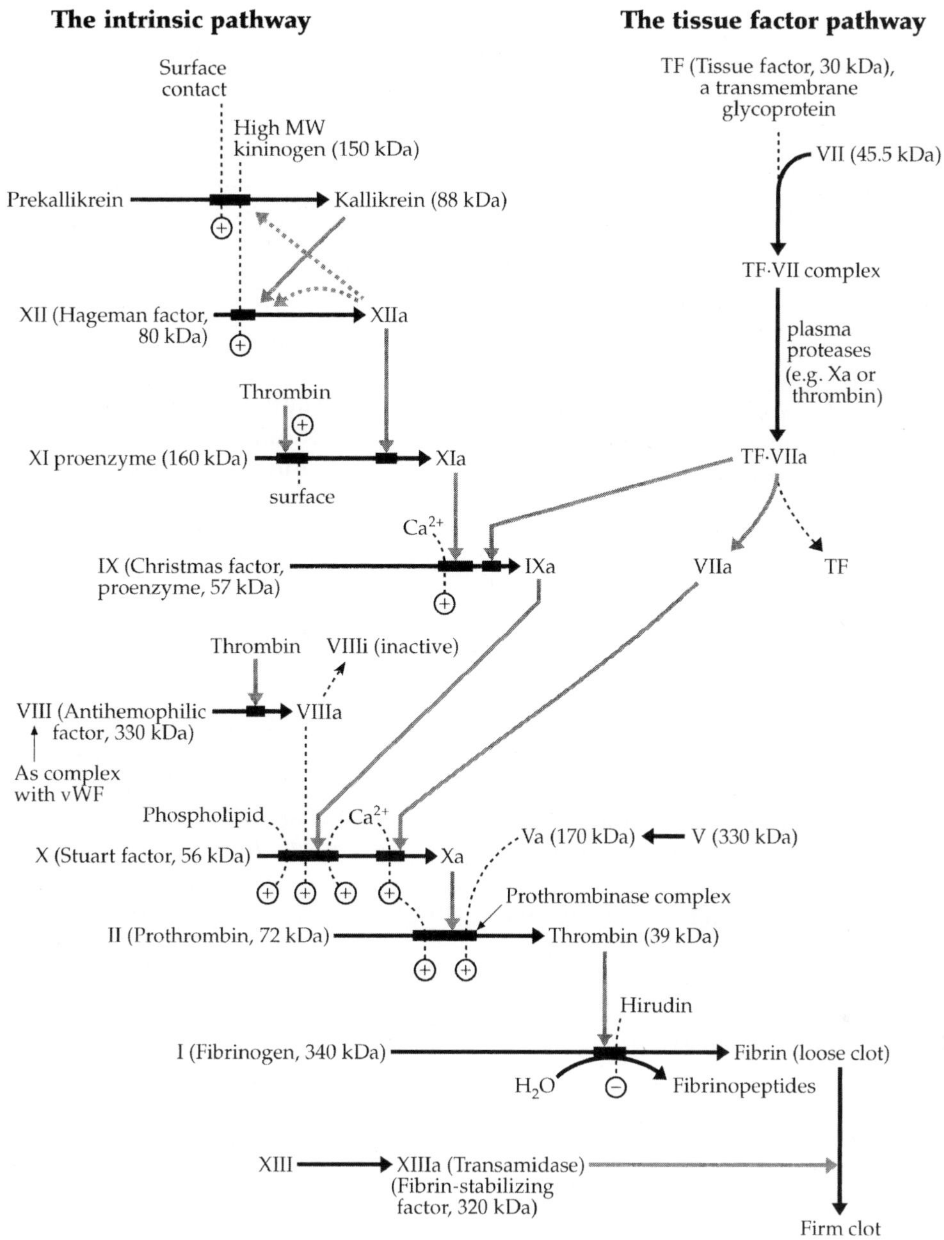

Figure 2–25. Major components of the human blood-clotting cascades. The site of action of the leech anticoagulant protein hirudin is also indicated. (From Metzler DE: Biochemistry, ed 2, Academic Press, San Diego, 2003.)

C. Terminology (Figure 2-26)
   1. Lung volume.
      a. Tidal volume.
      b. Inspiratory reserve volume.
      c. Expiratory reserve volume.
      d. Residual volume.
   2. Lung capacity.
      a. Inspiratory capacity.
      b. Functional residual capacity (FRC).
      c. Vital capacity.
      d. Total lung capacity.
   3. Dead space—does not participate in gas exchange.
      a. Anatomical dead space = conducting zone (see above).
      b. Physiological dead space—includes anatomical dead space and alveoli that do not participate in gas exchange.

D. Ventilation rate—volume of air moving in and out of the lungs per unit of time.
   1. Minute ventilation = tidal volume (mL) × breaths per minute.
   2. Alveolar ventilation = (tidal volume − dead space) × breaths per minute.

E. Mechanics and physics of respiration

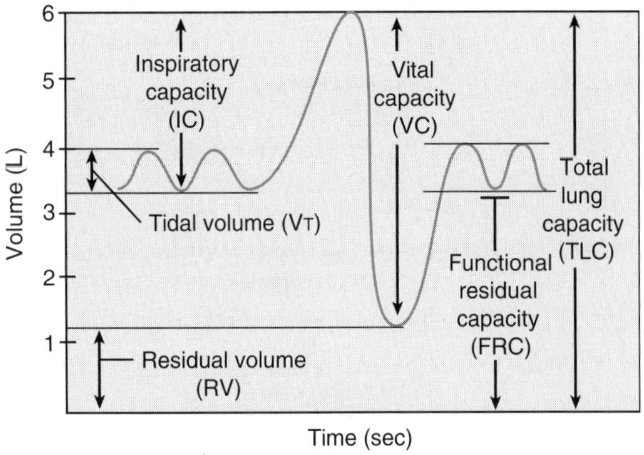

Figure 2–26. Tracing of lung volume changes during normal breathing and maximal inspiration. (From Berne RM, Levy MN: Principles of Physiology, ed 4, St. Louis, Mosby, 2006.)

1. Inspiration—primarily due to the contraction of the diaphragm. In heavy exercise, the external intercostal muscles and accessory muscles may be used.
2. Expiration—primarily passive by reverse pressure gradient between the lungs and atmosphere. In exercise, internal intercostals muscles and abdominal muscles may be used.
3. Compliance—distensibility of the system. Inversely related to elasticity. Relates the change in volume for a given change in pressure and also determines the effort needed to distend the lungs. (Compliance = δ V/P, where V = volume and P = pressure).
   a. Pressures to consider:
      (1) Atmospheric pressure = 760 mmHg.
      (2) Intra-alveolar pressure = pressure in the alveoli.
      (3) Intrapleural pressure = pressure in the pleural cavity which, since it is a closed sac surrounding the lung, is less than atmospheric pressure. Pressure here is referred to as *negative pressure*.
      (4) Boyles's Law states that when you increase the volume, the pressure decreases, and decreasing the volume increases the pressure.
   b. Factors that change lung compliance:
      (1) Emphysema increases lung compliance due to loss of elastic fibers. A higher FRC is present.
      (2) Fibrosis decreases lung compliance. A lower FRC exists.
4. Elastance—the reciprocal of compliance or the tendency of the lung to recoil.
   a. Collagen and elastic fibers provide elastance.
   b. Alveolar surface tension due to an aqueous film. Attraction between water molecules opposes the expansion of the lungs and tends to collapse the alveoli.
   c. Pulmonary surfactant decreases the surface tension in alveoli, increasing pulmonary compliance and reducing the tendency for the alveoli to collapse.
5. Relationship of pressure and resistance to airflow.
   a. Airflow is directly proportional to the pressure difference between the mouth/nose and the alveoli and is inversely proportional to the resistance of the airways. Q = δ P/R, where Q = flow.
   b. Airway resistance is primarily determined by changes in airway diameter (Poiseuille's Law). Changes in lung volume and air viscosity may also change resistance. Three factors must be considered:
      (1) Autonomic nervous system
         (a) Parasympathetic system causes constriction of smooth muscle and produces increased resistance.
         (b) Sympathetic system produces relaxation and decreases resistance.
      (2) Lung volume
         (a) High volume—more traction, less resistance.
         (b) Low volume—less traction, more resistance.
      (3) Viscosity of air
         (a) High density of gas increases resistance.
         (b) Low density (e.g., helium) decreases resistance.

F. Breathing cycle—summary
1. At rest
   a. Alveolar pressure = atmospheric pressure (no airflow since δ P is 0).
   b. Intrapleural pressure is negative due to the tendency of the lungs to collapse and chest wall to expand.
   c. Volume in lungs = FRC.
   d. Forces keeping alveoli open (transmural pressure gradient and surfactant) equal the forces promoting alveoli

to close (elasticity and alveolar surface tension).

2. Inspiration
   a. Diaphragm contracts, increasing thoracic volume and decreasing pressure in lungs.
   b. Change in airway and alveolar pressure (below atmospheric pressure) drives air into the lungs (tidal volume).
3. Expiration
   a. Elastic forces of the lungs compress air in alveoli.
   b. Alveolar pressure becomes greater than atmospheric pressure, forcing air out of the lungs.
   c. Volume remaining is FRC, and the volume expired is the tidal volume.

9.2 Gas Exchange and Transport

A. Gas exchange—occurs due to the ability of gases to move down partial pressure gradients.

1. Partial pressure = total pressure × fractional concentration of dissolved gas.
2. Partial pressure is the pressure that gas would exert if it occupied the total volume of the mixture.
3. The diffusion rates of gases depend upon the partial pressure differences across the alveoli and the surface area for diffusion (Figure 2-27).
   a. Pulmonary—capillary gas exchange
      (1) Oxygen moves from alveoli (Po_2 = 100 mmHg) to the pulmonary capillaries (Po_2 = 40 mmHg).
      (2) Carbon dioxide moves from the venous blood (Pco_2 = 46 mmHg) to the alveoli (Pco_2 = 40 mmHg).
   b. Tissue—capillary gas exchange
      (1) Oxygen moves from blood (Po_2 = 100 mmHg) into the cells (Po_2 ≤40 mmHg).
      (2) Carbon dioxide moves from the cells (Pco_2 > 46 mmHg) into the blood (Pco_2 = 40 mmHg).
4. Limitations to gas exchange
   a. Diffusion limited—gas exchange is limited by the diffusion process. Partial pressure is maintained, but exchange cannot occur.

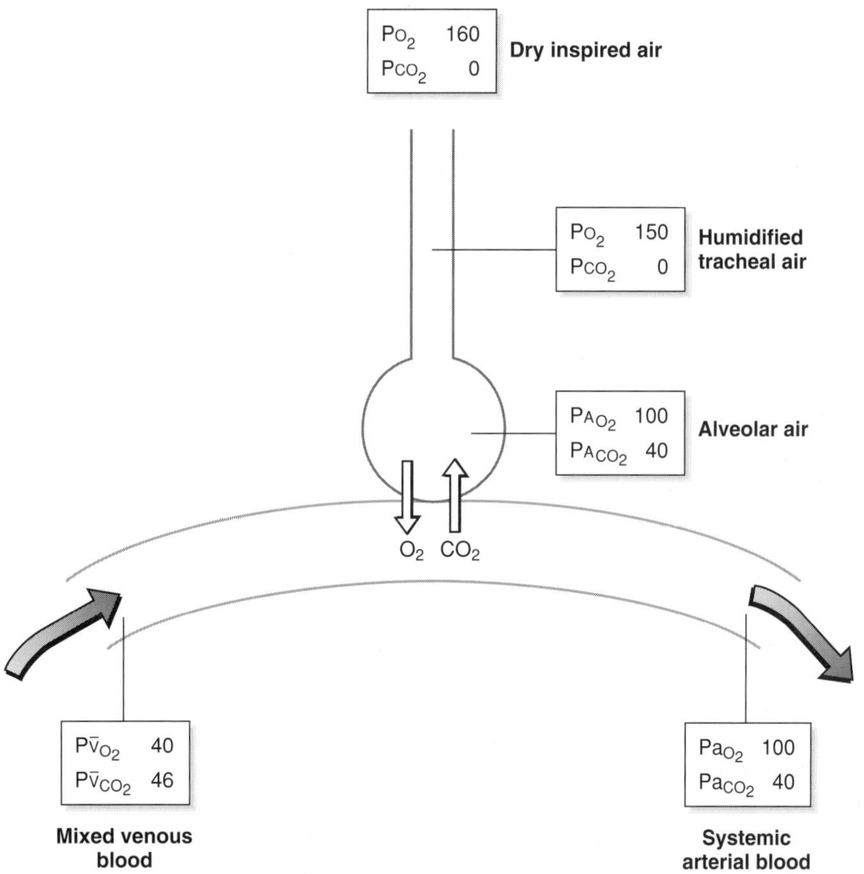

Figure 2–27. Values for Po_2 and Pco_2 in dry inspired air, humidified tracheal air, alveolar air, and pulmonary capillary blood.

(1) Fibrosis—alveolar membrane thickens, increasing the diffusion distance.
(2) Emphysema—surface area for diffusion is decreased.

b. Perfusion limited—gas exchange is limited by the flow rate through the pulmonary capillaries. Partial pressure is not maintained since equilibration occurs rapidly.

B. Gas transport

1. Oxygen—transported either dissolved or associated with hemoglobin.
   a. Dissolved oxygen (2%)—directly proportional to the PO_2 (approximately 0.3 mL/100 mL).
   b. Hemoglobin oxygen (98%)—responsible for most O_2 transport (20 mL/100 mL). Hemoglobin concentration determines the O_2 content of the blood.
   c. Hemoglobin–O_2 dissociation curve
      (1) Demonstrates the change in affinity of hemoglobin as each successive O_2 molecule binds to a heme site. This facilitates loading and unloading of oxygen as it is transported through the body.
         (a) Leaving the lungs, Hb is almost 100% saturated (bound to four heme groups). PO_2 is 100 mmHg. The high affinity of Hb at PO_2 >60 mmHg ensures Hb saturation at different atmospheric pressures.
         (b) In tissues (PO_2 = 40 mmHg), Hb releases O_2, leaving Hb about 75% saturated (oxygen reserve). At lower PO_2, the affinity of Hb for oxygen is less, facilitating the release to tissues.
      (2) Changes in hemoglobin–O_2 dissociation curve—reflect a change in affinity of hemoglobin for O_2.
         (a) Shift to right—decreased Hb affinity caused by:
            (i) Increases in PCO_2 or decreases in pH.
            (ii) Increases in temperature.
            (iii) Increases in 2,3-diphosphoglycerate (2,3-DPG) concentration (product of red blood cell [RBC] glycolysis).
         (b) Shift to the left—increased Hb affinity caused by:
            (i) Decreases in PCO_2 or increases in pH.
            (ii) Decreases in 2,3-DPG concentration.
            (iii) Fetal hemoglobin—does not bind 2,3-DPG.
            (iv) Carbon monoxide poisoning (carboxyhemoglobin).
         (c) Iron in its ferric state (Fe^{3+}); methemoglobin does not bind oxygen.
2. Carbon dioxide—transported in three forms (Figure 2-28).
   a. Dissolved CO_2—more soluble than O_2.
   b. Carbaminohemoglobin.
   c. Bicarbonate—90% of CO_2 transported in this form.
      (1) CO_2 produced in the tissues diffuses into the plasma and RBC.
      (2) RBC carbonic anhydrase catalyzes the formation of H_2CO_3, which dissociates into H^+ and HCO_3^-.
      (3) HCO_3 diffuses out of RBC (in exchange for Cl^-) and is transported to the lungs where, in RBC, CO_2 is regenerated catalyzed by carbonic anhydrase (reverse of reaction described in [2]).

9.3 Regulation

A. Ventilation/perfusion relationships

1. Pulmonary blood flow—pressure and resistance are much lower than systemic circulation. It is regulated primarily by hypoxic vasoconstriction (decreases blood flow due to poorly ventilated areas of the lung). Thromboxane A_2 from macrophages, leukocytes, and endothelial cells produces vasoconstriction. Prostacyclin is a potent vasodilator. Leukotrienes produce airway constriction.
2. Distribution of pulmonary blood flow—three zones due to gravitational effects:
   a. Zone I (apex)—highest V/Q (see later)
      (1) Lowest blood flow.
      (2) Arterial pressure < alveolar pressure (vessels partially collapsed).
   b. Zone II (middle)
      (1) Blood flow medium.
      (2) Arterial pressure > alveolar pressure > venous pressure.
      (3) Blood flow driven by difference between arterial pressure and alveolar pressure.

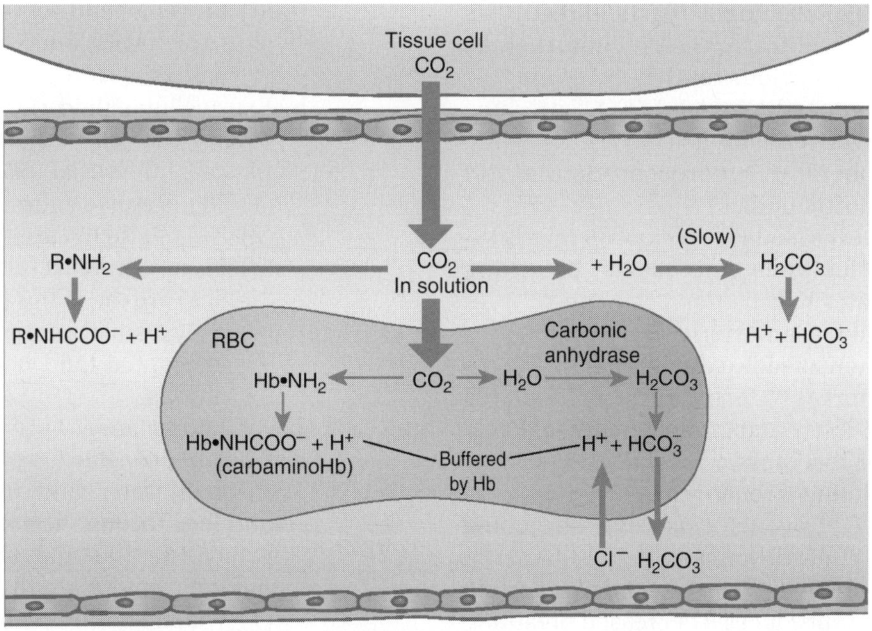

Figure 2–28. The three mechanisms of CO_2 transport in blood. As CO diffuses into capillary blood from peripheral tissues, it may slowly react with water to form carbonic acid, or with the amine side groups of plasma proteins to form carbamino compounds. However, the vast majority of CO diffuses into the red blood cells (RBCs), where it rapidly forms carbonic acid, a reaction catalyzed by carbonic anhydrase. The bicarbonate ions formed exchange with chloride ions in plasma because the erythrocyte membrane is readily permeable to small anions. As the hemoglobin loses its oxygen, it becomes more able to bind CO to its NH side groups to form carbaminohemoglobin compounds. (From Berne RM, Levy MN: Principles of Physiology, ed 4, St. Louis, Mosby, 2006.)

c. Zone III (base)—lowest V/Q (see later)
  (1) Blood flow highest.
  (2) Arterial pressure > venous pressure > alveolar pressure.
  (3) Blood flow driven by differences between arterial and venous pressures.

3. Ventilation/perfusion ratio—the ratio of alveolar ventilation (V) to pulmonary blood flow (Q).
  a. Normal V/Q = 0.8 (this is an average for all three zones).
    (1) Breathing frequency, tidal volume, and cardiac output are normal.
    (2) Po_2 (100 mmHg) and Pco_2 (40 mmHg) will be normal.
  b. V/Q is infinite—lack of perfusion (dead space), which can occur in pulmonary embolism.
  c. V/Q is high—reduced blood flow through the lung.
  d. V/Q is low—reduced alveolar ventilation.

B. Control of respiration
  1. CNS
    a. Medullary respiratory center (reticular formation)
      (1) Inspiratory center—controls the basic rhythm (frequency).
      (2) Expiratory center—inactive during quiet breathing but active during active breathing (exercise).
    b. Apneustic center (pons)
      (1) Stimulates inspiration.
      (2) Produces prolonged inspiration.
    c. Pneumotaxic center (pons)
      (1) Inhibits inspiration.
      (2) Limits tidal volume and respiratory rate.
    d. Cortex
      (1) Voluntary regulation of breathing.
      (2) Produces hyperventilation or hypoventilation.
  2. Chemoreceptors
    a. Central chemoreceptors (medulla)
      (1) Increased H^+
        (a) Acts directly on central chemoreceptors.
        (b) Stimulates breathing (hyperventilation).
      (2) Increased Pco_2
        (a) Diffuses into the cerebral spinal fluid, combines with H_2O to produce carbonic acid.

(b) Resulting H^+ acts directly on central chemoreceptors (see previous text).

(3) Reduced H^+ and CO_2 produce hypoventilation.

b. Peripheral chemoreceptors (carotid and aortic bodies)

(1) Decreased Po_2 (below 60 mmHg)—stimulates increased breathing rate.

(2) Increased arterial Pco_2—stimulates increased breathing rate.

(3) Increased arterial H^+—stimulates directly and independently of Pco_2.

c. Other receptors

(1) Hering–Breuer reflex

(a) Prevents excessive stretching of the lungs.

(b) Distention of smooth muscle produces a decreased breathing frequency.

(2) Mechanoreceptors

(a) Located in joints and muscles.

(b) Movement stimulates inspiratory center to increase respiration.

(c) Irritant receptors—located in epithelial cells of the lung. They are stimulated by noxious substances.

10.0 RENAL

A. Body fluids

1. Total body water (TBW) = about 60% of adult body weight. It is distributed in two major compartments:

a. Intracellular fluid (ICF)—within the cells = two thirds TBW.

(1) Mg^{2+} and K^+ are major cations.

(2) Proteins and organic phosphates (ATP, ADP, and AMP) are major anions.

b. Extracellular fluid (ECF)—all fluid outside of the cells = one third TBW (e.g., plasma, interstitial fluid,).

(1) Na^+ is major cation in ECF.

(2) HCO_3^- and Cl^- are major anions.

(3) Plasma proteins (albumin and globulins) are the major plasma proteins.

(4) Only a small amount of protein is in interstitial fluid under normal conditions.

2. Body fluid balance

a. Control of fluid volume—primarily through water and mineral retention and loss through the kidney. The basic principles essential to understanding fluid movement are the following:

(1) Volume of body fluid depends upon the amount of solute it contains.

(2) ICF and ECF are in osmotic equilibrium (290 mOsm/L). However, specific ion concentration does differ between compartments (see previous text).

(3) Equilibration between ICF and ECF occurs through fluid movement, not through the movement of osmotically active molecules.

b. Disturbances in body fluid occur under various conditions (Table 2-6).

B. Renal function

1. Overview of function

a. Regulatory function

(1) Composition of body fluids.

(2) Volume of body fluids.

b. Endocrine function

(1) Activation and secretion of vitamin D (1-25-dihdroxy-vitamin D_3).

Table 2–6. Disturbances of Body Fluids

Type	Example	ECF Volume	ICF Volume	Osmolarity	Hematocrit	Plasma Protein
Isosmotic volume contraction	Diarrhea	↓	N.C.	N.C.	↑	↑
Hyperosmotic volume contraction	Sweating; fever; diabetes insipidus	↓	↓	↑	N.C.	↑
Hyposmotic volume contraction	Adrenal isufficiency	↓	↑	↓	↑	↑
Isosmotic volume expansion	Infusion of isotonic NaCl	↑	N.C.	N.C.	↓	↓
Hyperosmotic volume expansion	High NaCl intake	↑	↓	↑	↓	↓
Hyposmotic volume expansion	SIADH	↑	↑	↓	N.C.	↓

ECF, Extracellular fluid; *ICF*, intracellular fluid; *NaCl*, sodium chloride; *N.C.*, no change; *SIADH*, syndrome of inappropriate antidiuretic hormone.
From Costanzo LS: Physiology, ed 3, WB Saunders, Philadelphia, 2004.

(2) Secretion of renin.
(3) Secretion of erythropoietin.

c. Excretory function
(1) Uric acid.
(2) Urea.
(3) Creatinine.
(4) Foreign substances/drugs.

2. Functional anatomy

a. Vasculature—composed of two sets of capillaries to filter and resorb/secrete plasma components.
(1) Renal arteries.
(2) Afferent arterioles.
(3) Glomerular capillaries.
(4) Efferent arterioles.
(5) Peritubular capillaries.
(6) Venules and renal veins.

b. Tubules
(1) Bowman's capsule.
(2) Proximal tubule.
(3) Loop of Henle.
(4) Distal tubule.
(5) Collecting ducts.

c. Accessory structures
(1) Ureters.
(2) Bladder.
(3) Urethra.

3. Renal activities

a. Renal blood flow—the volume of blood entering the renal artery (mL/min).
(1) The amount is directly proportional to the pressure difference between the renal artery and renal vein and indirectly proportional to resistance of the renal vasculature.
(2) Characterized by autoregulation between 100 to 200 mmHg blood pressure.
(3) Sympathetic stimulation and angiotensin II can alter RBF, increasing resistance and reducing RBF. This ultimately will result in a reduced GFR (see later).
(4) Measured by clearance of para-aminohippuric acid (PAH).

b. Glomerular filtration—the filtration across the glomerular capillaries and through the glomerular membrane, which normally is impermeable to protein. (Approximately 20% of the renal plasma flow is filtered by the glomerulus.)
(1) Glomerular filtration rate (GFR) = the rate at which tubular fluid is produced. This is dependent upon the following factors:
(a) Hydrostatic pressures (capillary pressure) in Bowman's capsule. This favors filtration.
(b) Colloid osmotic pressure in plasma. This opposes filtration.
(c) Colloid osmotic pressure in filtrate. This favors filtration when present.
(d) Bowman's hydrostatic pressure. This opposes filtration.
(e) Permeability of capillaries and glomerular membrane. May oppose or favor filtration.
(f) Renal blood flow. May oppose or favor filtration.
(2) Due to the combination of these factors, filtration is always favored along the entire length of the glomerular capillaries.
(3) GFR is measured by the clearance of inulin and creatinine, which are filtered but not resorbed or secreted by the renal tubules.

c. Tubular resorption—selective removal of filtered solutes from tubule back into the peritubule capillaries.
(1) May be either active (transporters in membranes) or passive (urea).
(2) All glucose is resorbed.
(a) Secondary active transport system in the proximal tubule, which depends upon the sodium gradient established by the Na^+-K^+-ATPase pump.
(b) Facilitated diffusion also occurs utilizing GLUT 1 and GLUT 2 carriers.
(c) Under normal conditions, all glucose is resorbed. However, the carrier proteins are saturable and specific. If the transport potential is exceeded (> T_{max}, transport maximum), glucose will appear in the urine.
(3) Most Na^+ is resorbed by an active transport system throughout the tubules. Na^+-K^+-ATPase pumps sodium out of the epithelial cells and, once in the interstitial space, establishes a concentration gradient for passive diffusion. Cl^- and water follow passively.

(a) Two thirds in the proximal tubule (not regulated).
(b) One quarter in the loop of Henle (not regulated).
(c) Remainder in the distal and collecting tubules (regulated by aldosterone).

(4) Half of the urea resulting from protein degradation is resorbed passively and the remainder excreted.
(a) Distal tubule and cortical and outer medullary collecting ducts are impermeable to urea and therefore do not contribute to resorption.
(b) Antidiuretic hormone (ADH) or vasopressin (see later) increases urea permeability in the inner medullary collecting ducts, and urea diffuses down a concentration gradient into the inner medulla.

(5) Most filtered K^+ is resorbed in the proximal tubule.

(6) Most filtered phosphate is resorbed in the proximal tubule and distal nephron. This is inhibited by parathyroid hormone (see Endocrinology section), leading to increased phosphate excretion.

(7) Most filtered calcium is passively resorbed in the proximal tubule and loop of Henle. Parathyroid hormone (PTH) increases Ca^{2+} resorption in the distal tubule.

(8) Most HCO_3^- is resorbed in the proximal tubule.
(a) Utilizes carbonic anhydrase as an intermediate step.
(b) Results in a net resorption of bicarbonate and sodium.
(c) At high levels of HCO_3^-, it is excreted.
(d) Increased P_{CO_2} increases bicarbonate resorption.

d. Tubular secretion—selective secretion of plasma constituents into the tubule for excretion in the urine.

(1) K^+ is passively secreted in the distal and collecting tubules by way of a K^+ Cl^- cotransporter pathway. This accounts for most of the K^+ appearing in the urine.
(a) Aldosterone (released due to elevated plasma K^+ or reduced plasma Na^+) stimulates the secretion of K^+ in exchange for Na^+ (see previous text).
(b) Acidosis will decrease K^+ secretion since H^+ will exchange for K^+. Alkalosis therefore will increase K^+ secretion.

(2) H^+ is excreted with urinary buffers.
(a) Inorganic phosphate is the major buffer involved with urinary excretion of acid.
(b) The net process results in the resorption of bicarbonate and secretion of H^+ as $H_2PO_4^-$ (titratable acid).
(c) NH_4^+ (produced from protein and phospholipid metabolism) is also secreted, resulting in an overall loss of H^+.

4. Renal clearance is the volume of arterial plasma that is completely cleared of a particular substance by the kidneys per minute.
a. A substance freely filterable but not secreted or resorbed can be used to measure GFR (inulin and creatinine).
b. A substance that is present in the plasma but not excreted has a clearance of 0. Under normal conditions, glucose has a plasma clearance of 0.

5. Corticopapillary osmotic gradient—changes in osmotic characteristics in the interstitial fluid of the kidney as you progress through the medulla to the pelvis of the kidney. This osmotic gradient established by the loop of Henle helps to resorb water from the distal ducts and collecting tubules in the presence of ADH (see previous text). This is also known as the *countercurrent mechanism*.
a. The gradient is established by selectively resorbing NaCl in the thick ascending limb by Na^+-K^+-$2Cl^-$ cotransporter.
b. Urea recycling and selective permeability of urea also add to the osmotic gradient in the inner medulla.

6. Osmoregulation—maintaining body fluid osmolarity of approximately 290 mOsm/L. This function is primarily under the control of the kidney.
a. Hypotonicity—produced when excess water is consumed (osmolarity < 290 mOsm/L).
(1) Inhibits osmoreceptors in hypothalamus.

(2) Decreases thirst and inhibits secretion of ADH (vasopressin) from posterior pituitary.
(3) Decreases circulating ADH, which results in decreased water permeability in the distal tubules and collecting ducts.
(4) Decreased water permeability results in decreased water resorption and increased urine volume (decreased urine osmolarity).
(5) Less water returned to the circulation returns plasma osmolarity to normal.

b. Hypertonicity—produced by deprivation of water or dehydration (osmolarity >290 mOsm/L).
(1) Stimulates osmoreceptors in hypothalamus.
(2) Stimulates thirst and secretion of ADH from posterior pituitary.
(3) Increased ADH increases water permeability in the distal tubules and collecting ducts.
(4) Increased water permeability results in increased water resorption and decreased urine volume (increased urine osmolarity).
(5) More water returned to the circulation returns osmolarity to normal.

7. Urination
a. Stretch receptors in the bladder initiate the micturition reflex.
(1) Sensory fibers enter the spinal cord and return to the bladder through parasympathetic fibers.
(2) Parasympathetic stimulation causes contraction of the bladder.
b. Voluntary relaxation of the external sphincter permits flow of urine through the external meatus.

8. Summary of terms in renal physiology (Tables 2-7 and 2-8).

10.1 Acid-Base Balance

A. Concerned with maintaining the normal H^+ concentration in body fluids. This is accomplished in three ways:
1. Intracellular and extracellular buffers
a. Buffers resist a change in pH.
b. Intracellular buffers
(1) Organic phosphates (e.g., ATP, ADP, glucose-1-phosphate).
(2) Proteins—hemoglobin and other proteins with a large number of acidic or basic groups.
c. Extracellular buffers
(1) Bicarbonate ion (HCO_3^-/CO_2).
(2) Phosphate ($HPO_4^{-2}/H_2PO_4^-$).
2. Excretion of CO_2 by respiratory mechanisms (rapid response).
3. Bicarbonate resorption and hydrogen ion excretion by the kidney (slow response).

B. Acid-base disorders
1. Metabolic acidosis

TABLE 2–7. COMMONLY USED ABBREVIATIONS IN RENAL PHYSIOLOGY

STRUCTURE	ABBREVIATION	MEANING	UNITS AND/OR NORMAL VALUE
Whole Kidney			
	C	Clearance	mL/min
	[U]	Concentration in urine	mg/mL
	[P]	Concentration in plasma	mg/mL
	$\dot{V}$	Urine flow rate	mL/min
	GFR	Glomerular filtration rate	120 mL/min
	RPF	Renal plasma flow	660 mL/min
	RBF	Renal blood flow	1200 mL/min
Single Nephron			
	[TF]	Concentration in tubular fluid	mg/mL
	$[TF/P]_x$	Concentration of x in tubular fluid relative to concentration of x in plasma	None
	$[TF/P]_{inulin}$	Concentration of inulin in tubular fluid relative to concentration of inulin in plasma	None
	$[TF/P]_x/[TF/P]_{inulin}$	Fraction of the filtered load remaining in tubular fluid or fractional excretion	None

From Costanzo LS: Physiology, ed 3, WB Saunders, Philadelphia, 2004.

TABLE 2–8. COMMONLY USED EQUATIONS IN RENAL PHYSIOLOGY

NAME	EQUATION	UNITS	COMMENTS
Clearance	$C_x = \frac{[U]_x \dot{V}}{[P]_x}$	mL/min	x is any substance
Clearance ratio	$\text{Clearance ratio} = \frac{C_x}{C_{inulin}}$	None	Also means fractional excretion of x
Renal plasma flow	$RPF = \frac{[U]_{PAH}\,\dot{V}}{[RA]_{PAH} - [RV]_{PAH}}$	mL/min	
Effective renal plasma flow	$\text{Effective RPF} = \frac{[U]_{PAH}\,\dot{V}}{[P]_{PAH}}$	mL/min	Underestimates RPF by 10%; equals C_{PAH}
Renal blood flow	$RBF = \frac{RPF}{1 - Hct}$	mL/min	1 – Hct is fraction of blood volume that is plasma
Glomerular filtration rate	$GFR = \frac{[U]_{inulin}\,\dot{V}}{[P]_{inulin}}$	mL/min	Equals C_{inulin}
Filtration fraction	$FF = \frac{GFR}{RPF}$	None	
Filtrated load	$\text{Filtered load} = GFR \times [P]_x$	mg/min	
Excretion rate	$\text{Excretion} = \dot{V} \times [U]_x$	mg/min	
Resorption or secretion rate	Resorption or secretion = Filtered load – excretion	mg/min	If *positive,* net resorption If *negative,* net secretion
Free-water clearance	$C_{H2O} = \dot{V} - C_{osm}$	mL/min	If *positive,* free water is excreted If *negative,* free water is resorbed

From Costanzo LS: Physiology, ed 3, WB Saunders, Philadelphia, 2004.
RA, Renal arteriole concentration; *RV*, renal veniole concentration.

a. Decreased HCO_3^- resulting in a decreased pH.
b. Causes:
   (1) Increased fixed (nonvolatile) acids (lactic acid).
   (2) Metabolic disorders (diabetic production of keto acids).
   (3) Decreased excretion of fixed acids.
   (4) Loss of bicarbonate (diarrhea).
c. Compensation
   (1) Increased respiration and loss of CO_2.
   (2) Increased H^+ loss by kidney.
   (3) Infusion of chemical buffers (medical intervention).

2. Metabolic alkalosis
   a. Increased HCO_3—resulting in increased pH.
   b. Causes
      (1) Loss of fixed acids (vomiting).
      (2) Gain of bicarbonate (ingestion of bicarbonate).
   c. Compensation
      (1) Retention of H^+ by kidney.
      (2) Retention of CO_2 (reduced respiration).
      (3) Infusion of buffers (medical intervention).
3. Respiratory acidosis—resulting in decreased pH
   a. Retention of CO_2.
   b. Caused by hypoventilation
      (1) Depression of respiratory center (medications/drugs).
      (2) Reduced respiratory muscle activity.
      (3) Lung disease.
   c. Compensation
      (1) Increased bicarbonate resorption in kidney.
      (2) Infusion of chemical buffers.
4. Respiratory alkalosis—resulting in increased pH
   a. Loss of CO_2.
   b. Caused by hyperventilation (anxiety, fever, poisons).
   c. Compensation.
      (1) Retention of H^+ by kidney.
      (2) Decreased respiration rate.
      (3) Infusion of chemical buffers.

C. Plasma anion gap = $[Na^+] - ([HCO_3^-] + [Cl^-])$ (Figure 2-29)

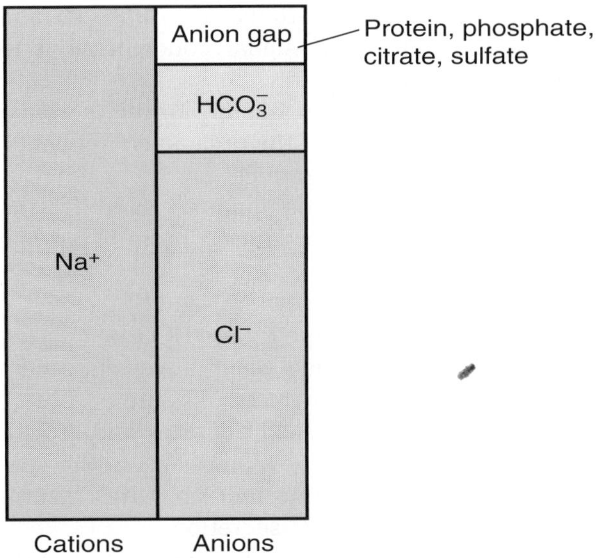

Figure 2–29. Anion gap of plasma.

11.0 ORAL PHYSIOLOGY

11.1 Taste

A. Anatomical considerations
   1. Taste receptors are modified epithelial cells (not neurons).
   2. Dissolved molecules interact with receptors; stimulate neurons that travel to the cortical gustatory area, hypothalamus, and limbic system.
   3. Pathways depend upon localization of receptors.
      a. Posterior one-third of tongue—glossopharyngeal and vagus nerves.
      b. Anterior two-thirds of tongue—facial nerve.

B. Taste discrimination (Figure 2-30)
   1. Coded by patterns of receptor activity.
   2. Five distinct categories of flavors have been identified. All receptors respond to varying degrees to these primary tastes.
      a. Sweet
         (1) Produced by certain organic molecules (e.g., glucose, saccharine, aspartame).
         (2) Utilize G proteins, which activate cAMP second messenger system.
         (3) Blockage of K^+ channels produce depolarization of receptor cell.
      b. Salt
         (1) Produced by chemical salts (e.g., NaCl, KCl).
         (2) Direct passage of ions through specialized channels is responsible for receptor depolarization.
      c. Sour
         (1) Produced by H^+ (acids).
         (2) Receptor stimulation results from the blockage of K^+ channels by H^+,

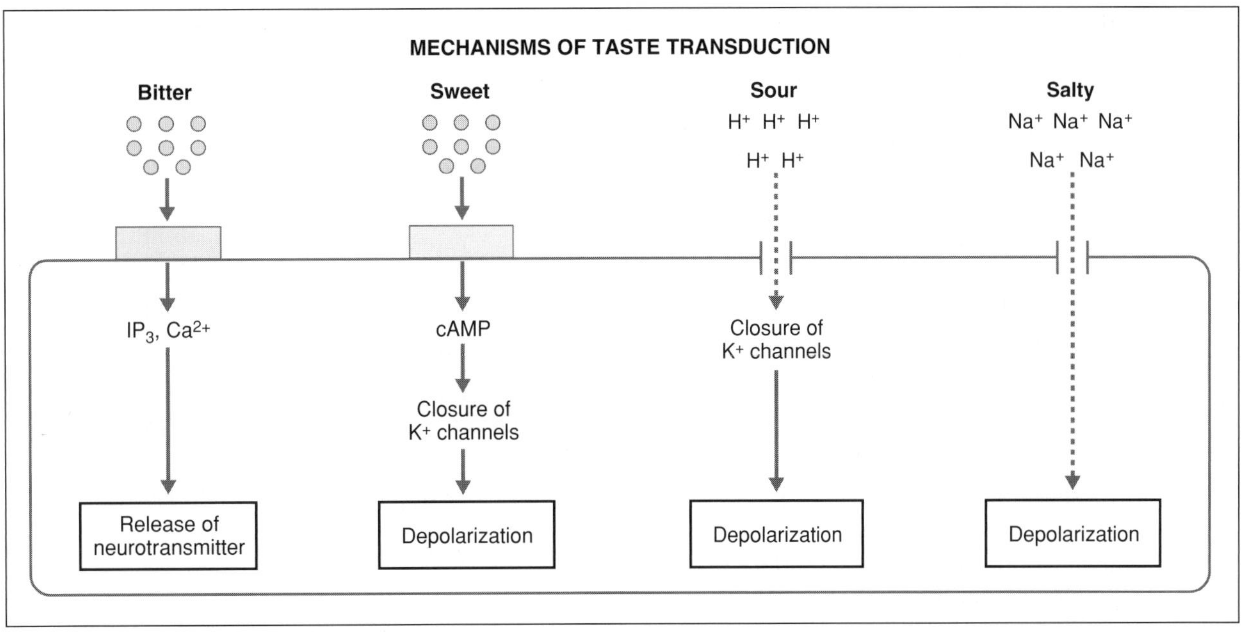

Figure 2–30. Mechanisms of taste transduction.

resulting in a reduced internal negativity and depolarization.

d. Bitter
  (1) Produced by a diverse range of compounds, including many poisonous substances. Few chemical similarities exist when one compares the bitter-tasting chemicals.
  (2) Taste G protein (gustducin) stimulated by the receptor activates a second messenger system to produce a depolarizing potential.

e. Umami (taste sensation from L-glutamate and aspartate)
  (1) Produced by amino acids, most notably glutamate.
  (2) Utilize G proteins, which activate a second messenger system responsible for receptor depolarization.

C. Taste abnormalities
1. Ageusia—absence of the sense of taste.
2. Hypogeusia—diminished taste sensation.
3. Dysgeusia—disturbed sense of taste.

11.1.1 Olfactory

A. Anatomical considerations
1. Olfactory epithelium contains receptors that are modified neurons.
2. Chemoreceptors on cilia of modified neurons send impulses to the olfactory bulb and subsequently to the thalamus, limbic system, and the frontal lobes of the CNS.
3. Transmission is through the olfactory nerve.

B. Smell discrimination
1. Thousands of receptors are available to detect odors.
2. Molecules bound to receptors activate G proteins that activate the cAMP second messenger system, which then opens Na^+ channels, depolarizing the receptor cell.
3. Coding for odor discrimination is determined by patterns of activity in the olfactory bulb glomeruli.

11.1.2 *Salivary Secretion*

A. Saliva
1. Salivary composition is dependent on the following structures:
  a. Salivary gland acini
    (1) Secrete a fluid similar in composition to plasma.
    (2) Fluid contains K^+, Na^+, Cl^-, and HCO_3^- in similar concentrations to plasma.
    (3) Also is responsible for the secretion of most of the organic components.
  b. Salivary gland ducts
    (1) Modify the fluid secreted by the acini to produce a more hypotonic fluid.
      (a) Reabsorb Na^+ and Cl^-.
      (b) Secrete K^+ and HCO_3^-.
      (c) Minimal water movement occurs in the ducts.
    (2) Secrete small peptides and growth factors.
    (3) Aldosterone increases Na^+ resorption and K^+ secretion.
    (4) As flow rate increases, less resorption and secretion occurs.
2. Composition (Figure 2-31)
  a. Inorganic components
    (1) Cations include Na^+, K^+.
    (2) Anions include Cl^-, HCO_3^-.
    (3) Additional electrolytes are $CaPO_4$, SCN^-, F^-, and $MgSO_4$.
  b. Organic components
    (1) Amylase—initiates starch digestion.
    (2) Lipase—initiates lipid digestion.
    (3) Proline-rich proteins (acidic and basic)
      (a) Stabilize calcium and hydroxyapatite (aid in supersaturation).
      (b) Play a role in pellicle formation and remineralization.

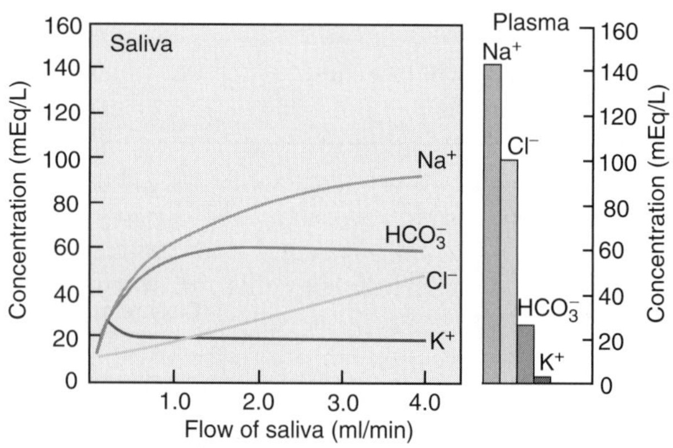

Figure 2–31. Average composition of parotid saliva as a function of salivary flow rate. Saliva is hypotonic to plasma at all flow rates. The bicarbonate (HCO_3^-) level in saliva exceeds that in plasma, except at very low flow rates. (Redrawn from Thaysen JH et al: Am J Physiol 178:155, 1954.)

(4) Histidine-rich proteins—aid in supersaturation of calcium
(a) Aid in supersaturation of calcium.
(b) May have antibacterial effect.
(c) May have antifungal effect .
(5) Tyrosine-rich proteins
(a) Aid in supersaturation of calcium.
(b) May have antimicrobial action.
(6) Cysteine-containing proteins (cystatins)
(a) Aid in supersaturation of calcium.
(b) May have antimicrobial activity.
(7) Mucous glycoproteins (mucins)—important for protection, lubrication, and oral clearance of microorganisms.
(8) Salivary peroxidase—catalyzes the oxidation of thiocyanate by H_2O_2 to produce highly reactive oxidizing agents.
(9) Lactoferrin—bacteriostatic due to its ability to bind iron.
(10) Secretory IgA
(a) Predominant immunoglobulin in saliva.
(b) Inhibits bacterial attachment.
(11) Lysozyme—strongly cationic antibacterial molecule.

c. Buffers
(1) HCO_3^-.
(2) Urea.
(3) Arginine-rich proteins.

3. Regulation occurs through both parasympathetic and sympathetic stimulation.
a. Parasympathetic (cranial nerves VII and IX)
(1) Muscarinic receptors.
(2) Second messengers (IP_3, diacylglycerol, and Ca^{2+}).
(3) Neuropeptides (vasoactive intestinal peptide [VIP] and substance P) are also released.
(4) Results in increased volume by increasing acinar and ductal cell transport and vasodilatation.
b. Sympathetic (superior cervical ganglion)
(1) β-adrenergic receptors.
(2) Second messenger (cAMP).
(3) Stimulation produces increased amounts of protein and low volume.

11.2 Mastication

Complex, highly co-ordinated activity that initiates digestion

A. Movements—characterized as a series of cyclical opening and closing activities involving several muscles that extend from ingestion to swallowing.
1. Muscle activity varies with the stage of mastication and can be interrupted by reflex activity (see below).
a. Jaw-opening muscles
(1) Mylohyoid.
(2) Digastric.
(3) Lateral pterygoid.
b. Jaw-closing muscles
(1) Temporalis.
(2) Masseter.
(3) Medial pterygoid.

B. Coordination of muscular activity occurs at the level of the brainstem.
1. Trigeminal sensory nucleus—receives sensory input via trigeminal nerve.
2. Trigeminal mesencephalic nucleus—contains afferent cell bodies of afferent fibers from muscle spindles of jaw-closing muscles and cell bodies of periodontal ligament, gingival, and palatal mechanoreceptors.
3. Trigeminal motor nucleus—contains motor neurons that control the muscles of mastication. Contain both gamma and alpha motor neurons.
4. Hypoglossal motor nucleus—controls muscles of the tongue.
5. Facial motor nucleus—controls the facial muscles.

C. Control of mastication
1. Brainstem activity
a. Responsible for rhythmic movements of mastication.
b. Reflex activity is coordinated in this area.
(1) Jaw-closing reflex (monosynaptic)
(a) Tapping the chin stretches muscle spindles in the jaw-closing muscles.
(b) Masseter and temporalis muscles contract after short latency.
(c) Stimulation of periodontal ligament and other orofacial receptors also produces a similar reflex.
(2) Jaw-opening reflex (polysynatic)—mechanical stimulation of periodontal ligament or other mechanoreceptors

stimulates jaw-opening muscles and inhibits jaw-closing muscles.
2. Cortical motor area
a. Responsible for modifications in masticatory motor neuron excitability.
b. Initiates tongue and orofacial movements.

11.3 Swallowing

A. Movements
1. Oral phase
a. Tongue forces bolus of food into the pharynx.
b. Bolus stimulates tactile receptors that initiate pharyngeal phase.
2. Pharyngeal phase
a. Palate is pulled forward, and pharyngeal folds move inward to prevent reflux into nasopharynx.
b. Larynx moves against epiglottis to prevent food from entering trachea and also opens upper esophageal sphincter.
c. Pharyngeal muscles contract to force bolus of food into the pharynx.
d. Peristaltic wave is initiated and respiration inhibited.
3. Esophageal phase
a. Peristalsis continues (controlled by swallowing center).
(1) Visceral motor neurons are parasympathetic.
(2) Neurons of myenteric plexus coordinate the motor activity.
b. Lower esophageal sphincter relaxes, mediated by vagal inhibitory fibers.
B. Coordination of swallowing occurs in the medulla (via vagus and glossopharyngeal nerves).
1. Initial (oral) phase is voluntary.
2. Pharyngeal and esophageal phase are involuntary.

12.0 DIGESTION

A. Functional considerations of the gastrointestinal tract
1. Histological considerations
a. Mucosa
(1) Mucous membrane—provides protection, secretions, and absorptive capacity.
(2) Lamina propria—contains blood vessels, nerves, and lymphoid tissue.
(3) Muscularis mucosa—contains smooth muscle.
b. Submucosa
(1) Larger vessels and nerves (Meissner's plexus).
(2) Connective tissue for distensibility and elasticity.
c. Muscularis externa
(1) Major smooth muscle layer in the GI tract.
(a) Inner circular layer.
(b) Outer longitudinal layer.
(2) Contains myenteric plexus (Auerbach's).
d. Serosa—important for lubrication and protection.
2. Neuroendocrine considerations
a. Basal electrical rhythm (BER)
(1) Fluctuations in membrane potentials.
(2) Influenced by mechanical, neural, and hormonal factors.
(3) Due to gap junctions, contraction occurs as a unit.
b. Intrinsic nerve plexuses—innervate exocrine, endocrine, and smooth muscle cells.
3. Extrinsic nerves (Figure 2-32)
a. Sympathetic nervous system—inhibitory.
b. Parasympathetic nervous system—stimulatory.
4. Gastrointestinal hormones
a. Released in response to local changes (also CNS activity).
b. Can be either stimulatory or inhibitory.
5. Gastrointestinal receptors
a. Chemoreceptors—sensitive to intestinal contents.
b. Mechanoreceptors—sensitive to tension and stretch of gastrointestinal tract.
c. Osmoreceptors—sensitive to osmotic qualities of intestinal contents.
6. Gastrointestinal reflexes
a. Short reflex—acts locally within the wall.
b. Long reflex—acts through the CNS through activation of the autonomic nervous system.
B. Oral cavity, pharynx, and esophagus (see Oral Physiology)

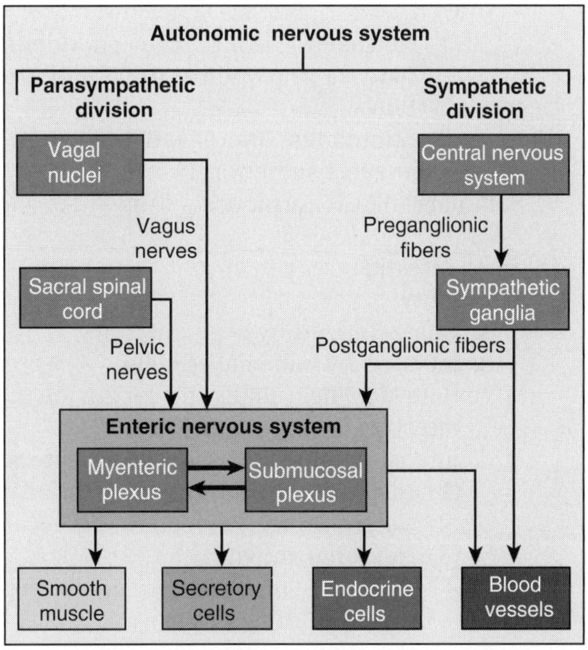

Figure 2–32. Major features of the autonomic innervation of the gastrointestinal tract. In most cases the autonomic nerves influence the functions of the gastrointestinal tract by modulating the activities of the neurons of the enteric nervous system. (Redrawn from Costa M, Furness JB: Br Med Bull 38:247, 1982.)

C. Stomach—function is storage, secretion and mixing
   1. Motility
      a. Characterized by spontaneous rhythmic depolarization and contractions.
      b. More powerful in antral area.
      c. Receptive relaxation mediated by vagus.
   2. Emptying—produced by factors acting through the enterogastric reflex (neuronal and endocrine)
      a. Inhibitory factors
         (1) Low pH in duodenum.
         (2) Fat in duodenum.
         (3) Hypertonicity in duodenum.
         (4) Distention of duodenum.
         (5) Sympathetic stimulation.
         (6) Intense pain.
      b. Stimulatory factors
         (1) Parasympathetic stimulation.
         (2) Increased volume and fluidity of gastric contents.
   3. Secretion
      a. Substances secreted
         (1) HCl (from parietal cells).
         (2) Pepsinogen (from chief cells).
         (3) Mucus.
         (4) Intrinsic factor.
         (5) Gastrin.
      b. Regulation
         (1) Cephalic phase
            (a) Vagally mediated.
            (b) Directly stimulates HCl, pepsinogen, and gastrin release.
         (2) Gastric phase
            (a) Acts via agents in the stomach.
            (b) Mediated via intrinsic nerves and vagus.
         (3) Intestinal phase
            (a) Acts via agents in the duodenum.
            (b) Gastrin released is stimulatory.
            (c) Cholecystokinin (CCK), secretin, and gastrin inhibitory peptide (GIP) are inhibitory.
         (4) Zollinger–Ellison syndrome—increased gastrin production due to pancreatic tumor.
   4. Digestion
      a. Carbohydrates continue to be digested due to the presence of salivary amylase.
      b. Protein digestion begins due to the conversion of pepsinogen to pepsin (active form is responsible for protein digestion into small peptides).
   5. Absorption of some substances
      a. Ethyl alcohol.
      b. Aspirin.

D. Liver
   1. Function
      a. Metabolism of nutrients
         (1) Helps regulate blood glucose, triglyceride, and cholesterol levels.
         (2) Metabolizes amino acids to provide additional sources of energy.
      b. Detoxification and degradation of organic compounds (drugs, hormones, waste products of metabolism).

c. Synthesis of essential proteins (e.g., clotting factors, albumin).
d. Storage of nutrients (e.g., glycogen, fat-soluble vitamins).
e. Activation of vitamin D.
f. Excretion of cholesterol and bilirubin via bile.

2. Bile
   a. Secreted by hepatocytes and stored in the gallbladder.
   b. Composition
      (1) Bile salts.
      (2) Cholesterol.
      (3) Lecithin.
      (4) Bilirubin.
   c. Water, bicarbonate, and salts are added by the duct cells.
   d. Involved in fat digestion (emulsion) and absorption.
   e. Most is resorbed (enterohepatic circulation).
   f. Stimuli for bile secretion
      (1) Chemical (primarily bile salts).
      (2) Hormonal/neuronal.
         (a) Secretin stimulates bicarbonate secretion from ducts.
         (b) CCK, gastrin, and vagal activity stimulate gallbladder contraction and relaxation of the sphincter of Oddi.
   g. Complications of bile secretion cause gallstones and obstructive jaundice.
   h. Bile acids cause Cl^- secretion (and Na/H_2O) in the intestine.

E. Pancreas
1. Endocrine secretion
   a. Insulin.
   b. Glucagon.
2. Exocrine secretion
   a. Proteolytic enzymes
      (1) Trypsinogen (activated by enterokinase).
      (2) Chymotrypsinogen (activated by trypsin).
      (3) Procarboxypeptidase (activated by trypsin).
   b. Pancreatic amylase.
   c. Pancreatic lipase.
   d. Bicarbonate.
3. Regulation of secretion
   a. Secretin
      (1) Released from the duodenal mucosa in response to low pH.
      (2) Stimulates increased bicarbonate secretion from pancreas.
   b. CCK
      (1) Released from the duodenal mucosa in response to fat and protein.
      (2) Stimulates increased pancreatic enzyme secretion.

F. Summary of GI hormones (Tables 2-9 and 2-10)

G. Small intestine
1. Motility
   a. Characterized by segmentation.
   b. Initiated by pacemaker cells.
   c. Rate declines along the length of the intestine.
   d. Intensity influenced by several factors
      (1) Distention.
      (2) Gastrin.
      (3) Neuronal activity
         (a) Parasympathetics increase segmentation.
         (b) Sympathetics decrease segmentation.
   e. Ileocaecal juncture—area between ileum and caecum.
      (1) Ileocaecal valve—normally closed, easily opened.
      (2) Ileocaecal sphincter—usually constricted.
2. Secretion
   a. Mucus—protection and lubrication.
   b. Salts—solubilize intestinal contents.
3. Digestion
   a. Fat—broken down to monoglycerides and fatty acids in the lumen under the influence of pancreatic lipase.
   b. Protein—broken down to small peptides and amino acids in the lumen due to the action of pancreatic enzymes. Intestinal brush border enzymes further hydrolyze peptide fragments to amino acids.
   c. Carbohydrates—broken down to disaccharides and monosaccharides in lumen (pancreatic amylase) and in intestinal brush border (disaccharidases). Deficiencies of enzymes required for carbohydrate digestion result in gastrointestinal disorders (lactose intolerance is the inability to metabolize lactose).
4. Absorption (Table 2-11)
   a. Fat—fatty acids and monoglycerides are absorbed passively (facilitated by bile). Triglycerides are synthesized within the epithelial cells. Chylomicrons

Table 2–9. Summary of Gastrointestinal Hormones

HORMONE	HORMONE FAMILY	SITE OF SECRETION	STIMULI FOR SECRETION	ACTIONS
Gastrin	Gastrin-CCK	G cells of the stomach	Small peptides and amino acids Distention of the stomach Vagal stimulation (GRP)	↑ Gastric H^+ secretion Stimulates growth of gastric mucosa ↑ Pancreatic enzyme secretion
Cholecystokinin (CCK)	Gastrin-CCK	I cells of the duodenum and jejunum	Small peptides and amino acids Fatty acids	↑ Pancreatic HCO_3^- secretion Stimulates contraction of the gallbladder and relaxation of the sphincter of Oddi Stimulates growth of the exocrine pancreas and gallbladder Inhibits gastric emptying
Secretin	Secretin-glucagon	S cells of the duodenum	H^+ in the duodenum Fatty acids in the duodenum	↑ Pancreatic HCO_3^- secretion ↑ Biliary HCO_3^- secretion ↓ Gastric H^+ secretion Inhibits trophic effect of gastrin on gastric mucosa
Gastric inhibitory peptide (GIP)	Secretin-glucagon	Duodenum and jejunum	Fatty acids Amino acids Oral glucose	↑ Insulin secretion from pancreatic β cells ↓ Gastric H^+ secretion

From Costanzo LS: Physiology, ed 3, WB Saunders, Philadelphia, 2004.

Table 2–10. Summary of Gastrointestinal Secretions

SECRETION	CHARACTERISTICS OF SECRETION	FACTORS THAT INCREASE SECRETION	FACTORS THAT DECREASE SECRETION
Saliva	High $[HCO_3^-]$ High $[K^+]$ Hypotonic α-Amylase and lingual lipase	Parasympathetic (prominent) Sympathetic	Sleep Dehydration Atropine
Gastric	HCL	Gastrin Acetylcholine Histamine	H^+ in the stomach Chyme in the duodenum Atropine Cimetidine Omeprazole
	Pepsinogen Intrinsic factor	Parasympathetic	
Pancreatic	High $[HCO_3^-]$ Isotonic	Secretin Cholecystokinin (CCK) (potentiates secretin) Parasympathetic	
	Pancreatic lipase, amylase, proteases	CCK Parasympathetic	
Bile	Bile salts Bilirubin Phospholipids Cholesterol	CCK (contraction of the gallbladder and relaxation of the sphincter of Oddi) Parasympathetic	Ileal resection

From Costanzo LS: Physiology, ed 3, WB Saunders, Philadelphia, 2004.

TABLE 2–11. SUMMARY OF MECHANISMS OF DIGESTION AND ABSORPTION OF NUTRIENTS

NUTRIENT	PRODUCTS OF DIGESTION	SITE OF ABSORPTION	MECHANISM
Carbohydrates	Glucose Galactose Fructose	Small intestine	Na^+-glucose cotransport Na^+-galactose cotransport Facilitated diffusion
Proteins	Amino acids Dipeptides Tripeptides	Small intestine	Na^+-amino acid cotransport H^+-dipeptide cotransport H^+-tripeptide cotransport
Lipids	Fatty acids Monoglycerides Cholesterol	Small intestine	Bile salts form micelles in the small intestine Diffusion of fatty acids, monoglycerides, and cholesterol into intestinal cells Reesterification in the cell to triglycerides and phospholipids Chylomicrons form in the cell (requiring apoprotein) and are transferred to lymph
Fat-soluble vitamins		Small intestine	Micelles form with bile salts and products of lipid digestion Diffusion into the intestinal cell
Water-soluble vitamins		Small intestine	Na^+-dependent cotransport
Vitamin B_{12}		Ileum	Intrinsic factor
Bile salts		Ileum	Na^+-salt acid cotransport
Ca^{2+}		Small intestine	Vitamin D–dependent Ca^{2+}-binding protein
Fe^{2+}	Fe^{3+} reduced to Fe^{2+}	Small intestine	Binds to apoferritin in the intestinal cell Binds to transferrin in blood

From Costanzo LS: Physiology, ed 3, WB Saunders, Philadelphia, 2004.

(lipoproteins and triglycerides) are extruded from the cell and pass into the lymphatic system.

b. Protein—amino acids and small peptides are absorbed and pass into the portal circulation. Amino acids are absorbed by a secondary active transport system.
c. Carbohydrates—monosaccharides are absorbed utilizing a cotransport system (secondary active transport mechanism with sodium). Fructose moves by facilitated diffusion.
d. NaCl and water
   (1) Active sodium and passive chloride transport occurs throughout the intestine.
   (2) Water moves due to osmotic pressure changes.
e. Vitamins
   (1) Both fat- and water-soluble vitamins are absorbed passively. Some specialized mechanisms exist.
   (2) Vitamin B_{12} absorption requires intrinsic factor from gastric mucosa.
f. Iron
   (1) Active transport from lumen into epithelial cells.
   (2) Reduced iron (ferrous) is more easily absorbed than oxidized form (ferric).
   (3) Absorption is enhanced by vitamin C.
   (4) Transferred in the blood by transferrin or stored within epithelial cells in the form of ferritin.
g. Calcium—primarily an active process stimulated by vitamin D and enhanced by parathyroid hormone, which increases activation of vitamin D.

H. Large intestine
   1. Motility
      a. Characterized by haustral contractions (slow, nonpropulsive contractions).
      b. Increased activity (mass movements) move contents to distal portion of intestine.
      c. Gastrocolic reflex—mass movement stimulated by gastrin release, often after a meal.
      d. Defecation reflex—distention of the rectum caused by mass movement of fecal material.

(1) Produces relaxation of smooth muscle of internal anal sphincter.
(2) Produces increased contraction of rectum and sigmoid colon.
(3) External sphincter relaxation is under voluntary control.

2. Secretion
   a. No digestive enzymes are secreted.
   b. Bicarbonate and mucus are produced for protective purposes.
3. Absorption
   a. Sodium is actively absorbed.
   b. Vitamin K is absorbed.
   c. Water is absorbed passively.

13.0 ENDOCRINES

13.1 Pituitary/Hypothalamus

Function in a coordinated fashion to regulate: growth; the thyroid, adrenal, and reproductive tissues; and overall osmolarity of body tissues.

A. Posterior lobe of pituitary
   1. Derived from neural tissue (integrated with the hypothalamus).
   2. Secretes ADH (vasopressin) and oxytocin.

B. Anterior lobe of pituitary
   1. Primarily a collection of endocrine cells that are stimulated or inhibited by hormones synthesized in the hypothalamus and delivered to the anterior pituitary by the hypothalamic-hypophyseal portal blood vessels.
   2. Secretes adrenocorticotropin hormone (ACTH), thyroid-stimulating hormone (TSH), growth hormone (GH), follicle-stimulating hormone (FSH), luteinizing hormone (LH), and prolactin.
   3. Pro-opiomelanocortin (POMC) is the prohormone, which, when hydrolyzed, produces ACTH, melanocyte-stimulating hormone (MSH), γ-lipotropin, and β endorphin.
   4. Hypothalamic-releasing hormones
      a. Thyrotropin-releasing hormone (TRH)—stimulates the release of TSH.
      b. Growth hormone-releasing hormone (GHRH)—stimulates the release of GH.
      c. Growth hormone-inhibiting hormone (somatostatin).
      d. Corticotropin-releasing hormone (CRH)—stimulates the release of ACTH and β endorphin.
      e. Prolactin-releasing hormone.
      f. Prolactin-inhibiting hormone (dopamine).

C. ADH (vasopressin)
   1. Responsible for regulation of body fluid osmolarity.
   2. Secreted in response to increased serum osmolarity, pain, nausea, hypoglycemia.
   3. Release inhibited by decreased serum osmolarity, ethanol, and atrial natriuretic peptide (ANP).
   4. Increases permeability of distal tubule and collecting ducts to increase water resorption and return osmolarity to normal (V_2 receptor). Also produces contraction of vascular smooth muscle (V_1 receptor).
   5. Diabetes insipidus—due to the failure of ADH to be secreted (central diabetes insipidus) or failure of renal duct cells to respond to ADH (nephrogenic diabetes insipidus).

D. Oxytocin
   1. Responsible for milk ejection from the lactating breast and uterine contraction during labor.
   2. Secreted in response to suckling, dilation of cervix, orgasm, and conditioned responses (sight, sound, or smell of the infant).
   3. Inhibited by opioids (endorphins).
   4. Produces contraction of the myoepithelial cells in mammary small ducts and rhythmic contraction of uterine smooth muscle.

E. ACTH
   1. Responsible for stimulating the conversion of cholesterol to pregnenolone, which serves as a precursor of adrenal steroids. Release is pulsatile and diurnal in nature.
   2. Secreted in response to stress, hypoglycemia, decreased blood cortisol, ADH, and serotonin.
   3. Release is inhibited by increased blood cortisol, opioids, and somatostatin.
   4. Activates cholesterol desmolase, which enhances pregnenolone synthesis. Upregulates ACTH receptors and produces hypertrophy and hyperplasia of adrenal tissue.
   5. Cushing disease results from ACTH hypersecretion.

F. TSH
   1. Responsible for regulating the growth of the thyroid gland and stimulating

the secretion of thyroid hormones (T_3 and T_4).
2. Secreted in response to TRH (from hypothalamus), which, in turn, is downregulated by T_3 and T_4.
3. Activates steps in the synthetic pathway of thyroid hormones and ultimate release.

G. Growth hormone
1. Important for normal growth and metabolism.
    a. Growth-promoting actions. (Most are mediated by release of somatomedin. Insulin-like growth factor [IGF] is the newer accepted name for somatomedin.)
        (1) Causes hypertrophy and hyperplasia.
        (2) Increases protein synthesis and organ growth.
        (3) Increases linear growth (bone thickness and length).
    b. Metabolic actions
        (1) Decreases glucose uptake and utilization (diabetogenic effect).
        (2) Increases lipolysis, increases fatty acids and insulin in blood.
2. Secreted in response to decreased glucose, fatty acids, fasting, exercise, stress, and sleep.
3. Inhibited by increased glucose, fatty acids, obesity, somatostatin, IGF, growth hormone, and pregnancy.
4. Gigantism, characterized by acromegaly and increased linear growth, is produced by growth hormone excess.

H. FSH
1. Responsible for stimulating granulosa cells to convert androstenedione to estrogens, which, in combination with FSH, result in a positive feedback to produce more estrogen. In males, FSH stimulates spermatogenesis and Sertoli cell function.
2. Secreted in response to gonadotropin-releasing hormone (GnRH) from the hypothalamus, which is released throughout life and becomes pulsatile at puberty.
3. Inhibited in males by testosterone and inhibin (glycoprotein secreted by Sertoli cells). In females, in the follicular phase, estradiol inhibits secretion of FSH; however, sharp increases in estradiol before ovulation stimulate FSH release. Progesterone inhibits FSH secretion.

I. LH
1. Responsible for stimulating Leydig cells to synthesize testosterone by increasing the activity of cholesterol desmolase (first step in steroidogenesis). Initiates ovulation, stimulates formation of the corpus luteum, and maintains steroid hormone production throughout the luteal phase of the menstrual cycle.
2. Secreted in response to GnRH and in midcycle by sharp increases in estradiol.
3. Inhibited in males by testosterone, which inhibits the release of GnRH and LH from the pituitary. In females, in the follicular phase, estradiol inhibits the secretion of LH. Progesterone inhibits LH secretion from the anterior pituitary.

J. Prolactin
1. Responsible for milk production and breast development.
2. Secreted in response to TRH, estrogen, breastfeeding, sleep, and stress.
3. Inhibited by dopamine, somatostatin, and prolactin (negative feedback).
4. High levels prevent ovulation by inhibiting the synthesis and release of GnRH.

13.2 Reproduction

A. Male reproductive system
1. Structure of testes
    a. Seminiferous tubules—responsible for sperm production.
    b. Sertoli cells
        (1) Provide nutrients for sperm.
        (2) Provide a barrier to the bloodstream to protect developing sperm.
        (3) Secrete fluid to assist sperm transport into epididymis.
    c. Leydig cells—site of synthesis and secretion of testosterone.
2. Testosterone
    a. Metabolism
        (1) Synthesized from cholesterol (stimulated by LH).
        (2) 17-β-hydroxysteroid dehydrogenase responsible for the final conversion of androstenedione to testosterone.
        (3) Small amounts of testosterone are converted to estrogen in some tissue.
        (4) Transported in plasma associated with sex steroid-binding globulin (which is increased by estrogen and decreased by androgens) and albumin.

(5) Synthesis is inhibited by feedback inhibition by testosterone on the release of LH from the pituitary and GnRH in the hypothalamus. Inhibin, released from the Sertoli cells, also inhibits FSH secretion.

b. Function
   (1) Development of male genital tract.
   (2) Development of primary and secondary sex characteristics.
   (3) Spermatogenesis.

3. Dihydrotestosterone
   a. Metabolism
      (1) Testosterone in some target tissues must be converted to dihydrotestosterone (active androgen in some tissues) by 5α-reductase.
      (2) Binds in a more stable fashion to DNA; thus is a more active androgen in some tissues.
   b. Function
      (1) Fetal differentiation of external genitalia.
      (2) Development of primary and secondary sex characteristics.
      (3) Growth of prostate.

4. Spermatogenesis—requires FSH and LH
   a. Mitotic division—spermatogonia to spermatocytes.
   b. Meiotic division—spermatocytes become haploid spermatids.
   c. Spermiogenesis—spermatids transformed into mature sperm.

B. Female reproductive system
1. Structure of ovary
   a. Cortex
      (1) Contains oocytes enclosed in follicles.
      (2) Responsible for steroid hormone synthesis.
   b. Medulla and hilum—remainder of ovary containing a mixture of cell types and blood vessels.
2. Estrogen and progesterone
   a. Metabolism
      (1) Synthesized by ovarian follicles.
      (2) Synthesized from cholesterol (stimulated by LH).
      (3) Pathway similar to steroid production in adrenal cortex and testes.
      (4) 3-β-hydroxysteroid dehydrogenase converts pregnenolone to progesterone.
      (5) Aromatase (stimulated by FSH) converts testosterone to 17-β-estradiol.
   b. Function (Tables 2-12 and 2-13)
3. Ovarian cycle
   a. Follicular phase
      (1) LH stimulates the conversion of cholesterol to androstenedione.
      (2) FSH stimulates the conversion of androstenedione to estrogens.
      (3) Estrogens and FSH (positive feedback) stimulate more estrogens, LH, and FSH receptors.
      (4) Elevated estradiol levels cause proliferation of the uterus.
      (5) FSH and LH levels are suppressed due to feedback of estradiol on the pituitary.
      (6) Since feedback inhibition of FSH is greater than LH, further follicular development does not occur.

TABLE 2–12. ACTIONS OF ESTROGENS ON TARGET TISSUES

Maturation and maintenance of uterus, fallopian tubes, cervix, and vagina
Responsible at puberty for the development of female secondary sex characteristics
Required for development of the breasts
Responsible for proliferation and development of ovarian granulosa cells
Upregulation of estrogen, progesterone, and LH receptors
Negative *and* positive feedback effects on FSH and LH secretion
Maintenance of pregnancy
Lowers uterine threshold to contractile stimuli
Stimulates prolactin secretion
Blocks action of prolactin on the breast

From Costanzo LS: Physiology, ed 3, WB Saunders, Philadelphia, 2004.

TABLE 2–13. ACTIONS OF PROGESTERONE ON TARGET TISSUES

Maintenance of secretory activity of uterus during luteal phase
Development of the breasts
Negative feedback effects on FSH and LH secretion
Maintenance of pregnancy
Raises uterine threshold to contractile stimuli during pregnancy

FSH, Follicle-stimulating hormone; *LH,* luteinizing hormone.
From Costanzo LS: Physiology, ed 3, WB Saunders, Philadelphia, 2004.

b. Ovulation
   (1) Burst of estrogen causes an LH surge and increased FSH secretion.
   (2) LH surge causes ovulation and completion of meiosis of the oocyte.
   (3) Estrogen secretion decreases.

c. Luteal phase
   (1) Due to the LH surge, the corpus luteum develops and begins synthesizing estradiol and progesterone.
   (2) These hormones cause feedback inhibition on the hypothalamus to reduce secretion of LH and FSH.
   (3) If fertilization does not occur, the corpus luteum degenerates. This results in a sharp decrease in estradiol and progesterone.
   (4) Under reduced hormonal stimulation, the endometrium is sloughed (menses).

4. Pregnancy
   a. If fertilization occurs, chorionic gonadotropin (CG) (from placenta) maintains the corpus luteum, which continues to secrete estradiol and progesterone.
   b. Continued elevated levels of estradiol and progesterone maintain the endometrium, stimulate breast development, and suppress follicular function.
   c. Progesterone also is responsible for reducing contractility of the uterus.

5. Parturition
   a. Oxytocin causes uterine contractions due to increased receptor sensitivity.
   b. The estrogen/progesterone ratio increases, which increases the sensitivity of the uterus to contractile sensitivity (fetal growth and uterine distention).
   c. Increased prostaglandin production and resulting increased intracellular calcium result in increased contractility.

13.3 Signaling Systems

A. General principles
1. Mechanisms of communication
   a. Endocrine—involve regulatory substances, which, when released, have effects on targets far removed from the endocrine cells.
   b. Paracrine—involve regulatory substances released from cells that are not immediately adjacent to the target cells but are sufficiently close to reach the target cell by diffusion.
   c. Autocrine—involve regulatory factors that act on that cell itself or neighboring identical cell.
   d. Neurocrine—involve regulatory factors released by neurons in the immediate vicinity of the target cells.
2. Classification of signaling systems
   a. Intracellular hormones
      (1) Lipophilic (nonpolar)—diffuse across membrane.
      (2) Bind to intracellular receptors forming complexes that bind to DNA (hormone response element), which activates gene transcription.
      (3) Binding domain stabilized by adjacent motifs called *zinc fingers.*
      (4) Transported in blood bound to plasma proteins.
      (5) Examples include steroid hormones, vitamin D, thyroid hormone, and carotenoids.
   b. Extracellular hormones (peptides and proteins)
      (1) Hydrophobic (polar)—cannot diffuse across membrane.
      (2) Bind to receptors on the cell surface and thereby activate second messenger systems.
      (3) Examples include insulin, epinephrine, glucagon, gastrin, pituitary hormones, and so forth.
3. G proteins—a family of proteins that bind to the inner aspect of the plasma membrane. G proteins bind to 7-transmembrane cell surface receptors and communicate the messages from these stimulated receptors to enzymes, which, in turn leads to the production of second messengers. These second messengers act on various cytoplasmic proteins. G proteins can also act on ion channels.
   a. Heterotrimeric in nature, having an α, β, and γ subunit.
   b. Alpha subunit—has GTPase activity.
      (1) Bound to GDP (G protein inactive).
      (2) Bound to GTP (G protein active).
   c. G proteins can either be stimulatory (G_s) or inhibitory(G_i).
   d. Cholera toxin modifies the G_s protein, resulting in a persistent stimulation of

adenylate cyclase and production of cAMP.

e. Pertussis toxin modifies G_i, preventing the adenylate cyclase system from being inhibited by G_i, also resulting in abnormally high levels of cAMP.

4. Mechanism of action
   a. Signaling systems that employ adenylate cyclase.
      (1) Examples: ACTH, LH, calcitonin, PTH, glucagon, β-adrenergic receptors.
      (2) Hormone binds to receptor, producing a conformational change on the α subunit to ultimately exchange the α_s-GDP complex with GTP.
      (3) α_s-GTP activates adenylate cyclase, which catalyzes the conversion of ATP to cAMP (α_s-GTP is inactivated by intrinsic GTPase).
      (4) cAMP activates protein kinase A, which phosphorylates intracellular proteins.
      (5) Phosphorylated proteins produce physiological activities within the cell.
      (6) cAMP is degraded to 5′ AMP by phosphodiesterase.
   b. Signaling systems that employ phospholipase C
      (1) Examples: TRH, GHRH, angiotensin II, oxytocin, α_1-adrenergic receptors.
      (2) Hormone binds to receptor and via G protein, activates phospholipase C.
      (3) Phospholipase C cleaves PIP_2 (phosphatidylinositol 4,5-diphosphate) to form inositol trisphosphate (IP_3) and diacylglycerol (DAG).
      (4) IP_3 binds to receptors on ER to produce Ca^{2+} release, and subsequent activation of additional molecules (calmodulin).
      (5) IP_3 is dephosphorylated by a cytoplasmic phosphorylase, thus inactivating the molecule.
   c. Signaling systems that employ tyrosine kinase
      (1) Examples: insulin, IGF-1.
      (2) Hormone binding results in changes that result in autophosphorylation of the receptor. (The enzyme, in this case, is a function possessed by the receptor itself.)
      (3) The phosphorylation triggers multiple cellular responses including:
         (a) Calcium influx.
         (b) Increased Na^+/H^+ exchange.
         (c) Amino acid and glucose uptake.
   d. Signaling systems that employ guanylate cyclase
      (1) Examples: atrial natriuretic peptide, nitric oxide.
      (2) Hormone binding results in the stimulation of guanylyl cyclase, which elevates the intracellular concentration of cGMP.
      (3) cGMP (second messenger) stimulates cGMP-dependent protein kinases (protein kinase G).

13.4 Pancreas/Parathyroid

A. Pancreatic hormones
   1. Insulin
      a. Structure and synthesis
         (1) A peptide consisting of two chains (α and β).
         (2) Synthesized as a prohormone and cleaved to produce the active hormone.
         (3) The cleaved peptide (C protein) is used as an indicator of β-cell function.
      b. Regulation of secretion
         (1) Stimulants
            (a) Increased concentrations of blood glucose, amino acids, fatty acids, and ketone bodies.
            (b) Oral glucose.
            (c) Increased levels of glucagons, growth hormone, cortisol, and GIP.
            (d) Increased potassium levels.
            (e) Cholinergic stimulation (vagal stimulation).
         (2) Inhibitors
            (a) Decreased blood glucose.
            (b) Fasting.
            (c) Exercise.
            (d) Somatostatin.
            (e) α-adrenergic agents.
      c. Mechanism of action
         (1) Receptor consists of four subunits (two α and two β subunits).

(a) α subunits are surface peptides that contain the recognition site for insulin.

(b) β subunits span the plasma membrane and have tyrosine kinase activity.

(2) Insulin binding to the receptor causes phosphorylation of the β subunits (autophosphorylation) and phosphorylation of target proteins, which have multiple effects within the cell.

(3) The insulin receptor complex is internalized, resulting in downregulation of its receptor (involved in decreased insulin sensitivity in obesity and type II diabetes).

(4) Glucose transporters are redistributed to the cell membrane, which results in increased transport of glucose into the cell.

d. Functions—facilitates the utilization of energy sources in the body. These activities are summarized in Figure 2-33.

2. Glucagon

a. Structure and synthesis

(1) Single polypeptide synthesized as a prohormone from α cells of the islets of Langerhan cells.

(2) Structurally related to other gastrointestinal hormones (secretin and GIP).

b. Regulation of secretion

(1) Stimulants

(a) Fasting and intense exercise.

(b) Reduced plasma glucose.

(c) Increased ingestion of amino acids.

(d) CCK.

(e) Acetylcholine.

(2) Inhibitors

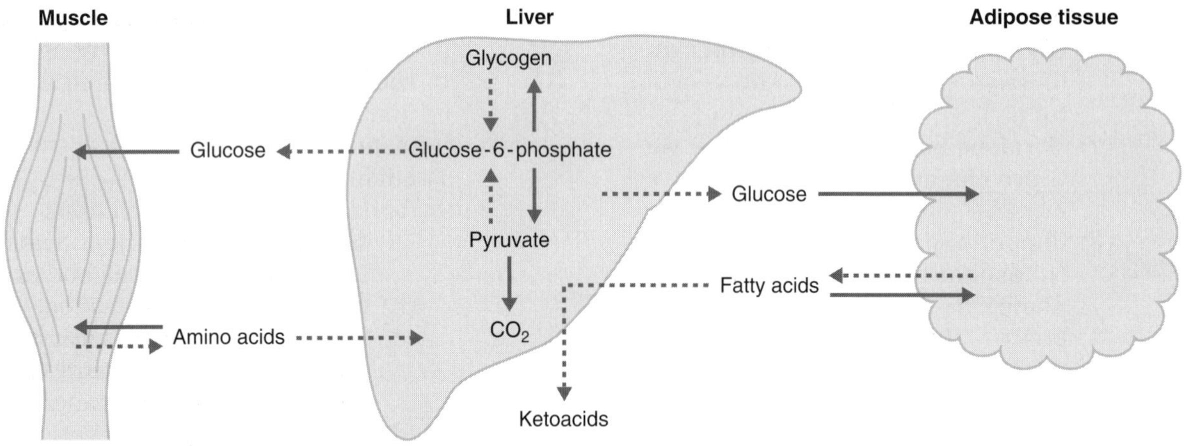

Nutrient	Effect of Insulin on Blood Level
Glucose	Decreased
Fatty acids	Decreased
Ketoacids	Decreased
Amino acids	Decreased

Figure 2–33. Effects of insulin on nutrient flow. *Solid arrows* indicate steps favored by insulin; *dashed arrows* indicate steps inhibited by insulin.

(a) Insulin and somatostatin.
(b) Increased plasma fatty acids and ketones.

c. Mechanism of action
(1) Cell membrane receptor activates adenylate cyclase utilizing the G protein, G_s.
(2) The cAMP produced activates protein kinase A, and protein kinase A catalyzes the phosphorylation of enzymes, which mediate the physiological effects.

d. Functions
(a) Increases glycogenolysis.
(b) Increases gluconeogenesis.
(c) Increases lipolysis.
(d) Increases ketone body production.
(e) Inhibits glycogenesis.

3. Somatostatin
a. Structure and synthesis
(1) Single polypeptide secreted by the δ cells of the islets of Langerhan cells.
(2) Secretion is stimulated by the ingestion of all nutrients (glucose, amino acids, and fatty acids) and glucagon.
(3) Secretion is inhibited by insulin.

b. Function
(1) Inhibits the secretion of insulin and glucagon.
(2) Serves to modulate the overall effects of a meal on the pancreatic release of insulin and glucagons.

B. Calcium-regulating hormones (PTH, calcitonin, and vitamin D)
1. Calcium balance—regulated by three organ systems
a. Bone—99% of calcium in the body (resorption regulated by PTH and calcitonin).
b. Kidney—filters and resorbs calcium (regulated by PTH).
c. Intestine—absorption regulated by 1,25-dihydroxycholecalciferol (active form of vitamin D).
(1) Net absorption and excretion is about 200 mg/day.
(2) Ionized calcium (Ca^{2+}) is the only biologically active form of the mineral.
(3) Hypocalcemia (low blood calcium)
(a) Symptoms include tetany, tiredness, and convulsions.
(b) Caused by renal failure and reduced 1,25-dihydroxycholecalciferol.

d. Hypercalcemia
(1) Symptoms include lethargy, depression, and cardiac arrhythmias.
(2) Caused by malignancy or hyperparathyroidism.

2. Parathyroid hormone (PTH)
a. Structure and synthesis
(1) Single chain polypeptide synthesized in the chief cell of the parathyroid gland.
(2) Synthesized as a prohormone and cleaved before release.

b. Regulation of secretion
(1) Stimulants
(a) Low serum calcium.
(b) Low serum magnesium.
(2) Inhibitors
(a) High serum calcium.
(b) High serum magnesium.
(c) Very low serum magnesium.

c. Mechanism of action
(1) Cell membrane receptor activates adenylate cyclase utilizing G_s (bone and kidney).
(2) In intestine, PTH enhances calcium absorption by activation of renal 1α hydroxylase to form 1, 25-dihydroxycholecalciferol, which, in turn, increases calcium absorption in the intestine.

d. Function—overall effect is to increase serum Ca^{2+} and decrease serum PO_4^{-3}.
(1) Bone
(a) Initially and rapidly activates PTH receptors on osteoblasts to increase bone formation.
(b) Long-term stimulation of osteoclasts to increase bone resorption mediated by cytokines.
(2) Kidney
(a) Inhibits phosphate reabsorption in proximal convoluted tubule.
(b) Stimulates Ca^{2+} reabsorption in the distal convoluted tubule.
(c) Overall effect is to increase the circulating levels of calcium and reduce the possibility of forming calcium complexes in ECF (reduces phosphate).
(3) Intestine—increases the absorption of calcium by activating vitamin D.

3. Calcitonin
   a. Structure and synthesis
      (1) Peptide synthesized in the thyroid gland by parafollicular cells.
      (2) Stored as a prohormone and secreted upon stimulation.
   b. Regulation for secretion—release is stimulated by increased plasma Ca^{2+}.
   c. Mechanism of action—inhibits osteoclastic activity.
   d. Function—overall effect is to prevent increases in plasma Ca^{2+}.
4. Vitamin D
   a. Structure and synthesis
      (1) Vitamin D (cholecalciferol) is obtained in the diet, but most is produced (from cholesterol) in the skin by exposure to sunlight. Unless it is activated by successive hydroxylation, it remains inactive.
      (2) Hydroxylation occurs in two organs
         (a) Liver hydroxylates cholecalciferol to form 25-hydroxycholecalciferol.
         (b) Kidney hydroxylates 25-hydroxycholecalciferol to 1,25-dihydroxycholecalciferol, which is physiologically active.
         (c) Kidney can also hydroxylate 25-hydroxycholecalciferol to 24, 25-hydroxycholecalciferol (inactive form).
   b. Regulation of synthesis (Figure 2-34)
      (1) Hydroxylation is regulated by negative feedback mechanisms, which depend upon plasma calcium levels and hormones responsible for regulating plasma concentration of calcium.
   c. Mechanism of action
      (1) Overall function of 1,25-dihydroxycholecalciferol is to increase plasma and phosphate concentrations in the blood. This is accomplished by stimulation of gene transcription and synthesis of new proteins in three tissues
         (a) Intestine
            (i) 1,25-dihydroxycholecalciferol induces the synthesis of calcium-binding proteins (calbindin D).
            (ii) Calcium also diffuses down an electrochemical gradient and is pumped into the circulation by Ca^{2+}-ATPase on the basolateral membrane.
            (iii) Phosphate absorption is also enhanced by 1,25-dihydroxycholecalciferol.
         (b) Kidney
            (i) 1,25-dihydroxycholecalciferol stimulates the reabsorption of both calcium and phosphate ions.

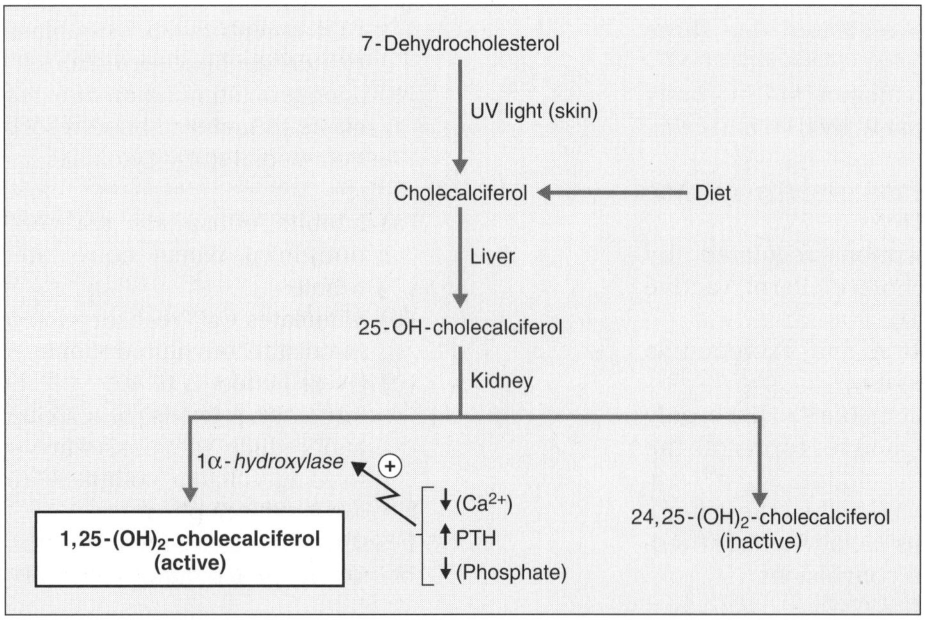

Figure 2–34. Steps involved in the synthesis of 1,25-dihydroxycholecalciferol.

(c) Bone
(i) 1,25-dihydroxycholecalciferol stimulates osteoclastic activity and bone resorption.

13.5 Adrenal/Thyroid

A. Thyroid hormone
1. Structure and synthesis
a. Iodide pump (trapping) is present in follicular cells. This pump is regulated by iodide levels in the body (low iodide stimulates the pump).
b. Iodide is oxidized and attached to tyrosyl residues of thyroglobulin (glycoprotein, which serves as the storage form of thyroid hormones).
c. Iodotyrosines are coupled to form either T_3 (three iodides) or T_4 (four iodides) and are stored in the peptide linkage (thyroglobulin).
d. The thyroglobulin is stored as colloid until stimulated to be secreted as T_3 (tri-iodothyronine) and T_4 (tetra-iodothyronine) by TSH.
2. Regulation of synthesis and secretion
a. All steps in the synthesis of thyroid hormone are stimulated by TSH.
b. Release of the hormone follows cleavage of thyroglobulin to deliver T_3 and T_4 to the circulation, where they are bound to plasma proteins.
c. Most T_4 is converted in liver and kidney to T_3 (more biological activity).
3. Mechanism of action—thyroid hormones act as a modulator of metabolism on virtually every organ in the body. They act by influencing gene expression.
a. Basal metabolic rate (increased)
(1) Increases oxygen consumption and body temperature.
(2) Due to increased activity of Na^+-K^+-ATPase activity.
b. Metabolism
(1) Potentiates the effects of other hormones on energy metabolism, resulting in increased glycogen breakdown, increased carbohydrate metabolism, and fat metabolism.
(2) Overall catabolic effect on protein metabolism.
c. Growth and development
(1) Act synergistically with growth hormone and somatomedins to promote bone growth.
(2) Required for the normal maturation of the CNS in children.
d. Cardiovascular, respiratory, and sympathomimetic
(1) Increased metabolism requires increased activity of respiratory and cardiovascular systems.
(2) Upregulation of β1-receptors by thyroid hormone mediates this response.

B. Adrenocortical (steroid) hormones
1. Structure and synthesis
a. Three classes of hormones are synthesized (all from cholesterol)
(1) Glucocorticoids (21 carbons).
(2) Mineralcorticoids (21 carbons).
(3) Androgens (19 carbons).
b. Rate-limiting step is the conversion of cholesterol to pregnenolone.
c. Due to compartmentalization of the synthetic enzymes, different zones of the adrenal gland specialize in synthetic activity.
(1) Zona glomerulosa (outermost zone)—secretes mineralcorticoids (aldosterone).
(2) Zona fasciculata (middle zone)—secretes mainly glucocorticoids (cortisol and corticosterone).
(3) Zona reticularis (innermost zone)—secretes adrenal androgens (DHEA and androstenedione).
2. Regulation of synthesis and secretion
a. Glucocorticoids
(1) Regulated exclusively by the hypothalamic–pituitary axis (CRH and ACTH).
(2) Pulsatile and diurnal in nature (highest in the morning).
(3) Glucocorticoids feed back negatively on hypothalamus (CRH) and anterior pituitary (ACTH).
(4) Cushing syndrome (excess secretion of adrenal hormones).
b. Aldosterone—regulated primarily by the renin-angiotensin system.
(1) Renin release in response to reduction in perfusion pressure or sodium depletion produces increased amount of angiotensin II.
(2) Angiotensin II acts upon the adrenal cortex to increase aldosterone secretion.

(3) Increased extracellular K^+ also increases aldosterone secretion by acting directly on the adrenal cells.

c. Androgens—regulated by the same mechanisms as glucocorticoids.

3. Actions of adrenocortical steroids (Table 2-14)

C. Adrenal medullary (catecholamines) hormones

1. Structure and synthesis
   a. Synthesized by a series of steps from tyrosine.
   b. Epinephrine (the methylated form of norepinephrine) is the major secretory product.
   c. The adrenal medulla is essentially a sympathetic ganglion, which has secretory cells instead of postganglionic neurons. The catecholamines are secreted directly into the bloodstream to play an important role in the "fight or flight" response.
2. Regulation of synthesis and secretion
   a. Catecholamines are stored in granules in chromaffin cells.
   b. Stimulation of the sympathetic nerve to the adrenal gland releases acetylcholine at ganglionic type receptors, which results in the release of catecholamines.
   c. Examples of stress-related factors that result in adrenal medullary secretion
      (1) Fear, anxiety, and excitement.
      (2) Trauma, pain.
      (3) Hypovolemia.
      (4) Hypoglycemia.
      (5) Hypothermia.
3. Mechanisms of action—although both epinephrine and norepinephrine are secreted from the adrenal medulla, epinephrine is the main catecholamine. β-adrenergic receptor stimulation tends to be the major response to adrenal medullary stimulation, even though epinephrine stimulates both α- and β-adrenergic receptors.
   a. α-receptor-mediated
      (1) Increased gluconeogenesis.
      (2) Decreased insulin secretion.
      (3) Increased vasoconstriction (splanchnic, renal, cutaneous, and genital).
      (4) Increased sphincter contraction (GI and urinary).
      (5) Dilation of pupils.
      (6) Increased sweating.
   b. β_1-receptor-mediated
      (1) Increased lipolysis and ketosis.
      (2) Increased cardiac contraction and rate.
      (3) Increased glycogenolysis.
   c. β_2-receptor-mediated
      (1) Increased insulin secretion.
      (2) Increased glucagon secretion.
      (3) Increased K^+ uptake by muscle.
      (4) Increased arteriolar dilation in cardiovascular muscle.
      (5) Increased muscle relaxation in bronchial wall, GI wall, and wall of the urinary bladder.

Table 2–14. Actions of Adrenocortical Steroids

ACTIONS OF GLUCOCORTICOIDS	ACTIONS OF MINERALOCORTICOIDS	ACTIONS OF ADRENAL ANDROGENS
Increase gluconeogenesis	Increase Na^+ resorption	Females: presence of pubic and axillary hair; libido
Increase proteolysis (catabolic)	Increase K^+ secretion	Males: same as testosterone
Increase lipolysis	Increase H^+ secretion	
Decrease glucose utilization		
Decrease insulin sensitivity		
Anti-inflammatory		
Immunosuppression		
Maintain vascular responsiveness to catecholamines		
Inhibit bone formation		
Increase GFR		
Decrease REM sleep		

From Costanzo LS: Physiology, ed 3, WB Saunders, Philadelphia, 2004.

SAMPLE QUESTIONS

1. ***Nonsteroidal anti-inflammatory agents are pain-relieving and anti-inflammatory. They are effective since they act to inhibit prostaglandin synthesis by:***
   A. Inhibiting fatty acid lipo-oxygenase activity.
   B. Inhibiting fatty acid-specific cyclo-oxygenase activity.
   C. Inhibiting fatty acid-specific hydroperoxidase activity.
   D. Inhibiting phospholipase A_2.
2. ***The synthesis of all steroid hormones involves which of the following compounds?***
   A. Pregnenolone.
   B. Progesterone.
   C. Aldosterone.
   D. Cortisone.
   E. Testosterone.
3. ***Lipid micelles are stabilized by which of the following?***
   A. Hydrophobic interactions.
   B. Hydrophilic interactions.
   C. Interactions of lipid and water.
   D. Interaction of hydrophobic lipid tails with hydrophobic domains of proteins.
4. ***Which one of the following carbohydrates is a ketose sugar?***
   A. Galactose.
   B. Fructose.
   C. Glucose.
   D. Mannose.
   E. Glyceraldehydes.
5. ***Mucopolysaccharidoses are hereditary disorders that are characterized by the accumulation of glycosaminoglycans in various tissues due to which of the following?***
   A. Overproduction (synthesis) of proteoglycans.
   B. Deficiency of one of the lysosomal, hydrolytic enzymes normally involved in the degradation of one or more of the glycosaminoglycans.
   C. The synthesis of abnormal proteoglycans.
   D. The synthesis of highly branched glycosaminoglycan chains.
6. ***Hydrolysis of which of the following compounds yields urea?***
   A. Ornithine.
   B. Argininosuccinate.
   C. Aspartate.
   D. Citrulline.
   E. Arginine.
7. ***The binding of epinephrine or glucagon to the corresponding membrane receptor has which of the following effects on glycogen metabolism?***
   A. The net synthesis of glycogen is increased.
   B. Glycogen phosphorylase is activated while glycogen synthase is inactivated.
   C. Glycogen phosphorylase is inactivated while glycogen synthase is activated.
   D. Both glycogen synthase and phosphorylase are activated.
   E. Both glycogen synthase and phosphorylase are inactivated.
8. ***When an enzyme is competitively inhibited, which of the following changes occur?***
   A. The apparent Km is unchanged.
   B. The apparent Km is decreased.
   C. V_{max} is decreased.
   D. V_{max} is unchanged.
9. ***Which compound is produced in the hexose monophosphate (pentose phosphate) pathway?***
   A. ATP.
   B. NADH.
   C. NADPH.
   D. Fructose 1,6-bisphosphate.
   E. Phosphoenolpyruvate.
10. ***During exercise, which of the following is decreased?***
    A. Oxidation of fatty acids.
    B. Glucagon release.
    C. Glycogenolysis.
    D. Lipogenesis.
11. ***Increased formation of ketone bodies during fasting is a result of which of the following?***
    A. Increased oxidation of fatty acids as a source of fuel.
    B. Decreased formation of acetyl CoA in the liver.
    C. Decreased levels of glucagon.
    D. Increased glycogenesis in muscle.
12. ***Which of the following enzymes found in the liver is involved in gluconeogenesis during the postabsorptive state?***
    A. Glucose 6-phosphate dehydrogenase.
    B. 6-phosphogluconate dehydrogenase.
    C. Glucose 6-phosphatase.
    D. Glucokinase.

13. ***In which one of the following tissues is glucose transport into the cell* unaffected *by insulin?***
   A. Skeletal muscle.
   B. Liver.
   C. Adipose tissue.
   D. Smooth muscle.
14. ***Which of the following genetic diseases that results from a deficiency in the liver enzyme that converts phenylalanine to tyrosine?***
   A. Albinism.
   B. Homocystinuria.
   C. Porphyria.
   D. Phenylketonuria.
15. ***If the molar percentage of guanine in a human DNA is 30%, what is the molar percentage of adenine in that molecule?***
   A. 10%.
   B. 20%.
   C. 30%.
   D. 40%.
   E. 50%.
16. ***Which of the following phrases best describes restriction enzymes?***
   A. Site-specific endonucleases.
   B. Enzymes that regulate RNA.
   C. Nonspecific endonucleases.
   D. Topoisomerases.
17. ***The coenzyme that serves as an intermediate carrier of one-carbon units in the synthesis of nucleic acids is which of the following?***
   A. Ascorbic acid.
   B. Tetrahydrofolic acid.
   C. Biotin.
   D. Pyridoxine.
18. ***Following the production of Okazaki fragments, which of the following is required to close the gap between the fragments?***
   A. DNA ligase.
   B. DNA polymerase.
   C. RNA polymerase.
   D. Reverse transcriptase.
19. ***Which of the following is not involved in the process of gene cloning?***
   A. DNA polymerase.
   B. DNA ligase.
   C. RNA polymerase.
   D. Restriction endonuclease.
20. ***Vitamin K serves as a coenzyme for:***
   A. The enzymatic hydroxylation of proline to 4-hydroxyproline.
   B. The carboxylation of inactive prothrombin to form active prothrombin.
   C. The synthesis of nucleic acids.
   D. Protein synthesis.
21. ***Chondroitin sulfate is a major component of which of the following?***
   A. Bacterial cell walls.
   B. Mucin.
   C. IgA.
   D. Cartilage.
   E. Hair.
22. ***Which of the following amino acids is positioned at every third residue in the primary structure of the helical portion of the collagen-α chains?***
   A. Glycine.
   B. Glutamate.
   C. Proline.
   D. Lysine.
   E. Hydroxyproline.
23. ***Which of the following is not involved in the process of mineralization?***
   A. Matrix vesicles.
   B. Amelogenins.
   C. Fluoride.
   D. Phosphoryns.
24. ***ATP is utilized directly for each of the following processes* except:**
   A. Accumulation of Ca^{2+} by the sarcoplasmic reticulum.
   B. Transport of Na^{+} from intracellular to extracellular fluid.
   C. Transport of K^{+} from extracellular to intracellular fluid.
   D. Transport of H^{+} from parietal cells into the lumen of the stomach.
   E. Transport of glucose into muscle cells.
25. ***Both active transport and facilitated diffusion are characterized by which of the following?***
   A. Transport in one direction only.
   B. Hydrolysis of ATP.
   C. Transport against a concentration gradient.
   D. Competitive inhibition.
26. ***Which of the following statements regarding the autonomic nervous system (ANS) is true?***
   A. The third cranial nerve (the oculomotor nerve) carries sympathetic fibers to the smooth muscles of the eye.
   B. The facial and the glossopharyngeal cranial nerves carry the parasympathetic preganglionic fibers for the autonomic innervation to the salivary glands.
   C. The parasympathetic nervous system innervates primarily striated muscle in the body.
   D. The parasympathetic nervous system is organized for diffuse activation and responses.
27. ***Which of the following responses is due to the stimulation of α-adrenergic receptors?***
   A. Slowing of heart rate.
   B. Constriction of blood vessels in skin.
   C. Increased gastrointestinal motility.
   D. Increased renal blood flow.
28. ***Which of the following is a property of C fibers?***
   A. Have the slowest conduction velocity of any nerve fiber type.
   B. Have the largest diameter of any nerve fiber type.
   C. Are afferent nerves from muscle spindles.
   D. Are afferent nerves from Golgi tendon organs.
   E. Are preganglionic autonomic fibers.

29. *The participation of calcium in the contraction of skeletal muscle is facilitated or associated with which of the following?*
A. Calcium release from sarcoplasmic reticulum.
B. Calcium binding to the myosin heads.
C. Active transport of calcium out of longitudinal tubules.
D. Uptake of calcium by T-tubules.

30. *Calcium that enters the cell during smooth muscle excitation binds with which of the following?*
A. Calmodulin.
B. Inactive myosin kinase.
C. Troponin.
D. Myosin.
E. Actin.

31. *Which of the following does not affect the muscle tension produced during contraction?*
A. The extent of motor-unit recruitment.
B. The proportion of each single motor unit that is stimulated to contract.
C. The number of muscle fibers contracting.
D. The frequency of stimulation.

32. *The pressure in a capillary in skeletal muscle is 37 mmHg at the arteriolar end and 16 mmHg at the venular end. The interstitial pressure is 0 mmHg. The colloid osmotic pressure is 26 mmHg in the capillary and 1 mmHg in the interstitial fluid. The net force producing fluid movement across the capillary wall is which of the following ?*
A. 1 mmHg out of the capillary.
B. 3 mmHg out of the capillary.
C. 12 mmHg out of the capillary.
D. 3 mmHg into the capillary.

33. *A patient has a heart rate of 70 bpm. Her EDV (end-diastolic volume) is 140 mL. Her ESV (end-systolic volume) is 30 mL. Calculate the CO (cardiac output) of this individual.*
A. 9800 mL.
B. 2100 mL.
C. 7700 mL.
D. 15,400 mL

34. *The velocity of blood flow _____.*
A. Is higher in the capillaries than the arterioles
B. Is higher in the veins than in the venules
C. Is higher in the veins than in the arteries
D. Falls to zero in the descending aorta during diastole

35. *Which of the following does not occur to compensate for a fall in blood pressure below normal values?*
A. Increased cardiac output.
B. Increased stroke volume.
C. Increased heart rate.
D. Decreased total peripheral resistance.

36. *CO_2 generated in the tissues is carried in venous blood primarily in which form?*
A. CO_2 in the plasma.
B. H_2CO_3 in the plasma.
C. HCO_3^- in the plasma.
D. CO_2 in the red blood cells.
E. Carboxyhemoglobin in the red blood cells.

37. *Which of the following is the most significant stimulant of the respiratory center?*
A. Decreased blood oxygen tension.
B. Increased blood hydrogen ion concentration.
C. Decreased blood hydrogen ion concentration.
D. Increased blood carbon dioxide tension.

38. *The primary factor determining the percent of hemoglobin saturation is:*
A. Blood PO_2.
B. Blood PCO_2.
C. Diphosphoglycerate concentration.
D. The temperature of the blood.
E. The acidity of the blood.

39. *For which of the following substances would you expect the renal clearance to be the lowest, under normal conditions?*
A. Urea.
B. Creatinine.
C. Sodium.
D. Water.
E. Glucose.

40. *The process of active sodium transport in the ascending limb of the loop of Henle is absolutely essential for which of the following processes?*
A. Regulation of chloride excretion.
B. Regulation of pH in extracellular fluid.
C. Regulation of aldosterone excretion.
D. Regulation of water excretion.

41. *Hypertension (long-term) will be compensated by which of the following renal mechanisms?*
A. Increased circulating ADH (vasopressin).
B. Increased sympathetic activity.
C. Decreased circulating aldosterone.
D. Increased circulating angiotensin II.

42. *Which of the following statements regarding tubular secretion in the kidney is true?*
A. The secretion of K^+ increases when a person is in acidosis.
B. The secretion of H^+ increases when a person is in alkalosis.
C. It is a process that transports substances from the filtrate to the capillary blood.
D. It accounts for most of the K^+ in the urine.

43. *Which of the following statements regarding salivary secretion is true?*
A. In general, saliva is more hypertonic than plasma.
B. As salivary flow increases, bicarbonate concentration decreases.
C. As salivary flow increases, ionic concentration increases.
D. Salivary secretion is regulated primarily by hormonal stimulation.

44. ***Which of the following is the predominant immunoglobulin in whole saliva?***
    A. Secretory IgA.
    B. Secretory IgG.
    C. Secretory IgM.
    D. Secretory IgB.
45. ***The pancreas produces enzymes that are responsible for the digestion of dietary compounds. Which of the following foods would* not *be digested by enzymes synthesized and secreted by the pancreas?***
    A. Carbohydrates.
    B. Lipids.
    C. Vitamins.
    D. Protein.
46. ***Which of the following statements regarding the hormone secretin is true?***
    A. It is responsible for activating chymotrypsinogen.
    B. It stimulates the release of pancreatic secretion rich in bicarbonate.
    C. It stimulates the release of pancreatic enzymes.
    D. It stimulates the contraction of the gallbladder to release bile.
47. ***Phospholipase C is an enzyme that plays an important role in the production of second messengers, which produce intracellular responses. Which two second messengers are produced through the action of this enzyme?***
    A. cAMP and tyrosine kinase.
    B. Acetylcholine and histidine.
    C. Adenylate cyclase and protein kinase.
    D. 1,2-diacylglycerol and inositol 1,4, 5-trisphosphate.
48. ***Hormones secreted by the posterior pituitary gland include which of the following?***
    A. Prolactin.
    B. Follicle-stimulating hormone.
    C. Luteinizing hormone.
    D. Vasopressin.
49. ***The effects of which one of the following hormones are not mediated through cAMP?***
    A. Estrogen.
    B. Glucagon.
    C. Epinephrine.
    D. Norepinephrine.
50. ***A scientist has discovered a new peptide hormone. He thinks it acts through the second messenger system, which utilizes cAMP. If this is true, which of the following substances should* decrease *the response of this new peptide hormone in cells?***
    A. Adenylate cyclase.
    B. Monoamine oxidase inhibitors.
    C. Phosphodiesterase.
    D. Aspirin.
51. ***Which of the following proteoglycans is present in extracellular space?***
    A. Hyaluronic acid.
    B. Keratan sulfate.
    C. Chondroitin sulfate.
    D. Dermatan sulfate.
    E. Heparin.
52. ***Porphyrins use which amino acid in their synthesis?***
    A. Alanine.
    B. Phenylalanine.
    C. Cysteine.
    D. Glycine.
53. ***Which of the following is an essential amino acid?***
    A. Tyrosine.
    B. Tryptophan.
    C. Proline.
    D. Serine.
    E. Alanine.
54. ***Aspartame contains aspartic acid and which of the following amino acids?***
    A. Phenylalanine.
    B. Leucine.
    C. Isoleucine.
    D. Lysine.
    E. Proline.
55. ***Which of the following is the end product of purine degradation in humans?***
    A. Urea.
    B. Uric acid.
    C. Adenosine.
    D. Xanthine.
56. ***Which of the following participates in both fatty acid biosynthesis and β-oxidation of fatty acids?***
    A. Malonyl CoA.
    B. FAD.
    C. Acetyl CoA.
    D. NAD^+.
57. ***The rate-limiting enzyme in glycolysis is which of the following?***
    A. Fructose bisphosphatase.
    B. Phosphofructokinase.
    C. Phosphoglucose isomerase.
    D. Glucokinase.
58. ***The coenzyme essential for normal amino acid metabolism is _____.***
    A. Biotin
    B. Tetrahydrofolate
    C. Pyridoxal phosphate
    D. Niacin
59. ***Which of the following metabolic activities is increased 1 hour after a meal (during the absorptive state)?***
    A. Glycogenolysis.
    B. Oxidation of free fatty acids.
    C. Glucagon release.
    D. Glycolysis.

60. ***Which of the following coenzymes are involved in the metabolism of pyruvate to acetyl CoA?***
A. Thiamin pyrophosphate, lipoic acid, FAD, NAD, and coenzyme A.
B. NAD, tetrahydrofolate, lipoic acid, FAD, and vitamin B_{12}.
C. Mg^{2+}, FAD, nicotinamide adenine dinucleotide, and biotin.
D. Coenzyme A, niacin, FAD, and ascorbic acid.

61. ***Relative or absolute lack of insulin in humans would result in which one of the following reactions in the liver?***
A. Increased glycogen synthesis.
B. Increased gluconeogenesis.
C. Decreased glycogen breakdown.
D. Increased amino acid uptake.

62. ***Which one of the following is elevated in plasma during the absorptive period (compared to the postabsorptive state)?***
A. Chylomicrons.
B. Acetoacetate.
C. Lactate.
D. Glucagon.

63. ***Insulin produces which of the following changes in mammalian cells?***
A. Increase in liver glycogen production.
B. Increase in blood glucose concentration.
C. Decrease in the transport of glucose into muscle.
D. Increase in the transport of glucose into the brain .

64. ***Which of the following describes the function of RNA polymerase?***
A. Translates DNA into protein.
B. Terminates transcription.
C. Removes introns during transcription.
D. Synthesizes RNA 5′→3′.

65. ***Analysis of DNA fragments (probing) is possibly due to which of the following properties of DNA?***
A. Phosphodiester bonds.
B. Complimentary strands.
C. Protein binding.
D. Western blotting.

66. ***The amount of cytosine will be equal to the amount of guanine in which of the following molecules?***
A. DNA.
B. RNA.
C. DNA and RNA.
D. mRNA.

67. ***What is the correct general structure of the backbone of DNA and RNA?***
A. Sugar-base–sugar.
B. Bases linked through phosphodiester linkages.
C. Bases linked through hydrogen bonds.
D. Sugars linked through phosphodiester linkages.

68. ***The conversion of information from DNA into mRNA is called which of the following?***
A. Translation.
B. Transcription.
C. Transduction.
D. Transformation.

69. ***Which of the following mineralized tissues have the greatest percentage of inorganic material?***
A. Enamel.
B. Dentin.
C. Bone.
D. Calculus.

70. ***Each of the following describes collagen except one. Which is the*** **exception?**
A. Most abundant protein in the body.
B. Modifications to procollagen occur in the extracellular matrix.
C. Incorporates hydroxyproline into the molecule by tRNA.
D. Hydroxylation of proline requires vitamin C and molecular oxygen.

71. ***Hydroxyapatite _____.***
A. Is weakened if fluoride is substituted for some of the hydroxyl ions
B. Is a noncrystalline structure
C. If containing carbonate ion becomes more soluble
D. Is composed of calcium and phosphate in a 1:1 ratio

72. ***The type of collagen characteristically found in cartilage is which of the following?***
A. Type I.
B. Type II.
C. Type III.
D. Type IV.

73. ***Which process transports amino acids across the luminal surface of the epithelia that lines the small intestine?***
A. Simple diffusion.
B. Primary active transport.
C. Cotransport with sodium ion.
D. Cotransport with chloride ion.

74. ***Cell membranes typically contain the following compounds*** **except:**
A. Phospholipids
B. Proteins
C. Cholesterols
D. Triacylglycerols
E. Sphingolipids

75. ***Monoamine oxidase (MAO) _____.***
A. Inactivates reduced steroid derivatives
B. Is not associated with nerves
C. Inactivates catecholamines by oxidative deamination
D. Is located in the synapse where it inactivates the neurotransmitter acetylcholine

76. *Which one of the following does not release acetylcholine?*
A. Sympathetic preganglionic fibers.
B. Sympathetic postganglionic fibers that innervate the heart.
C. Parasympathetic postganglionic fibers to effector organs.
D. Parasympathetic preganglionic fibers.

77. *Where are the temperature control centers located?*
A. Cerebellum.
B. Hypothalamus.
C. Medulla.
D. Cerebral cortex.

78. *The energy for skeletal muscle contraction is derived from which of the following processes?*
A. Calcium release from sarcoplasmic membranes and binding to troponin.
B. Cleavage of ATP by the myosin head.
C. Membrane sodium-potassium ATPase pump.
D. Sodium influx during the action potential.

79. *Muscle spindle stretching when the patellar tendon is tapped produces which of the following responses?*
A. Muscle contraction within muscle where the spindles are located.
B. Increased sympathetic stimulation of the spindles.
C. A reduction in the number of afferent impulses entering the spinal cord.
D. An inhibition of the stretch reflex.

80. *The gamma motor neurons control which of the following?*
A. Muscle spindles.
B. Iris of the eye.
C. Voluntary muscle fibers.
D. Pyloric sphincter.

81. *Which of the following would be expected to raise blood pressure?*
A. A drug that inhibits the angiotensin II-converting enzyme and thus the production of angiotensin II (ACE inhibitors).
B. A drug that inhibits the synthesis of nitric oxide.
C. A drug that blocks vasopressin receptors.
D. Increased stimulation of the carotid baroreceptor.

82. *Which of the following ions has a higher intracellular concentration compared to the extracellular fluid?*
A. Na^+.
B. K^+.
C. Cl^-.
D. HCO_3^-
E. Ca^{2+}.

83. *All of the following local chemical factors will cause vasodilatation of the arterioles,* except:
A. Decreased K^+
B. Increased CO_2
C. Nitric oxide
D. Decreased O_2
E. Histamine release

84. *Increasing the radius of arterioles will increase which of the following?*
A. Systolic blood pressure.
B. Diastolic blood pressure.
C. Viscosity of the blood.
D. Capillary blood flow.

85. *In which of the following might arterial blood pressure be abnormally high?*
A. Ventricular fibrillation.
B. Acute heart failure.
C. Anaphylactic shock.
D. Increased intracranial pressure.

86. *A major function of surfactant is to increase which of the following?*
A. Pulmonary compliance.
B. Alveolar surface tension.
C. The work of breathing.
D. The tendency of the lungs to collapse.

87. *The minimum volume of air that remains in the lungs after a maximal expiration is termed the _____.*
A. Tidal volume
B. Functional residual capacity
C. Residual volume
D. Vital capacity

88. *The center that provides output to the respiratory muscles is located in the _____.*
A. Pons
B. Medulla
C. Cerebral cortex
D. Cerebellum
E. Hypothalamus

89. *Aldosterone _____.*
A. Stimulates Na^+ reabsorption in the distal and collecting ducts
B. Is secreted by the juxtaglomerular apparatus
C. Stimulates K^+ absorption in the distal tubule
D. Stimulates bicarbonate reabsorption in the proximal tubule

90. *What happens to net fluid filtration in the glomerulus when plasma protein concentration is decreased?*
A. Net filtration (ultrafiltration) increases.
B. Net filtration (ultrafiltration) decreases.
C. Net filtration remains unchanged.
D. Net filtration ceases.

91. *Which of the following factors would result in decreased glomerular filtration rate?*
A. A fall in plasma protein concentration.
B. An obstruction of the tubular system which would increase capsular hydrostatic pressure.
C. Vasodilation of the afferent arterioles.
D. Inulin administration.

92. ***Which of the following statements regarding tubular reabsorption is true?***
A. Most calcium filtered is passively reabsorbed and not regulated under any conditions.
B. Most urea is reabsorbed passively and is unaffected by regulatory mechanisms.
C. Glucose is reabsorbed by secondary active transport and facilitated diffusion.
D. Most filtered phosphate is reabsorbed in the collecting ducts and is unaffected by regulatory mechanisms.

93. ***Which of the following processes is* not *a true component of swallowing?***
A. Closure of the glottis.
B. Involuntary relaxation of the upper esophageal sphincter.
C. Movements of the tongue against the palate.
D. Esophageal peristalsis.

94. ***Which of the following statements regarding the regulation of gastrointestinal motility is true?***
A. Sympathetic stimulation inhibits motility.
B. Parasympathetic stimulation inhibits motility.
C. Gastrointestinal motility is not influenced by the central nervous system (CNS).
D. Gastrointestinal motility is not influenced by hormones.

95. ***Which one of the following statements regarding the regulation of gastrointestinal function is true?***
A. The main sympathetic nerve supply to the digestive tract is the vagus.
B. In general, sympathetic stimulation is excitatory to digestive activity.
C. Salivary secretion is stimulated by both branches of the autonomic nervous system, although not to the same degree.
D. Parasympathetic stimulation of the salivary glands produces a saliva rich in mucus.

96. ***Which of the following factors will not influence the rate at which a meal will leave the stomach?***
A. Acidification of the duodenum.
B. Increasing the tonicity of the intestine.
C. Saline in the duodenum.
D. Lipid in the intestine.

97. ***Which of the following forms of thyroid hormone is most readily found in the circulation?***
A. Tri-iodothyronine (T_3).
B. Thyroxine (T_4).
C. Thyroglobulin.
D. TSH.

98. ***A hormone acts to stimulate its neighboring cell to divide. This hormone would best be described as belonging to which category of hormones?***
A. Paracrine.
B. Autocrine.
C. Endocrine.

99. ***Blood levels of progesterone are highest during _____.***
A. The follicular phase of the ovarian cycle
B. The luteal phase of the ovarian cycle
C. Ovulation
D. Menstruation

100. ***Glucagon will decrease which of the following?***
A. Glycogenolysis.
B. Gluconeogenesis.
C. Glycogenesis.
D. Blood glucose.

3

Microbiology and Pathology

JEAN YANG

OUTLINE

1.0 IMMUNOLOGY AND IMMUNOPATHOLOGY

The human body's immune system is an elegant and elaborate process involving two types of immunity. In general, the body's first defense mechanism against infection includes anatomic (e.g., skin, mucosal membranes) or physiologic (e.g., temperature, low pH) barriers. When a pathogen invades this physical barrier, the body has two different types of immune responses: the innate (nonspecific) immune response and the acquired (specific/adaptive) immune response. Innate immunity is the body's early defense to any kind of bodily injury, including trauma or infection. Since this nonspecific immune response has a limited ability to recognize specific antigens, it generally reacts to most pathogens in the same manner. When the innate immune response fails to effectively combat invading pathogens, the body mounts an acquired immune response. Acquired immunity, however, involves a highly sophisticated recognition of foreign structures. This ability to learn to identify specific structures allows the body's defenses to act quickly and efficiently in killing specific pathogens.

1.1 Host Defense Mechanisms

A. Anatomical barriers
   1. Skin
      a. Acts as a physical barrier to external pathogens.
      b. Langerhans cells—dendritic cells that are found in the stratum spinosum layer and are important in their ability to initiate the immune system.
      c. Acidic environment of pH 3 to 5 retards growth of microbes.
   2. Mucosal membranes
      a. Line the gastrointestinal, respiratory, and urogenital tracts.
      b. There are a variety of protective mechanisms. For instance, in the stomach and vaginal tract the pH remains low, discouraging microbial growth. The pulmonary mucosa contains cilia and secretes mucus, clearing the air that enters the respiratory tract.
      c. Lysozyme is an important antimicrobial enzyme that is secreted in saliva and tears.

B. Physiologic barriers
   1. Temperature—raised body temperature (i.e., fever) inhibits growth of some pathogens.
   2. Low pH—acidic pH of the stomach kills most ingested micro-organisms.

C. Innate immune response
   1. Acute inflammation
      a. Early immune response to injury or infection includes:
         (1) Edema—caused by the increased vascular permeability of endothelial cells. Initially, the arterioles briefly vasoconstrict. This is followed by vasodilation and increased permeability of the endothelium. Fluid then moves from the circulation into the interstitial tissue, resulting in hyperemia and local edema. These actions are described by the four classic signs of inflammation: tumor (swelling), rubor (redness), calor (heat), and dolor (pain).
         (2) Complement activation (discussed later in the complement system section).
         (3) Release of inflammatory mediators by polymorphonuclear leukocytes or neutrophils, basophils, and mast cells.
         (4) Activation of natural killer cells, which resemble cytotoxic T cells. They act to destroy cells primarily infected with viruses or tumors.
      b. Possible outcomes of acute inflammation:
         (1) Complete resolution.
         (2) Scarring.
         (3) Abscess formation. Clinically, if the abscess spreads into the soft tissues, a cellulitis develops. Two dental-significant formations of cellulitis include Ludwig's angina and cavernous sinus thrombosis.
            (a) Clinically, if the abscess spreads into the soft tissues, a cellulitis develops.
            (b) Two dental-significant formations of cellulitis include Ludwig's angina and cavernous sinus thrombosis.
   2. Chronic inflammation
      a. Usually a more moderate inflammatory response that persists.
      b. Mediators of chronic inflammation include mononuclear leukocytes or macrophages, plasma cells, and lymphocytes.
      c. Example in dentistry: a periapical lesion that persists at the root apex for many years due to continual stimulation of pathogens from inside the tooth.
   3. Granulomatous inflammation
      a. A form of chronic inflammation, characterized by the formation of granulomas.
      b. Granulomas are areas that the immune system "walls off" if phagocytes fail to destroy foreign particles or microbes present in it.
      c. Inflammatory mediators include a dense concentration of macrophages, fibroblasts, lymphocytes, and (less frequently) plasma cells. The continuous activation of macrophages induces them to attach to one another, assuming an epithelium-like (epithelioid) appearance; they may also fuse with each other to form multinucleated giant cells.
      d. Two types of granulomas:
         (1) Granulomas associated with infectious diseases. Examples include:
            (a) Tuberculosis (*Mycobacterium*) infections—granulomas found in infected areas are called *tubercles* and often display central caseous necrosis.
            (b) Fungal infections (*Cryptococcus, Histoplasma, Coccidioides*).
            (c) Syphilis (*Treponema pallidum*)—granulomas seen during syphilis infections are called *gumma.*
            (d) Cat scratch disease.
         (2) Granulomas associated with foreign bodies
            (a) Examples: foreign particles (glass, metals), surgical sutures, and so forth.

D. Acquired immune response
   1. Immunologic attributes of the acquired immune response:
      a. Specificity (antibody recognition can be as specific as a single amino acid).
      b. Diversity (antibodies can recognize billions of unique structures).
      c. Memory (i.e., memory B cells).
      d. Self/non-self recognition (i.e., major histocompatibility complex).
   2. There are two types of specific immune responses: cell–mediated immunity, which is mediated by T cells, and humoral immunity, which is mediated by antibodies that are produced by B cells.
   3. Cell-mediated immunity

a. Is mediated by T cells.
b. Since T cells cannot directly recognize antigens, antigens must be processed and presented to them by antigen-presenting cells (APCs), such as macrophages, dendritic cells, B cells, and endothelial cells. APCs digest the antigens into small peptides and present them with a class II MHC molecule to the CD4 receptor on the helper T cell. This activates the helper T cells to release cytokines that cause inflammation and the activation of other T cells, B cells, and macrophages (Figure 3-1).

4. Humoral immunity (antibody-mediated immunity)
   a. This branch of the specific immune response serves two purposes:
      (1) To target antigens—the aggregation of antibodies produced by B cells on an antigen specifically identifies, neutralizes, and opsonizes the antigen, making it easier to phagocytize.
      (2) Serves as a memory function—allows the immune system to more efficiently recognize and destroy microbes from previous exposure or infection.
   b. Antigens are first recognized by macrophages or directly by B cells. Like cell-mediated immunity, the macrophage will process and present the antigens to helper T cells. This causes them to secrete cytokines, interleukin-4 (IL-4), and interleukin-5 (IL-5), which results in B-cell stimulation and growth, thus resulting in the production of specific antibodies against the antigen presented (Figure 3-2).

1.1.1 *Wound healing*

A. Primary wound healing
   1. Describes the repair of two well-apposed edges, such as surgical incisions.
   2. Timeline of cellular events:
      a. First 24 hours—formation of a fibrin clot. Fibronectin, an adhesive molecule found in plasma and on cell surfaces, forms crosslinks to stabilize the clot. PMNs or neutrophils migrate to the injured site.
      b. Day 1 to 2—basal cells begin to proliferate (i.e., undergo mitosis) to close the epidermal defect.
      c. Day 3—proliferation of basal cells continues. Granulation tissue forms at the injured site. Macrophages replace PMNs. Fibroblasts appear and secrete proteoglycans and type III collagen. Neovascularization begins.
      d. End of the first week—formation of a scar. Fibroblasts and microphages continue to clean up and remodel the area. Fibroblasts secrete type I collagen. The vascularization and cellular infiltrate largely disappear.
   3. Secondary wound healing
      a. Describes repair of a larger wound with margins that are not well-apposed.
      b. Cellular events are similar to primary wound healing except that more granulation tissue is formed and there is a larger inflammatory response. Also, the duration of healing is longer.

1.1.2 Immune effector cells

A. T cells
   1. Important regulators of the immune response.

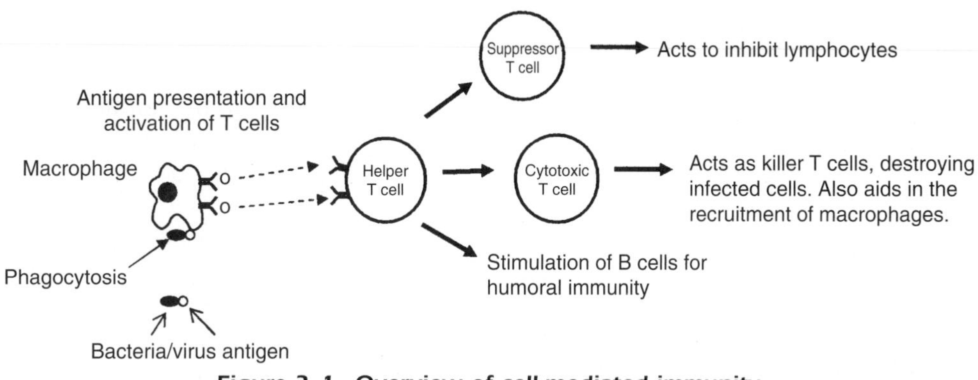

Figure 3–1. Overview of cell-mediated immunity.

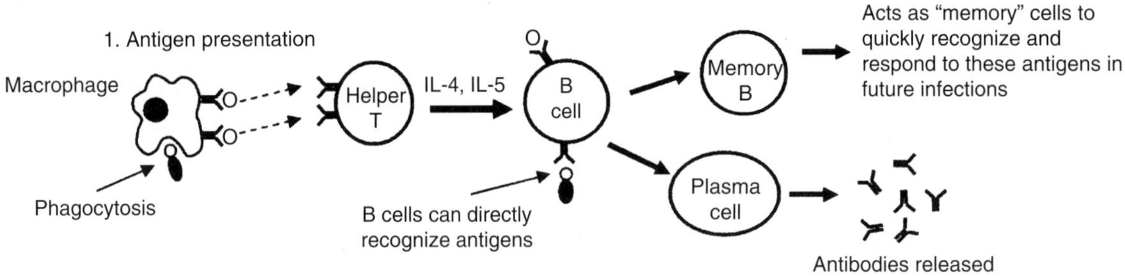

Figure 3–2. Overview of humoral immunity.

2. Involved in both cell-mediated and humoral immunity.
3. Play a role in type IV delayed hypersensitivity reactions.
4. Can be categorized by their function, namely, regulatory or effector. The regulatory function is primarily mediated by helper T cells, which have CD4 surface receptors. The effector function is primarily mediated by cytotoxic and suppressor T cells, which contain CD8 surface receptors:
   a. CD4—helper T cells
      (1) Recognize class II MHC molecules on antigen-presenting cells.
      (2) Mainly for the recognition of bacterial antigens.
      (3) Regulatory functions include:
         (a) Stimulate B cells to develop into antibody-producing plasma cells.
         (b) Stimulate CD8 cells to become activated cytotoxic T cells.
         (c) Stimulate the actions of macrophages during delayed hypersensitivity reactions.
   b. CD8—cytotoxic and suppressor T cells
      (1) Recognize class I MHC molecules on antigen-presenting cells.
      (2) Function mainly in recognition of viral or neoplastic antigens.
      (3) Cytotoxic functions are carried out by:
         (a) Releasing perforans—destroy cell membranes.
         (b) Inducing apoptosis—programmed cell death.
   c. T cell maturation occurs in the thymus. There are three developmental stages:
      (1) Immature: $CD4^-CD8^-$, a double-negative cell that expresses neither CD4 nor CD8.
      (2) Less mature: $CD4^+CD8^+$, a double-positive cell that expresses both CD4 and CD8.
      (3) Mature: $CD4^+CD8^-$ or $CD4^-CD8^+$, a single-positive cell that expresses either CD4 or CD8.

B. B lymphocytes
   1. Involved in the humoral immune response.
   2. Perform two important functions:
      a. Responsible for the production and secretion of antibodies.
      b. Are antigen-presenting cells. Antigens are recognized by surface immunoglobulins.
   3. Activated B cells differentiate into:
      a. Plasma cells—produce and release monoclonal antibodies.
      b. Memory B cells—circulate for long periods of time and are able to respond quickly to re-exposures.

C. Mononuclear cells—monocytes (in blood) and macrophages (in tissues)
   1. Produced in the bone marrow.
   2. Important functions include:
      a. Phagocytosis—defense against microbes, removal of cellular debris or breakdown products.
      b. Cytokine production.
      c. Act as antigen-presenting cells.
   3. When monocytes enter tissues, they mature into macrophages.
   4. The body has an extensive network of macrophages known as the *reticuloendothelial system.* These macrophages are fixed and serve different functions, depending on their tissue location. Examples include:
      a. Dust cells and heart–failure cells in the lungs.
      b. Kupffer cells in the liver.
      c. Mesangial cells in the kidney.

d. Macrophages in the lymph nodes.
e. Splenocytes in the spleen.
f. Microglia in the CNS.
g. Histocytes in connective tissues.

5. The presence of macrophages indicates chronic inflammation.
6. Phagocytosis
   a. Occurs in three stages:
      (1) Migration and attachment to site of injury/infection.
      (2) Ingestion—formation of a phagosome.
      (3) Killing—release of enzymes to destroy ingested microbe.
   b. Phagocytosis is a process that initiates with the formation of a membrane-bound vacuole (phagosome) around the foreign particle or microbe. The phagosome then fuses with a lysosome, which contains many degradative enzymes, resulting in the formation of a phagolysosome. This process results in the destruction of the microbe.

D. Mast cells
1. Contain surface antigen receptors, including IgE. IgE plays an important role in type I immediate hypersensitivity reactions.
2. Contain dense granules with inflammatory mediators, including:
   a. Histamine. There are two receptors that bind histamine:
      (1) H1 receptors—cause increased permeability and vasodilation in capillaries. Also cause bronchoconstriction in the lungs.
      (2) H2 receptors—play a role in gastric acid and pepsin secretion.
   b. Slow-reacting substance of anaphylaxis (SRS-A)
      (1) A leukotriene.
      (2) Actions include bronchoconstriction in the lungs.
      (3) May play an important role as a mediator of asthmatic bronchoconstriction.

1.1.3 Cytokines

A. Cytokines are inflammatory mediators that are released by a variety of cells, such as macrophages or lymphocytes, to regulate immune responses. *Think of them as the words that immune cells use to communicate with each other.*

B. Cytokines secreted from lymphocytes are also called *lymphokines*.

C. Types of cytokines:
1. Interleukins (ILs)
   a. Are mediators that affect lymphocytes.
   b. A summary of important interleukins is shown in Table 3-1.
2. Interferons (INFs)
   a. Are mediators that are important for antiviral immunity.
   b. A summary of important interferons is shown in Table 3-2.

D. Prostaglandins (PGs) and leukotrienes (LTs)—mediators of the inflammatory response. PGs and LTs are metabolites of arachidonic acid. They are produced by the cyclo-oxygenase and the lipoxygenase pathway, respectively (Figure 3-3). General actions of these cytokines include vasoconstriction, bronchoconstriction, and increased inflammatory activity.

1.1.4 Complement System

A. Consists of a group of nearly 30 preformed serum and membrane proteins found in blood serum or on cell surfaces. They become activated through protease activity in a cascading order.

TABLE 3–1. IMPORTANT INTERLEUKINS AND THEIR ACTIONS

CYTOKINE	SOURCE	ACTIONS
IL-1	Macrophages	Stimulate cell activity or production of mediators in a variety of cells, including lymphocytes, macrophages, and endothelial cells. They also cause fever.
IL-2	Helper T cells	Activate helper and cytotoxic T cells.
IL-3	Activated T cells	Stimulate production of RBCs in bone marrow.
IL-4	Helper T cells	Stimulate B cell growth and production of IgE and IgG.
IL-5	Helper T cells	Stimulate B cell differentiation into plasma cells, activity of eosinophils, and production of IgA.

TABLE 3–2. IMPORTANT INTERFERONS AND THEIR ACTIONS

CYTOKINE	SOURCE	ACTIONS
INF-α	Leukocytes	Inhibit viral growth
INF-β	Fibroblasts	Inhibit viral growth
INF-γ	Helper T cell	Strong activator of macrophages, important in cell-mediated immunity

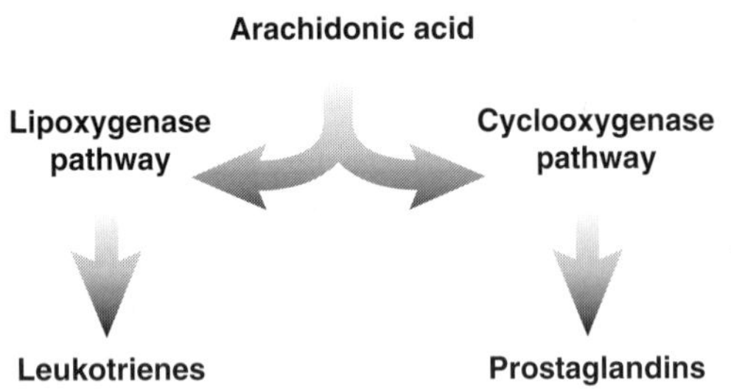

Figure 3–3. Cyclo-oxygenase and lipoxygenase pathways.

B. Main function is to generate reaction products that enhance antigen clearance and stimulate an inflammatory response. It achieves this by the following actions:
   1. Lysis of foreign body by formation of membrane attack complexes (C5–C9).
   2. Opsonization—specific complement proteins (C3b), or opsonins, bind to the surfaces of microbes or foreign particles to encourage their phagocytosis.
   3. Chemotaxis of inflammatory mediators—C5a acts to recruit inflammatory cells (i.e., neutrophils) to the site of injury/infection.
   4. Production of anaphylatoxins (C3a, C4a, and C5a)—act to stimulate mast cells in releasing mediators (histamine), resulting in increased vascular permeability (edema), vasodilation, and bronchoconstriction.

C. The complement cascade: two pathways (Figure 3-4):
   1. The alternative pathway—complement becomes activated by direct contact with the microbe or injured site. C3 binds directly to the surface antigen, activating the complement system.
   2. The classical pathway—antibodies first bind to the surface antigen present on the microbe or injured site. Complement (C1) will then bind onto the antibody, activating the complement cascade.
   3. The end product of both pathways is the same—the formation of a membrane attack complex. This complex forms directly on the surface of the microbe, "punches a hole in it," and results in cell or microbe lysis.

1.1.5 Immunoglobulins (Antibodies)

A. Antibody effector functions include:
   1. Neutralization—by binding directly to the antigen, the antibody neutralizes the antigen by preventing it from further interaction with other cells.
   2. Opsonization—when antibodies bind to an antigen, they act as opsonins to help facilitate with host phagocytosis or complement activation.
   3. Activation of the complement system.

B. Antibodies can also cause agglutination of antigens (i.e., antigens clump together). The classic example of this is blood typing, where blood type is determined by agglutination of RBCs to specific agglutins.

C. Immunoglobulin classes
   1. IgG
      a. 75% of antibodies.

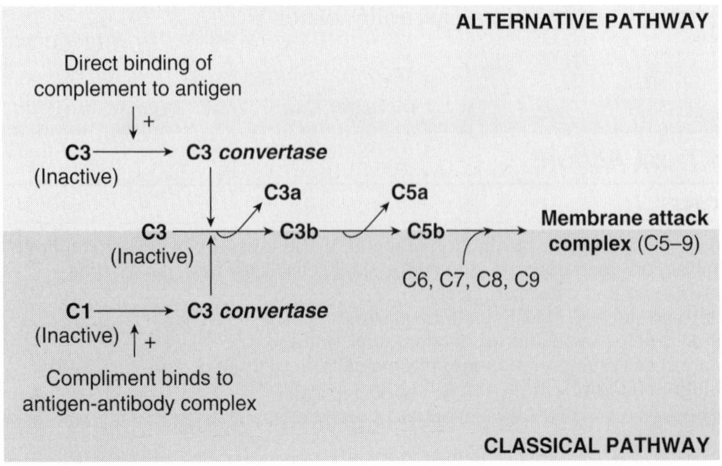

Figure 3–4. Complete cascade.

b. Associated with the secondary immune response. (Note: IgM responds first.)
c. Important for its actions against microbes.
d. Major actions:
(1) Activates complement.
(2) Acts as an opsonin to encourage phagocytosis of bacteria.
(3) The only antibody that can cross the placenta and is present in newborns.
e. IgG's ability to activate complement suggests that it likely plays a role in the pathogenesis of adult periodontitis.

2. IgA
a. 15% of antibodies.
b. Important for the immunity of mucous membranes.
c. Found in mucosal secretions of the genitourinary, intestinal, and respiratory tracts. It is also found in tears, saliva, and colostrum.
d. Major action—prevents adhesion of microbes to mucous membranes by binding surface antigens.

3. IgM
a. 9% of antibodies.
b. Associated with the body's primary immune response. It is the first antibody to arrive at the site of injury/infection.
c. Important for its actions against microbes.
d. Major actions:
(1) The most efficient Ig activator of the complement system.
(2) Acts as an antigen receptor for B cells.

4. IgD
a. 0.2% of antibodies.
b. Major actions unknown.
c. May act as an antigen receptor for B cells and induce the activation of B cells by the antigen.

5. IgE
a. 0.004% of antibodies.
b. Important in its role in type I hypersensitivity reactions.
c. Acts as antigen receptors for granulocytes, including basophils and mast cells, and stimulates their degranulation.

1.2 Hypersensitivity

Hypersensitivity reactions are characterized by exaggerated immune responses that result in injury. There are four types of hypersensitivity reactions.

A. Type I immediate hypersensitivity
1. Antibody mediator: IgE.
2. A hyperresponse of the immune system caused primarily by the production and accumulation of IgE antibody.
3. The accumulation of IgE requires prior sensitization or exposure to a specific allergen. Reexposure of the allergen causes it to bind to IgE receptors on mast cells, resulting in large releases of inflammatory mediators.
4. Two subtypes:
a. Atopic allergies
(1) Are limited to specific target tissue or organ.
(2) Family members display a strong hereditary predisposition to allergy sensitization, which may result from a genetic defect affecting the regulation of the IgE response.
(3) Important examples:
(a) Asthma
(i) Primary inflammatory mediator: SRS-A.
(ii) Symptoms include bronchoconstriction and edema in the lower respiratory tract.
(b) Hay fever (allergic reaction)
(i) Primary inflammatory mediator: histamine.
(ii) Symptoms include rhinitis, teary eyes, and respiratory congestion.
b. Anaphylaxis
(1) Primary inflammatory mediator: histamine.
(2) Allergen binding of IgE causes a very large release of histamine, which can result in anaphylactic shock, a life-threatening condition that includes severe bronchoconstriction and low blood pressure.
(3) Treatment: epinephrine (vasoconstrictor, bronchodilator), antihistamines.

B. Type II antibody-dependent cytotoxic hypersensitivity
1. Antibody mediators: IgG and IgM.
2. The binding of antibodies to cell membrane antigens activates the complement system, resulting in the formation of a membrane attack complex and cell death. Antibodies can also mediate cell destruction by antibody-dependent, cell-mediated cytotoxicity.
3. Important examples:
a. Erythroblastosis fetalis.

b. Blood transfusion reactions.

C. Type III immune-complex mediated hypersensitivity

1. Antibody mediator: IgG.
2. Antigen–antibody interactions result in the formation of immune complexes. These complexes become trapped along the vascular walls, activating complement and the immune response. Damage to the blood vessel walls occurs primarily from phagocytosis of the immune complex by the cells of the reticuloendothelial system.
3. Important examples:

a. Arthus reaction

(1) A localized type III reaction.

(2) Injection of an antigen into a patient who already has a high level of circulating antibody (IgG), usually resulting from repeated exposure, leads to formation of localized immune complexes.

(3) Symptoms include severe swelling and hemorrhaging within a few hours after exposure.

b. Serum sickness

(1) A generalized type III reaction.

(2) Systemic injection of drug serum (i.e., specific antigens) causes the formation of immune complexes throughout the microvasculature.

(3) Symptoms typically develop within days or weeks after exposure and can include fever, hives, lymphadenopathy, and arthritis.

c. Other examples of generalized type III reactions:

(1) Rheumatoid arthritis—an autoimmune disease with chronic inflammation of the joints.

(2) Systemic lupus erythematosus.

(3) Although the specific antigen is unknown, immune complexes have been found to be deposited in inflamed areas.

D. Type IV delayed (cell-mediated) hypersensitivity

1. There are no antibody mediators. Helper T cells are the main mediators in delayed hypersensitivity.
2. Antigens are presented by antigen-presenting cells to helper T cells. The activated helper T cells release cytokines to activate the immune response, including stimulating macrophages to increase their release of lytic enzymes. Note: the leakage of these enzymes may result in tissue damage.
3. Symptoms may appear days after exposure (i.e., delayed).
4. Important examples:

a. Contact dermatitis.

(1) Mediated by haptens. Haptens are small proteins that have antigenic properties They are unable to initiate an immune response by themselves, unless they can join with a larger body protein.

(2) Examples include poison ivy or oak, reactions to cosmetics, drugs (penicillin), and so forth.

b. Tuberculin (PPD) test—skin test, used to test for *M. tuberculosis* exposure.

c. Rejection of skin graft.

1.3 Immunopathology

A. Bruton's agammaglobulinemia

1. Characterized by a deficiency or very low levels of antibodies.
2. Results from a failure of B cells to differentiate, leading to a decreased concentration of plasma cells and antibody production.
3. Cell-mediated immunity is unaffected.
4. Recurrent bacteria-related (pyogenic) infections are common in these patients.
5. Treatment: administration of IgG.

B. Transient hypogammaglobulinemia

1. Seen in infants.
2. There is a decreased amount of antibodies present due to slow antibody production.
3. Treatment: administration of IgG after the first 6 months.

C. DiGeorge's syndrome

1. Characterized by a deficiency of T cells.
2. Results from a failure of the third and fourth brachial (pharyngeal) pouches to develop normally, leading to a lack of thymus and parathyroid development. Mandibular development is also affected.
3. Symptoms include:

a. Tetany—caused by hypoparathyroidism hypocalcemia.

b. Recurrent viral and fungal infections.

D. Severe combined immunodeficiency (SCID)

1. Characterized by a deficiency in both T cells and B cells.
2. Severe, recurrent, opportunistic infections are common in infants.
3. Treatment: bone marrow transplantation or gene therapy.

E. Angioedema
   1. Acquired angioedema is caused by a deficiency of the complement inhibitor, C1-INH, which inhibits the conversion of C1 to C1 esterase. Note: angioedema can also be caused by allergic reactions and may be seen in patients taking certain medications, such as angiotensin-converting enzyme (ACE) inhibitors.
   2. Symptoms include diffuse, soft tissue swellings in the face, extremities, and pelvic area.
   3. Can be life-threatening.

F. Chronic granulomatous disease
   1. Results from neutrophils with a defective NAPDH oxidase system. This affects the ability of neutrophils to kill microorganisms, since they are unable to produce superoxide radicals.
   2. Chronic bacterial infections and the formation of granulomas are common.
   3. Genetic transmission: X-linked.

G. Autoimmune diseases
   1. Systemic lupus erythematosus (SLE or lupus)
      a. Exact cause is unknown.
      b. More common in female patients.
      c. Characterized by the presence of antinuclear antibodies (ANAs). Common ANA findings include anti-DNA, anti-RNA, and anti-Sm antigen. ANAs can form immune complexes in the microvasculature of many organ systems, including:
         (1) Skin—causing characteristic butterfly rash along the malar and nose area.
         (2) Joints—causing arthritis-like symptoms.
         (3) Kidney—most significant problem because it can lead to kidney failure.
         (4) Heart—increased risk of endocarditis due to vegetations found on heart valves.
      d. Raynaud's phenomenon may be seen in patients. This describes when a patient's fingertips or toes become white and blue upon exposure to cold temperatures, due to a decrease in blood flow. Note: Raynaud's phenomenon is also seen in patients with CREST syndrome (calcinosis, Raynaud's syndrome, esophageal dysmotility, sclerodactyly, and telangiectasia) or acrosclerosis.
   2. Scleroderma (systemic sclerosis)
      a. Exact cause is unknown.
      b. Abnormal deposition of collagen leads to the development of fibrosis in certain organs, which can result in organ failure.
      c. Raynaud's phenomenon is common in these patients. Other symptoms may include dysphagia, dyspnea, and myocardial fibrosis.
      d. Oral findings include microstomia, or decreased opening of the mouth.

2.0 GENERAL MICROBIOLOGY

2.1 Biology of Micro-Organisms

2.1.1 Bacteria

A. Growth of bacteria—can be divided into four phases (Figure 3-5):
   1. Phase 1: lag phase—period when bacteria are metabolically active but are not reproducing.
   2. Phase 2: log phase—period when bacteria grow exponentially, via rapid cell division (binary fission, when a parent cell divides into two separate cells). This exponential growth results in a very rapid increase of the number of bacteria present. Note: penicillins act on this phase.
   3. Phase 3: stationary phase—occurs when the bacteria have reached a steady state (i.e., reproduction rate = death rate) due

Figure 3–5. Bacterial growth curve.

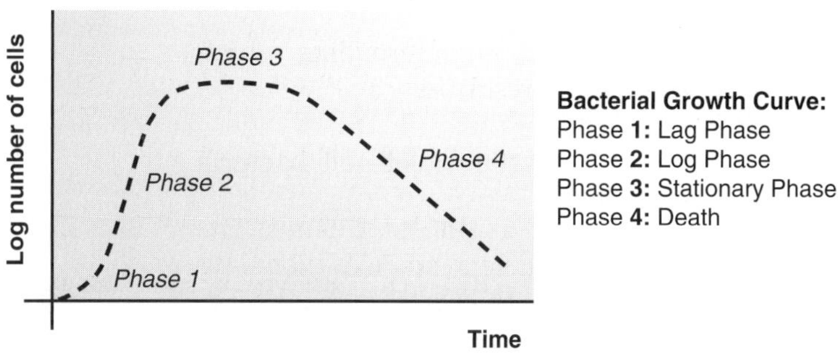

to nutrient depletion and/or toxic byproducts produced.

4. Phase 4: death—as resources decrease and toxic waste increases, bacteria begin to die.

B. Classification of bacteria

1. Classification by oxygen metabolism
   a. Oxygen metabolism in bacteria results in the formation of two toxic molecules: hydrogen peroxide (H_2O_2) and a free radical superoxide (O^-_2).
   b. Since both of these molecules are toxic, bacteria utilizing oxygen for growth require the presence of two enzymes to neutralize their effects. H_2O_2 is catalyzed by superoxide dismutase; O^-_2 is catalyzed by catalase (Figure 3-6).
2. Classification by oxygen requirement
   a. Aerobes: require oxygen for growth.
   b. Facultative anaerobes: do not require oxygen for growth but utilize it when it is present.
   c. Anaerobes: cannot grow in the presence of oxygen.
   d. Note: supragingival plaque consists of mostly aerobes and facultative anaerobes; subgingival plaque consists mostly of anaerobes.
3. Classification by shape
   a. Cocci—round, circular shape. For example:
      (1) Diplococci—occur in pairs.
      (2) Streptococci—occur in chains.
      (3) Staphylococci—occur in clusters.
   b. Bacilli—rod-shaped.
   c. Spirochetes—spiral-shaped.
   d. Pleomorphic—bacteria that appear with different, inconsistent shapes.

C. Classification by gram-staining

1. General characteristics of gram-staining:
   a. Used for identification purposes.
   b. Divides most bacteria into two groups:
      (1) Gram-positive bacteria—will stain a blue color.
      (2) Gram-negative bacteria—will stain a red color.
   c. May be useful in determining which antibiotic to prescribe.
2. Stain protocol
   a. Stain with crystal violet—all bacteria stain blue.
   b. Iodine solution—all bacteria retain blue color.
   c. Rinse with acetone or ethanol—gram-negative bacteria, with their thin walls, will lose their blue color. Gram-positive bacteria retain the blue color.
   d. Stain with safranin—gram-negative cells stain red. Gram-positive remain blue.

D. Classification by acid-fast staining

1. Used mostly for mycobacteria—which cannot be gram-stained.
2. Stain protocol
   a. Stain with carbolfuchsin—all bacteria stain red.
   b. Wash with acid alcohol.
   c. Stain with methylene blue—mycobacteria will retain the red color, while other bacteria will stain blue.

2.2 Bacterial Cell Walls and Their External Surfaces

All bacteria are surrounded by a cell wall except *Mycoplasma*. They only have a cell membrane.

A. Cell wall—a multilayered structure located external to the cytoplasmic membrane

1. Cell wall characteristics of gram-positive bacteria:
   a. A thick peptidoglycan layer.
   b. The peptidoglycan backbone consists of alternating *N*-acetylmuramic acid (NAM) and *N*-acetylglucosamine (NAG).
   c. Contains teichoic acid, which is antigenic, outside the peptidoglycan.
2. Cell wall characteristics of gram-negative bacteria:
   a. A thin peptidoglycan layer.
   b. In the space between the outer and cytoplasmic membranes, certain species contain enzymes called *β-lactamases,* which degrade penicillins and other β-lactam drugs.
   c. Lipopolysaccharide (LPS or endotoxin).
      (1) Found in the outer membrane.
      (2) Causes an immune response by activating macrophages, B cells, and complement.
      (3) The toxicity of LPS is attributed to presence of lipid A.

Superoxide radical: $2O^-_2 + 2H^+ \rightarrow H_2O_2 + O_2$ catalyzed by superoxide dismutase

Hydrogen peroxide: $2H_2O_2 \rightarrow 2H_2O + O_2$ catalyzed by catalase

Figure 3–6. Equations for the neutralization of H_2O_2 and O^-_2 in bacteria by superoxide dismutase and catalase.

(4) O antigen—the outer membrane of the LPS. Often used for identification purposes.
(5) Found in dental plaque and gingival inflammation.

3. Cell wall characteristics of acid-fast bacteria:
   a. An unusual cell wall with a high concentration of mycolic acid, which results in its ability to resist decolorization with acid-alcohol (i.e., such cells are acid-fast); thus, they cannot be gram-stained.
   b. Characteristic of mycobacteria (e.g., *Mycobacterium tuberculosis*)

B. Specialized structures outside the cell wall
1. Capsule
   a. A gelatinous layer that surrounds the cell walls of certain bacteria. Generally made of polysaccharides, although the composition varies depending on species.
   b. Functions
      (1) Are antiphagocytic—prevent phagocytosis by macrophages.
      (2) For identification purposes—quelling reaction: when the polysaccharide capsules are treated with antiserum, they swell, allowing them to be identified.
      (3) May play a role in the adherence of the bacteria to certain tissues (i.e., caries on the tooth surface).
2. Spores
   a. Spores allow certain bacteria to survive through unfavorable environmental conditions.
   b. They have a thick, outer layer, and it has been suggested that their resistance may be related to dipicolinic acid, a calcium chelator.
   c. Spore-forming bacteria include those from the genus *Bacillus* and *Clostridium*.
3. Flagella—a long, whiplike appendage that promotes mobility of bacteria.
4. Pilli (fimbriae)—hairlike filaments that mediate attachment of bacteria.

2.2.1 Viruses

A. General characteristics
1. Basic structure: nucleocapsid—consists of a capsid, or protein coat, and the viral genome, or its nucleic acid (DNA or RNA).
2. Some viruses also acquire an outer envelope from the infected host cell. Enveloped viruses are normally more sensitive to environmental conditions than are nonenveloped viruses.
3. Viruses are obligate intracellular parasites and require other organisms for metabolism and reproduction.

B. Replication or growth cycle—seven stages:
1. Attachment—the virus binds to the host cell via specific surface proteins.
2. Penetration—the virus enters the host cell by receptor-mediated endocytosis, translocation of the entire virus across the plasma membrane, or by fusing its viral envelope with the host membrane.
3. Uncoating of the viral genome—the viral nucleic acid separates from its outer protein coat.
4. Early viral protein synthesis—the virus may use its own enzymes or host enzymes to first produce proteins needed for viral genome replication.
5. Late viral protein synthesis—structural proteins for the capsid are produced.
6. Assembly of virion—the newly synthesized viral genomes and capsid proteins are assembled.
7. Release—progeny virions may be released from the host cell by:
   a. Host cell lysis—newly formed viruses are released via lysis of the host cell, leading to host cell death. Note: in cultured cells, the lysis of host cells following viral infections leaves patterns of cytopathic effects (CPUs). CPUs may be used for identification purposes.
   b. Budding—viruses obtain their outer envelope from the plasma membrane of the host cell. The host membrane contains surface proteins (antigens) or spikes, which the budding virion also acquires onto its outer envelope (Figure 3-7).

C. Detection of viral growth (Figure 3-8)
1. Eclipse period—the period of time when the virus is actively replicating within the host cell. No progeny virions are assembled.
2. Latent period—time between the initial viral infection to when the virus can be detected.

D. Viral–bacterial interactions
1. Bacteriophages—viruses that infect bacteria.

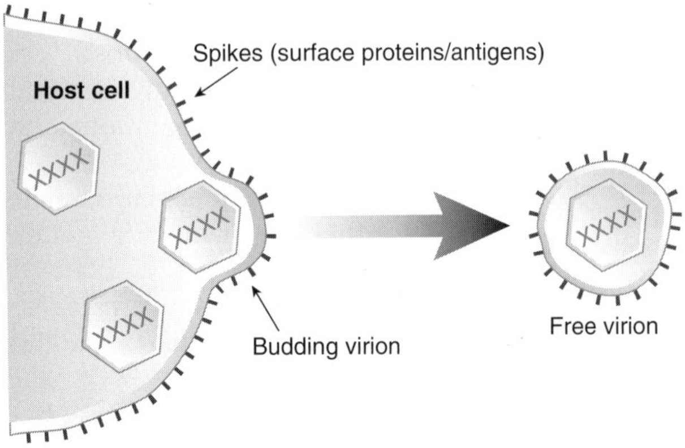

Figure 3–7. Viral budding.

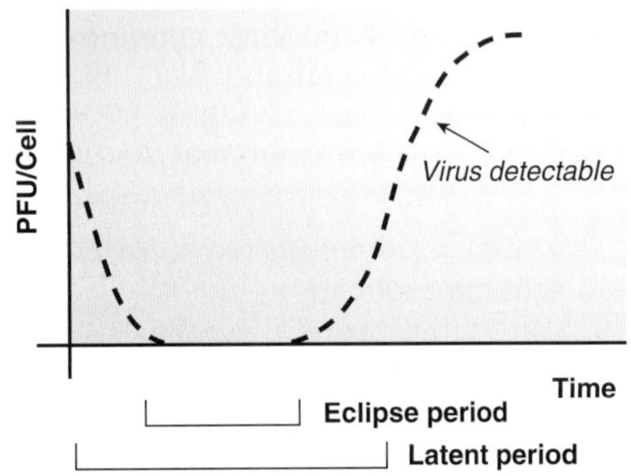

Figure 3–8. Viral growth curve. PFU, Plaque-forming units.

a. Virulent phage—the release of new bacteriophages results in lyses of the host bacteria.
b. Temperate phage—after infection, the host bacteria is not lysed.

2. Lysogeny—a bacteriophage-infected bacteria that retains its normal functioning. New characteristics developed in the lysogenic bacteria, as a result of the infection, are called *lysogenic conversions*.

2.2.2 Fungi

A. General characteristics
1. Fungi are eukaryotic cells.
2. Many fungi are thermally dimorphic (i.e., they can exist as two distinct forms: molds or yeasts). Molds grow as long filaments in a free-living state at ambient temperatures. Yeasts grow as single cells in host tissues at body temperature.
3. Spores—some fungi are spore-producing. This form allows them to survive extreme environmental conditions. It may also play a role in the transmission of fungal infections.
4. Medically significant spores
   a. Blastospores—formed by budding.
   b. Chlamydospores—have thick walls, making them more resistant to environmental changes.
   c. Arthrospores—formed from the ends of hyphae.
   d. Sporangiospores—formed by molds.

B. Immune response
1. Fungal infections generally initiate a type IV delayed hypersensitivity reaction.
2. Formation of granulomas in response to a fungal infection is common.

2.3 Antimicrobials

2.3.1 Antibiotics

A. Inhibitors of bacterial cell wall synthesis
1. Penicillins
   a. Bactericidal.
   b. Action: inhibits transpeptidase, the enzyme that catalyzes the final crosslinking step in synthesis of peptidoglycan, a component of the bacterial cell wall.
   c. Adverse reactions to penicillin include hypersensitivity (allergic) reactions (anaphylaxis, skin rashes), seizures, and platelet dysfunction.
   d. Types of penicillins:
      (1) Natural penicillins
         (a) Effective against gram-positive bacteria and gram-negative cocci. Limited effect against gram-negative bacilli bacteria.
         (b) Are susceptible to β-lactamases.
         (c) Include penicillin G and penicillin V.
      (2) Extended-spectrum penicillins
         (a) More effective against gram-negative bacilli, as compared to natural penicillins.
         (b) Are susceptible to β-lactamases.
         (c) Include amoxicillin and ampicillin.
      (3) Penicillinase-resistant penicillins (antistaphylococcal penicillins)
         (a) Resistant to degradation by β-lactamases.
         (b) Used for treatment of certain strains of *Staphylococcus aureus* that produce penicillinase.
         (c) Include cloxacillin, dicloxacillin, methicillin, nafcillin, and oxacillin.

2. Cephalosporins
   a. Bactericidal.
   b. Broad-spectrum antibiotics.
   c. There are four generations of cephalosporins, with expanded coverage with increasing generation.
   d. Action: similar to penicillins, but they are more resistant to β-lactamases than are penicillins.
   e. Adverse reactions include a disulfiram-like reaction with some cephalosporins when alcohol is consumed.
   f. Although cephalosporins are structurally similar to penicillin, patients who are allergic to penicillin have a 10% chance of being hypersensitive to cephalosporins.
   g. Include cephalexin, cefadroxil, and cefazolin.
3. Other inhibitors of cell wall synthesis
   a. Bacitracin
      (1) For topical use only.
      (2) Is highly nephrotoxic if given systemically.
   b. Vancomycin
      (1) Is produced by *Streptococcus orientalis*.
      (2) Effective against gram-positive bacteria.
      (3) Has a limited effect against gram-negative bacteria (*Flavobacterium* is the exception).
      (4) Used for multidrug-resistant bacteria (e.g., methicillin-resistant *Staphylococcus aureus*) or treatment of endocarditis.

B. Inhibitors of protein synthesis
1. Aminoglycosides
   a. Bactericidal.
   b. Mechanism of action: blocks 30S ribosomal subunit to inhibit protein synthesis.
   c. They are effective against aerobic bacteria but are ineffective against anaerobic bacteria because they require oxygen for transport into bacteria. They are also useful against many gram-negative rods, tuberculosis (streptomycin), and enterococci (gentamicin).
   d. Are administered by IV or intramuscular injection.
   e. Adverse reactions include:
      (1) Ototoxicity (via damage to CN VIII), which may result in deafness.
      (2) Nephrotoxicity, which may result in permanent kidney damage.
   f. Include streptomycin, gentamicin, and tobramycin.
2. Tetracycline
   a. Bacteriostatic.
   b. Action: blocks 30S ribosomal subunit to inhibit protein synthesis.
   c. Broad-spectrum antibiotic that targets gram-positive and gram-negative bacteria and other micro-organisms, such as *Rickettsiae*, mycoplasma, and *Chlamydiae*.
   d. Adverse reactions include:
      (1) Hepatotoxicity, which may result in severe damage to the liver, especially in pregnant women.
      (2) Tooth discoloration in developing teeth. It should be avoided in pregnant women or young children.
3. Macrolides
   a. Bacteriostatic.
   b. Action: blocks 50S ribosomal subunit to inhibit synthesis of proteins.
   c. Effective in treating mostly gram-positive bacterial infections.
   d. Adverse reactions include ototoxicity and GI problems.
   e. Includes erythromycin and clarithromycin.
4. Clindamycin
   a. Bacteriostatic; can be bacteriocidal at higher concentrations.
   b. A semisynthetic derivative of lincomycin.
   c. Action: blocks 50S ribosomal subunit to inhibit synthesis of proteins.
   d. Effective in treating anaerobic gram-positive or gram-negative bacteria, including *Bacterioides fragilis* and *Fusobacterium*.
   e. Adverse reaction: pseudomembranous colitis, which is caused by the overgrowth of *Clostridium difficile* in the gut.
5. Chloramphenicol
   a. A broad-spectrum antibiotic that is effective against gram-positive and gram-negative, aerobic, and anaerobic bacteria.
   b. Used as a last resort due to its toxicity and its possible severe adverse reactions.
   c. Adverse reactions include reversible anemia, aplastic anemia, and gray baby syndrome, which can lead to death.

C. Inhibitors of folate synthesis
  1. Both humans and bacteria require folate for the synthesis of DNA precursors. Unlike bacteria, humans are unable to synthesize their own folic acid; they rely on exogenous folate, via diet or vitamins, to fulfill their requirement for folate. Since bacteria are able to produce their own folic acid; therefore, sulfa drugs have a selective effect on them.
  2. Sulfonamides (sulfa drugs)
    a. Bacteriostatic.
    b. Action: are synthetic analogs of para-aminobenzoic acid (PABA). Sulfonamides competitively inhibit and block the metabolic pathway of folic acid synthesis in bacteria.
    c. Adverse reactions include hemolytic anemia in patients with glucose 6-phosphate dehydrogenase deficiency.

D. Inhibitors of DNA replication
  1. Quinolones
    a. Bactericidal.
    b. Action: inhibit DNA gyrase (topoisomerase).
    c. Include ciprofloxacin.

2.3.2 Chlorhexidine

1. Broad antimicrobial spectrum.
2. The only FDA-approved mouthwash that has been shown to decrease supragingival plaque and gingival inflammation associated with gingivitis.
3. Actions:
  a. Chlorhexidine will bind to oral tissues (tooth, mucosa), salivary pellicle, and bacteria, resulting in a persistent, cumulative, antimicrobial effect.
  b. After rinsing, some of the chlorhexidine will remain in the mouth. It is gradually released over time.

2.4 Sterilization and Disinfection

A. Sterilization
  1. The removal of all micro-organisms, including spores, from a substance.
  2. A summary of sterilization techniques is listed in Table 3-3.

B. Disinfection
  1. Eliminates most micro-organisms but does not include the removal of bacterial spores and some viruses and fungi.
  2. Example: sodium hypochlorite—a surface disinfectant
    a. Mechanism of action: oxidative destruction of cells.
    b. Advantages: it is a broad-spectrum agent and is inexpensive. It is commonly used as an intracanal irrigant during root canal therapy.
    c. Disadvantages: it is toxic to tissues.

C. Antiseptics
  1. A disinfectant that can be applied to skin.
  2. Antiseptic agents are summarized in Table 3-4.

TABLE 3–3. SUMMARY OF STERILIZATION TECHNIQUES

	MECHANISM OF ACTION	TEMPERATURE OR TIME REQUIRED	ADVANTAGES	DISADVANTAGES
Dry heat	Coagulation of proteins	160° C for 2 hrs	Noncorrosive to metal	Longer time than moist heat
		171 °C for 1 hr	Simple method	Can damage heat-sensitive items
Moist heat (autoclave)	Denatures proteins	Wrapped instruments: 121 °C (250 °F)/15 psi for 15 minutes	Short time	Can damage heat-sensitive items
		Unwrapped (flash cycle) instruments: 134 °C (270 °F)/30 psi for 3 minutes	Very effective and dependable	
Ethylene oxide gas	An alkylating agent that denatures nucleic acids (DNA) and proteins	1–12 hrs	Good for heat-sensitive or moisture-sensitive items	Very toxic Flammable Long time
2% glutaraldehyde	An alkylating agent that denatures nucleic acids (DNA) and proteins	12 hrs	Good for heat-sensitive or moisture-sensitive items Noncorrosive to metals	Very toxic Long time Expensive

TABLE 3–4. SUMMARY OF ANTISEPTICS AND THEIR ACTIONS

	MECHANISM OF ACTION	ADVANTAGES	DISADVANTAGES
2% tincture of iodine	Disruption of cell membranes	Most effective antiseptic	—
Alcohol (70% ethanol)	Dissolution of lipids in cell membranes Denatures proteins	Low toxicity Effective against most vegetative bacteria, fungi, and viruses Noncorrosive to metals	Limited contact time due to quick evaporation Decreased action against microbes in dried blood or saliva
Quaternary ammonium compounds	Cationic detergents that disrupt cell membranes		Are inactivated by anionic detergents Limited antiseptic effect
Formaldehyde	Denatures/precipitates proteins		Toxic
Soaps, detergents	Anionic compounds that physically remove microbes	Generally low toxicity	Limited antiseptic effect

3.0 MICROBIOLOGY AND PATHOLOGY OF SPECIFIC INFECTIOUS DISEASES

3.1 Bacterial

3.1.1 Cocci-Shaped, Gram-Positive Bacteria

A. *Streptococcus* species
   1. General characteristics
      a. Cocci-shaped; observed in lines.
      b. Gram-positive.
      c. Facultative anaerobes.
      d. Hemolytic classification:
         (1) α-hemolytic—incomplete lysis of red blood cells.
            (a) Appears in the green zone.
            (b) α-hemolytic bacteria include *S. viridans*, *S. mutans*, *S. sanguis and S. salivarius.*
            (c) These bacteria, such as *S. viridans,* are the most common organisms causing subacute endocarditis.
         (2) β-hemolytic—complete lysis of red blood cells.
            (a) Appear in the clear zone.
            (b) β-hemolytic *Streptococcus* are further divided into Lancefield groups A through U.
            (c) β-hemolytic bacteria include group A (*S. pyogenes*) bacteria.
         (3) γ-hemolytic—nonlysis of red blood cells.

B. *Streptococcus pyogenes*
   1. Hemolytic class: β.
   2. Virulent factors:
      a. M protein—an important virulent factor.
      b. DNAse—cleaves DNA.
      c. Erythrogenic toxin—causes scarlet fever rash.
      d. Streptolysin O/S (hemolysin)—causes lysis of red and white blood cells.
      e. Streptokinase (fibrinolysin)—dissolves fibrin in blood clots by cleaving plasminogen to increase levels of plasmin.
      f. Hyaluronidase—spreading factor that breaks down hyaluronic acid, increasing the bacterium's ability to spread.
      g. Exotoxin A—causes necrotizing fascitis by rapidly destroying tissue.
   3. Diseases include pharyngitis (i.e., strep throat), rheumatic fever following a strep infection, scarlet fever, impetigo, glomerulonephritis following a strep infection, toxic shock syndrome, and necrotizing fascitis.

C. *Streptococcus viridans*
   1. Hemolytic class: α.
   2. Diseases: endocarditis, caries.

D. *Streptococcus pneumoniae*
   1. Hemolytic class: α.
   2. Virulent factors:
      a. Polysaccharide capsule—prevents phagocytosis.
      b. Pneumolysin—a cytolytic toxin.
      c. IgA protease—hydrolyzes IgA to aid in its ability to colonize along the respiratory mucosa.
   3. Diseases:
      a. Pneumonia—the most common cause of bacterial pneumonia.
      b. Meningitis.
      c. Otitis media—the most common cause of otitis media in infants older than 2 months.

4. Dental significance:
   a. Streptococci are the most common bacteria in the mouth.
   b. They are cariogenic bacteria for several reasons, including:
      (1) They lower the pH to promote the demineralization of enamel, which begins between pH 1 and 5, by producing lactic acid.
      (2) They provide a structural component for plaque by producing dextrans. The streptococci surface contains glycosyl transferase. This enzyme cleaves glucose and fructose from sucrose to form dextrans and fructans, respectively (Figure 3-9).
   c. They provide food for bacteria growth by their production of fructans (levans) from fructose.
   d. They contribute to the adhesion of bacteria to the tooth surface by the production of fructans.
   e. *S. mutans* is the most cariogenic. It contains a polysaccharide glycocalyx coating that allows it to stick firmly to surfaces.
   f. *S. sanguis* is the most common *Streptococcus* isolated from the mouth.
   g. Streptococci are commonly present in Ludwig's angina.

E. *Staphylococcus aureus*
   1. General characteristics
      a. Cocci-shaped; arranged in grape-like clusters.
      b. Gram-positive.
      c. Part of normal skin, mucous membranes flora.
      d. Causes suppurative or pus-forming (pyogenic) infections, mostly in the form of abscesses.

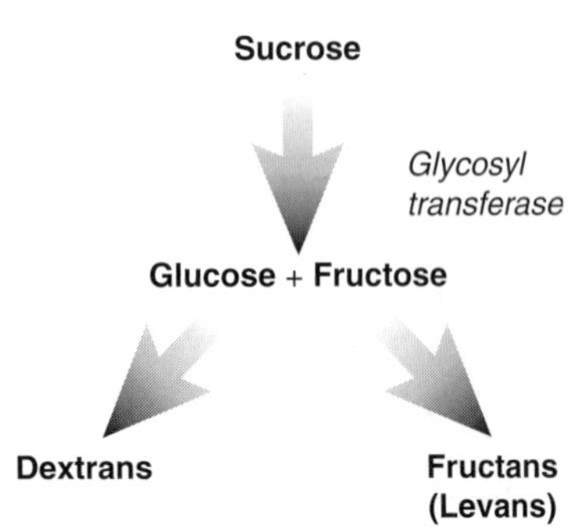

Figure 3–9. The breakdown of sucrose by *Streptococci's* glycosyl transferase.

   2. Virulent factors:
      a. Protein A—found in its cell wall. It inhibits complement fixation by binding to the Fc portion of IgG, resulting in decreased phagocytosis and opsonization. It can also elicit a hypersensitivity reaction and damage platelets.
      b. Coagulase—clots blood (*S. aureus*).
      c. Staphylokinase (fibrinolysin)—dissolves blood clots by cleaving plasminogen to increase levels of plasmin.
      d. Hyaluronidase—spreading factor that breaks down hyaluronic acid, increasing its ability to spread.
      e. β–lactamases (penicillinase, β-hemolysin,)—inactivate penicillin by degrading β-lactam ring. Note: some modified penicillins (penicillinase-resistant penicillins) are resistant to β–lactamases and are therefore more effective in treating penicillinase-producing staphylococci (e.g., Augmentin).
      f. Toxins—all are exoproteins that can behave as superantigens.
         (1) Enterotoxin—causes food poisoning (vomiting, diarrhea).
         (2) Exfoliatin—causes "scalded skin" syndrome, an exfoliative dermatitis in children.
         (3) Toxic shock syndrome toxin.
            (a) Diseases include food poisoning, endocarditis, and impetigo.
            (b) It is often related with death following viral respiratory infections, such as influenza.

3.1.2 Rod-Shaped, Gram-Positive Bacteria

A. *Corynebacterium diphtheriae*
   1. General characteristics
      a. Contains granules that stain metachromatically. Note: in the laboratory, methylene blue stain is used to reveal metachromic granules in bacteria; it stains the cell blue and the granules red.
      b. Consists of a fibrin pseudomembrane.
   2. Virulent factors:
      a. Only bacteria that have been infected with a bacteriophage carrying the DNA that codes for the diphtheria toxin, are pathogenic.
      b. The diphtheria toxin acts to block elongation factor-2 during translation, inhibiting protein synthesis.

3. Vaccine: toxoid that is part of the DPT vaccine.

B. *Lactobacillus* species
1. General characteristics
   a. Produce lactic acid.
   b. Part of normal gut, mouth, and vaginal flora.
      (1) It is the main source of lactic acid in the vagina and responsible for keeping its pH low.
      (2) *L. casei* has been found in deep dental caries.

3.1.3 Spore-Forming, Gram-Positive Bacteria

A. *Bacillus anthracis*
1. General characteristics
   a. Rod-shaped.
   b. Aerobic.
2. Virulent factors:
   a. Spores—which allow it to survive in the soil for years. Humans can be infected by spores on animal products. The portals of entry include the skin, mucous membranes, and the respiratory tract.
   b. Exotoxin with three characteristics: edema factor, protective antigen, and lethal factor.
   c. Its aerosol transmission and ability to produce a lethal exotoxin unfortunately make it a choice for bioterrorism.
3. Disease: anthrax
   a. Two types:
      (1) Cutaneous anthrax—10% fatal. Clinically observed as a skin lesion or pustule with a dark (eschar) scab. Inflammation will be present around the lesion.
      (2) Pulmonary anthrax (wool-sorter's disease)—50% fatal. Quick onset of fever, muscle pain, respiratory distress, and hemorrhaging lymph nodes leading to necrosis and cyanosis.
   b. Vaccine: purified protective antigen.

B. *Clostridium* species (*C. tetani, C. botulinum, C. perfringens, C. difficile*)
1. General characteristics
   a. Rod-shaped.
   b. Anaerobic.
2. Virulent factors:
   a. Produce some of the most potent exotoxins that have been identified.
   b. Hyaluronidase—an enzyme that breaks down hyaluronic acid, increasing its ability to spread.
3. *C. tetani*
   a. Spores are commonly found in soil.
   b. Exotoxin: tetanus toxin (tetanospasmin)—a neurotoxin that inhibits the transmission of glycine from motor neurons in the CNS.
   c. Disease: tetanus (lockjaw)
      (1) Tetanus toxins usually enter the body through an open wound.
      (2) Symptoms include painful muscle contractions, trismus, and the spasm of facial muscles. These symptoms continue until death occurs by exhaustion or respiratory failure.
   d. Treatment: antitoxins are given to bind unbound toxins, an example of passive-active immunity. Antibiotics (penicillin G) should also be administered as well as surgical debridement of the infected site.
   e. Vaccine: consists of tetanus toxoid and should be given about every 10 years. It is part of the DPT vaccine. It can also be administered post-infection.
4. *C. botulinum*
   a. Spores are commonly found in canned foods that have been improperly sterilized or in undercooked foods.
   b. Exotoxin: botulinum toxin
      (1) A neurotoxin that inhibits the transmission of acetylcholine (Ach) in peripheral nerves, leading to loss of motor function.
      (2) The most potent toxin known.
   c. Disease: botulism
      (1) Symptoms include muscle weakness and paralysis, cranial nerve impairment, diplopia, dysphagia and speech impairment, respiratory failure, and death.
   d. Treatment: trivalent antitoxins are given, along with respiratory support. These antitoxins are immunoglobulins that act to neutralize the toxins.
   e. Infant botulism—occurs when an infant becomes infected after ingesting spores. Recovery occurs without intervention.
5. *C. perfringens*
   a. Spores are commonly found in soil.
   b. Live bacteria are part of the normal gut and vaginal flora.

c. Exotoxin: α–toxin or lecithinase. This toxin destroys cell membranes by causing cell lysis.
d. Contains collagenase.
e. Disease: gas gangrene (myonecrosis).
(1) Occurs around an improperly treated wound.
(2) Gas is produced around the infected site by degradative enzymes released after cell lysis. Clinically, pain, swelling, and cellulitis may be observed. Shock and death may ensue from large amounts of tissue destruction.
f. Treatment: antibiotics (penicillin) should be administered, as well as surgical debridement and removal of the infected tissues.

C. *Actinomycetes* species
1. General characteristics
a. Gram-positive. Some species may contain mycolic acids in their cell walls, allowing them to stain acid-fast.
b. Anaerobic.
c. Part of normal gut and mouth flora.
d. Contain sulfur granules, which can be observed as yellow specks in purulent exudates.
e. Have branch-like projections that make their appearance similar to fungi.
2. Diseases
a. Root surface caries.
b. Actinomycosis—an endogenous, suppurative infection caused by *A. israelii*. It commonly occurs in the cervicofacial area ("lumpy jaw") and can spread to form abscesses or sinus tracts after minor trauma or dental work.

3.1.4 Gram-Negative Bacteria

Enteric gram-negative bacteria are a family of gram-negative, rod-shaped bacteria that are residents of the enteric tract.

A. General characteristics
1. Gram-negative.
2. Rod-shaped.
3. Facultative anaerobes.
4. May be part of normal gut flora.
5. Exchange of genetic material is common, causing the formation of new strains.
6. Produce exotoxins, known as *enterotoxins*.
7. Surface antigens are used to aid in the identification of strains. These include K antigen (capsular antigen), O antigen (somatic antigen), and H antigen (flagella antigen).
a. *Escherichia coli*
(1) Surface traits: O antigen, H antigen, flagella, and pili.
(2) Virulent factors:
(a) Capsule—aids in the evasion of host phagocytosis.
(b) Pili—aids in the attachment of *E. coli* to the intestinal surface.
(c) Enterotoxin—which it releases after attachment, clinically causing diarrhea.
(3) The most common cause of cystitis and "traveler's diarrhea."
b. *Pseudomonas aeruginosa*
(1) Surface traits: flagella, pili, slime layer.
(a) Virulent factors:
(i) Produce fluorescent pigments contained in metachromatic granules. Wounds infected with *P. aeruginosa* therefore display a bluish-green color.
(b) Are able to survive in inhospitable environments, which makes it difficult to eliminate them from hospitals and clinics.
(2) Infections are a problem for immunocompromised patients. Common infections include wound infections (especially in burn patients), urinary tract infections, pneumonia in cystic fibrosis patients, and septicemia.
c. *Proteus*
(1) Surface trait: O antigen.
(2) Virulent factors:
(a) Very motile.
(b) Produces urease, which hydrolyzes urea to ammonia.
(3) Disease: cystitis.
d. *Salmonella*
(1) Surface traits: cell wall O antigen, flagella, H antigen, and capsular Vi.
(2) Diseases: enterocolitis, septicemia, and enteric/typhoid fevers. Note: enterocolitis infections should not be treated with antibiotics. This

could prolong the patient's symptoms. Usually, the diseases are self-limiting.

e. *Shigella*
   (1) Surface trait: O antigen.
   (2) Virulent factor: some strains produce neurotoxins.
   (3) Disease: enterocolitis or bacterial dysentery.

f. *Vibrio cholerae*
   (1) Surface traits: O antigen, pili.
   (2) Virulent factors:
      (a) Pili—aids in its ability to attach to the intestinal surface.
      (b) Releases an enterotoxin, known as *choleragen*. Clinically, choleragen causes diarrhea.
   (3) Disease: cholera or diarrhea.

g. *Helicobacter pylori*
   (1) Surface trait: flagella.
   (2) Virulent factors:
      (a) Is unique in its ability to thrive in the gastric mucosa overlying gastric mucous cells in the stomach.
      (b) Produces urease, which converts urea to ammonia and carbon dioxide. The ammonia produced neutralizes acid in the stomach, increasing the gastric pH.
      (c) Has been detected in dental plaque and saliva.
   (3) Disease: chronic gastritis and peptic ulcers. There is an increased risk for developing some stomach cancers, including adenocarcinoma and non-Hodgkin's lymphoma.

h. *Bacteroides*
   (1) Bacterial colonies display black pigmentation.
   (2) Diseases:
      (a) Periodontal disease, including pregnancy gingivitis.
      (b) Endogenous infections through mucosal openings.
      (c) The most common organism found in severe anaerobic infections.
   (3) *Bacteroids* with dental significance include *B. melaninogenicus, B. corrodens,* and *B. forsythus*.

3.1.4.1 Other Gram-Negative Bacteria

A. *Haemophilus influenzae*
   1. Rod-shaped.
   2. Encapsulated.
   3. Virulent features:
      a. LPS (endotoxin), IgA protease, capsule.
   4. Disease:
      a. Meningitis—leading cause in children.

B. *Bordetella pertussis*
   1. Rod-shaped.
   2. Virulent features:
      a. Pertussis toxin, hemagglutinin, pili, capsule.
   3. Transmission—airborne droplets. The bacteria colonize on the cilia of epithelial cells, causing decreased cilia activity and cell death.
   4. Disease:
      a. Whooping cough (pertussis).
   5. Vaccine:
      a. Killed bacteria or purified proteins (part of the DPT vaccine).

C. *Porphyromonas gingivalis*
   1. Rod-shaped.
   2. Anaerobic.
   3. Colonies display black pigmentation.
   4. Associated with periodontal disease and dental abscesses.

D. *Neisseria meningitidis*
   1. Cocci-shaped.
      a. Virulent features:
         (1) LPS (endotoxin), IgA protease, capsule.
      b. Transmission:
         (1) Bacteria in the infected air droplets colonize on the mucosal membranes of the nasopharynx and then enter the bloodstream to specific sites (e.g., meninges, joints).
      c. Disease:
         (1) Meningitis. It is the leading cause of meningitis in people aged 6 to 60.

E. *Neisseria gonorrhoreae*
   1. Cocci-shaped.
   2. Virulent factors:
      a. LPS (endotoxin).
         (1) IgA protease—hydrolyzes IgA, which would otherwise block its attachment to the mucosal surface.
      b. Pili—an important feature because it is antiphagocytic and mediates its attachment to the mucosal epithelium.

3. Disease: gonorrhea
   a. The second most common sexually transmitted disease (STD) in the United States. (The most common STD in the United States is chlamydia.)
   b. Although it is commonly asymptomatic, symptoms include urethritis and genital infections.
   c. Consequences include pelvic inflammatory disease and sterility.
   d. Transmission of disease to infants can occur within the birth canal, causing severe ophthalmia that can lead to blindness.

3.1.4.2 Role of Gram-Negative Bacteria in Periodontal Disease

A. Etiology of periodontal disease: bacterial plaque
   1. Consists of 95% bacteria.
   2. Bacterial types in supragingival plaque will differ depending on diet and saliva composition. Diet and saliva do not affect the makeup of bacteria in subgingival plaque. Subgingival plaque consists mostly of rod-shaped, gram-negative anaerobic bacteria and spirochetes.

B. Plaque and calculus formation—three phases:
   1. Formation of a salivary pellicle—salivary glycoproteins coat the tooth surface, forming a pellicle. This allows plaque to stick to enamel (i.e., bacteria are able to colonize on the pellicle). Plaque usually develops within 24 hours.
   2. Plaque maturation—an organized bacteria colonization of the pellicle in the following order: gram-positive, cocci bacteria (mostly *Streptococci*) will colonize the pellicle first. Dextrans produced from these bacteria form the structural component of plaque. These bacteria are followed by gram-negative, rod-shaped anaerobic bacteria, such as *Bacteroides, Fusobacterium, Porphyromonas,* and *Prevotella*, and finally by filament-type bacteria such as *Actinomyces*.
   3. Plaque mineralization (calculus formation)—mineralization of plaque occurs when it becomes supersaturated with calcium and phosphates from saliva. It then mineralizes to form calculus.

3.1.5 Acid-fast Bacteria

A. Mycobacteria species
   1. General characteristics
      a. Rod-shaped.
      b. Aerobic.
      c. Cannot be gram-stained due to their waxy cell walls, which contain mycolic acids. Must use acid-fast staining for diagnosis.
   2. *Mycobacterium tuberculosis*
      a. Infects reticuloendothelial cells, including macrophages. Since oxygen is required for metabolism, the infection usually occurs in oxygen-rich areas, such as the lungs and kidney.
      b. Cord factor, a surface glycolipid, contributes to its pathogenicity.
      c. Disease: tuberculosis
         (1) There is a higher prevalence of this disease in lower socioeconomic and immunocompromised individuals.
         (2) Disease states:
            (a) Primary tuberculosis—asymptomatic. A fibrous nodule may result at the site of infection. Less than 5% of those infected progress to the active disease state.
            (b) Secondary tuberculosis—reactivation of disease, often due to compromised immunity.
            (c) Miliary tuberculosis—when infection disseminates through the vascular system.
         (3) Important characteristics:
            (a) The host responds to contain the infection by forming granulomas, known as *tubercles,* often with the presence of central caseous necrosis and multinucleated giant cells.
            (b) Ghon complex—the calcified scar that remains following the primary infection; it usually includes the primary lung lesion and its regional lymph node.
         (4) Purified protein derivative (PPD) skin test:
            (a) Tests for a delayed hypersensitivity reaction to certain *M. tuberculosis* proteins.
            (b) A positive result signifies active disease or a previous infection. Further tests, such

as chest radiograph and lab cultures, are needed to make a diagnosis.

(5) Treatment: isoniazid, rifampin, pyrazinamide, and ethambutol are among the choices (in combination).

3. *Mycobacterium leprae*—causes leprosy (Hansen's disease).

B. Spirochetes

1. *Treponema pallidum*

a. Disease: syphilis

(1) A sexually transmitted disease that occurs in three stages:

(a) Primary syphilis—an asymptomatic, firm ulcer, known as a *chancre,* forms at the site of the initial infection. The chancre will resolve on its own. Oral lesions may be present. They are most commonly seen on the lips, although they may also be present intraorally.

(b) Secondary syphilis—after a few months, the infection spreads, and signs of a systemic illness, such as fever, malaise, headache, musculoskeletal pain, and lymphadenopathy are observed. Common signs include a diffuse maculopapular rash (notably on the palms and soles), papules on the skin or mucus membranes, and genital lesions (condylomata lata). These lesions are very infectious and will resolve on their own.

(c) Tertiary syphilis—about a third of those infected who were never treated will progress to this stage. Symptoms include the formation of granulomas (known as *gummas*), cardiovascular damage leading to heart failure or an atherosclerotic aneurysm of the ascending aorta, and CNS impairment.

(2) Treatment: antibiotic therapy (penicillin G).

b. Congenital syphilis

(1) Transmission of the disease to infants can occur within the birth canal. This can lead to severe infection, birth defects, or death.

(2) Important signs and symptoms:

(a) Hutchinson's incisors of the anterior teeth and Mulberry molars of the posterior teeth.

(b) Deafness and blindness from interstitial keratitis may also occur.

3.1.6 Chlamydial and Rickettsial Organisms

A. *Chlamydiae* bacteria

1. General characteristics

a. Although they are considered bacteria, they are obligate intracellular parasites (i.e., they rely on a host cell to grow and reproduce).

b. Unique cell cycle—begins when the extracellular, spore-like elementary body enters the cell and transforms into a larger, metabolically active reticulate body. It then undergoes repeated binary fission to form daughter elementary bodies, which are then released.

2. *Chlamydia trachomatis*

a. Predominately invades mucous epithelial cells.

b. Diseases: trachoma, genital infections, inclusion conjunctivitis.

c. The most common sexually transmitted disease in the United States.

d. Although it is commonly asymptomatic, symptoms include nongonococcal urethritis, genital or respiratory infections, and conjunctivitis.

e. Consequences include pelvic inflammatory disease, sterility, and salpingitis.

f. Transmission of disease to infants can occur within the birth canal, causing inclusion conjunctivitis and/or pneumonia.

g. Treatment: antibiotic therapy. Sulfonamides, macrolides (azithromycin), and tetracycline are among the choices.

B. Rickettsiae bacteria

1. General characteristics

a. Rod-shaped.

b. Gram-negative but are difficult to stain.

c. They are obligate, intracellular bacteria and thus cannot be cultured on laboratory media.

d. Disease transmission usually occurs via arthropod vectors such as ticks, lice, and fleas.

e. Mainly invade vascular endothelium and smooth muscle cells, causing blood vessel inflammation and necrosis.
2. *Rickettsia rickettsii*—causes Rocky Mountain spotted fever. This disease is transmitted by ticks and results in a hemorrhagic rash and hemorrhagic spots.
3. *Rickettsia prowazekii*
   a. Causes typhus fever. It is transmitted by lice and, depending on the severity of disease, symptoms can range from a mild rash to skin necrosis and internal organ hemorrhages.
   b. *R. prowazekii* can remain latent in the host and re-emerge years later. This reactivation is also known as *recrudescent typhus* or *Brill-Zinsser disease.*

3.2 Viral

3.2.1 DNA viruses

A. Herpesviruses family
1. Herpesviruses are known to cause latent infections (recurrence of disease after a latent period of time).
2. Basic virion structure: double-stranded DNA, a capsid, a glycoprotein envelope, and a nuclear membrane, which is obtained via budding. Note: Herpesviruses derive their virion envelopes from the host nuclear membrane, not the host plasma membrane.
3. Herpes simplex virus type I (HSV-I)
   a. Primary herpetic gingivostomatitis
      (1) Caused by the initial exposure to HSV-I.
      (2) Most often transmitted through saliva.
      (3) Usually occurs in children.
      (4) Symptoms include fever, malaise, and small ulcerations in the mouth. Commonly asymptomatic.
   b. Acute herpetic gingivostomatitis
      (1) Usually occurs in children.
      (2) Symptoms are more severe and painful than in primary herpetic gingivostomatitis. Numerous yellowish vesicles form and ulcerate within the oral cavity. The gingiva appears erythematous. Systemic symptoms involve fever, malaise, irritability, and regional lymphadenopathy.
   c. Adult recurrence
      (1) Following the primary infection, the virus remains latent in sensory nerve ganglia. Reactivation occurs at the site of initial infection or in adjacent areas innervated by the infected nerve.
      (2) The most common site of recurrence in adults is along the vermilion border of the lips, known as *herpes labialis* (cold sores). Infection of the eye (herpetic conjunctivitis) is also common.
3. Treatment: Acyclovir, a nucleoside analog—an example of a competitive inhibitor. It acts to inhibit viral DNA synthesis and replication. Clinically, it does not cure the disease but often decreases the duration of symptoms and amount of viral shedding.
4. Herpes simplex virus type II (HSV-II)
   a. Disease: genital herpes
      (1) A sexually transmitted disease.
      (2) Symptoms begin as flu-like symptoms, followed by severe genital itching and the formation of painful vesicles that ulcerate. Infectious individuals may be asymptomatic.
      (3) Transmission of disease to infants can occur within the birth canal and may result in CNS impairment, conjunctivitis, or vesicle formation at the site of infection.
5. Varicella-zoster virus (VZV)
   a. Disease: chicken pox as the primary disease; zoster (shingles) as the recurrent form.
      (1) Symptoms include a general vesicular rash. Infected children are highly contagious.
      (2) The administration of aspirin is contraindicated in this and in other childhood viral infections. Aspirin given to infected children increases the incidence of Reye's syndrome, which can cause encephalitis and liver impairment.
      (3) VZV will remain latent in the dorsal spinal ganglia. Reactivation of the disease, known as *zoster,* usually occurs at times of reduced immunity. It travels along the dermatome of the infected nerve.
      (4) Treatment: acyclovir or famciclovir.
      (5) Vaccine: live, attenuated virus.

6. Epstein-Barr virus
   a. Diseases:
      (1) Mononucleosis ("kissing disease")
         (a) Transmitted through saliva.
         (b) Infects B cells and can remain latent in them after symptoms have resolved.
         (c) Symptoms include pharyngitis, fever, lymphadenopathy, and lethargy. Splenomegaly may also occur. Spontaneous recovery usually occurs in 2 to 3 weeks.
         (d) Laboratory findings include lymphocytosis and the presence of atypical T lymphocytes and heterophile antibodies.
      (2) Burkitt's lymphoma and a B-cell lymphoma that usually occurs in Africa.
         (a) Affects the posterior maxilla and/or mandible.
         (b) Histologic evaluation reveals a characteristic starry-sky appearance.
      (3) Hairy leukoplakia—presents as white, hyperkeratotic lesions found on the tongue. Most often seen in immunocompromised patients.
      (4) Nasopharyngeal carcinoma.
7. Cytomegalovirus (CMV, HHV-5)
   a. Most CMV infections are asymptomatic in healthy individuals. Symptomatic CMV infections are commonly seen in immunocompromised patients.
   b. Symptoms may include mononucleosis-like symptoms.
   c. CMV can remain latent in lymphocytes or salivary glands cells.
   d. Treatment: ganciclovir or foscarnet, for severe infections in AIDS patients.
8. Human herpes virus 8 (HHV-8)
   a. Disease: Kaposi's sarcoma:
      (1) A malignant tumor that mainly affects immunocompromised patients. It is more commonly found in Africa.
      (2) Signs and symptoms include plaque-like or nodular skin and oral lesions. Internal organs may also be affected.

B. Poxvirus family
   1. Basic virion structure: double-stranded DNA, a capsid, and envelope.
   2. It is one of the largest and most complex viruses known.
   3. Smallpox virus (variola virus)—causes smallpox. This is the only disease that has been completely eradicated as a result of vaccination.

C. Adenoviruses
   1. Basic virion structure: double-stranded DNA and a capsid surrounded by fibers, which aid in its attachment to the host cell.
   2. Diseases include respiratory illnesses (especially in children), conjunctivitis, and pharyngitis.

D. *Papovavirus* family
   1. Basic virion structure: double-stranded, circular DNA and a capsid.

E. *Human papillomavirus* (HPV)
   1. Basic virion structure: double-stranded, circular DNA and a capsid.
   2. Diseases include papillomas, or warts, and cervical cancer.

3.2.2 RNA viruses

A. Orthomyxoviruses
   1. Influenza virus:
      a. Basic virion structure: single-stranded RNA, capsid, envelope. Also contains an RNA-dependent RNA polymerase.
      b. Envelope—covered with spikes or peplomers. These peplomers contribute to their pathogenicity and can also be used for identification purposes. The spikes consist of two proteins: neuraminidase (which aids in the attachment to host cell via specific receptors) and hemagglutinin (which causes the agglutination of RBCs).
      c. Influenza viruses are known to show small or large changes in the antigenicity of their hemagglutinin and neuraminidase proteins (i.e., undergo antigenic change), which sometimes can result in a new strain of virus. This property contributes to their capacity to cause devastating epidemics.
      d. Influenza can be classified as influenza A, B, and C.
      e. Disease: flu
         (1) Servere consequences of a flu infection include:
            (a) Reye's syndrome—a rare but serious reaction that can lead to encephalitis and liver impairment. Aspirin given to children with flu-like symptoms increases

the incidence of Reye's syndrome.
(b) May also lead to meningitis in young children.
(2) Treatment:
(a) Amantadine or rimantadine. They act to prevent viral replication and are only effective against Influenza A. Their effects are greater when given prophylactically, but they can also be administered for treatment.
(b) Ribavirin—a nucleoside analog that is effective against both influenza A and B. It acts to inhibit viral DNA and RNA replication.
(3) Vaccine: killed virus, usually consisting of two A strains and one B strain.

B. Paramyxoviruses
1. Basic virion structure: single-stranded negative RNA, helical nucleocapsid. No icosahedral capsid, enveloped.
2. Contain an RNA-dependent RNA polymerase.
3. Their general structures resemble the structure of orthomyxoviruses except that they are usually larger in size, have different surface proteins, and have nonsegmented genomes.
4. Measles virus
a. Disease: measles (rubeola).
b. Transmitted via respiratory droplets.
c. Symptoms: the infection begins with flu-like symptoms. Koplik spots (bright erythematous patches with a white, central dot surrounded by bluish rings) appear along the buccal mucosa and are virtually diagnostic of the disease. A maculopapular rash will follow, covering most of the body.
d. Vaccine: live, attenuated virus that is part of the MMR vaccine.
5. Mumps virus
a. Disease: mumps.
b. Transmitted via respiratory droplets.
c. Symptoms: infection begins with flu-like symptoms followed by infection and swelling of the salivary glands, with the parotid gland most commonly affected. Orchitis, or testicular inflammation, may be present in males.
d. Consequences include orchitis (testicular inflammation) in postpubertal males. If bilateral, sterility may occur. Meningitis, and loss of hearing may occur in children.
e. Vaccine: Live, attenuated virus that is part of the MMR vaccine.
6. Respiratory syncytial virus
a. Its virion surface proteins cause infected cells to fuse.
b. Diseases: it is a major cause of lower respiratory infections, including pneumonia and bronchiolitis, in infants.
7. Parainfluenza viruses
a. Diseases: It is the the second most common cause of viral respiratory infections, including croup, in children.

C. Togaviruses family
1. Basic virion structure: single-stranded RNA, a capsid and an envelope with surface proteins, including hemagglutinin.
2. Rubella virus
a. Disease: rubella (German measles).
b. Transmitted via respiratory droplets.
c. Symptoms: infection begins with flu-like symptoms and lymphadenopathy, followed by a rash that then progressively spreads from the head and neck to the rest of the body.
d. Transmission of disease from an infected mother to her fetus can cause birth defects including heart disease, cataracts, deafness, and brain impairments.

D. Picornavirus family
1. Basic virion structure: single-stranded positive RNA, icosahedral capsid. No envelope is present.
2. Rhinoviruses—cause of the common cold.
3. Poliovirus
a. Transmission: fecal-oral route.
b. Disease: poliomyelitis.
(1) Symptoms of polio range from completely asymptomatic to CNS impairment leading to paralysis. Note: the virus preferentially replicates in the motor neurons of the anterior horn of the spinal cord; thus, the death of those cells leads to muscle paralysis.
(2) Outbreaks rarely occur in the Western world due to successful vaccinations.
(3) Two vaccines are available:

(a) Salk vaccine—consists of a killed virus that is given intravenously.

(b) Sabin vaccine—consists of a live, attenuated virus that is administered orally.

4. Hepatitis A—discussed later in the hepatitis viruses section.
5. Coxsackievirus (group A and group B)
   a. Basic virion structure: double-stranded RNA and a capsid. Also contains an RNA polymerase.
   b. Diseases caused by coxsackievirus A
      (1) Herpangina ("summer illness")—presents with intraoral ulcerating vesicles that are seen only in the posterior portion of the mouth, including the uvula, anterior pillars, oropharynx, and soft palate. Symptoms also include fever and sore throat.
      (2) Hand-foot-and-mouth disease—vesicles, like those seen in herpangina, are seen on the oral mucosa or tongue and are not limited to the posterior portion of the mouth. Vesicles are also found on the hands and feet.
   c. Diseases caused by coxsackievirus B
      (1) Pleurodynia, myocarditis, and pericarditis

E. Reovirus family
1. Rotavirus
   a. Basic virion structure: segmented, double-stranded RNA and capsid. The virion contains an RNA-dependent RNA polymerase, which is required because human cells lack this enzyme and therefore cannot synthesize mRNA from an RNA template.
   b. The most common cause of gastroenteritis in children.

F. Human immunodeficiency virus (HIV)
1. Part of the Retroviridae family (i.e., it is a retrovirus).
2. Basic virion structure
   a. The nucleocapsid contains single-stranded RNA and three enzymes: reverse transcriptase, integrase, and protease.
   b. An exterior consists of two glycoproteins, gp120 and gp41, which are imbedded in the lipid bilayer. This lipid bilayer was obtained from the host cell via budding.
3. Virion characteristics
   a. The HIV genome includes:
      (1) *gag gene*—codes for core proteins.
      (2) *pol gene*—codes for its three enzymes.
      (3) *env gene*—codes for its two envelope glycoproteins.
   b. HIV enzymes
      (1) Reverse transcriptase—reverse transcription of RNA to viral DNA.
      (2) Integrase—responsible for integrating viral DNA into host DNA.
      (3) Protease—responsible for cleaving precursor proteins.
4. Pathogenicity
   a. HIV mainly infects CD4 lymphocytes, or helper T cells. Its envelope protein, gp120, binds specifically with CD4 surface receptors. After entry, viral RNA is transcribed by reverse transcriptase to viral DNA and integrated into the host DNA. New virions are synthesized and released by lysis of the host cell.
   b. The predominant site of HIV replication is lymphoid tissues.
   c. Although HIV mainly infects CD4 helper T cells, it can bind to any cell with a CD4 receptor, including macrophages, monocytes, lymph node dendritic cells, and a selected number of nerve cells. Macrophages are the first cells infected by HIV.
5. HIV infection versus acquired immunodeficiency syndrome (AIDS).
   a. AIDS describes an HIV-infected person who has one of the following conditions:
      (1) A CD4 lymphocyte count of less than 200.
      (2) The person is infected with an opportunistic infection or other AIDS-defining illness, including (but not limited to) tuberculosis, recurrent pneumonia infections, or invasive cervical cancer.
   b. The cause of death in an AIDS patient is most likely due to an opportunistic infection.
6. Common opportunistic infections associated with AIDS:
   a. Pneumonia caused by *Pneumocystis jiroveci (carinii)*.

b. Tuberculosis.
c. Periodontal disease—severe gingivitis, periodontitis, ANUG, necrotizing stomatitis.
d. Candidiasis.
e. Oral hairy leukoplakia (EBV).
f. Kaposi's sarcoma (HHV-8).
g. Recurrent VZV infections.
h. Condyloma acuminatum or verruca vulgaris (warts, HPV)—less common.
i. CMV infections.
j. Disseminated herpes simplex, herpes zoster.
k. Hodgkin's, non-Hodgkin's lymphoma.

7. Laboratory diagnosis of HIV
   a. ELISA test—detects HIV antibodies. False negatives do occur.
   b. Western blot—detects HIV proteins. There is a 99% accuracy rate when both the ELISA test and Western blot are used to diagnose HIV infection.
   c. PCR—more sensitive; can amplify and identify the virus at an early stage.
8. Treatment
   a. Inhibitors of reverse transcriptase.
      (1) Nucleoside analogs
         (a) Inhibit viral replication via competitive inhibition.
         (b) Examples: zidovudine (AZT), didanosine, lami- vudine, stavudine.
      (2) Nonnucleoside inhibitors.
         (a) Act by binding directly to reverse transcriptase.
         (b) Examples: nevirapine, delavirdine.
   b. Protease inhibitor.
   c. "Triple cocktail" therapy—often consists of two nucleoside inhibitors and a protease inhibitor.

G. Hepatitis viruses—this group of viruses causes hepatitis, a disease affecting the liver.
1. General characteristics of hepatitis.
   a. The general presentation of hepatitis is the same regardless of the infecting virus; however, the time and severity of symptoms may differ.
   b. Symptoms of hepatitis include fever, anorexia, malaise, nausea, jaundice, and brown-colored urine.
   c. Complications of a hepatitis infection include cirrhosis, liver failure, and hepatorenal failure.
   d. A summary of these viruses is shown in Table 3-5.
2. Hepatitis A virus.
   a. Symptoms last 2 to 4 weeks.
   b. There is no risk of developing chronic hepatitis in the future.
   c. Incubation period is short, lasting 2 to 6 weeks.
   d. Laboratory diagnosis: ELISA test for IgM antibody.
   e. Vaccine: killed virus.
   f. Prevention: serum immunoglobulins are available.
3. Hepatitis B virus ("serum hepatitis").
   a. Symptoms last 2 to 4 weeks, but may be asymptomatic.
   b. Incubation period: ranges from 4 to 26 weeks, but averages 6 to 8 weeks.
   c. The hepatitis B viral structure has also been named the *Dane particle*.
   d. Infection increases the risk for hepatocellular carcinoma.
   e. Laboratory assay of hepatitis B antigens and antibodies:
      (1) HBsAg—present only in acute infection or chronic carriers.
      (2) HBsAb—detectable only after 6 months post-initial infection. HBsAb is present in chronic infections or vaccinated individuals. Note: HBsAb is also being produced during acute infections and in chronic carriers; however, it is not detectable via current laboratory methods.

Table 3–5. Summary of Hepatitis Viruses

	GENOME	FAMILY	TRANSMISSION
Hepatitis A	ssRNA	Picornavirus	Oral–anal
Hepatitis B	dsDNA	Hepadnavirus	Sexual contact Blood (needles) Perinatal
Hepatitis C	ssRNA	Flavivirus	Sexual contact Blood (needles)
Hepatitis D	ssRNA	Deltavirus	Sexual contact Blood (needles)
Hepatitis E	ssRNA	Calicivirus	Oral–anal

ss, Single stranded, *ds,* double stranded.

(3) HBcAg—present in either acute or chronic infection.
(4) HBeAg—present when there is active viral replication. It signifies that the carrier is highly infectious.
(5) HBeAb—appears after HBeAg. It signifies that the individual is not as contagious.

f. Vaccine: contains HBsAg.
g. Prevention: immunoglobulins (HBsAb) are available.

4. Hepatitis C virus.
   a. 90% of blood transfusion-related hepatitis is caused by hepatitis C.
   b. 50% progress to chronic disease.
   c. Increased risk for hepatocellular carcinoma.
   d. Incubation period: ranges from 2 to 26 weeks, but averages 8 weeks.
   e. Treatment and prevention: α-interferon is used to treat chronic hepatitis C. There is currently no vaccine available.
5. Hepatitis D virus—can only infect cells previously infected with hepatitis B.
6. Hepatitis E virus—a high mortality rate in infected pregnant women.

Quick lists of disease-causing organisms

A. Top four viruses that cause respiratory disease in children
   1. RSV—most common
   2. Parainfluenza
   3. Rhinovirus
   4. Adenovirus
B. Common viral causes of pharyngitis
   1. Coxsackievirus
   2. Adenovirus
   3. Picornaviruses
   4. Orthomyxoviruses
   5. EBV
C. Leading causes of meningitis
   1. *E. coli*—in neonates
   2. *H. influenzae*—in infants and children
   3. *N. meningitis*—in young adults
   4. *S. pneumoniae*—in older adults
D. Common causes of nosocomial infections
   1. *Escherichia coli*
   2. *Staphylococcus aureus and S. epidermidis*
   3. *Streptococcus faecalis*
   4. *Pseudomonas aeruginosa*
   5. *Klebsiella pneumoniae*
   6. *Enterobacter* spp.
   7. *Candida* spp.
E. Microorganisms that can affect fetus of an infected mother
   1. Rubella
   2. Herpes
   3. HIV
   4. Syphilis
   5. Toxoplasmosis
   6. CMV

3.3 Vaccines

A. Bacterial vaccines
   1. Active immunity—vaccines that contain killed bacteria or inactive bacterial products, such as capsular polysaccharides, toxoids, or purified proteins.
   2. Passive immunity—vaccines that contain preformed immunoglobulins or antitoxins. Can be used for either the treatment or prevention of certain bacterial diseases.
   3. A summary of bacterial vaccines is shown in Table 3-6.

TABLE 3–6. BACTERIAL VACCINES

	CAPSULAR POLYSACCHARIDES	TOXOIDS	KILLED BACTERIA OR PURIFIED PROTEINS	IMMUNOGLOBULINS (PASSIVE IMMUNITY)
S. pneumoniae	X	—	—	—
N. meningitides	X	—	—	—
H. influenzae	X	—	—	—
C. diphtheriae	—	X	—	X
C. tetani	—	X	—	X
B. pertussis	—	—	X	—
C. botulinum				X

B. Viral vaccines
   1. Active immunity—vaccines that contain live, attenuated viruses; killed viruses; or viral products such as surface antigens. As compared to the other vaccines, immunity from live virus vaccines usually lasts longer.
   2. Passive immunity—vaccines that contain preformed immunoglobulins
   3. A summary of viral vaccines is shown in Table 3-7.

3.4 Prions

Although prions are not considered to be microbes and are currently under investigation, they can be disease-causing molecules.

A. General characteristics
   1. Basically, they are infectious protein particles (atypical virus-like agents).
   2. They do not contain nucleic acid.
   3. Are more resistant to inactivation by radiation or heat than viruses, but can be inactivated by hypochlorite and autoclaving.
   4. They exist in two forms: an abnormal prion consists of a β-pleated sheet, and a normal prion consists of an α-helical structure.
   5. Pathogenesis: the abnormal prion is able to induce a structural change in the normal prion, so that it also becomes an abnormal prion with a β-pleated sheet.
   6. Transmission: includes inoculation or ingestion of nervous tissue containing the abnormal prion.

B. Diseases caused by prions include Creutzfeldt-Jakob disease, a severe degenerative brain disease caused by the ingestion of beef from a cow infected with mad cow disease.

3.5 Fungal

3.5.1 Cutaneous Mycoses (Skin Fungi)

A. Dermatophytes
   1. Dermatophytes are cutaneous fungi that mainly infect keratinized skin, hair, and nails.
   2. Three genera: *Microsporum*, *Trichophyton*, and *Epidermophyton*.
   3. Disease: tinea
      a. This group of diseases is classified according to the organ affected.
      b. These diseases are summarized in Table 3-8.

3.5.2 Subcutaneous Mycoses

Subcutaneous mycoses are caused by fungi that grow in soil and are introduced into subcutaneous tissue through trauma.

A. Sporotrichosis
   1. Dimorphic fungi (*Sporothrix schenckii*) found on vegetation and usually introduced into skin via thorn punctures.

Table 3–7. Viral Vaccines

	LIVE, ATTENUATED VIRUS	KILLED VIRUS	VIRAL ANTIGENS	IMMUNOGLOBULINS (PASSIVE IMMUNITY)
MMR	X	—	—	—
Measles				
Mumps				
Rubella				
VZV	X	—	—	X
Adenoviruses	X	—	—	—
Hepatitis A	—	X	—	X
Hepatitis B	—	—	X	X
Poliovirus	X	X	—	—
Influenza		X	—	—
Smallpox virus	X	—	—	—
Rabies virus	—	X	—	X

TABLE 3–8. SUMMARY OF DISEASES CAUSED BY DERMATOPHYTES

DISEASE	ORGAN(S) AFFECTED	DERMATOPHYTES RESPONSIBLE		
		MICROSPORUM	TRICHOPHYTON	EPIDERMOPHYTON
Tinea pedis (athlete's foot)	Feet	—	X	X
Tinea capitis	Hair, skin	X	X	—
Tinea cruris (jock itch)	Groin	—	X	X
Tinea corporis*	Entire body*	X	X	X
Tinea unguium	Nails	—	X	—
Tinea barbae	Bearded areas	—	X	—

* Tinea corporis—common signs are circular (ring-shaped) lesions.

2. Symptoms include local pustule or ulcer with nodules that form along draining lymphatics.

B. Chromomycosis
   1. Soil fungi (*Cladosporium*).
   2. Symptoms include wartlike lesions with crusting abscesses that extend along the affected lymphatic vessel.

C. Mycetoma
   1. Soil fungi (*Petriellidium*) enters through wounds on the feet, hands, or back.

3.5.3 Opportunistic Fungi

A. *Aspergillus* (molds)
   1. Found mostly on rotten vegetables.
   2. Transmission is via airborne conidia.
   3. Virulent factor: aflatoxin, which inhibits transcription by binding to DNA.
   4. It is also a carcinogen that can lead to cancer of the liver.
   5. Causes three forms of lung infection:
      a. Allergic bronchopulmonary aspergillosis—characterized by the formation of bronchial mucous plugs in the lungs. Asthma-like symptoms are mediated by a high IgE *Aspergillus* antibody titer.
      b. Aspergilloma—when *Aspergillus* colonize (form "fungus balls") in lung cavities without invasion.
      c. Invasive aspergillosis—*Aspergillus* infection that spreads to other organs. Usually occurs in immunocompromised patients.
   6. Common species include *A. fumigatus, A. flavusa*, and *A. niger*.

B. *Candida albicans*
   1. Found in the normal gut, oral, and vaginal flora.
   2. *C. albicans* may be seen in three forms:
      a. As yeast cells.
      b. Pseudohyphae—not a true hyphae but an elongated form.
      c. Chlamydospores—the only fungal species to be observed in this form.
   3. Disease: candidiasis (thrush).
      a. Overgrowth occurs in immunocompromised patients.
      b. Also occurs with angular cheilitis.
      c. Appears as white patches along the buccal mucosa, palate, or tongue that wipe off when rubbed.
      d. Treatment includes nystatin or imidazole-derived drugs, such as ketoconazole.

3.5.4 Systemic Fungus

A. General characteristics
   1. Most are spore-forming and are transmitted via inhalation of airborne spores.
   2. Express dimorphism: exists as yeasts, when causing systemic infections, and molds, when found in the soil.
      a. *Coccidioides immitis*
         (1) Spore: arthrospores.
         (2) Disease: coccidioidomycosis, valley fever (in San Joaquin Valley of California), or desert rheumatism (in Arizona).
         (3) Usually asymptomatic, but flu-like symptoms may be present.

(4) Treatment: amphotericin B.

b. *Blastomyces dermatitidis*
   (1) Spore: conidia.
   (2) Disease: blastomycosis.

c. *Histoplasma capsulatum*
   (1) Spore: two asexual spores—tuberculate macroconidia and microconidia.
   (2) Disease: histoplasmosis.
   (3) Note: histoplasmosis may clinically resemble tuberculosis because its yeast cells are often found in macrophages.
   (4) Treatment: usually no therapy is necessary; oral ketoconazole may help with progressive lung lesions.

3.5.5 Molds

A. General characteristics
   1. Are spore-forming and are transmitted via inhalation of airborne spores.
   2. Have a tendency to invade blood vessel endothelium in the paranasal sinuses, bronchi, or intestines. This results in a loss of blood supply, leading to infarction and tissue necrosis.
   3. Affect immunocompromised patients.
   4. Diseases: mucormycosis, phycomycosis, and zygomycosis.

3.5.6 Protozoa

A. *Plasmodium*—causes malaria, which is transmitted by mosquitos.

B. *Trichomonas vaginalis*—causes trichomoniasis, which is characterized by inflammation of the vagina, prostate, or urethra.

C. *Entamoeba histolytica*—causes intestinal dysentery.

D. *Cryptosporidium*—causes cryptosporidiosis, which clinically presents as diarrhea. It often affects immunocompromised (AIDS) patients; however, there are also occasional outbreaks of infections in swimming pools.

E. *Toxoplasma gondii*
   1. Causes toxoplasmosis. Infection is usually asymptomatic in healthy people but it can pose a problem for immunocompromised patients.
   2. It is transmitted by ingesting its cyst (oocyst), which is found in cat feces or undercooked lamb or pork.
   3. It can cross the placental barrier and cause severe neonatal disease or death of the fetus.
   4. It is the most common cause of encephalitis in AIDS patients.

4.0 SYSTEMIC PATHOLOGY

4.1 Cardiovascular Pathology

Bacterial endocarditis

Endocarditis is an infection of the endocardium of the heart, most often affecting the heart valves.

A. Acute endocarditis
   1. Most commonly caused by *Staphylococcus aureus*.
   2. It occurs most frequently in intravenous drug users, where it usually affects the tricuspid valve.

B. Subacute endocarditis
   1. Most commonly caused by less virulent organisms, such as intraoral *Streptococcus viridans* that can be introduced systemically via dental procedures.
   2. Pathogenesis: occurs when a thrombus or vegetation forms on a previously damaged or congenitally abnormal valve. These vegetations contain bacteria and inflammatory cells. Complications can arise if the thrombus embolizes, causing septic infarcts. Other complications include valvular dysfunction or abscess formation.
   3. Symptoms can remain hidden for months.
   4. Valves affected (listed most to least common):
      a. Mitral valve (most frequent).
      b. Aortic valve.
      c. Tricuspid (except in IV drug users, where the tricuspid valve is most often affected).

Atherosclerosis

A. Caused by the formation of plaques in medium to large vessels. In arteriosclerosis, the same process affects arterioles and smaller arteries. The plaques eventually calcify, resulting in rigidity and distortion of the arterial walls.
   1. The plaques mainly consist of cholesterol, foam cells, and calcium. The main complications that can arise from these plaques are:
      a. Calcification of the plaque—the plaques eventually calcify, resulting in

rigidity and distortion of the arterial walls.
   b. Thrombus formation, producing obstructive disease.
   c. Embolization of the plaque.
   d. Vessel narrowing, leading to ischemia of peripheral tissues.
2. Arteries affected include abdominal aorta (most common), coronary arteries, the circle of Willis, the internal carotid, and the popliteal arteries.
3. Risk factors include:
   a. Advanced age.
   b. Male sex.
   c. Smoking.
   d. Hypertension.
   e. Hypercholesterolemia (abnormally high LDL).
   f. Diabetes mellitus.
4. Complications
   a. Vessel narrowing, leading to ischemia of peripheral tissues.
   b. Formation of a thrombus and embolus, leading to acute arterial occlusion.

Ischemic heart disease (IHD), angina pectoris

A. The clinical presentation of IHD is angina (chest pain). It is caused by partial or complete interruption of arterial blood flow to the myocardium.
   1. Most often caused by coronary artery disease (CAD).
      a. CAD/IHD is the leading cause of death for both men and women in the United States.
      b. The decrease in cardiac oxygen supply is caused by the formation of atherosclerotic plaques in the coronary arteries. This limits the rate of blood flow and may result in the acute cessation of circulation in the event of a plaque rupture.
      c. Risk factors: same as those for atherosclerosis, as previously listed.
   2. Three types of angina:
      a. Stable angina—arteries are approximately 70% occluded; pain occurs with physical exertion.
      b. Unstable angina—prolonged or recurrent pain at rest. Often results in a myocardial infarction (MI).
      c. Variant or Prinzmetal's angina—intermittent chest pain at rest. It is less common than other forms. Decreased oxygen occurs via vasospasm of coronary arteries.

Myocardial infarction (MI)—heart attack

A. Ischemia versus MI: as previously discussed, ischemia is a reversible mismatch between the supply and demand of oxygen. Infarction is an irreversible mismatch that results in cell death caused by the lack of blood flow (oxygenation). For instance, chest pain caused by ischemia can be relieved by administering nitroglycerin (a vasodilator) to the patient. If the patient has an MI, the pain will not be relieved with nitroglycerin.
   1. MIs most commonly occur when a coronary artery is occluded by a thrombus generated in an atherosclerotic artery.
   2. Symptoms include:
      a. Chest pain, shortness of breath.
      b. Diaphoresis (sweating), clammy hands.
      c. Nausea, vomiting.
   3. Consequences:
      a. Death (one third of patients).
      b. Arrhythmias (most common *immediate* cause of death).
      c. Congestive heart failure.
      d. Myocardial rupture, which may result in death from cardiac tamponade.
      e. Thrombus formation on infarcted tissue; may result in systemic embolism.

Congestive heart failure (CHF)

A. Left-sided CHF
   1. May result from nearly any heart disease affecting the left ventricle (e.g., ischemic heart disease, hypertension, valvular disease).
   2. Common signs and symptoms include:
      a. Dyspnea (shortness of breath) exacerbated by exertion.
      b. Paroxysmal nocturnal dyspnea.
      c. Orthopnea.
      d. Tachypnea.
      e. Pleural effusion.
      f. Consequences include pulmonary edema.
B. Right-sided CHF
   1. The most common cause of right heart failure is left heart failure. It uncommonly occurs in isolation. Other causes include left-sided lesions (mitral stenosis),

pulmonary hypertension, cardiomyopathy, and tricuspid or pulmonary valvular disease.
2. Frequently presents with peripheral edema, especially in the ankles and feet (i.e., dependent edema), enlarged liver or spleen, and distention of the neck veins.

Valvular disease

A. Generally, there are three types:
   1. Stenosis—fibrotic, stiff, and thickened valves, resulting in reduced blood flow through the valve.
   2. Regurgitation or valvular insufficiency—valves are unable to close completely, allowing blood to regurgitate.
   3. Prolapse—"floppy" valves; may occur with or without regurgitation. The most common valvular defect.

B. Rheumatic fever—before antibiotic therapy, this was the most common cause of valvular disease.
   1. Usually preceded by a group A streptococci respiratory infection; for example, strep throat.
   2. All three layers of the heart may be affected. The pathologic findings include Aschoff bodies, which are areas of focal necrosis surrounded by a dense inflammatory infiltration.
   3. Most commonly affects the mitral valve, resulting in mitral valve stenosis, regurgitation, or both.

C. Acute pericarditis
   1. Characterized by inflammation of the pericardium.
   2. Causes include:
      a. Viral infection.
      b. Bacterial infection, including *Staphylococcus, Pneumococcus.*
      c. Tuberculosis.
      d. MI.
      e. Systemic lupus erythematosus.
      f. Rheumatic fever.
   3. Signs and symptoms include:
      a. Pericardial friction rub on cardiac auscultation.
      b. Angina.
      c. Fever.
   4. Consequences include constrictive pericarditis, which results from fusion and scarring of the pericardium. This may lead to the restriction of ventricular expansion, preventing the heart chambers from filling normally.

Cardiac tamponade

A. Caused by accumulation of fluid in the pericardium. This severe condition can quickly impair ventricular filling and rapidly lead to decreased cardiac output and death.
   1. Signs and symptoms include:
      a. Hypotension.
      b. Jugular venous distention.
      c. Distant heart sounds.

4.2 Respiratory Pathology

A. Pulmonary infections
   1. Bacterial pneumonia
      a. Is an inflammatory process of infectious origin affecting the pulmonary parenchyma.
   2. Bacterial infections include:
      a. *Streptococcus pneumoniae* (most common).
      b. *Staphylococcus aureus.*
      c. *Haemophilus influenzae.*
      d. *Klebsiella pneumoniae.*
      e. Anaerobic bacteria from the mouth (aspiration of oral secretions).
   3. Viral infections include:
      a. Influenza.
      b. Parainfluenza.
      c. Adenoviruses.
      d. Respiratory syncytial virus.
      e. Note: viruses can also cause pneumonia. Infection of the interstitial tissues, or interstitial pneumonia, is commonly associated with these types of infections.
      f. Common symptoms include fever, dyspnea, and a productive cough (Box 3-1).
      g. Two types:
         (1) Lobar pneumonia
            (a) Infection may spread through entire lobe(s) of lung. Intra-alveolar exudates result in dense consolidations.
            (b) Typical of *S. pneumoniae* infections.
         (2) Bronchopneumonia
            (a) Infection and inflammation spread through distal airways, extending from the bronchioles and alveoli. A patch distribution

Box 3–1. Diseases that Produce a Productive Cough

Pneumonia
Lung abscess
Tuberculosis
Chronic bronchitis
Bronchiectasis
Bronchogenic carcinoma

involving one or more lobes is observed.

(b) Typical of *S. aureus*, *H. influenzae*, and *K. pneumoniae* infections.

4. Lung abscess—localized area of suppuration.
   a. Causes include:
      (1) Complication of bacterial pneumonia (e.g. *Staphylococcus*) infection or bronchiectasis.
      (2) Aspiration of anaerobic bacteria from the mouth.
      (3) Bronchial obstruction (often by cancer).
   b. May be seen in patients with impaired gag reflex (e.g., patients under general anesthesia, alcoholics).
   c. Common symptoms include a productive cough with a foul odor, cyanosis, and dyspnea.
5. Tuberculosis
   a. Caused by *Mycobacterium tuberculosis.*
   b. For progression of disease and disease states, refer to the microbiology section.
   c. Common symptoms include weight loss, anorexia, fever, night sweats, a productive cough, and hemoptysis.
   d. Treatment: multidrug therapy with drugs such as rifampin, ethambutol, and isoniazid.

B. Obstructive lung diseases
   1. Chronic obstructive pulmonary diseases (COPD).
      a. Chronic bronchitis
         (1) Caused by narrowing and obstruction of the respiratory airways.
         (2) Characterized by hypersecretion of mucus, leading to a chronic productive cough that must be present for at least 3 successive months for over 2 consecutive years.
         (3) Is associated with smoking.
         (4) Consequences include:
            (a) Cor pulmonale—right-sided hypertrophy of the heart.
            (b) Bronchogenic carcinoma—squamous metaplasia of the bronchial epithelium.
         (5) Chronic pulmonary congestion may lead to:
            (a) Thickening of the alveolar wall.
            (b) Hemosiderosis. Results from macrophages engulfing extravasated RBCs from destroyed vessels. These cells thus contain iron.
      b. Emphysema
         (1) Caused by the destruction of alveolar walls by proteases, including elastase, that are released by inflammatory cells.
         (2) Effect of smoking: α_1-antitrypsin is normally present in the lung to inhibit the actions of elastase. Smoking inhibits the actions of α_1-antitrypsin and thus increases the number of inflammatory cells present (Figure 3-10).
         (3) Lungs show decreased elasticity.
         (4) Two types:
            (a) Centrilobular emphysema—affects bronchioles of the upper lobes of the lungs. Causes include smoking.
            (b) Panacinar emphysema—affects the entire lung. Causes include a hereditary α_1-antitrypsin deficiency.
      c. Bronchiectasis

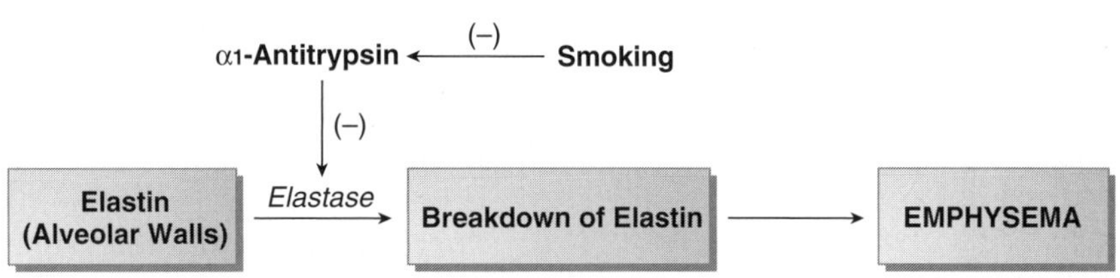

Figure 3–10. Pathogenesis of emphysema: role of elastase, α-1 antitrypsin, and smoking.

(1) Characterized by permanent dilation of bronchi caused by chronic lung infections with inflammation and necrosis of the bronchial wall.
(2) Common symptoms include a productive cough with a foul odor, hemoptysis, and recurrent lung infections that may lead to lung abscesses.

d. Asthma
(1) An obstructive lung disease characterized by narrowing of the airways. Inflammation of the airways is a major component of asthma.
(2) Common symptoms are dyspnea, wheezing on expiration, and coughing.
(3) Two types:
(a) Extrinsic (allergic, atopic) asthma
(i) An atopic allergy caused by a type I immediate hypersensitivity immune reaction to an allergen.
(ii) Seen in children, adults.
(b) Intrinsic (nonallergic) asthma
(i) Not caused by an allergic reaction.
(ii) Mostly seen in adults.

C. Pneumoconioses—are environmentally related lung diseases that result from chronic inhalation of various substances.
1. Silicosis (stone mason's disease)
a. Inhalant: silica dust.
b. Associated with extensive fibrosis of the lungs.
c. Patients have a higher susceptibility to tuberculosis infections.
2. Asbestosis
a. Inhalant: asbestos fibers.
b. Associated with the presence of pleural plaques.
c. Consequences include:
(1) Mesothelioma (malignant mesothelial tumor).
(2) Bronchogenic carcinoma.
3. Anthracosis
a. Inhalant: carbon dust.
b. Usually not as harmful as silicosis or asbestosis.
c. Associated with the presence of macrophages containing carbon.

D. Other lung diseases
1. Sarcoidosis
a. More common in African-Americans.
b. Associated with the presence of noncaseating granulomas.
2. Cystic fibrosis
a. Transmission: caused by a genetic mutation (nucleotide deletion) on chromosome 7, resulting in abnormal chloride channels.
b. The most common hereditary disease in Caucasians.
c. Genetic transmission: autosomal recessive.
d. Affects all exocrine glands. Organs affected include lungs, pancreas, salivary glands, and intestines. Thick secretions or mucous plugs are seen to obstruct the pulmonary airways and intestinal tracts.
e. Is ultimately fatal.
f. Diagnostic test: sweat test—sweat contains increased amounts of chloride.
3. Atelectasis
a. Characterized by collapse of the alveoli.
b. May be caused by a deficiency of surfactant and/or hypoventilation of alveoli.

4.3 Gastrointestinal and Hepatobiliary Pathology

A. Salivary gland pathology
1. Sjögren's syndrome
a. An autoimmune disease of the salivary and lacrimal glands.
b. Autonuclear antibodies (ANAs) against salivary ducts may be seen.
c. Triad of symptoms include:
(1) Xerostomia—from decreased saliva production.
(2) Keratoconjunctivitis sicca (dry eyes)—from decreased tear production.
(3) Rheumatoid arthritis.
(4) Enlargement of the salivary or lacrimal glands, known as Mikulicz syndrome, may also be observed.
d. Histologically, a dense infiltration of the gland by lymphocytes is observed.
(1) Warthin's tumor (papillary cystadenoma lymphomatosum)—a benign tumor of the parotid glands.
(2) Pleomorphic adenoma
(a) The most common salivary gland tumor.
(b) Is benign.
(c) Prognosis is good after proper surgical excision.

2. Mucoepidermoid carcinoma
   a. One of the most common malignant salivary gland tumors.
   b. Most commonly occurs in the parotid glands.
   c. Prognosis of tumor depends on grade and stage of disease.

B. Esophagus pathology
1. Mallory-Weiss syndrome
   a. Characterized by lacerations (tears) in the esophagus.
   b. Most commonly occurs from vomiting (alcoholics).
   c. A related condition, known as *Boerhaave syndrome*, occurs when the esophagus ruptures, causing massive upper GI hemorrhage.
2. Esophageal varices
   a. The formation of varices (collateral channels) occurs from portal hypertension. Causes of portal hypertension include blockage of the portal vein or liver disease.
   b. Rupture of esophageal varices results in massive hemorrhage into the esophagus and hematemesis.
   c. Common in patients with liver cirrhosis.
3. Gastroesophageal reflux disease (reflux esophagitis)
   a. Caused by the reflux of gastric contents (juices) into the lower esophagus.
   b. One of the most common GI disorders.
   c. Symptoms include dysphagia and substernal pain (heartburn).
   d. Although chronic or severe reflux disease is uncommon, consequences of these conditions can lead to Barrett's esophagus, development of a stricture, or hemorrhage.
   e. Treatment: diet control, antacids, and medications that decrease the production of gastric acid (e.g., H_2 blockers).
4. Barrett's esophagus
   a. A complication of chronic gastroesophageal reflux disease.
   b. Histologic findings include the replacement of squamous epithelium with metaplastic columnar epithelium.
   c. Complications include increased incidence of esophageal adenocarcinoma, stricture formation, or hemorrhage (ulceration).

C. Stomach pathology
1. Peptic ulcers
   a. Commonly associated with *Helicobacter pylori* infections or the long-term use of NSAIDs.
   b. Most common complication is hemorrhage. Note: it is not a precursor lesion of carcinoma of the stomach.
   c. Symptoms include epigastric pain that may worsen when eating.

D. Exocrine pancreas pathology
1. Acute pancreatitis
   a. Caused by early activation of pancreatic enzymes, resulting in autodigestion of the pancreas.
   b. Predisposed by excess of alcohol intake or biliary tract disease (gallstones).
   c. Laboratory tests show an increase in serum lipase and amylase and a decrease in calcium.
   d. Symptoms include severe abdominal pain.

E. Liver pathology
1. Jaundice
   a. Characterized by yellowness of tissues, including skin, eyes, and mucous membranes.
   b. Caused by excess conjugated and/or unconjugated serum bilirubin.
   c. Types and causes include:
      (1) Hepatocellular jaundice—caused by liver diseases such as cirrhosis and hepatitis.
      (2) Hemolytic jaundice—caused by hemolytic anemias.
      (3) Obstructive jaundice—caused by blockage of the common bile duct either by gallstones (cholelithiasis) or carcinomas involving the head of the pancreas.
2. Cirrhosis
   a. Characterized by abnormal hepatic architecture with excessive scarring and nodule formation.
   b. Most commonly caused by alcoholism. Other causes may include viral hepatitis, biliary obstruction, hemochromatosis, drugs and chemical agents, and Wilson's disease.
   c. Clinical findings include:
      (1) Portal hypertension.
      (2) Formation of arteriovenous shunts including esophageal varices.
      (3) An increase in serum transaminases, including AST (SGOT) and AST (SGPT).

- d. Associated with an increased incidence of hepatocellular carcinoma.
3. Wilson's disease
   - a. Caused by a decrease in ceruloplasmin, a serum protein that binds copper, resulting in metastatic copper deposits.
   - b. Common organs affected include:
     - (1) Liver, leading to cirrhosis.
     - (2) Basal ganglia.
     - (3) Cornea, where Kayser-Fleischer rings (greenish rings around the cornea) are observed.
4. Hepatitis—refer to microbiology section.

F. Small bowel pathology

1. Malabsorption syndromes
   - a. A common clinical symptom of all malabsorption syndromes is steatorrhea. There is also a decrease of nutrients absorbed, including fat-soluble vitamins.
   - b. Celiac sprue
     - (1) Characterized by malabsorption and mucosal lesions of the small intestines.
     - (2) Caused by an allergy to gluten (wheat, rye).
     - (3) Histologically, the intestinal villa may appear flat or blunted.
     - (4) Symptoms include weight loss, weakness, and diarrhea.
     - (5) Complications include T cell lymphomas.
   - c. Crohn's disease
     - (1) A chronic inflammatory bowel disease.
     - (2) Histologically characterized by:
       - (a) A textured, cobblestone appearance of the intestinal mucosa caused by submucosal edema with elevation of surviving mucosa.
       - (b) Presence of transmural chronic inflammation and edema.
       - (c) Noncaseating granulomas.
2. Peutz-Jeghers syndrome
   - a. Disease is characterized by dark, freckle-like spots that appear on the skin, lips, and oral mucosa. Intestinal polyps are also present.
   - b. Genetic transmission: autosomal dominant.

G. Large bowel pathology

1. Hirschsprung's disease
   - a. A congenital disease.
   - b. Caused by a section of aganglionic colon, which failed to develop normally due to the absence of ganglion cells). This results in bowel obstruction and distention of the bowel proximal to the affected area.
2. Ulcerative colitis
   - a. An inflammatory bowel disease.
   - b. Caused by chronic inflammation and ulceration of the colon and rectum.
   - c. Histologically characterized by the presence of chronic inflammation and crypt abscesses.
   - d. Symptoms include chronic, bloody diarrhea.
   - e. Complications include:
     - (1) Toxic megacolon.
     - (2) Colon cancer.
     - (3) Perforation of the colon.

4.4 Genitourinary Pathology

A. Renal pathology

1. Glomerulonephritis
   - a. Characterized by inflammation of the glomerulus.
   - b. Characterized by following clinical manifestations:
     - (1) Nephrotic syndrome (nephrosis)
       - (a) Most often caused by glomerulonephritis.
       - (b) Laboratory findings include:
         - (i) Proteinuria (albuminuria) and lipiduria—proteins and lipids are present in urine.
         - (ii) Hypoalbuminemia—decreased serum albumin due to albuminuria.
         - (iii) Hyperlipidemia—especially an increase in plasma levels of low-density lipoproteins and cholesterol.
       - (c) Symptoms include severe edema, resulting from a decrease in colloid osmotic pressure due to a decrease in serum albumin.
     - (2) Nephritic syndrome
       - (a) Characterized by inflammatory rupture of the glomerular capillaries, leaking blood into the urinary space.
       - (b) Classic presentation: poststreptococcal glomerulonephritis. It occurs after a group A, β-hemolytic *Streptococcus* infection (e.g., strep throat.)
       - (c) Caused by autoantibodies forming immune complexes in the glomerulus.
       - (d) Clinical manifestations: oliguria, hematuria, hypertension, edema,

and azotemia (increased concentrations of serum urea nitrogen and creatine).

2. Polycystic kidney disease
   a. Characterized by the formation of cysts and partial replacement of renal parenchyma.
   b. Genetic transmission: autosomal dominant.
   c. Clinical manifestations: hypertension, hematuria, palpable renal masses, and progression to renal failure. Commonly associated with berry aneurysms.
3. Nephrosclerosis
   a. Disease of the renal arteries.
   b. Clinical manifestations:
      (1) Benign (arterial) nephrosclerosis
         (a) Caused by the formation of atherosclerotic plaques in the renal artery.
         (b) Results in narrowing of the arterioles.
      (2) Malignant nephrosclerosis
         (a) Caused by malignant hypertension. Common signs of malignant hypertension include severe hypertension, retinal hemorrhages, and hypertrophy of the left ventricle.
         (b) Results in inflammatory changes in the vascular walls, which may lead to rupture of the glomerular capillaries.
4. Renal tubule diseases
   a. Acute tubular necrosis
      (1) Characterized by impaired kidney functions due to the destruction of the renal tubule epithelium.
      (2) Caused by a variety of conditions that lead to ischemia of the renal tubules, usually resulting from renal tubular injury or problems with vascular flow. It can also be induced by ingesting toxins or drug-related toxicity (e.g., gentamicin).
      (3) The most common cause of acute renal failure.
      (4) Is a reversible condition, although it can be fatal.
   b. Pyelonephritis
      (1) A bacterial infection that affects the renal tubules, interstitium, and renal pelvis.
      (2) One of the most common renal diseases.
      (3) Usually caused by gram-negative, rod-shaped bacteria that are part of the normal flora of the enteric tract. Most commonly caused by *Escherichia coli*, followed by *Proteus*, *Klebsiella*, and *Enterobacter*.
      (4) The infecting bacteria are usually from the patient's own enteric flora—an example of an endogenous infection.
      (5) Usually associated with a urinary tract infection (acute pyelonephritis) or involved with another precipitating condition, such as obstruction (chronic pyelonephritis).
   c. Fanconi's syndrome
      (1) Characterized by the failure of the proximal renal tubules to resorb amino acids, glucose, and phosphates.
      (2) May be inherited or acquired.
      (3) Clinical manifestations include glycosuria, hyperphosphaturia, hypophosphatemia, aminoaciduria, and systemic acidosis.

B. Urinary tract pathology
1. Nephrolithiasis, urolithiasis
   a. Formation of calculi (calcium stones) in the kidney (nephrolithiasis) or urinary tract (urolithiasis).
   b. Commonly associated with hyperparathyroidism.
   c. Signs and symptoms include urinary tract obstruction, severe pain, and pyelonephritis.
   d. Note: an enlarged prostate can also cause urinary tract obstruction in males.
2. Urinary tract infection
   a. Most often caused by gram-negative, rod-shaped bacteria that are normal residents of the enteric tract, especially *Escherichia coli*.
   b. Clinical manifestations: frequent urination, dysuria, pyuria (increased PMNs), hematuria, and bacteriuria.
   c. May lead to infection of the urinary bladder (cystitis) or kidney (pyelonephritis).

4.5 Blood-Lymphatic Pathology

A. Disorders of primary hemostasis
1. General characteristics of disorders of primary hemostasis (due to problems of blood vessels or platelets):
   a. Occur early in life.

b. Unlike secondary hemostasis, bleeding occurs in more superficial areas such as skin and mucous membranes rather than in secondary hemostasis.
c. Signs include petechiae.
d. Can be caused by vascular and platelet abnormalities or alterations in the plasma proteins required for adhesion of platelets to vascular subendothelium.
e. Laboratory findings include prolonged bleeding time, as seen in platelet disorders.

2. Vascular abnormalities
   a. Scurvy
      (1) Caused by a vitamin C deficiency leading to decreased synthesis of collagen. Note: vitamin C is necessary for the formation of collagen via hydroxylation of lysine and proline.
      (2) Symptoms include:
         (a) Delayed wound healing.
         (b) Petechiae and ecchymosis.
         (c) Gingival bleeding, swelling, and ulcerations.
3. Platelet abnormalities
   a. Thrombocytopenia
      (1) Characterized by a decreased number of platelets.
      (2) The most common type of bleeding disorder.
      (3) Can be caused by a number of diseases, such as irradiation, acute leukemia, disseminated intravascular coagulation (DIC), or idiopathic thrombocytopenic purpura (ITP).
   b. Thrombocytopenic purpura
      (1) Idiopathic: An autoimmune disease characterized by the presence of autoantibodies against platelets, resulting in the removal of platelets by splenic macrophages.
      (2) May also be drug-induced.

B. Disorders of secondary hemostasis
1. General characteristics of disorders of secondary hemostasis (due to problems with clotting factors):
   a. Symptoms occur later in life.
   b. As compared to disorders of primary hemostasis, bleeding occurs in deeper areas and larger vessels (i.e., joint spaces).
   c. Laboratory findings include abnormal:
      (1) Partial thromboplastin time (PTT)—measures the intrinsic and common clotting pathway (i.e., tests all coagulation factors except factor 7).
      (2) Prothrombin time (PT)—measures the extrinsic pathway.
      (3) Does not affect the bleeding time.
2. Hemophilia
   a. Caused by a deficiency of particular clotting factor(s).
   b. All types of hemophilia affect the intrinsic pathway of the clotting cascade.
   c. Signs and symptoms include:
      (1) Prolonged PTT.
      (2) Continuous bleeding from cuts or trauma, which can lead to excessive blood loss.
      (3) Bleeding into joint cavities (hemarthroses) and muscle.
   d. Two types:
      (1) Hemophilia A (classic hemophilia)
         (a) Caused by a deficiency of factor 8 (antihemophilic factor).
         (b) Transmission: sex-linked recessive—only occurs in males; however, females can be carriers.
      (2) Hemophilia B (Christmas disease)
         (a) Caused by a deficiency of factor 9 (plasma thromboplastin).
         (b) Transmission: sex-linked recessive—only occurs in males; however, females can be carriers.
         (c) Lower incidence rate than hemophilia A.
3. Vitamin K deficiency
   a. Causes include malnutrition and malabsorption of fats.
   b. A decrease in clotting factors 2, 7, 9, and 10 and prothrombin is observed.
   c. Prolonged PT.

C. Disorders of both primary and secondary hemostasis
1. von Willebrand's disease
   a. Characterized by a defective von Willebrand's factor (vWF). Defective vWF affects both primary hemostasis by affecting platelet adhesion to endothelium, and secondary hemostasis, by a defective factor 8.
   b. Genetic transmission: autosomal dominant. It is the most common hereditary bleeding disorder.
2. Liver disease—disease of the liver results in a decreased production of coagulation factors and therefore can lead to problems with hemostasis.

3. Disseminated intravascular coagulation—a condition in which clots form throughout the vasculature. This uses up all available clotting factors and platelets, resulting in problems with bleeding.

4.6 Lymphoproliferative Diseases

4.6.1 Leukemia

A. General characteristics
   1. Leukemia is characterized by the uncontrolled proliferation of an abnormal, monoclonal cell. The bone marrow and peripheral blood become saturated with blasts or blast-like cells, which results in a decreased production of normal RBCs, WBCs, and platelets in the bone marrow.
   2. General signs and symptoms:
      a. Recurrent infections secondary to a decreased numbers of normal WBC production.
      b. Severe anemia, pallor, and fatigue secondary to a decrease in RBC production.
      c. Bleeding problems secondary to a decreased platelet production, which exhibits signs such as petechiae.
   3. Uncontrolled growth of leukemic cells causes leukocytosis and accumulation of leukemic cells in other organs, including the spleen (splenomegaly), liver (hepatomegaly), and lymph nodes (lymphadenopathy).
   4. Oral manifestations:
      a. Spontaneous bleeding from mucous membranes.
      b. Gingival hyperplasia (Box 3-2).
      c. Mucosal ulcerations.

B. Acute leukemias
   1. General characteristics
      a. Rapid onset of symptoms occur most often in children or patients older than 60.
      b. Consists of proliferation of immature blast cells.

Box 3–2. Causes of Gingival Hyperplasia

1. Lymphoproliferative diseases
2. Medications, such as:
   Calcium channel blockers
   Phenytoin (Dilantin)
   Cyclosporin

   2. Signs and symptoms:
      a. Constitutional symptoms: fever, weakness, fatigue.
      b. Pallor from severe anemia.
      c. Bone and joint pain.
      d. Lymphadenopathy—enlarged lymph nodes.
   3. Acute lymphocytic or lymphoblastic leukemia
      a. Predominantly occurs in children.
      b. Most common malignancy in children.
      c. Blood smear: lymphoblasts appear as null cells.
      d. Prognosis is good with high cure rates.
   4. Acute myelogenous leukemia
      a. Mostly occurs in adults.
      b. Most malignant leukemia (responds poorly to therapy).
      c. Blood smear: Auer rods may be observed in blast cells.

C. Chronic leukemias
   1. General characteristics
      a. Consists of proliferation of mature cells (differentiated cells).
      b. Usually less severe than the acute form.
      c. Signs and symptoms are similar to those found in acute leukemia, except for a slower and more gradual onset. Weight loss is common.
   2. Chronic myelogenous leukemia
      a. Characterized by the proliferation of myeloid cells (precursor cells of erythrocytes, granulocytes, and platelets).
      b. Associated with the Philadelphia chromosome, which results from translocation of chromosomes 9 and 22.
      c. Signs and symptoms include prominent splenomegaly and modestly enlarged liver and lymph nodes.
      d. Occurs during middle age.
   3. Chronic lymphocytic leukemia
      a. The most common leukemia.
      b. Least malignant type of leukemia.
      c. Characterized by the proliferation of abnormal B lymphocytes, which cannot produce antibodies. The patient is more susceptible to bacterial infections.
      d. Mostly seen in older adults (> 60).
      e. Blood smear: lymphoblasts may appear as smudge cells.

4.6.2 Lymphomas

A. Hodgkin's disease
   1. Characterized by enlarged lymph nodes and the presence of Reed-Sternberg cells

(multinucleated giant cells) in lymphoid tissues.

2. Disease spreads from lymph node to lymph node in a contiguous manner.
3. Enlarged cervical lymph nodes are most commonly the first lymphadenopathy observed.
4. The cause is unknown.
5. Occurs before age 30.
6. Prognosis of disease depends largely on the extent of lymph node spread and systemic involvement.

B. Non-Hodgkin's lymphoma
1. Characterized by tumor formation in the lymph nodes.
2. Tumors do *not* spread in a contiguous manner.
3. Most often caused by the proliferation of abnormal B cells.
4. Occurs after age 40.
5. Example: Burkitt's lymphoma
   a. Commonly associated with an Epstein-Barr virus (EBV) infection and a genetic mutation resulting from the translocation of the *C-myc* gene from chromosome 8 to 14.
   b. The African type occurs in African children and commonly affects the mandible or maxilla.
   c. In the United States, it most commonly affects the abdomen.
   d. Histologically, the tumor displays a characteristic "starry-sky" appearance.

4.7 Plasma Cell Pathology

A. Multiple myeloma
1. Plasma cell neoplasm that results in the proliferation of monoclonal plasma cells. These tumor cells produce nonfunctional immunoglobulins.
2. Laboratory findings include:
   a. Monoclonal IgG spike.
   b. Bence-Jones proteins found in urine.
3. Radiographic findings: characteristic "punched-out" radiolucencies in bones.

4.8 Endocrine

A. Thyroid pathology
1. Hypothyroidism
   a. General signs and symptoms:
      (1) A decreased metabolism, resulting in weight gain and retarded growth.
      (2) Enlarged face, tongue, eyelids, larynx, and hands.
      (3) Mental and physical slowness.
      (4) Decreased heart rate.
      (5) Sensitivity to cold temperature.
      (6) Goiter.
   b. Clinical manifestations:
      (1) Hashimoto's thyroiditis—an autoimmune disease in which antibodies attack the thyroid gland, causing direct injury to the thyroid.
      (2) Myxedema—hypothyroidism in adults.
         (a) Most commonly caused by treatment for hyperthyroidism such as surgery, irradiation, or drug therapy.
         (b) Iodine deficiency.
      (3) Cretinism—hypothyroidism in children.
         (a) Causes include embryologic malformation and iodine deficiency.
         (b) Clinical findings include mental retardation and dwarfism.
         (c) Oral findings include macroglossia, prolonged retention of primary teeth, and delayed eruption of permanent teeth.
2. Hyperthyroidism (thyrotoxicosis)
   a. General signs and symptoms:
      (1) Increased metabolism, resulting in weight loss.
      (2) Irritability, nervousness, and tremor.
      (3) Tachycardia, often with arrhythmia and palpitation.
      (4) Goiter.
      (5) Oral findings include early loss of primary teeth and early eruption of permanent teeth.
   b. Clinical manifestations:
      (1) Graves' disease
         (a) An autoimmune disease in which antibodies bind to the thyroid-stimulating hormone (TSH) receptor, resulting in constant stimulation for the release of triiodothyronine (T3) and thyroxine (T4).
         (b) General signs include exophthalmos or protrusion of eyeballs.

(2) Plummer's disease
(a) May be caused by a nodular growth or adenoma of the thyroid.
(b) Clinical signs are similar to Graves' disease, except no exophthalmos is present.

c. Dental significance: caution is required when administering anesthesia with epinephrine to patients with uncontrolled or undiagnosed hyperthyroidism. Epinephrine may cause the patient to develop a thyrotoxic crisis.

B. Parathyroid pathology
1. Hyperparathyroidism
a. General characteristics include:
(1) Hypercalcemia—high levels of serum calcium.
(2) Hypophosphatemia—low levels of serum phosphate.
(3) Increased alkaline phosphatase (Box 3-3).
(4) Osseous changes, including:
(a) Extensive loss of bone density.
(b) Metastatic calcifications.
(c) Kidney stones.
(5) Radiographic findings of bone include a "ground glass" appearance.
b. Clinical manifestations:
(1) Primary hyperparathyroidism—most commonly caused by a parathyroid adenoma.
(2) Secondary hyperparathyroidism—usually occurs as a result of chronic renal disease or kidney failure. During renal disease, active vitamin D is not produced, leading to low levels of calcium being absorbed from the intestinal tract. This low level of calcium chronically activates the parathyroid to release the parathyroid hormone (PTH), resulting in hyperparathyroidism.

2. Hypoparathyroidism
a. Most commonly caused by accidental surgical removal of the parathyroid gland during thyroid surgery.
b. May be associated with DiGeorge's syndrome, but this is rare.
c. General findings:
(1) Hypocalcemia or low levels of serum calcium.
(2) Increased neuromuscular excitability and tetany due to hypocalcemia.

C. Pituitary gland pathology
1. Growth hormone (GH) deficiency
a. Causes of a decreased level of GH include:
(1) Decreased secretion of growth hormone-releasing hormone (GHRH) from the hypothalamus.
(2) Decreased secretion of GH from the anterior pituitary, also known as *pituitary dwarfism*.
(3) Decreased response of cells to GH.
b. Clinical manifestation: dwarfism
(1) General signs and symptoms include:
(a) Abnormally short height (failure to thrive).
(b) Smaller maxilla and mandible.
(c) Delayed eruption of permanent teeth.

2. Excessive production of growth hormone
a. Gigantism
(1) Occurs if the increase in GH occurs before the epiphyseal plates have fused.
(2) Clinical signs include abnormally tall height, enlarged mandible.
b. Acromegaly
(1) Occurs if the increase in GH occurs after the epiphyseal plates have fused.
(2) Clinical signs include gradual enlargement of the hands, feet, and skull. Patients may find that shoes, gloves, dentures, and such have become too small.

3. Diabetes insipidus
a. Characterized by a deficiency of antidiuretic hormone (ADH).
b. Symptoms include polyuria and polydipsia.

4. Sheehan's disease

Box 3–3. Diseases that Can Cause an Increase in Alkaline Phosphatase

Hyperparathyroidism
Paget's disease
Osteosarcoma
Multiple myeloma
Prostate cancer

a. Characterized by the lack of anterior pituitary functioning, resulting in a decreased secretion of follicle-stimulating hormone (FSH), luteinizing hormone (LH), TSH, adrenocorticotropic hormone (ACTH), and so forth.
b. Caused by necrosis of the anterior pituitary after a complicated childbirth.

D. Adrenal (suprarenal) gland pathology
1. Adrenal medulla pathology
a. Pheochromocytoma
(1) A benign tumor formed from adrenal chromaffin cells. Ten percent become malignant. Note: if the adrenal tumor is formed from extra-adrenal chromaffin cells, it is known as a *paraganglioma*.
(2) Tumor secretions result in increased epinephrine and norepinephrine.
(3) Associated syndromes include Sturge-Weber syndrome and multiple endocrine neoplasia (MEN) type IIa and type IIb.
(4) General signs and symptoms include:
(a) Secondary hypertension.
(b) Increased heart rate, palpitations.
b. Neuroblastoma
(1) A malignant catecholamine-producing tumor formed from immature medullary cells.
(2) Most common malignant tumor found in children.
(3) Tumor secretions result in increased epinephrine and norepinephrine.
(4) Characterized by amplification of the *N-myc* oncogene.
2. Adrenal cortex pathology
a. Addison's disease—primary adrenocortical deficiency
(1) Characterized by a decrease in steroid hormone secretion by the adrenal cortex. This results in an increase in production of ACTH from the anterior pituitary. (Another form of Addison's disease is due to abnormally low secretory rates of ACTH.)
(2) Clinical findings from decreased cortisol production include:
(a) Darker pigmentation in certain areas (e.g., skin, mucosa) results from increased secretion of melanin by melanocyte that are stimulated by melanocytes-stimulating hormone (MSH). The increased levels of MSH result from an increased ACTH production.
(b) Poor response to stress.
(c) Anemias, GI disturbances, hypotension, and weakness.
(3) Oral findings include dark pigmentation on the tongue, palate, gingiva, and mucosa.
(4) Treatment: cortisol or other steroid therapy.
b. Cushing's disease—refer to Pituitary Gland Pathology.

E. Endocrine pancreas pathology—diabetes mellitus
1. General characteristics of diabetes mellitus
a. Characterized by hyperglycemia (abnormally high levels of blood glucose).
b. Hallmark symptoms:
(1) Polyuria—frequent urination.
(2) Polydipsia—constant thirst.
(3) Polyphagia—frequent intake of food.
c. Complications include:
(1) Retinopathy.
(2) Nephropathy.
(3) Peripheral neuropathy.
(4) Cardiovascular disease—leading cause of death for diabetic patients.
(5) Oral complications of uncontrolled diabetes include:
(a) Increased periodontal disease.
(b) Increased susceptibility to *Candidiasis*.
2. Two types of diabetes mellitus:
a. Type I diabetes.
(1) Also known as juvenile-onset or insulin-dependent diabetes mellitus (IDDM).
(2) Caused by autoimmune destruction of pancreatic β-cells, resulting in a complete absence of insulin production.
(3) The disease usually presents before the age of 25.
(4) Characterized by severe hyperglycemia and ketoacidosis (ketoacidosis is uncommon in noninsulin-dependent diabetes [NIDDM] patients). Untreated

ketoacidosis may result in diabetic coma.

(5) Treatment: requires insulin and diet control.

b. Type II diabetes

(1) Also known as adult-onset or NIDDM.

(2) Caused by a decreased sensitivity of peripheral insulin receptors to insulin, insulin receptor dysfunction, or a decreased production of insulin. Unlike in IDDM, insulin is still produced.

(3) Occurs later in life, usually after the age of 40.

(4) Is commonly seen in obese patients.

(5) It is more prevalent than IDDM.

(6) Treatment: diet control. May or may not require insulin or other hypoglycemic agent (e.g., glucophage and glyburide).

3. Diabetic shock—seen in patients who do not consume enough carbohydrates following an insulin injection. This results in an abnormally low level of glucose in the blood.

4.9 Musculoskeletal

A. Bone pathology

1. Osteoporosis

a. Characterized by a decrease in bone mass.

b. Causes include:

(1) A change in serum calcium/phosphorus or vitamin D that may result from an endocrine (parathyroid) disorder.

(2) A decreased level of estrogen, leading to increased bone loss. This condition is also known as *postmenopausal osteoporosis*.

(3) Physical inactivity.

(4) Hypercorticism.

(5) Hyperthyroidism.

c. Complications include compression fractures, which commonly occur.

2. Vitamin D deficiency

a. Vitamin D deficiency results in the failure of new bone to mineralize, leading to abnormal growth of epiphyseal plates and growth retardation.

b. Two types:

(1) Osteomalacia—vitamin D deficiency in adults. Characterized by defective calcification of osteoid matrix.

(2) Rickets—vitamin D deficiency in infants and children. Characterized by inadequate calcification and increased thickness in epiphyseal growth plates, resulting in skeletal deformities.

c. Oral findings include:

(1) A delayed eruption of teeth.

(2) Abnormal formation of dentin.

3. Scurvy

a. Caused by vitamin C (ascorbic acid) deficiency, leading to impaired osteoid matrix formation.

b. Clinical findings include:

(1) Subperiosteal hemorrhage.

(2) Osteoporosis.

(3) Note: the epiphyseal cartilage is not replaced by osteoid.

4. Osteogenesis imperfecta ("brittle bone" disease)

a. Caused by the defective formation of type I collagen.

b. Characterized by fragile (brittle) bones and a deformed skeleton.

c. Symptoms include fractures and blue ocular sclerae.

d. Oral findings include dentinogenesis imperfecta.

5. Osteopetrosis (Albers-Schönberg disease or marble bone disease)

a. Caused by abnormal osteoclasts. This results in defective bone remodeling (i.e., abnormally low bone resorption) and increased bone density, which may invade into bone marrow space.

b. Causes severe defects in infants, including:

(1) Anemia and infections—caused by decreased bone marrow.

(2) Blindness, deafness, paralysis of facial muscles—caused by the narrowing of cranial nerve foramina.

(3) Is life-threatening.

(4) Oral findings include delayed eruption of teeth.

c. Disease is less severe in adults

6. Paget's disease (osteitis deformans)

a. Characterized by abnormal bone remodeling leading to distortion of bone architecture.

b. Laboratory findings include increased serum alkaline phosphatase.
c. Radiographic findings include a characteristic "cotton wool" appearance.
d. Complications include:
(1) Osteosarcoma.
(2) Fractures.
(3) Heart disease.
(4) Deafness or blindness.
e. Oral findings include:
(1) Development of spaces between teeth.
(2) Common complaint of edentulous patients is that "dentures no longer fit!"

7. Osteomyelitis
a. An infection of bone.
b. Most commonly caused by *Staphylococcus aureus* and streptococci.
c. Clinical findings include pain and systemic signs of infection (i.e., fever, malaise).

8. Fibrous dysplasia
a. Caused by replacement of normal bone with an irregular bone containing fibrous connective tissue.
b. Radiographic findings include a characteristic "ground glass" appearance.
c. Three types:
(1) Monostotic—affects one bone (most common). Usually asymptomatic.
(2) Polyostotic (Jaffe type)—affects more than one bone.
(3) McCune-Albright's syndrome—polyostotic fibrous dysplasia with other systemic manifestations, including café au lait spots (brown macules) and endocrine abnormalities such as precocious puberty.

9. Osteochondroses
a. Most often caused by osteonecrosis of the epiphyseal plates or the ossification centers in bone. This results in the reossification and sclerosis of the affected areas.
b. Occurs in children and adolescents; most commonly in adolescent boys who play sports.
c. Clinical manifestations include:
(1) Legg-Calvé-Perthes disease—affects epiphyseal plates of the femur.
(2) Osgood-Schlatter disease—affects tibial tuberosity (i.e., knee).
(3) Scheuermann's disease—affects vertebral endplates.

10. Langerhans cell granulomatosis (histocytosis X)
a. A group of diseases that are caused by the proliferation of Langerhans' cells (previously known as *histocytes*).
b. Most commonly causes bone lesions; however, other tissues can be affected.
c. Histologic findings include Langerhans' cells containing Birbeck granules and eosinophils.
d. Three types:
(1) Letterer-Siwe disease—an acute, disseminated form that is fatal in infants.
(2) Hand-Schüller-Christian disease—a chronic, disseminated form that has a better prognosis than Letterer-Siwe disease. It usually presents before the age of 5 and is characterized by a triad of symptoms:
(a) Bone lesions—found in skull, mandible (loose teeth).
(b) Exophthalmos.
(c) Diabetes insipidus.
(3) Eosinophilic granuloma of bone—a localized, least severe form of the three. Lesions may heal without treatment.
(a) Most commonly occurs in young adults.
(b) Lesions in the mandible may cause loose teeth.

B. Bone malignancies
1. Osteosarcoma (osteogenic sarcoma)
a. Most common true primary bone tumor. Note: the most common bone tumor is metastatic carcinoma. The most common primary bone tumor is multiple myeloma.
b. Findings include an increased serum alkaline phosphatase and radiographic observation of Codman's triangle (lifting of the periosteum by the tumor).
c. Occurs in children and adolescents.
2. Ewing's sarcoma
a. Extremely anaplastic, small-cell malignant tumor.
b. Commonly found in long bones (femur) or pelvis.

c. Usually occurs before age 20.
d. Symptoms include intermittent pain, fever, and swelling.

C. Cartilage pathology
1. Achondroplasia
a. Caused by delayed or abnormal growth of cartilage, leading to a shortened bone growth (skeleton).
b. Characterized by short stature (dwarfism) with shortened extremities.
c. Oral findings include mandibular prognathism.
2. Osteochondroma
a. Bony growths surrounded by cartilage.
b. The most common benign tumor of the bone.
c. Usually occurs before age 30.
d. Most often found at the distal ends of long bones.
3. Chondrosarcoma
a. A malignant cartilaginous tumor.
b. Peak incidence occurs in men aged 30 to 60.
c. The second most common primary bone tumor occuring in bone, excluding multiple myeloma. Osteosarcoma is the most common.
d. Sites of origin usually include the pelvis, spine, scapula, or femur.

D. Joint pathology
1. Rheumatoid arthritis
a. Cause is autoimmune in nature.
b. More common in women aged 20 to 50.
c. Characterized by inflammation of the synovial membrane. Granulation tissue, known as *pannus*, will form in the synovium and expand over the articular cartilage. This causes the destruction of the underlying cartilage and results in fibrotic changes and ankylosis. Scarring, contracture, and deformity of the joints may occur.
d. Clinical symptoms include swollen joints. It can affect any joint in the body.
2. Osteoarthritis
a. Most common arthritis.
b. Cause is unknown.
c. Higher incidence in women, usually after age 50.
d. Characterized by degeneration of the articular cartilage and the formation of osteophytes (bony spurs) at the margins of affected areas.
e. Clinical signs and symptoms include:
(1) Stiff and painful joints affecting joints in the hand (phalangeal joints) and weight-bearing joints.
(2) Heberden's nodes—nodules at the distal interphalangeal joint.
(3) Bocard's nodes—nodules at the proximal interphalangeal joint.

E. Muscle pathology
1. Myasthenia gravis
a. An autoimmune disease caused by autoantibodies to acetylcholine receptors at the neuromuscular junctions.
b. Characterized by muscle weakness or the inability to maintain long durations of muscle contractions; this worsens during exercise but recovers after rest.
c. Affects various muscle groups, including:
(1) Eyes—diplopia, ptosis.
(2) Neck—dysphagia, problems swallowing or speaking.
(3) Extremities—arms and legs.
d. Treatment: cholinesterase inhibitors (neostigmine), anti-immune therapy.
2. Muscle tumors
a. Rhabdomyoma—benign tumor of skeletal muscle.
b. Leiomyoma
(1) Benign tumor of smooth muscle.
(2) Most common tumor found in women.
(3) Usually affects the uterus, although it can occur anywhere.
c. Rhabdomyosarcoma
(1) Malignant tumor of skeletal muscle.
(2) Most common sarcoma found in children.
(3) Usually affects head and neck region—orbit, nasal cavity, and nasopharynx.

4.10 Skin Pathology

4.10.1 Skin Lesions

A. Seborrheic keratosis
1. A round, brown-colored, flat wart.
2. Most often seen in middle-aged to older adults.
3. A benign lesion.

B. Verruca vulgaris
1. Commonly known as *warts*.
2. Caused by the human papillomavirus (HPV).

3. Warts can be seen on skin or as an oral lesion (vermilion border, oral mucosa, or tongue).
4. Transmitted by contact or autoinoculation.
5. A benign lesion.

C. Actinic keratosis
1. Dry, scaly plaques with an erythematous base.
2. Similar to actinic cheilosis, which occurs along the vermilion border of the lower lip.
3. Caused by sun damage to the skin.
4. Dysplastic lesion, may be premalignant.

D. Nevus
1. Commonly known as *moles*.
2. A benign, pigmented tumor of melanocytes, found deep within connective tissue.
3. Types of skin nevi:
   a. Junctional nevus—found in the epidermis. It is the only type of nevus that may be considered to be premalignant.
   b. Compound nevus—found in both the epidermis and underlying dermis.
   c. Intraepidermal nevus—found in the dermis.

E. Psoriasis
1. Characterized by skin lesions that appear as scaly, white plaques.
2. Caused by rapid proliferation of the epidermis.
3. Autoimmune pathogenesis; exact mechanism is unclear.

F. Keloids
1. Characterized by a progressively enlarging scar.
2. Caused by an abnormal accumulation of collagen at the site of injury.
3. More common in African-Americans.

4.10.2 Skin Diseases with Oral Manifestations

A. Erythema multiforme
1. Erythematous, ulcerative lesions on the skin and oral mucosa.
2. Skin lesions are round and have a bull's-eye or target-like appearance.
3. Can be caused from an allergic reaction.
4. In severe cases, known as Stevens-Johnson syndrome, lesions are seen on the skin, oral mucosa, eye, and genital area.
5. Treatment: corticosteroids in severe cases.

B. Pemphigus
1. Ulcerative lesions on the skin and oral mucosa.
2. An autoimmune disease in which patients have autoantibodies against hemidemosomal attachment of epidermis cells.
3. Histologically characterized by acantholysis, in which epidermal cells appear to detach and separate from each other, as seen by Tzanck smears.
4. Can be life-threatening if untreated.
5. A positive Nikolsky sign is observed. Because of sloughing of the epidermis, a red blister forms after pressure is applied to affected skin.
6. Treatment: corticosteroids.

C. Pemphigoid
1. Ulcerative lesions on the skin and oral mucosa.
2. An autoimmune disease in which patients have autoantibodies against basal cells (desmosome attachment to the basement membrane).
3. Histologically, the entire epithelium appears to separate from the connective tissue. There is no acantholysis.
4. A positive Nikolsky sign is observed.
5. Complications include blindness, due to ocular lesions present in some patients.
6. Treatment: corticosteroids.

D. Lichen planus
1. Skin lesions appear as a cluster of purple-colored papules. Oral lesions are characterized by intersecting white lines known as *Wickham's striae*, most often seen along the buccal mucosa.
2. Histologically characterized by saw-tooth rete ridges and the presence of Civatte bodies.
3. It is generally self-limiting and resolves spontaneously 1 to 2 years after onset; however, the oral lesions may persist for years.

E. Peutz-Jeghers syndrome
1. Lesions appear as small, melanotic, and freckle-like. They can be found on the skin, oral mucosa, lips, feet, and hands.
2. May also present with intestinal polyps, which may develop into a gastrointestinal carcinoma.
3. Genetic transmission: autosomal dominant.

4.11 Genetic Diseases

A. Lysosomal (lipid) storage diseases
1. Genetic transmission: autosomal recessive.
2. This group of diseases is characterized by a deficiency of a particular lysosomal

enzyme. This results in an accumulation of the metabolite, which would have otherwise been degraded by the presence of normal levels of this specific enzyme.

3. Diseases include:
   a. Gaucher's disease
      (1) Deficient enzyme: glucocerebrosidase.
      (2) Metabolite that accumulates: glucocerebroside.
      (3) Important cells affected: macrophages.
   b. Tay-Sachs disease
      (1) Deficient enzyme: hexosaminidase A.
      (2) Metabolite that accumulates: G_{M2} ganglioside.
      (3) Important cells affected: neurons.
      (4) Symptoms include motor and mental deterioration, blindness, and dementia.
      (5) Common in the Ashkenazi Jews.
   c. Niemann-Pick disease
      (1) Deficient enzyme: sphingomyelinase.
      (2) Metabolite that accumulates: sphingomyelin.
      (3) Important cells affected: neurons.

B. Glycogen storage diseases (glycogenoses)
   1. Genetic transmission: autosomal recessive.
   2. This group of diseases is characterized by a deficiency of a particular enzyme involved in either glycogen production or degradative pathways.
   3. Diseases include:
      (1) von Gierke disease (type I)
         (a) Deficient enzyme: glucose-6-phosphatase.
         (b) Major organ affected by the buildup of glycogen: liver.
      b. Pompe disease (type II)
         (1) Deficient enzyme: α-glucosidase (acid maltase).
         (2) Major organ affected by the buildup of glycogen: heart.
      c. Cori disease (type III)
         (1) Deficient enzyme: debranching enzyme (amylo-1,6-glucosidase).
         (2) Organs affected by the buildup of glycogen: varies between the heart, liver, or skeletal muscle.
      d. Brancher glycogenosis (type IV)
         (1) Deficient enzyme: branching enzyme.
         (2) Organs affected by the buildup of glycogen: liver, heart, skeletal muscle, and brain.
      e. McArdle syndrome (type V)
         (1) Deficient enzyme: muscle phosphorylase.
         (2) Major organ affected by the buildup of glycogen: skeletal muscle.

C. Connective tissue diseases
   1. Marfan's syndrome
      a. Genetic transmission: autosomal dominant.
      b. Characterized by a defective microfibril glycoprotein, fibrillin.
      c. Clinical findings include tall stature, joints that can be hyperextended, and cardiovascular defects, including mitral valve prolapse and dilation of the ascending aorta.
   2. Ehlers-Danlos syndrome
      a. Genetic transmission: autosomal dominant or recessive.
      b. This group of diseases is characterized by defects in collagen.
      c. Clinical findings include hypermobile joints and highly stretchable skin. The skin also bruises easily. Oral findings include Gorlin's sign and possible temporomandibular joint (TMJ) subluxation. The oral mucosa may also appear more fragile and vulnerable to trauma.

D. Birth defects and chromosome abnormalities
   1. General chromosome abnormalities
      a. The normal human cell contains 46 chromosomes, including 22 homologous pairs of autosomes and one pair of sex chromosomes (XX for female and XY for male). A somatic cell is diploid, containing 46 chromosomes. Gametes are haploid, containing 23 chromosomes.
         (1) Aneuploidy
            (a) Any deviation in the number of chromosomes, whether fewer or more, from the normal haploid number of chromosomes.
            (b) Nondisjunction—a common cause of aneuploidy. It is the failure of chromosomes to pass to separate cells during meiotic or mitotic cell division.
            (c) Often seen in malignant tumors.
         (2) Deletion: loss of a sequence of DNA from a chromosome.

(3) Translocation: the separation of a chromosome and the attachment of the area of separation to another chromosome.

2. Abnormalities in chromosome number
   a. Trisomy 21 (Down syndrome)
      (1) The most common chromosomal disorder.
      (2) A disorder affecting autosomes. It is generally caused by meiotic nondisjunction in the mother, which results in an extra copy of chromosome 21 or trisomy 21.
      (3) Risk increases with maternal age.
      (4) Clinical findings include mental retardation and congenital heart defects. There is also an increased risk of developing acute leukemia and an increased susceptibility to severe infections.
      (5) Oral findings include macroglossia, delayed eruption of teeth, and hypodontia.
   b. Trisomies 18 and 13
      (1) Trisomy 18 (Edwards syndrome): characterized by an extra copy of chromosome 18. Oral findings include micrognathia.
      (2) Trisomy 13 (Patau's syndrome): characterized by an extra copy of chromosome 13. Oral findings include cleft lip and palate.
      (3) Meiotic nondisjunction is usually the cause of an extra chromosome in both of these trisomies.
      (4) Clinical findings for both of these trisomies are usually more severe than trisomy 21. Most children with these diseases die within months after being born due to manifestations such as congenital heart disease.
   c. Klinefelter's syndrome
      (1) One of the most common causes of male hypogonadism.
      (2) Characterized by two or more X chromosomes and one or more Y chromosomes. Typically, there are 47 chromosomes with the karyotype of XXY.
      (3) The cause is usually from meiotic nondisjunction.
      (4) Clinical findings include atrophic and underdeveloped testes, gynecomastia, tall stature, and a lower IQ.
   d. Turner's syndrome
      (1) One of the most important causes of amenorrhea.
      (2) Characterized by having only one X chromosome, with a total of 45 chromosomes and a karyotype of XO.
      (3) Clinical findings include underdeveloped female genitalia, short stature, webbed neck, and amenorrhea. Affected females are usually sterile. Unlike other chromosomal disorders, this one is usually not complicated by mental retardation.
   e. Treacher Collins syndrome (mandibulofacial dysostosis)
      (1) Genetic transmission: autosomal dominant.
      (2) A relatively rare disease that results from abnormal development of derivatives from the first and second branchial arches.
      (3) Clinical findings include underdeveloped zygomas and mandible and deformed ears. Oral findings include cleft palate and small or absent parotid glands.

4.12 Nervous System

4.12.1 Infections

A. Bacterial meningitis (pyogenic, suppurative infections)
   1. Common causes include:
      a. *Escherichia coli* in newborns.
      b. *Haemophilus influenzae* in infants and children.
      c. *Neisseria meningitides* in young adults.
      d. *Streptococcus pneumoniae* and *Listeria monocytogenes* in older adults.
   2. Clinical findings include severe headache, irritability, fever, and a stiff neck.
      a. A spinal tap shows CSF fluid that is cloudy or purulent and is under increased pressure. There is also an increase in protein and a decrease in glucose levels.
   3. Can be fatal if left untreated.

B. Viral meningitis
   1. Can be caused by many different viruses, including cytomegalovirus, herpes virus, rabies, and HIV.
   2. CSF fluid from a spinal tap differs from that seen in a bacterial infection. It shows

mononuclear cells, higher levels of protein, and normal levels of glucose.

C. Demyelinating and degenerative diseases
   1. Multiple sclerosis
      a. A demyelinating disease that primarily affects myelin (i.e. white matter). This affects the conduction of electrical impulses along the axons of nerves. Areas of demyelination are known as *plaques*.
      b. The most common demyelinating disease.
      c. Onset of disease usually occurs between ages 20 and 50; slightly more common in women.
      d. Disease can affect any neuron in the central nervous system, including the brainstem and spinal cord. The optic nerve (vision) is commonly affected.
   2. Amyotrophic lateral sclerosis (Lou Gehrig's disease)
      a. Characterized by the rapid degeneration of motor neurons in the spinal cord and corticospinal tracts.
      b. More common in men in their 50s.
      c. Clinically, the disease results in rapidly progressive muscle atrophy due to denervation. Other symptoms include fasciculations, hyperreflexia, spasticity, and pathologic reflexes. Death usually occurs within a few years from onset, usually by respiratory failure or infection.
   3. Alzheimer's disease
      a. The most common cause of dementia in older people.
      b. Characterized by degeneration of neurons in the cerebral cortex.
      c. Histologic findings include amyloid plaques and neurofibrillary tangles.
      d. Clinically, the disease takes years to develop and results in the loss of cognition, memory, and the ability to communicate. Motor problems, contractures, and paralysis are some of the symptoms at the terminal stage.
   4. Parkinson's disease
      a. Characterized by the degeneration of neurons in the basal ganglia, specifically the substantia nigra and striatum.
      b. Histologic findings in affected neurons include Lewy bodies.
      c. Clinically, the disease affects involuntary and voluntary movements. Tremors are common. Symptoms include pin-rolling tremors, slowness of movements, muscular rigidity, and shuffling gait.
   5. Huntington's disease
      a. Causes dementia.
      b. Genetic transmission: autosomal dominant.
      c. Characterized by the degeneration of striatal neurons, affecting cortical and basal ganglia function.
      d. Clinically, the disease affects both movement and cognition and is ultimately fatal.

5.0 GROWTH DISTURBANCES

5.1 Neoplasms—Etiology, Epidemiology, and Biology

A. Neoplasms are new and abnormal growths in which cell multiplication is uncontrolled and progressive. These tumors can be benign or malignant.

B. Benign versus malignant tumors
   1. Malignant neoplasms (cancer) are invasive (able to infiltrate past the basement membrane into adjacent tissues) and are able to metastasize to other related or nonrelated parts of the body. Benign tumors are self-limiting, expansive, noninvasive tumors that do not metastasize. They can, however, be harmful if their growth impinges on surrounding structures. Generally, the names of tumors end with "oma."
   2. Benign tumors—general characteristics:
      a. Rate of growth: slow. Regression of the lesion is possible.
      b. Are usually surrounded by a capsule made of condensed connective tissue.
      c. It is uncommon for them to recur after surgical resection.
      d. Histologic features:
         (1) Are highly differentiated cells that resemble normal cells.
         (2) Contain small nuclei.
         (3) Low nuclear–cytoplasmic ratio.
         (4) Low mitotic activity.
   3. Malignant tumors—general characteristics:
      a. Nomenclature: malignant neoplasms are named according to their presumed cellular origin and their histologic appearance. For example, a tumor of epithelial origin (carcinoma) that is observed in a glandular growth pattern is called an *adenocarcinoma*.
      b. General names of malignant tumors:

(1) Carcinoma—develops from epithelial cells.
(2) Sarcoma—develops from mesenchymal cells.
(3) Lymphoma—develops from lymphoid cells.
(4) Teratoma—develops from all three developmental germ layers.

c. Rate of growth varies from slow to rapid.
d. There is no distinct capsule.
e. May recur after surgical resection.
f. Histologic features:

(1) Anaplasia—there is a loss of differentiation in these cells.
(2) Pleomorphism—cells and their nuclei can appear in various forms and shapes.
(3) Karyomegaly—contain large nuclei.
(4) Hyperchromatism—dark staining nuclei.
(5) High nuclear–cytoplasmic ratio.
(6) High mitotic activity.
(7) May be aneuploidy (have an abnormal number of chromosomes).

C. Premalignant tumors—noninvasive neoplasms that may carry a risk for developing into a malignant cancer.

1. Dysplasia—considered a cancer precursor wherein cells appear abnormal in appearance and organization, although the risk of developing into a malignant tumor varies. In other words, it is a lesion with the potential to invade, but has not yet invaded. It can be reversible.
2. Hyperplasia—an abnormal increase in the number of normal cells that leads to the enlargement of an organ or tissue. Can be benign or malignant.
3. Metaplasia—when one type of adult tissue is replaced by another type of tissue.
4. Carcinoma in situ—when anaplastic cells are confined within the epithelium of origin. There is no invasion of the basement membrane. The likelihood of invasive growth is presumed to be high.

D. Carcinogenesis—both environmental and genetic factors may contribute to the formation of neoplasms.

1. Environmental factors include:

a. Geographic location—has been shown that where a person lives can affect the likelihood of developing certain types of cancer. For example, people living in Japan are eight times more likely to die of stomach cancer than people living in the United states.
b. Chemical factors—examples include smoking and asbestos.
c. Radiation—an example includes ultraviolet (UV) radiation from the sun, which increases risk for squamous cell carcinoma (SCC) and basal cell carcinoma (BCC).
d. Viral infections—example: links between HPV and cervical cancer, and hepatitis B and hepatocellular carcinoma.

2. Genetic factors—the genes that have been identified in neoplasms are all related to the regulation of normal cell proliferation. There are two types:

a. Oncogenes—genes that promote cell proliferation. This can result from:

(a) Point mutations—a gene mutation resulting from a change in a single base pair.
(b) Gene amplification—when extra copies of a chromosomal sequence are produced.
(c) Promoter insertion—insertion of a retroviral promoter into the host to increase gene expression.

b. Tumor suppressor genes—genes that encode for proteins whose normal function is to suppress cell proliferation. Mutations in these genes can inhibit these proteins, causing increased and uncontrolled cell proliferation. Possible causes of mutations in these genes include:

(a) Point mutations.
(b) Frameshift mutations—a deletion or insertion of genes that are not a multiple of three base pairs.
(c) Deletions—removal of a DNA sequence.
(d) Translocations—genes are duplicated at another location in the genome. Note: translocation of a chromosome involves the separation of a chromosome and the attachment of the area of breakage to another chromosome.

Specific neoplasms

For lymphoproliferative diseases and other neoplasms, refer to the specific sections in the systemic pathology section.

A. Oral cancer: squamous cell carcinoma
   1. SCC is the most common oral cancer, accounting for 90% of the cases. It is a tumor of keratinocytes.
   2. It carries a poor prognosis.
   3. Males are two times more likely to be affected than females, especially in men older than the age of 50.
   4. Metastasis of oral SCC most commonly spreads via the lymphatic system to the cervical lymph nodes.
   5. Risk factors include:
      a. Smoking or chewing tobacco.
      b. Excessive alcohol consumption.
      c. Nutritional deficiencies (iron, vitamin A).
   6. High-risk sites:
      a. Lower vermilion border of the lip—most common oral site.
      b. Lateral border and ventral surface of the tongue—most common intraoral site.
      c. Floor of the mouth.
      d. Soft palate.
      e. Tonsillar pillars.
      f. Buccal mucosa.

B. Skin cancer—the most common type of cancer in the United States.
   1. Squamous cell carcinoma
      a. A tumor of keratinocytes.
      b. Is related to sun-exposed skin, or UV radiation.
      c. Males are more commonly affected than females.
      d. Commonly occurs as an indurated, crusting ulcer with raised margins.
      e. Risk of metastasis is lower than intraoral SCC.
   2. Basal cell carcinoma (BCC)
      a. A tumor of basal cells.
      b. Involves sun-exposed areas, frequently the head and neck.
      c. Most common type of skin cancer.
      d. Carries a good prognosis because it metastasizes slowly.
      e. BCCs are seen in patients diagnosed with nevoid basal cell carcinoma syndrome (Gorlin-Goltz syndrome). This disease is characterized by the presence of BCCs, odontogenic keratocysts (OKCs), bone abnormalities, and calcifications of the cranium.
   3. Malignant melanoma
      a. A tumor of melanocytes.
      b. The most severe form of skin cancer.
      c. May appear intraorally, but these findings are rare.

C. Bronchogenic carcinoma (lung cancer)
   1. The leading cause of cancer-related death in men and women.
   2. Most important risk factor: smoking.
   3. Types of lung cancer include:
      a. SCC—the most common form.
      b. Adenocarcinoma—is becoming more common. Occurs in the peripheral portion of the lung.
      c. Small (oat) cell carcinoma—the most malignant form of lung cancer, which involves rapid metastatic spread. It carries the worst prognosis.
   4. Sites of distant metastasis include the brain, bones (bone marrow), liver, and adrenal gland.

D. Colon and rectal cancer
   1. Most common form: adenocarcinoma.
   2. Sigmoid colon or rectal areas are the most frequently involved areas.
   3. Often develops from villous adenomas.
   4. Common symptoms include blood in stools and rectal bleeding.

E. Breast cancer
   1. Most common form: adenocarcinomas arising from the ductal epithelium.
   2. The second most common cause of cancer-related deaths in women.
   3. Approximately 50% of tumors have estrogen-receptor proteins.
   4. Risk increases with age, positive family history, obesity, early menarche, and late menopause or pregnancy.

F. Prostate cancer
   1. Most common form: adenocarcinomas arising from the glandular epithelium.
   2. The second most common cause of cancer-related deaths in men.
   3. Laboratory findings include:
      a. Higher levels of prostate-specific antigen (PSA).
      b. Increased serum alkaline phosphatase.

Sample Questions

1. ***All of the following cells are associated with chronic inflammation* except *one. Which one is the* exception?**
   A. Macrophages.
   B. Neutrophils.
   C. T lymphocytes.
   D. B lymphocytes.
   E. Plasma cells.
2. ***Dust cells can be found in the ____.***
   A. Brain
   B. Heart
   C. Lungs
   D. Liver
   E. Spleen
3. ***Which of the following mediators aid in the killing of intracellular bacteria?***
   A. Histamine.
   B. Interleukin-2.
   C. Catalase.
   D. IgG.
   E. Lysozyme.
4. ***The class of antibodies that plays an important role in type I hypersensitivity reactions is ____.***
   A. IgA
   B. IgD
   C. IgE
   D. IgG
   E. IgM
5. ***DiGeorge's syndrome is characterized by a deficiency of ____.***
   A. B lymphocytes
   B. T lymphocytes
   C. Both B and T lymphocytes
   D. Antibodies
   E. Complement inhibitor
6. ***Which of the following is the* most common *cause of subacute endocarditis?***
   A. *Staphylococcus aureus.*
   B. *Staphylococcus epidermidis.*
   C. *Streptococcus viridans.*
   D. *Streptococcus pyogenes.*
   E. *Streptococcus pneumoniae.*
7. ***Aschoff bodies are observed in which of the following conditions?***
   A. Acute myelogenous leukemia.
   B. Pheochromocytoma.
   C. Osteopetrosis.
   D. Rheumatic fever.
   E. Scleroderma .
8. ***Endotoxin consists of ____.***
   A. Lipopolysaccharide
   b. M protein
   c. Hyaluronidase
   d. Lactic acid
   e. Coagulase
9. ***All of the following conditions are commonly associated with a group A, β-hemolytic streptococci infection* except *one. Which one is the* exception?**
   A. Scarlet fever.
   B. Toxic shock syndrome.
   C. Pharyngitis.
   D. Endocarditis.
   E. Impetigo.
10. ***Karyotyping can be used to diagnose which of the following diseases?***
    A. Klinefelter's syndrome.
    B. Multiple myeloma.
    C. Niemann-Pick disease.
    D. Pemphigus.
    E. Peutz-Jeghers syndrome.
11. ***In pemphigus, autoantibodies are directed against which of the following structures?***
    A. Acetylcholine receptor.
    B. Sarcomere.
    C. Epidermis.
    D. Thyroid follicle.
    E. Lysosomes.
12. ***Which of the following is a major complication of chronic bronchitis?***
    A. Myxedema.
    B. Pneumothorax.
    C. Emphysema.
    D. Pernicious anemia.
    E. Malignant transformation.
13. ***Which of the following cells are defective in chronic granulomatous disease?***
    A. Neutrophils.
    B. Lymphocytes.
    C. Plasma cells.
    D. Killer T cells.
    E. Macrophages.
14. ***Which of the following describes cells that are abnormal in appearance and may become premalignant?***
    A. Aplasia.
    B. Dysplasia.
    C. Karyomegaly.
    D. Pleomorphism.
    E. Metaplasia.
15. ***The HIV virus binds directly to the surface receptors of CD4 lymphocytes with ____.***
    A. Reverse transcriptase
    B. Integrase
    C. Hemagglutinin
    D. Glycoprotein 120
    E. Protease

16. ***Which of the following microbes is the* most *common cause of gastroenteritis in children?***
    A. Reoviruses.
    B. Picornaviruses.
    C. Togaviruses.
    D. Paramyxoviruses.
    E. Orthomyxoviruses.
17. ***A cotton wool appearance may be used to describe the radiograph of a patient with _____.***
    A. Osteopetrosis
    B. Osteitis deformans
    C. Peutz-Jeghers syndrome
    D. Seborrheic keratosis
    E. Osteogenesis imperfecta
18. ***An autoclave sterilizes dental instruments by causing which of the following?***
    A. Coagulation of proteins.
    B. Denaturing of proteins.
    C. Precipitation of nucleic acids.
    D. Disruption of cell membranes.
    E. Dissolution of lipids.
19. ***Ehlers-Danlos syndrome is a disease affecting _____.***
    A. Bone
    B. Connective tissue
    C. Muscle
    D. Joints
    E. Glycogen synthesis
20. ***An increase in alkaline phosphatase may be seen in all of the following conditions* except *one. Which one is the* exception?**
    A. Hyperparathyroidism.
    B. Osteoporosis.
    C. Osteitis deformans.
    D. Adenocarcinoma of the prostate.
    E. Multiple myeloma.
21. ***The* most *common cause of death in diabetic patients is _____.***
    A. Peripheral neuropathy
    B. Pancreatic cancer
    C. Cardiovascular disease
    D. Kidney failure
    E. Opportunistic infections
22. ***Neuraminidase is produced by _____.***
    A. Influenza virus
    B. Hepatitis C viruses
    C. Human immunodeficiency virus
    D. Measles virus
    E. Rubella virus
23. ***Which of the following skin lesions is* most *likely premalignant?***
    A. Verruca vulgaris.
    B. Keloids.
    C. Seborrheic keratosis.
    D. Actinic keratosis.
    E. Compound nevus.
24. ***The* most *prominent mechanism of spread of the hepatitis A virus is by which of the following routes?***
    A. Oral-anal.
    B. Respiratory.
    C. Sexual contact.
    D. Perinatal.
    E. Insect vectors.
25. ***Accumulation of fluid in the pericardium occurs* most often *with which of the following conditions?***
    A. Unstable angina.
    B. Cardiomyopathy.
    C. Myocarditis.
    D. Acute pericarditis.
    E. Tamponade.
26. ***The* most *common cause of pyelonephritis is _____.***
    A. *Staphylococcus aureus*
    B. *Vibrio cholerae*
    C. *Escherichia coli*
    D. *Helicobacter pylori*
    E. *Bordetella pertussis*
27. ***Polycystic kidney disease is* most *commonly associated with _____.***
    A. Renal cell carcinoma
    B. Peripheral neuropathy
    C. Urolithiasis
    D. Berry aneurysm
    E. Non-Hodgkin's lymphoma
28. ***Squamous cell carcinoma is the most common oral cancer. It is a tumor of _____.***
    A. Melanocytes
    B. Basal cells
    C. Fibroblasts
    D. Keratinocytes
    E. Macrophages
29. ***Tinea pedis, which is commonly known as athlete's foot, is a fungal infection that is caused by the following dermatophyte(s):***
    A. *Microsporum*
    B. *Trichophyton*
    C. *Epidermophyton*
    D. Both A and B
    E. Both B and C
30. ***Fibrotic and thickened heart valves that result in a reduction of blood flow through the valve characterize which of the following?***
    A. Stenosis.
    B. Regurgitation.
    C. Insufficiency.
    D. Prolapse.
    E. Ischemia.
31. ***Cystic fibrosis is a hereditary disorder that results from defective _____.***
    A. Collagen
    B. Lysosomal enzymes
    C. Chloride channels
    D. Fibrillin
    E. Myelin

32. ***The most common mutation accounting for the pathogenesis of trisomy 21 is _____.***
    A. Chromosome translocation
    B. Meiotic nondisjunction
    C. Mitotic nondisjunction
    D. Single deletion
    E. X-linked inheritance
33. ***An endocrine disorder that causes an early loss of primary teeth and the early eruption of secondary teeth is _____.***
    A. Myxedema
    B. Hashimoto's thyroiditis
    C. DiGeorge's syndrome
    D. Plummer's disease
    E. Dwarfism
34. ***Which of the following is* not *a feature of poststreptococcal glomerulonephritis?***
    A. Hematuria.
    B. Hypertension.
    C. Edema.
    D. Polyuria.
35. ***The most common cause of osteomyelitis is _____.***
    A. *Streptococcus pyogenes*
    B. *Staphylococcus aureus*
    C. *Lactobacillus casei*
    D. *Pseudomonas aeruginosa*
    E. *Escherichia coli*
36. ***All of the following are histopathologic features of malignant cells* except *one. Which one is the* exception?**
    A. Anaplasia.
    B. Pleomorphism.
    C. Aneuploidy.
    D. Large nuclei.
    E. Low nuclear-cytoplasmic ratio.
37. ***Which of the following best describes anaplastic cells that have not invaded the basement membrane and are confined within their epithelium of origin?***
    A. Dysplasia.
    B. Hyperplasia.
    C. Metaplasia.
    D. Sarcoma.
    E. Carcinoma in situ.

Test items 38–42 refer to the following testlet.

A 43-year-old man presents for an emergency dental appointment complaining of a burning sensation in his mouth. Upon examination, white plaques are observed along the oral mucosa. The patient otherwise appears healthy. There is no history of systemic illness, but the patient did state that he had a blood transfusion more than 10 years ago following a car accident. The doctor referred the patient to emergency room for further tests.

38. ***Upon further evaluation, the doctor requests an HIV and hepatitis test. The laboratory performed both an ELISA test and Western blot, revealing that the patient is HIV-positive. The Western blot is used to identify which of the following?***
    A. Antibodies.
    B. DNA.
    C. RNA.
    D. Proteins.
    E. Plaque-forming units.
39. ***Given the patient's history, if the patient was later diagnosed with active hepatitis, which of the following would most likely be the causative agent?***
    A. Hepatitis A.
    B. Hepatitis B.
    C. Hepatitis C.
    D. Hepatitis D.
    E. Hepatitis E.
40. ***Which of the following would the doctor likely prescribe for the patient's intraoral infection?***
    A. Amoxicillin.
    B. Vancomycin.
    C. Ciprofloxacin.
    D. Nystatin.
    E. Chlorhexidine.
41. ***All of the following molecules may be found within the nucleocapsid of an HIV virus* except *one. Which one is the* exception?**
    A. Reverse transcriptase.
    B. Integrase.
    C. Neuraminidase.
    D. Protease.
    E. Ribonucleic acid.
42. ***The patient is referred to an infectious disease specialist and placed on "triple therapy." Two years later, the patient is admitted to the emergency room with a dry cough and shortness of breath. His temperature is 101 degrees F. The most likely cause of the patient's pneumonia is _____.***
    A. *Staphylococcus aureus*
    B. *Haemophilus influenzae*
    C. *Pneumocystis jiroveci (carinii)*
    D. *Klebsiella pneumoniae*
    E. *Streptococcus pneumoniae*

Test items 43–45 refer to the following testlet.

A mother brings her 6-year-old daughter in for an examination because she noticed brown macules on her daughter's leg. The macules have jagged edges but do not appear raised. The mother is worried that her daughter may have a malignancy. After further evaluation and tests, the macules are identified as café au lait spots.

43. ***Café au lait spots are seen in conjunction with polyostotic fibrous dysplasia and endocrine abnormalities in which of the following disorders?***
A. McCune-Albright's syndrome.
B. Stevens-Johnson syndrome.
C. Marfan's syndrome.
D. Gorlin-Goltz syndrome.
E. Peutz-Jeghers syndrome.

44. ***The patient's radiographs could be described as having what type of characteristic appearance?***
A. Cotton wool.
B. Ground glass.
C. Cobweb.
D. Soap bubble.
E. Starry sky.

45. ***A bone biopsy was taken from the patient. Which of the following would* most *likely be observed under the microscope?***
A. A dense inflammatory infiltrate.
B. Fibrous tissue.
C. Pleomorphic cells.
D. Metastatic calcifications.
E. Giant cells.

Test items 46–49 refer to the following testlet.

A 6-year-old boy presents with a history of severe epistaxis. For the past 3 years the patient has experienced these nose bleeds, often without any apparent cause. The patient is otherwise in good health, but his mother has noticed that he "bruises easily." Laboratory tests are ordered.

46. ***The laboratory test results show a normal PT but a prolonged PTT. A prolonged PTT test suggests that the patient has an abnormality affecting which component of the coagulation cascade?***
A. Activation of platelets.
B. Activation of thromboplastin.
C. Activation of plasminogen.
D. Intrinsic pathway .
E. Extrinsic pathway.

47. ***The diagnosis of hemophilia A is made. This disease is caused by a deficiency of _____.***
A. Factor V.
B. Factor VII.
C. Factor VIII.
D. Factor IX.
E. Factor X.

48. ***Which of the following describes the hereditary transmission of this disease?***
A. Autosomal dominant.
B. Autosomal recessive.
C. X-linked.
D. It is not genetically transmitted.

49. ***The clinical presentation of hemophilia B is indistinguishable from hemophilia A. Which of the following best describes the laboratory method needed to distinguish these two conditions?***
A. Bleeding time.
B. Assay of coagulation factor levels.
C. Assay of von Willebrand's factor.
D. Blood smear.
E. Platelet count.

50. ***An infection by which of the following bacteria may result in the formation of gummas?***
A. *Mycobacterium tuberculosis.*
B. *Neisseria gonorrhoreae.*
C. *Treponema pallidum.*
D. *Bordetella pertussis.*
E. *Streptococcus pyogenes.*

51. ***Which of the following receptors are recognized by CD8 lymphocytes?***
A. Class I MHC molecules.
B. Class II MHC molecules.
C. Surface IgE.
D. Surface IgM.
E. Histamine receptor.

52. ***Which of the following cytokines stimulate B lymphocytes to differentiate into plasma cells?***
A. IL-1.
B. IL-2.
C. IL-3.
D. IL-4.
E. IL-5.

53. ***All of the following symptoms are mediated by antibodies* except *one. Which one is the* exception?**
A. Arthus reaction.
B. Tuberculin reaction.
C. Asthma.
D. Erythroblastosis fetalis.
E. Serum sickness.

54. ***Which of the following is released by mast cells after antigen binding?***
A. IgE.
B. Lysozyme.
C. IL-4.
D. Leukotriene.
E. Interferon.

55. ***Symptoms of a myocardial infarction include all of the following* except *one. Which one is the* exception?**
A. Angina.
B. Diaphoresis.
C. Fever.
D. Vomiting.
E. Dyspnea.

56. ***A positive quelling reaction can be observed in bacteria with a _____.***
A. Thick peptidoglycan layer
B. Capsule
C. Flagella
D. Cell wall that contains teichoic acid
E. Glycocalyx coating

57. ***Which of the following groups of micro-organisms produce dipicolinic acid?***
   A. *Actinomycetes.*
   B. *Histoplasma.*
   C. *Streptococcus.*
   D. *Staphylococcus.*
   E. *Clostridium.*
58. ***Which of the following consists of glucose molecules linked together that act as the structural component of plaque?***
   A. Fructose.
   B. Sucrose.
   C. Levans.
   D. Dextrans.
   E. Fructans.
59. ***The most common cause of bacterial meningitis in newborns is _____.***
   A. *Staphylococcus aureus*
   B. *Streptococcus pneumoniae*
   C. *Escherichia coli*
   D. *Haemophilus influenzae*
   E. *Listeria monocytogenes*
60. ***All of the following can be found in the cell wall of a gram-negative bacterium* except *one. Which one is the* exception?**
   A. Endotoxin.
   B. A thin peptidoglycan layer.
   C. Lipopolysaccharide.
   D. Teichoic acid.
   E. O antigen.
61. ***What type of vaccine is used for* Clostridium tetani?**
   A. Capsular polysaccharides.
   B. Toxoids.
   C. Killed bacteria.
   D. Immunoglobulins.
   E. No vaccine is available.
62. ***The class of antibodies that plays an important role in mucosal immunity is _____.***
   A. IgA
   B. IgD
   C. IgE
   D. IgG
   E. IgM
63. ***The presence of which of the following in a patient's serum indicates that the patient is a highly infectious hepatitis B carrier?***
   A. HBsAg.
   B. HBsAb.
   C. HBcAg.
   D. HBeAg.
   E. HBeAb.
64. ***All of the following microbes listed are associated with infections secondary to an HIV infection* except *one. Which one is the* exception?**
   A. *Pneumocystis jiroveci (carinii).*
   B. Epstein-Barr virus.
   C. Coxsackievirus.
   D. *Mycobacterium tuberculosis.*
   E. *Candida albicans.*
65. ***Rheumatoid arthritis is characterized by inflammation of the _____.***
   A. Articular capsule
   B. Articular cartilage
   C. Cortical bone
   D. Perichondrium
   E. Synovium
66. ***The most common form of breast cancer is _____.***
   A. Adenocarcinoma
   B. Teratoma
   C. Follicular lymphoma
   D. Sarcoma
   E. Carcinoma
67. ***Which of the following antimicrobials is bacteriostatic and inhibits protein synthesis in bacteria?***
   A. Streptomycin.
   B. Penicillin V.
   C. Ciprofloxacin.
   D. Cephalexin.
   E. Tetracycline.
68. ***Which of the following may be observed in a child diagnosed with rickets?***
   A. Dark pigmentation on the oral mucosa.
   B. Early eruption of teeth.
   C. Hutchinson's incisors.
   D. Abnormal dentin.
   E. Macroglossia.
69. ***In 2% glutaraldehyde, which of the following times is minimally sufficient for achieving sterilization?***
   A. 15 minutes.
   B. 1–2 hours.
   C. 6 hours.
   D. 12 hours.
70. ***An 8-year-old boy presents with macroglossia and delayed eruption of his primary teeth. Of the following choices, which one is most likely?***
   A. Plummer's disease.
   B. Osteochondroses.
   C. Cretinism.
   D. Wilson's disease.
   E. Mallory-Weiss syndrome.
71. ***Which of the following bacteria would be expected to first colonize onto plaque?***
   A. *Streptococci.*
   B. *Bacteroides.*
   C. *Fusobacterium.*
   D. *Actinomyces.*
   E. *Prevotella.*
72. ***The hereditary transmission of Peutz-Jeghers syndrome is _____.***
   A. Autosomal dominant
   B. Autosomal recessive
   C. Sex-linked dominant
   D. Sex-linked recessive
   E. Not genetically transmitted

73. ***Which of the following structures is the*** **most** ***common site for oral cancer?***
A. Soft palate.
B. Lateral border of the tongue.
C. Lower lip.
D. Floor of mouth.
E. Buccal mucosa.

74. ***The presence of Auer rods in a peripheral blood smear suggests which of the following conditions?***
A. Acute lymphocytic leukemia.
B. Acute lymphoblastic leukemia.
C. Acute myelogenous leukemia.
D. Chronic lymphocytic leukemia.
E. Hodgkin's lymphoma.

75. ***Complications of Barrett's esophagus include all of the following*** **except** ***one. Which one is the*** **exception?**
A. Varices.
B. Stricture.
C. Hemorrhage.
D. Adenocarcinoma.
E. Ulceration.

76. ***The presence of M-protein antibodies suggests immunity to infection by which type of bacteria?***
A. *Streptococcus pyogenes.*
B. *Streptococcus viridans.*
C. *Streptococcus sanguis.*
D. *Staphylococcus aureus.*
E. *Lactobacillus casei.*

77. ***Hemorrhagic infarction and tissue necrosis suggest which of the following?***
A. Aspergillosis.
B. Blastomycosis.
C. Histoplasmosis.
D. Mucormycosis.
E. Toxoplasmosis.

78. ***Which of the following is usually*** **least** ***malignant?***
A. Acute lymphoblastic leukemia.
B. Acute lymphocytic leukemia.
C. Acute myelogenous leukemia.
D. Chronic lymphocytic leukemia.
E. Chronic myelogenous leukemia.

79. ***Bronchogenic carcinoma is a complication most characteristic of which of the following conditions?***
A. Silicosis.
B. Asbestosis.
C. Anthracosis.
D. Sarcoidosis.
E. Bronchiectasis.

80. ***Which of the following disorders is*** **least likely** ***to be included in the differential diagnosis of a patient with jaundice?***
A. Hepatitis.
B. Hemolytic anemia.
C. Cholelithiasis.
D. Glomerulonephritis.
E. Carcinoma of the pancreas.

81. ***A productive cough may be seen in all of the following conditions*** **except** ***one. Which one is the*** **exception?**
A. Pneumonia.
B. Lung abscess.
C. Bronchiectasis.
D. Asthma.
E. Bronchogenic carcinoma.

82. ***Antinuclear antibodies are seen in the serum samples from patients with _____.***
A. Hypogammaglobulinemia
B. Chronic granulomatous disease
C. Systemic lupus erythematosus
D. Multiple myeloma
E. Pheochromocytoma

83. ***Nephrolithiasis is*** **most** ***likely to be associated with which of the following conditions?***
A. Hyperparathyroidism.
B. Myxedema.
C. Pyelonephritis.
D. Wilson's disease.
E. Thrombocytopenia.

84. ***An infant diagnosed with osteopetrosis has dysfunctional _____.***
A. Chondrocytes
B. Osteoblasts
C. Osteoclasts
D. Fibroblasts
E. Lymphocytes

85. ***All of the following factors play a role in the virulence of the microbe that causes whooping cough*** **except** ***one. Which one is the*** **exception?**
A. IgA protease.
B. Hemagglutinin.
C. Exotoxin.
D. Capsule.
E. Pili.

86. ***T-cell lymphoma is most likely to occur in a patient with which of the following conditions?***
A. Chronic granulomatous disease.
B. Myasthenia gravis.
C. Osteochondroma.
D. Wilson's disease.
E. Celiac sprue.

Test items 87–92 refer to the following testlet.

A 60-year-old homeless man who lives in a community shelter presents with history of coughing for the past 6 months. He has a slight fever, hemoptysis, and productive cough with a yellowish sputum discharge. After further examination and tests, the patient is diagnosed with active tuberculosis.

87. When the sputum samples were taken to the laboratory, what test did the doctor order to be performed to help make the diagnosis?
A. Gram stain.
B. Acid-fast stain.
C. Spore stain.
D. PPD test (tuberculin test).
E. Voges-Proskauer test.

88. After 2 weeks, the bacterial cultures came back from the lab confirming the initial diagnosis, positively identifying the organism* Mycobacterium tuberculosis. M. tuberculosis *is known to infect which of the following cells?
A. Fibroblasts.
B. Basal cells.
C. Type I pneumocytes.
D. Macrophages.
E. Erythrocytes.

89. Which of the following is a glycolipid found on the surface of* M. tuberculosis *that plays a role in its pathogenesis?
A. Cord factor.
B. O antigen.
C. Protein A.
D. Exotoxin A.
E. Lecithinase.

90. Since the patient was living in a homeless shelter, the tuberculin test was administered to all of the staff and residents living at the shelter. This test is based on a delayed type hypersensitivity reaction that is mediated by ____.
A. Only IgG
B. IgG and IgM
C. IgE
D. T cells and macrophages
E. Mast cells and basophils

91. Which of the following is the* most appropriate *drug used in combination therapy for tuberculosis to treat the patient?
A. Amoxicillin.
B. Clindamycin.
C. Cephalosporin.
D. Tetracycline.
E. Rifampin.

92. After 3 weeks, the patient was feeling "much better" and was discharged from the hospital, although he remained on his drug therapy for another 6 months. Which of the following* best *describes the calcified scar that later formed in the affected lung parenchyma and hilar lymph node?
A. Gumma.
B. Chancre.
C. Metastatic calcifications.
D. Tubercle.
E. Ghon complex.

Test items 93–97 refer to the following testlet.

A 55-year-old man presents with malaise and dyspnea. He has a low-grade fever and reports that his shortness of breath has increased steadily over the past week and a half. He has a history of rheumatic fever and denies ever using recreational drugs. He is currently being treated by a dentist for full mouth reconstruction.

93. Upon further examination, a heart murmur was detected. Given the patient's past medical history, which heart valve is* most likely *affected?
A. Mitral valve.
B. Tricuspid valve.
C. Aortic valve.
D. Pulmonary valve.

94. Before the patient's development of rheumatic fever, he likely suffered from which of the following conditions?
A. Cystitis.
B. Pharyngitis.
C. Food poisoning.
D. Thrombocytopenia.
E. Meninigitis.

95. After further evaluation and tests, the patient is diagnosed with subacute endocarditis. If the infecting microbe was cultured in the laboratory, the results would most likely show that this microbe is positive for ____.
A. α-hemolysis
B. β-hemolysis
C. γ-hemolysis
D. Coagulase
E. Lecithinase

96. Which of the following is the most likely complication that may occur from the vegetations forming on the patient's defective heart valve?
A. Myocardial infarction.
B. Hemorrhage.
C. Petechiae.
D. Cor pulmonale.
E. Embolus.

97. After the diagnosis is made, the patient is immediately placed on high-dose, IV antibiotics. One of the antibiotics that is administered to the patient is streptomycin, an aminoglycoside. The antimicrobial effect of streptomycin is to inhibit the synthesis of ____.
A. The bacterial cell wall
B. Folate
C. Proteins
D. Nucleic acids
E. β-lactamase

Test items 98–100 refer to the following testlet.

A 3-year-old African girl presents in the emergency room with a palpable mass in her lower right mandible. She is currently in the United States visiting relatives with her parents. Her mom claims that a few days ago she noticed a growing mass in her daughter's jaw. There appears to be slight swelling around the area, although it is painless and not tender to the touch. After further examination, a biopsy was taken, and the diagnosis of Burkitt's lymphoma was made.

98. Burkitt's lymphoma is a malignancy that affects which of the following cells?

A. Macrophages.
B. T lymphocytes.
C. B lymphocytes.
D. Neutrophils.
E. Keratinocytes.

99. The pathology report reveals a characteristic pattern of tumor cells that is classically associated with Burkitt's lymphoma. Which of the following describes this histopathologic pattern?

A. Honeycomb.
B. Cobweb.
C. Cotton wool.
D. Sun ray.
E. Starry sky.

100. The African form of Burkitt's lymphoma has been linked to the Epstein-Barr virus. This virus is also responsible for which of the following diseases?

A. Mononucleosis.
B. Shingles.
C. Chicken pox.
D. Kaposi's sarcoma.
E. Herpangina.

4

Dental Anatomy and Occlusion

MAJOR M. ASH, JR AND STANLEY J. NELSON

OUTLINE

1. Introduction to Dental Anatomy
2. Development of Human Dentitions
3. Chronology of Primary Dentition
4. Morphology of Primary Teeth
5. Chronology of Permanent Dentition
6. Morphology of Permanent Teeth
7. Development of Dental Occlusions
8. Occlusal Contact Relations and Mandibular Movements
9. Anatomy, Physiology, and Function of the Temporomandibular Joint
10. Masticatory Muscles
11. Masticatory System and Role of Occlusion

This section is a review of those basic courses in dental anatomy and occlusion important for a foundation in the study and practice of dentistry. The coverage of these subjects is not exhaustive but should reflect what fundamental information has already been covered early in the dental curriculum. Insofar as possible, the material is based on an evidence-based paradigm that is consistent with the highest level of external evidence, recognizing that the application of such evidence has to be based on appropriate clinical expertise as well as meeting the needs of individual patients. The test questions should be viewed as a learning experience. The basis for answers may be found as needed in the attached references.

1.0 INTRODUCTION TO DENTAL ANATOMY

Dental anatomy requires special terminology and nomenclature for communication, for learning, and for clinical and insurance record keeping in the dental office. The term *dental anatomy,* as used here, is an inclusive term for considering the morphological features of the human primary and permanent dentitions, including their pulp cavities and root canals; pertinent information about the development, calcification, and eruption/emergence of the teeth; and the clinical relevance of these odontological features to their function and esthetics.

There are tables in this section that provide information on the dimensions and chronologies of the teeth and, in context, referral to frequency variations in eruption sequences, number of roots and root canals, and variations in tooth size and form. It should be recognized that collections of samples that make up these data come largely from Euro-American populations, sometimes limited because of the problem of obtaining data from other populations, access to in utero material, and statistical methods of incorporating diverse data into a common table derived from various sources. For example, prevalence data on a major anatomical variant of the two-rooted mandibular (i.e., one with an additional distolingual and third root) suggest real differences between specific populations as to the prevalence of this variant of the mandibular first molar, which is of special interest for endodontic therapy. Differences in data on tooth eruption and tooth dimensions may not appear to be significant; however, differences in data found in various textbooks and journals need to be addressed. An example of such differences may be seen in the answers to some of the questions. Sexual, racial, and individual variations in dentofacial patterns reinforce the need to carefully consider interceptive extraction or space-regaining therapy for each patient because of the unpredictability of crowding behavior during the transition from mixed to permanent dentition. The effect of racial origin should be considered when using dental sclerosis as a means of age determination in forensic cases.

A. Terminology

It is not unusual in the literature to find that more than one term is used to describe a particular dentition (e.g., *primary* or *deciduous* dentition, and *permanent* or *succedaneous* dentition, recognizing that the term deciduous can mean "not permanent, transitory," and the term permanent does not indicate necessarily that all the teeth that succeed the primary dentition will not be lost because of disease or injury. In context, both terms for each dentition should present no problem; however, consistent use of a term is important and should reflect the requirements or traditions of a particular journal, dental association, or specialty.

The term *occlusion* can be defined simply as the contact relationship of the teeth in function and parafunction. The contacting interface between the teeth of opposing dental arches may be considered from the standpoint of a static, functional, or parafunctional morphological tooth contact relationship. It should be kept in mind that such relationships reflect a number of factors concerned with the development and stability of occlusion.

It also must be recognized that changes do occur in terminology; however, they occur in the literature over time, and the reader must be aware of some of the past as well as newer terms that may conceptually relate somewhat differentially to the same aspect of occlusion (e.g., working side contacts [older term] versus laterotrusive contacts [newer term]); therefore, the literature may exhibit several terms that reflect various conceptual views of occlusal relationships. For example, in the Glossary of Dental Terms for the National Board Dental Exam, *centric relation* is defined conceptually as a position of the mandible with the condyles in a specified location that is independent of tooth contact; however, also included is a synonym for centric relation—*retruded contact position*. The term *retruded* has related historically to a concept of centric relation and occlusal contact in which the condyles were thought to be in a most retruded position (Figure 4-1, *A*) compared to the position of the condyles that is now currently held (Figure 4-1, *B*).

B. Formulas for human and nonhuman dentitions

The number and denomination of mammalian teeth are expressed in formulas that reflect the differences between human dentitions and nonhuman dentitions. The denomination of each tooth may be represented by the first letter in its name (I for *I*ncisor, C for *C*anine, P for *P*remolar, and M for *M*olar). A notation expressing the number of such teeth in the upper and lower jaws follows these denominations. The formulae include one side only. The dental formula (10 teeth on one side) for the primary/deciduous dentition in humans is indicated as:

$$\mathrm{I}\,\frac{2}{2}\;\mathrm{C}\,\frac{1}{1}\;\mathrm{M}\,\frac{2}{2} = 10$$

Similarly, a dental formula for the permanent/succedaneous human dentition reflects the addition of two maxillary and mandibular premolars, and the addition of one maxillary and one mandibular third molar. The dental formula (16 teeth on one side) for the human permanent dentition is indicated as:

$$\mathrm{I}\,\frac{2}{2}\;\mathrm{C}\,\frac{1}{1}\;\mathrm{P}\,\frac{2}{2}\;\mathrm{M}\,\frac{3}{3} = 16$$

The dental practitioner is expected to be able to differentiate the human dentition from the more common nonhuman dentitions. On occasion it is necessary to communicate with veterinarians and, in some instances, with attorneys dealing with bite wounds and the identification of human and animal remains in forensic matters. The formula (21 teeth on one side) for a dog (collie) is indicated as:

$$\mathrm{I}\,\frac{3}{3}\;\mathrm{C}\,\frac{1}{1}\;\mathrm{P}\,\frac{4}{4}\;\mathrm{M}\,\frac{2}{3} = 21$$

It is not unusual for dentists to be interested in some of the morphological traits used in anthropo-

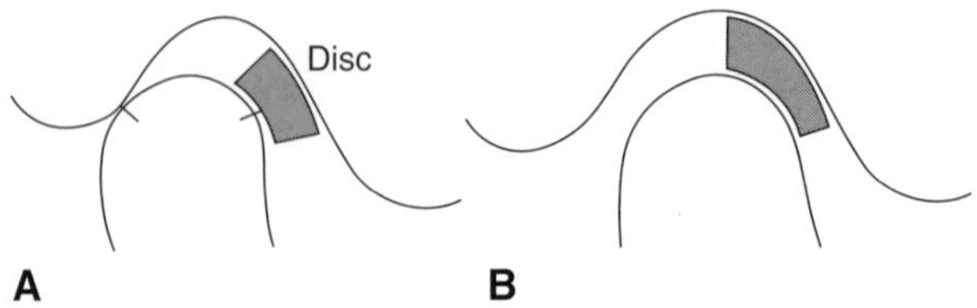

Figure 4–1. A, Most retruded position of the condyles (bilaterally). B, Condyles (bilaterally) in most superior-anterior position, resting on the posterior slopes of the articular eminences with the discs properly interposed. (From Ash MM, Ramfjord SP: Occlusion. Philadelphia: WB Saunders, 1995.)

logical studies (e.g., Carabelli's trait, peg-shaped incisors, enamel extensions, and shoveling). Because of keyboard limitations, notations in anthropological tables are often limited to di_1, di_2, dc, dm_1, and dm2 for the deciduous dentition, and to I_1, I_2, C, P_1, P_2, M_1, M_2, and M_3 for the succedaneous dentition.

C. Terms of orientation

Terms of orientation in dental anatomy generally relate to indicate place, direction, and extent, including such terms as *mesial, distal, facial, buccal, lingual,* and a*nterior/posterior* as shown in Figure 4-2. Abbreviations related to tooth orientation include: *B,* buccal; *D,* distal; *DB,* distobuccal; *M,* mesial; *MB,* mesiobuccal; *L,* lingual; *DL,* distolingual; *ML,* mesiolingual; *MM,* mesiomarginal; *CR,* cusp ridge. Abbreviations related to permanent tooth identification in tables include: *CI,* central incisor; *LI,* lateral incisor; *C,* canine; P_1, P_2, first and second premolars; M_1, M_2, M_3, first, second, and third molars. All the teeth can be identified by one or more numbering systems. The universal system to be considered later is used in this text except where otherwise indicated.

D. Anatomical landmarks

A labiolingual section of a maxillary central incisor (Figure 4-3) shows several of the landmarks relative to the tooth and periodontium.

Anatomical landmarks include such terms as *crown, root, apex, incisal edge, cervical line, pulp chamber, pulp horn, pulp (root) canal, fissure, cusp, apex,* and *bifurcation (furcation)* as indicated in Figure 4-4, *A, B.*

The primary and permanent teeth are divided for discussion purposes into the crown and root, which is a division marked on the tooth surface by the *cervical line.* This line is the junction between the enamel covering the crown of the tooth and the cementum covering the root. It is referred to as the *cementoenamel junction (CEJ).* It may occur in several forms: (a) the enamel overlapping the cementum; (b) an end-to-end approximating

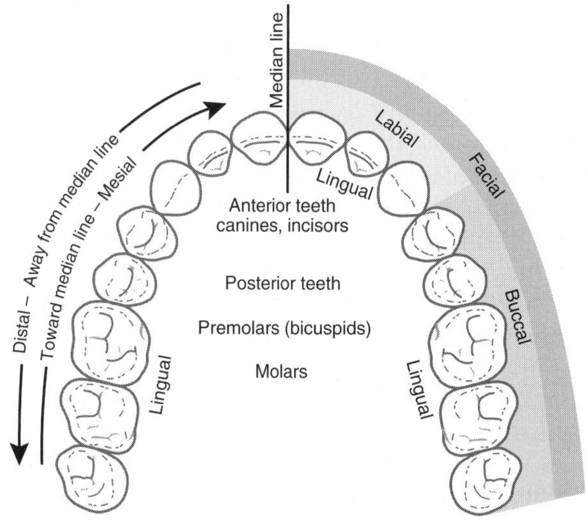

Figure 4–2. Directional orientation terms.

Figure 4–3. Faciolingual (labiolingual) section of a permanent maxillary first molar showing tooth and supporting structures.

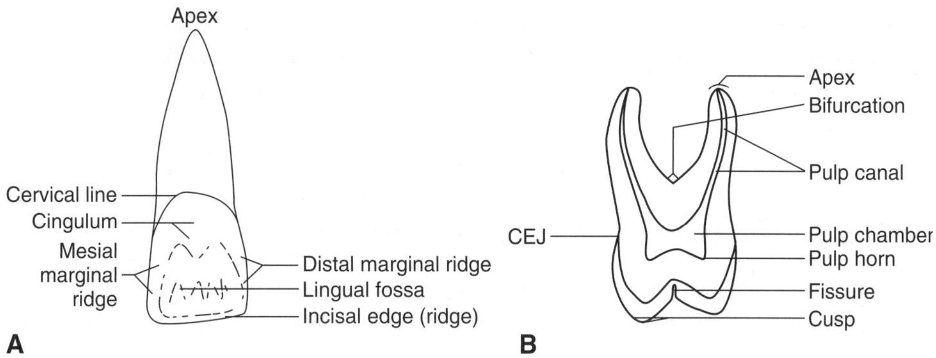

Figure 4-4. Anatomical landmarks. **A**, Anterior tooth. **B,** Posterior tooth.

junction; (c) the absence of connecting enamel and cementum so that the dentin is an external part of the surface of the root; and (d) an overlapping of the enamel by the cementum. These different junctions have clinical significance in the presence of disease (e.g., gingivitis, recession of the gingiva with exposure of the CEJ, depth of gingival crevice and level of attachment of the supporting periodontal fibers [Figure 4-3]; cervical sensitivity, caries, and erosion; and placement of margins of dental restorations).

1. Cementoenamel junction
   a. The CEJ is a significant landmark for probing the depth of the gingival crevice and the level of the attachment of periodontal fibers to the cementum in the presence of periodontal diseases. Using a periodontal probe (Figure 4-5, *A*), it is possible to relate the position of the gingival margin and the level of attachment to the CEJ (Figure 4-5, *B*).
   b. The clinician should be able to envision the CEJ of each tooth and relate it to areas of risk (e.g., pathologically deepened crevice and loss of attachment or an enamel projection into the bifurcation of a mandibular molar [Figure 4-5, *C*]). Enamel projections into buccal and lingual bifurcations are considered to increase vulnerability to the advance of periodontal disease. Thus, the CEJ (and its *location* and *nature*) is more than a descriptive term used simply to describe some aspect of tooth morphology; the CEJ has clinical significance.
   c. The distance from the alveolar bone or alveolar bone crest to the CEJ or enamel is about 1.5 mm in a normal periodontium.
2. Occlusal landmarks—all landmarks on a tooth should be recognized and identified by name. The landmarks on Figures 4-6 include the following:
   a. Cusp
   b. Buccocervical ridge
   c. Cingulum

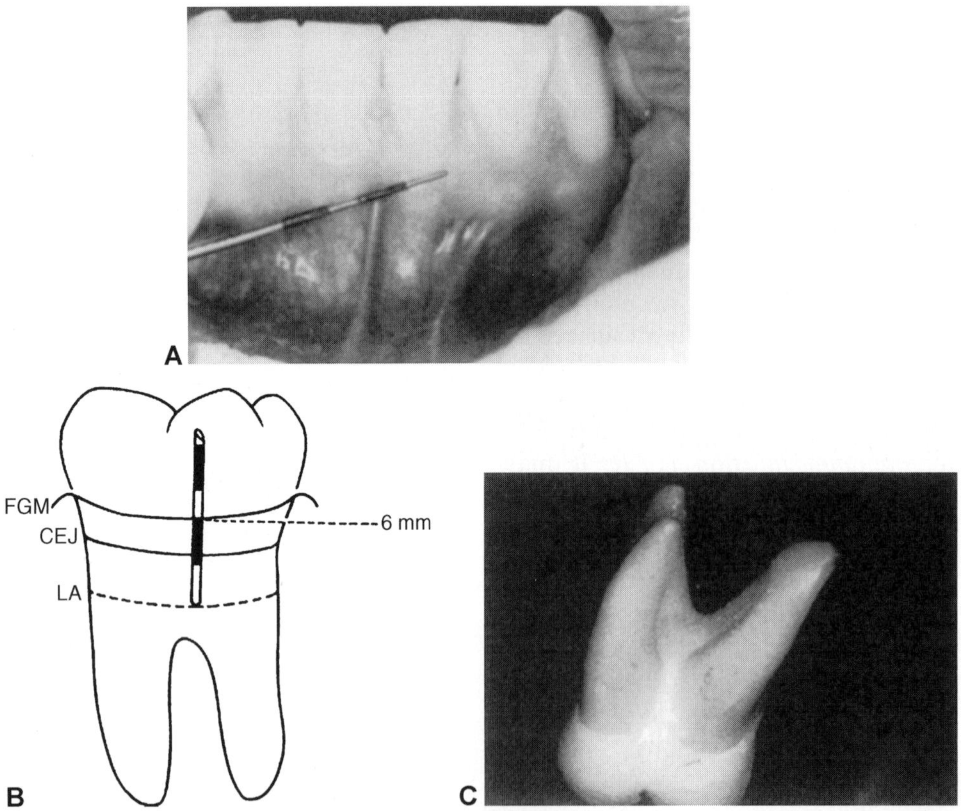

Figure 4–5. A, Periodontal probe with 3-mm increments for measuring depth of gingival crevice or level of periodontal attachment. B, The distance from the free gingival margin *(FGM)* to the tip of probe at the level of attachment *(LA)* indicates the depth of the pathologically deepened crevice of 6 mm and a loss of attachment of 3+ mm relative to the cementoenamel junction *(CEJ)*. C, Enamel projection into the bifurcation of a mandibular molar. (From Ash MM, Nelson SJ: Wheeler's Dental Anatomy, Physiology and Occlusion [8th edition]. Philadelphia: WB Saunders, 2003.)

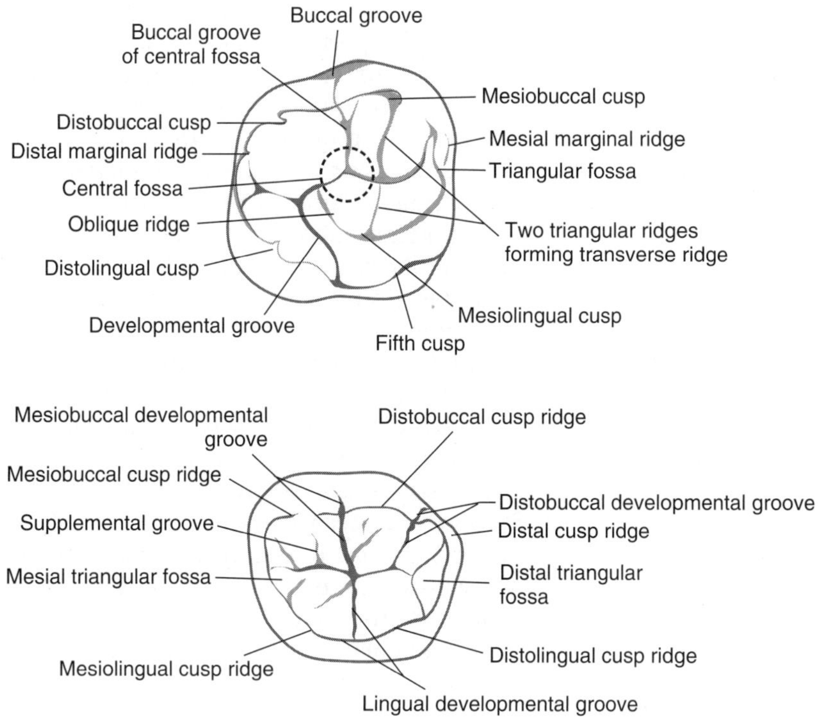

Figure 4–6. Occlusal landmarks on maxillary and mandibular molars.

d. Marginal ridge
e. Fossa
f. Oblique ridge
g. Developmental groove
h. Transverse ridge
i. Supplemental groove
j. Triangular ridge

It is necessary to know how morphological features relate to contact relations in functional jaw movements and in jaw closure (e.g., the occlusal contact relation of the mesial buccal cusp of the right mandibular first molar with the central fossa of the maxillary right first molar when the mandible is closed into the maximal intercuspal [clenching] position). These and other morphological features, as well as the positions of the teeth, may be related to the development of occlusal stability and oral motor behavior as the occlusion develops.

E. Tooth numbering systems

Practitioners need to be able to designate easily (using an acceptable tooth identification system) which tooth or teeth are being considered for diagnosis and treatment, and to be able to indicate the identity of a tooth or teeth in dental and insurance records. Thus, in the dental office the dentist, the hygienist, the dental assistant, and the front office assistant have to be knowledgeable about the tooth identification system used in their office and systems used elsewhere for purposes of referral and for reading pertinent professional literature.

1. Universal system

In 1968 the American Dental Association recommended the universal numbering system; however, because it does not have universal usage, there are calls to change it. Even so, the notation of one letter for each tooth in the primary dentition and one number for each tooth in the permanent dentition has made its use favored in the United States. An overview of the primary dentition and its universal numbering is shown in Figure 4-7. A simplified scheme to show the letter notations for the 20 primary teeth in four quadrants follows:

Midsagittal Plane

Right	A	B	C	D	E	F	G	H	I	J	Left
	T	S	R	Q	P	O	N	M	L	K	

As shown, the right maxillary central incisor is indicated with the letter *E*. Similarly, the left mandibular left central incisor is indicated with the letter *O*. There is no provision for supernumerary teeth. An overview of the permanent dentition and its universal numbering is shown in Figure 4-8.

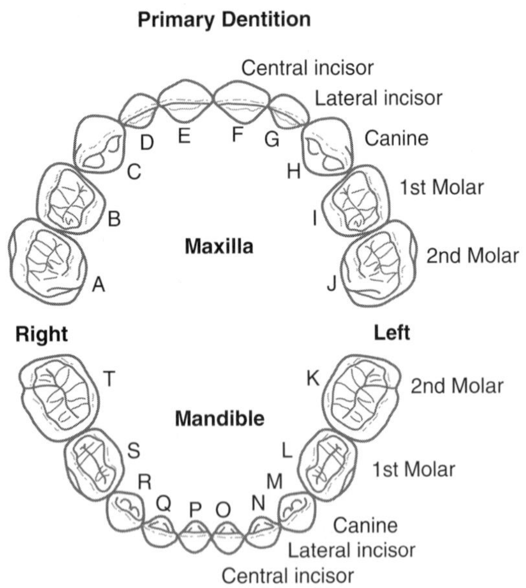

Figure 4–7. Letters used in identifying the primary teeth.

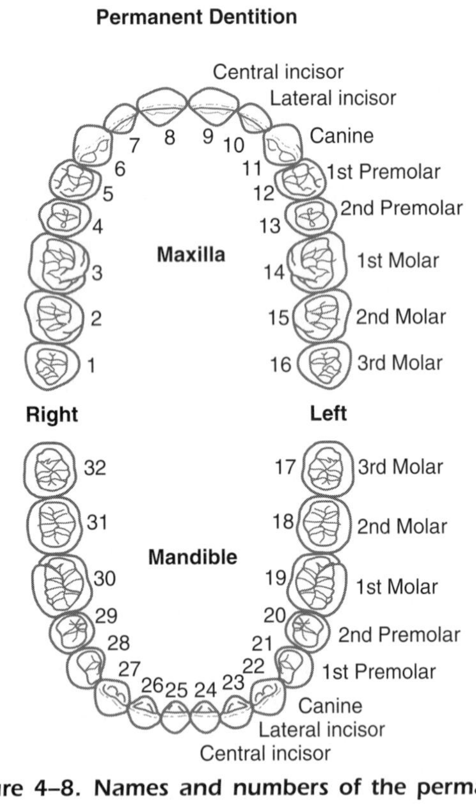

Figure 4–8. Names and numbers of the permanent teeth used in the universal numbering system.

A simplified notation scheme for the permanent dentition follows:

1	2	3	4	5	6	7	8	9	10	11	12	13	14	15	16
32	31	30	29	28	27	26	25	24	23	22	21	20	19	18	17

A single number is used to represent each tooth in the permanent dentition (normally 32 teeth). For example, the right maxillary first molar is indicated in the universal system with the number *3* and the left mandibular first molar as *19*. There is no provision for numbering supernumerary teeth, nor specific indications for missing teeth that have been replaced with restorative treatment. However, there have been suggestions for such additions.

2. Symbolic system

Credit for a symbolic system for tooth numbering is given to two dentists and can be referred to as the Zsigmondy/Palmer notation system. However, in the United States the system is usually indicated as the Palmer system. In this symbolic system the arches are divided into four quadrants, as shown in the following depiction of the entire primary dentition. The Palmer notation for the primary dentition follows:

E	D	C	B	A	A	B	C	D	E
E	D	C	B	A	A	B	C	D	E

For a single tooth, such as the primary maxillary right central incisor, the designation is A|. For the maxillary left central incisor, the notation is given as |A. This numbering system presents difficulties when an appropriate font is not available for keyboard recording of these notations.

The Palmer notation for the permanent dentition divides the arches into four quadrants with eight or more teeth in each quadrant. With a complement of 32 teeth, the entire dentition would appear as follows:

8	7	6	5	4	3	2	1	1	2	3	4	5	6	7	8
8	7	6	5	4	3	2	1	1	2	3	4	5	6	7	8

The notation for the right permanent maxillary central incisor is 1|. The notation for the right permanent maxillary first molar would be 6|. The Palmer notation system is used frequently in the orthodontic literature.

3. FDI system

The Fédération Dentaire Internationale (FDI) recommends a two-digit system for both the primary and permanent dentitions. This system has been adopted by the World Health Organization (WHO) and is accepted by other organizations and in research and public health journals. The FDI system of notation for the primary dentition follows:

Upper right					Upper left				
55	54	53	52	51	61	62	63	64	65
85	84	83	82	81	71	72	73	74	75
Lower right					Lower feft				

Numeral *5* indicates the right maxillary quadrant; number *6,* the left maxillary quadrant; number *7,* the left mandibular quadrant; and number *8,* the right mandibular quadrant. Teeth for each quadrant are numbered from *1* to *5,* beginning with the central incisors. Hence, the right and left maxillary central incisors of the primary dentition would be numbered *51,* and *61,* respectively, and the left and right mandibular central incisors as *71* and *81,* respectively. The FDI system for the permanent dentition follows:

Upper right								Upper left							
18	17	16	15	14	13	12	11	21	22	23	24	25	26	27	28
48	47	46	45	44	43	42	41	31	32	33	34	35	36	37	38
Lower right								Lower feft							

In the permanent dentition, the first digit indicates the quadrant and the second digit the tooth in that quadrant. Quadrant indication numbers are: the right maxillary quadrant is *1,* the left maxillary quadrant is *2,* the left mandibular quadrant is *3,* and the right mandibular quadrant is *4.* The teeth in each quadrant are numbered from *1* to *8.* Hence, the right maxillary central incisor is indicated by the double digit *11* (pronounced one-one, not eleven); the left maxillary central incisor as *21*; the left mandibular central incisor as *31*; and the right mandibular central incisor as *41.* For several reasons it is important that practitioners know the FDI system, including its use in the international literature.

2.0 DEVELOPMENT OF HUMAN DENTITIONS

Knowledge of the development of the teeth and their emergence in the oral cavity is applicable to clinical practice as well as to other areas of interest such as anthropology, demography, forensics, and paleontology, which will be referred to only briefly here. Although the bibliography can be used to broaden the scope of reader interest, only those areas considered to be basic for the practice of dentistry will be reviewed here.

A. Morphogenesis of the teeth

The interactive mechanisms of patterning, morphogenesis, and cytodifferentiation during organogenesis have been covered in Oral Embryology. Tooth development involves interactions between epithelium and mesenchyme, with the formation of a bud-like epithelial structure that becomes convoluted into a *cap* and *bell* stage. Subsequently, epithelial and mesenchymal cells such as *dental papilla* differentiate into enamel-secreting ameloblasts and dentin-secreting odontoblasts. These stages of early tooth development are well-defined histologically; however the formation of different shapes of teeth (morphogenesis) and their correct position in the jaws (patterning) have only recently demonstrated the importance of molecular genetics and signaling pathways in tooth morphogenesis.

These intercellular signaling networks are composed of proteins, including ligands, receptors, and transcription factors. The outcome of these intricate mechanisms during the development of the teeth generally leads to the right shape of teeth in the right place; however, morphological variability and dental malformations do occur, which may be of significant clinical importance.

B. Timing of human dentitions development

The timing of chronological events in the development of the dentitions has been historically difficult to ascertain because of the lack of adequate documentation of the sources of information. Tables of dental chronologies reflect an abbreviated version of a long history of accumulated successive compilations and revisions of chronologies of the primary teeth, which is also true for the permanent dentition. It is recognized that such chronologies have some deficiencies in population sampling and collection methods, and that incorporating revised data based on making critical choices from available sources is not without methodological errors. Recent partial chronologies of dental development reflect the use of statistical methods that provide three different types of formation data: age of attainment chronologies based on tooth emergence, age of prediction chronologies based on being in a stage of development, and maturity assessment scales used to assess whether a subject of known age is ahead of or behind when compared with a reference population. These types of chronologies are used when more precise information about a particular aspect of dental development is needed for research and surgical procedures.

1. Dental age

Dental age is usually based on the formation or emergence of the teeth, as well as simply counting the number of teeth, the presence of permanent teeth, and the amount of root resorption of the primary teeth. Thus, looking into the mouth and noting which teeth are present is a simple way to approximate the age of young children and adolescents. The dentition may be considered to be the best physiological indicator of chronological age in juveniles.

C. Eruption/emergence of the teeth

The term *eruption* has been defined historically as the emergence of the tooth into the oral cavity; however, it has recently been considered to mean continuous tooth movement from the dental tooth bud to occlusal contact. Thus, the term *emergence* is thought to be more specific for the emergence of the teeth through the alveolar gingiva.

3.0 CHRONOLOGY OF PRIMARY DENTITION

The *primary dentition* (Figure 4-9) is considered to be clinically complete when the second primary molars are in occlusion at about the mean age of 29 months, keeping in mind that the completion of the roots of the canines occurs at about 3.25 years of age. The emergence of the permanent first molars signals the start of the *mixed dentition* period, which is considered to have been completed when all the primary teeth are lost and only the succeeding permanent (succedaneous) teeth are present.

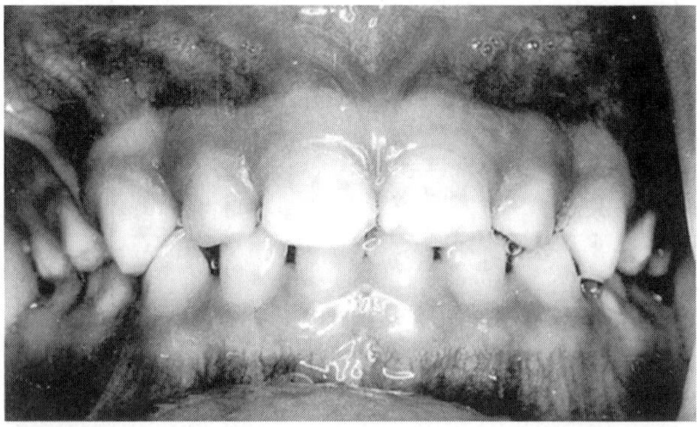

Figure 4–9. Primary dentition in a 5-year-old child. (From Ash MM, Ramjford SP: Occlusion. Philadelphia: WB Saunders, 1995.)

The chronology of the primary dentition is summarized in Table 4-1. The universal numbering system for the primary teeth is used, as well as general indications of primary incisors, canine, and molars i1, i2, C, m1, and m2. The dimensions for the primary dentition are given in Table 4-2.

TABLE 4–1. CHRONOLOGIES OF THE PRIMARY DENTITION

TOOTH		FIRST EVIDENCE OF CALCIFICATION (WEEKS IN UTERO)	CROWN COMPLETED (MONTHS)	EMERGENCE (MEAN AGE) (MONTHS)	ROOT COMPLETED (YEARS)
Upper					
i1	E, F	14	1½	10	1½
i2	D, G	16	2½	11	2
C	C, H	17	9	19	3¼
m1	B, I	15	6	16	2½
m2	A, J	19	11	29	3
			Maxillary Teeth		
		Right	**A B C D E | F G H I J**	**Left**	
			T S R Q P | O N M L K		
			Mandibular Teeth		
Lower					
i1	P, O	14	2½	8	1½
i2	Q, N	16	3	13	1½
C	R, M	17	9	20	3¼
m1	S, L	15½	5½	16	2¼
m2	T, K	18	10	27	3

From: Ash MM, Nelson SJ: Wheeler's Dental Anatomy, Physiology, and Occlusion (8th edition). Philadelphia: WB Saunders, 2003.

TABLE 4–2. MEASUREMENTS OF THE PRIMARY TEETH*

		CROWN HEIGHT	ROOT LENGTH	MD CROWN DIAMETER	LL CROWN DIAMETER	MD CERVIX DIAMETER	LL CERVIX DIAMETER
Maxillary Teeth			A B C D E | F G H I J				
CI	E | F	6.0	10.0	6.5	5.0	4.5	4.0
LI	D | G	5.6	11.4	5.1	4.0	3.7	3.7
C	C | H	6.5	13.5	7.0	7.0	5.1	5.5
m1	B | I	5.1	10.0	7.3	8.5	5.2	6.9
m2	A | J	5.7	11.7	8.2	10.0	6.4	8.3
Mandibular Teeth			T S R Q P | O N M L K				
CI	P | O	5.0	9.0	4.3	4.0	3.0	3.5
LI	Q | N	5.2	10.0	4.1	4.0	3.0	3.5
C	R | M	6.0	11.5	5.0	4.8	3.7	4.0
m1	S | L	6.0	9.8	7.7	7.0	6.5	5.3
m2	T | K	5.5	11.3	9.9	8.7	7.2	6.4

* Average measurements (in mm) adapted from Black GV (Cited by Ash MM, Nelson SJ: Wheeler's Dental Anatomy, Physiology, and Occlusion (8th edition). Philadelphia: WB Saunders, 2003). *MD* = mesiodistal; *LL* = labiolingual
A | J to T | *K* = universal numbering system for primary teeth.

4.0 MORPHOLOGY OF PRIMARY TEETH

A detailed coverage of the individual morphology of the primary teeth is beyond the scope of this review, and the reader is invited to consider the material in the bibliography. However, it is anticipated that the present coverage of those aspects of morphology for identification and function of the primary dentition will provide a reminder of the important details that have already been considered in the dental curriculum.

A. Schematic views of primary dentition

Schematic views of the primary dentition are shown in Figure 4-10. Illustrated are the labial and facial surfaces as well as the occlusal incisal views of the incisors and canines. Occlusal views of first and second primary molars are provided in Figure 4-11.

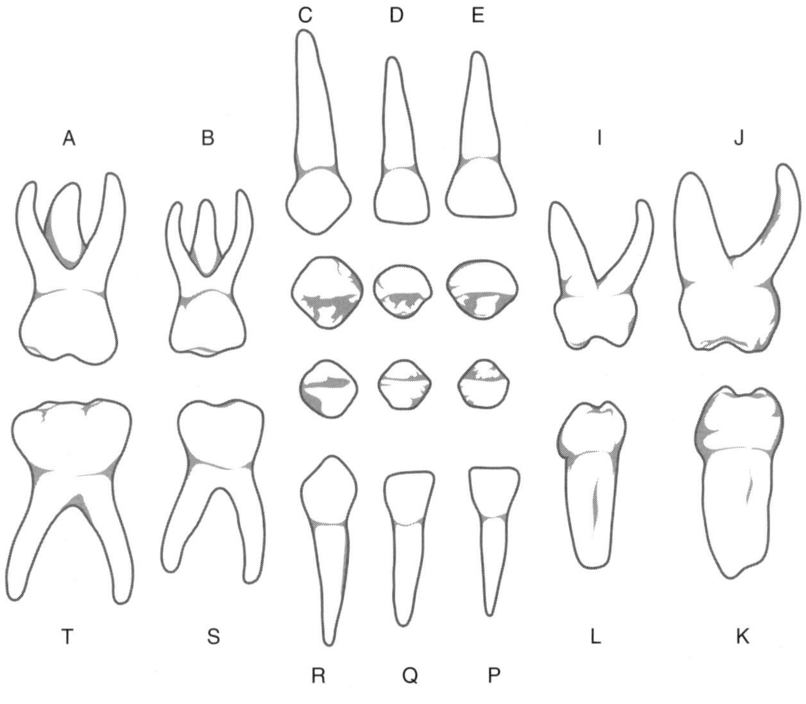

Figure 4–10. Schematic illustration of primary teeth. Primary right molars (buccal aspect): **B,** maxillary first molar; **A,** maxillary second molar; **S,** mandibular first molar; **T,** mandibular second molar. Primary right maxillary teeth, (facial/labial aspect); **C,** maxillary canine; **D,** maxillary lateral incisor; **E,** maxillary central incisor. Primary right mandibular teeth; **P,** mandibular central incisor; **Q,** mandibular lateral incisor; **R,** mandibular canine. Primary teeth between the anterior teeth depict the incisal aspect of the central incisors, lateral incisors, and canines. Primary left molars (mesial aspect); **I,** maxillary first molar; **J,** maxillary second molar; **K,** mandibular second molar; **L,** mandibular first molar.

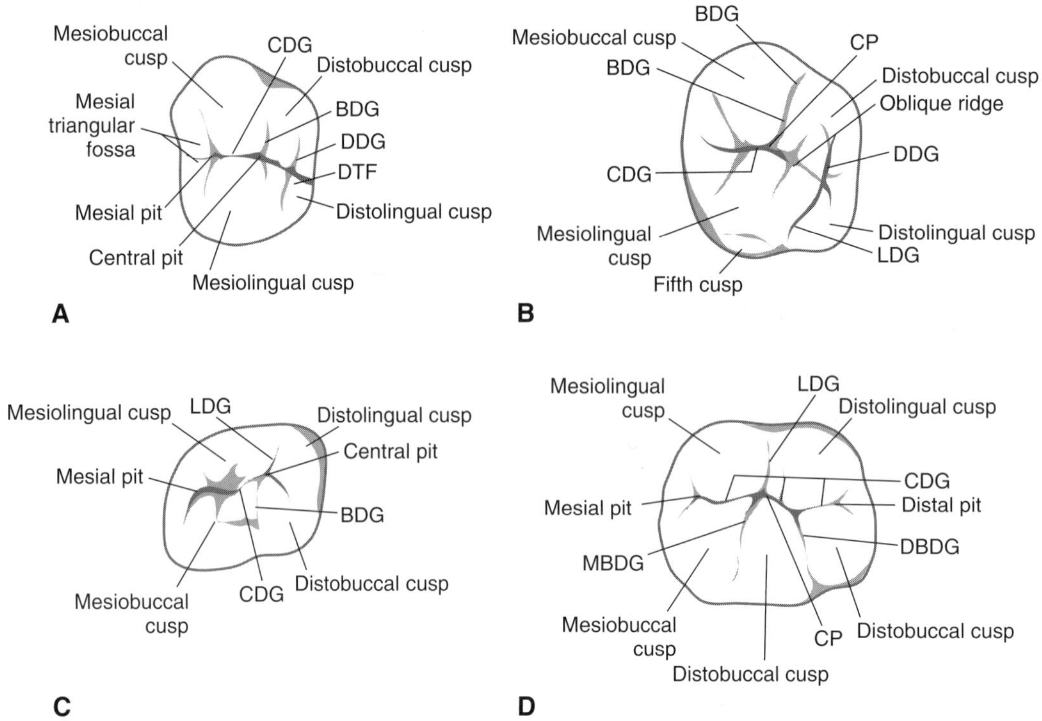

Figure 4–11. Primary molars. Occlusal views. **A,** Maxillary first molar: *CDG, BDG, DDG, DTF,* central, buccal, and distal developmental grooves. **B,** Maxillary second molar: *CP,* central pit; *CDG, BDG, LDG, DDG:* central, buccal, lingual, and distal developmental grooves. **C,** Mandibular first molar: *BDG, CDG, LDG:* buccal, central, and lingual developmental grooves. **D,** Mandibular second molar: *CP,* central pit; *CDG, LDG, MBDG, DBDG:* central, lingual, mesiobuccal, and distobuccal developmental grooves.

B. Identification characteristics of primary teeth—the primary teeth compared to the permanent teeth have the following identifying differences.
   1. General characteristics:
      a. Smaller in overall size and crown dimensions.
      b. Whiter in color than permanent teeth.
      c. Markedly more prominent cervical ridges.
      d. Molar roots widely flared, especially maxillary molars.
      e. Molar roots thin, ribbon-shaped; wider buccolingually.
      f. Root trunks narrow or absent.
      g. Crowns frequently abraded.
      h. Large pulp chambers.
      i. Thinner enamel covering.
      j. Roots often partially resorbed.
   2. Some identifying characteristics of primary maxillary and mandibular first molars:
      a. Maxillary first primary molar
         (1) Three roots.
         (2) Generally three cusps (occasional small distolingual cusp).
         (3) Prominent buccal cervical ridge (buccal mesial half).
         (4) Buccal height of contour is at cervical third of crown.
         (5) Lingual height of contour is at middle third of crown.
         (6) Mesiobuccal root size is wider buccolingually than distobuccal root. Lingual root is longest, most divergent.
         (7) Mesiobuccal cusp is largest.
         (8) Smallest molar mesiodistally.
         (9) Distal marginal ridge thin and poorly developed.
      b. Mandibular first primary molar
         (1) Two roots.
         (2) Four cusps.
         (3) Rhomboidal occlusal outline.
         (4) Mesiobuccal cusp is largest and best-developed.
         (5) Very prominent buccal cervical ridge along the mesial half of the buccal surface.
         (6) Buccal height of contour on cervical third of the crown; lingual height on middle third.

5.0 CHRONOLOGY OF PERMANENT DENTITION

The permanent dentition of 32 teeth is completed by 18 to 25 years of age, as indicated in Table 4-3. Such a table suggests the complexity of bringing together all the biological mechanisms at the right time and place to provide the appropriate relationships between tooth form and jaw movements, tooth form, and supporting structures of the teeth, and the alignment of the teeth and their contact relationships with adjacent teeth and opposing teeth in opposing arches, all in such a way as to stabilize the occlusion and protect the supporting structures of the teeth. The dimensions for the permanent dentition are provided in Table 4-4.

TABLE 4–3. CHRONOLOGIES OF PERMANENT TEETH

	TOOTH	FIRST EVIDENCE OF CALCIFICATION	CROWN COMPLETED (YEARS)	EMERGENCE (ERUPTION) (YEARS)	ROOT COMPLETED (YEARS)
CI	8, 9	3–4 mo	4–5	7–8	10
LI	7, 10	10–12 mo	4–5	8–9	11
C	6, 11	4–5 mo	6–7	11–12	13–15
P1	5, 12	1½–1¾ yr	5–6	10–11	12–13
P2	4, 13	2–2¼ yr	6–7	10–12	12–14
M1	3, 14	At birth	2½–3	6–7	9–10
M2	2, 15	2½–3 yr	7–8	12–13	14–16
M3	1, 16	7–9 yr	12–16	17–21	18–25

Maxillary Teeth

Right	**1**	**2**	**3**	**4**	**5**	**6**	**7**	**8**	**9**	**10**	**11**	**12**	**13**	**14**	**15**	**16**	**Left**
	32	**31**	**30**	**29**	**28**	**27**	**26**	**25**	**24**	**23**	**22**	**21**	**20**	**19**	**18**	**17**	

Mandibular Teeth

	TOOTH	FIRST EVIDENCE OF CALCIFICATION	CROWN COMPLETED (YEARS)	EMERGENCE (ERUPTION) (YEARS)	ROOT COMPLETED (YEARS)
CI	24, 25	3–4 mo	4–5	6–7	9
LI	23, 26	3–4 mo	4–5	7–8	10
C	22, 27	4–5 mo	6–7	9–10	12–14
P1	21, 28	1¼–2 yr	5–6	10–12	12–13
P2	20, 29	2¼–2½ yr	6–7	11–12	13–14
M1	19, 30	At birth	2½–3	6–7	9–10
M2	18, 31	2½–3 yr	7–8	11–13	14–15
M3	17, 32	8–10 yr	12–16	17–21	18–25

After Ash MM, Nelson SJ: Wheeler's Dental Anatomy, Physiology, and Occlusion (8th edition). Philadelphia: WB Saunders, 2003.

TABLE 4–4. DIMENSIONS OF PERMANENT TEETH*

	CROWN LENGTH	ROOT LENGTH	CROWN MD	DIAMETER FL†	CURVATURE M	CURVATURE D
Maxillary Teeth						
Central incisor	10.5	13.0	8.5	7.0	3.5	2.5
Lateral incisor	9.0	13.0	6.5	6.0	3.0	2.0
Canine	10.0	17.0	7.5	8.0	2.5	1.5
1st premolar	8.5	14.0	7.0	9.0	1.0	0.0
2nd premolar	8.5	14.0	7.0	9.0	1.0	0.0
First molar	7.5	B 12, L 13	10.0	11.0	1.0	0.0
Second molar	7.0	B 11 L 12	9.0	11.0	1.0	0.0
Third molar	6.5	11	8.5	10.0	1.0	0.0
Mandibular Teeth						
Central incisor	9.0	12.5	5.0	6.0	3.0	2.0
Lateral incisor	9.5	14.0	5.5	6.0	3.0	2.0
Canine	11.0	16.0	7.0	7.5	2.5	1.0
1st premolar	8.5	14.0	7.0	7.5	1.0	0.0
2nd premolar	8.0	14.5	7.0	8.0	1.0	0.0
First molar	7.5	14.0	11.0	10.5	1.0	0.0
Second molar	7.0	13.0	10.5	10.0	1.0	0.0
Third molar	7.0	11.0	10.5	9.5	1.0	0.0

* Average measurements in millimeters

† FL = faciolingual, buccolingual, labiolingual

Adapted from Ash MM, Nelson SJ: Wheeler's Dental Anatomy, Physiology, and Occlusion (8th edition). Philadelphia: WB Saunders, 2003.

6.0 MORPHOLOGY OF PERMANENT TEETH

A schematic representation of the permanent dentition is shown in Figure 4-12. The teeth of each side of the arches are indicated with their universal system numbers.

A. Incisors—some type traits and other characteristics
B. Canine—some type and arch traits and other characteristics
C. Premolars—type traits and other characteristics
D. Maxillary molars—type traits and other characteristics
E. Mandibular molars—type traits and other characteristics
F. Relationship of roots to the maxillary sinus and to the inferior dental canal

The relationship between the roots of the maxillary teeth and the sinus is important in root canal therapy, oral surgery, and sinus lift procedures for implants. The first and second maxillary molars are generally of particular interest, especially with alveolar extension of the maxillary sinus, because of the possibility of perforating the sinus membrane during tooth removal and during placement of implants. Perforation with root canal instrumentation is also a risk to be evaluated closely.

The position of the mandibular molars, especially the third molar, is important because of the proximity of the roots and imbedded third molars to the inferior dental (mandibular) canal (IDC) and the inferior alveolar nerve (IAN). Radiographic indicators of risk of exposure of IAN after mandibular third molar extraction includes darkening of roots, interruption of the white lines of the canal, diversion of the canal, and narrowing of the tooth root.

Table 4–5. Some Type and Arch Traits and Other Characteristics

	CI 8, 9	LI 7, 10	CI 24, 25	LI 23, 26
Pulp horns	Facial view, 3	Usually 2	1 or none	Variable
MI angle	Sharp right angle	Slight rounding	Sharp right angle	Some rounding
DI angle	Slight rounding	Distinct round	Sharp right angle	More rounded
Mesial profile	Straight	Slight rounding	Straight	Straight
Distal profile	Nearly round	Distinct round	Straight	Straight
Incisal outline	Straight	Straight	Straight	Slight DL twist
Proximal contacts				
Mesial	Incis(al) third	Incis/middle third	Incis third	Incis third
Distal	Incis/mid third	Mid(dle) third	Incis third	Incis third
Curve at CEJ				
Mesial	3.5 mm	3.0 mm	3.0 mm	3.0 mm
Distal	2.5 mm	2.0 mm	2.0 mm	2.0 mm
Contour height				
Facial/lingual	Cervical third	Cervical third	Cervical third	Cervical third
Pulp canal(s)	1	1	1, possibly 2	1

	CANINES 6, 11	CANINES 22, 27
Pulp horns	1	1
Facial aspect		
Proximal contacts		
Mesial	Junction of incisal/mid third	Incisal third
Distal	Middle third	Middle third
Mesial aspect	Wider mesiodistally	Narrower, longer
Lingual aspect	Deeper lingual fossae	Flat lingual surface
Marginal ridges	Pronounced; 2 fossae	Parallel or slight convergence
Cingulum	Large; centered MD	Smaller; possibly off-center distally
Lingual pits/grooves	Common	None
Incisal aspect	Marked asymmetry of < asymmetry Halves	Distal cusp mesial/distal Ridge rotated
Incisal/proximal	Cusp tip may be at or cusp tip lingual to root	Views labial to root axis line
CEJ curvature	2.5 mm (mesial)	1.0 mm (distal)
Contour height	0.5 mm	<0.5 mm
Facial/lingual	Cervical third	Cervical third

	FIRST PREMOLARS 5, 12	SECOND PREMOLARS 4, 13	FIRST PREMOLARS 21, 28	SECOND PREMOLARS 20, 29
Buccal/facial view				
Buccal cusps	Pointed	Obtuse	Pointed	More obtuse
Cusp tip	Tipped distally	Tipped mesially	Middle axis	Middle axis
Crown margins	Bulging	Narrow	Prominent	Prominent
Proximal contacts	MD, mid third	MD, mid third	MD, mid third	MD, mid third
Mesial BC ridge	Longer than D	Shorter than D	Shorter than D	M and D similar
Crown symmetry	Bilateral asymmetry	Symmetrical	Bilateral symmetry	Bilateral symmetry
Outline	Trapezoid	Trapezoid	Trapezoid	Trapezoid
Lingual view	All buccal crown profile visible	None of buccal profile visible	Most of buccal profile visible	None of buccal profile visible
Occlusal surface	Little visible	None visible	Mostly visible	Little visible
Mesial aspect	Transverse ridge	Transverse ridge	Transverse ridge	No transverse ridge
ML groove	None	None	Usually present	None
MM ridge groove	Usually present	Not present	Not present	Not present
MM ridge root(s)	Horizontal usually 2, BL	Horizontal	Inclined apically	Horizontal
		Single	Single	Single
Occlusal view				
Table outline	Trapezoidal (see Fig. 4-12)	Rectangular (see Fig. 4-12)	Triangle/diamond (see Fig. 4-12)	Square/round
Groove/pit pattern				
Y groove pattern	Longer	Shorter	No central pit	Central pit
Supplemental grooves	Absent	Present		
	Rare	Frequent		

	FIRST MOLARS 3, 14	SECOND MOLARS 2, 15	THIRD MOLARS 1, 17
Facial aspect	Widest of three	Intermediate width	Smallest width
DB cusp height	Same as MB cusp	DB slightly shorter	DB much shorter
MB root apex	In line with MB cusp	In line with center tip of crown	MB/DB fused, in line with crown center
Occlusal view			
Crown outline	Square/rhomboid (see Fig. 4-12)	More rhomboidal (see Fig. 4-12)	Triangle/heart-shaped (see Fig. 4-12)
Lobes 5 4 3–4			
Lingual aspect			
DL cusp	Largest	Smaller width/height	Usually missing
Lingual root	Widest MD	Narrower	Narrowest
Dimensions:			

	FIRST MOLARS 19, 30	SECOND MOLARS 18, 31	THIRD MOLARS 17, 32
Facial view			
Cusps	5-MB, DB, D, ML, DL	4-MB, DB, ML, DL	4-MB, DB,ML, DL
Buccal grooves	2	1	
Roots	Wide separation	Closer together, fused, short, marked relatively vertical distal inclination	
Lingual view	Visible buccal profiles/ profiles/surfaces	Profiles/surfaces proximal surfaces not visible	Not visible
Occlusal outline	Hex-, pentagonal rectangular	Heart-shaped/ovoid	
Groove(s)	Y pattern + 4 pattern	No pattern	

7.0 DEVELOPMENT OF DENTAL OCCLUSIONS

The development of occlusion involves three time frames (i.e., time of emergence and contacting of the primary teeth, period of the mixed dentition with emergence and contacting of permanent teeth, and the time when the rest of the permanent teeth emerge and make occlusal contact). The factors that determine the size of the teeth and dimensions of the jaws and provide room for succedaneous teeth relate to the orderly transition

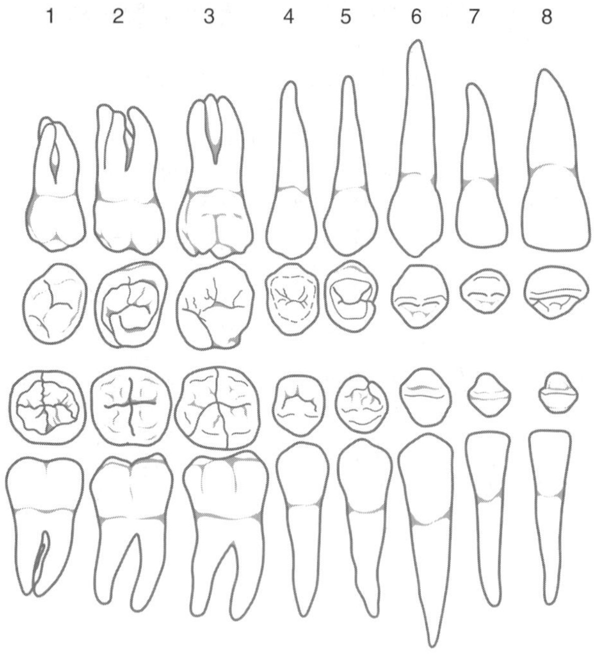

Figure 4–12. Schematic representations of the permanent teeth of the right side.

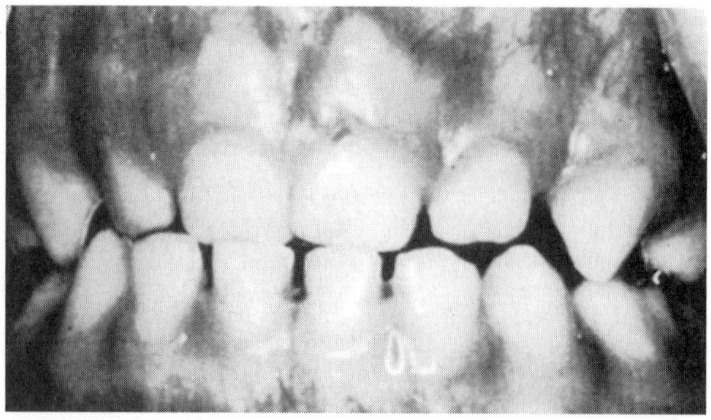

Figure 4–13. Primary dentition showing spacing that generally suggested a low probability of crowding in the permanent dentition. (From Ash MM, Nelson SJ: Wheeler's Dental Anatomy, Physiology, and Occlusion [8th edition]. Philadelphia: WB Saunders, 2003.)

from the primary dentition through the mixed dentition to the permanent dentition and its completion. For example, the chances for crowding in the permanent dentition based on the available spaces between the primary teeth (>6 mm) would be none; however, for 3 to 5 mm of spacing in the primary dentition, the chances of crowding are 1 in 5. If the primary teeth are crowded, there is a 1:1 chance of crowding of the permanent dentition. Among other factors, the availability of interdental spaces in the primary dentition is dependent on tooth size and dimension of the arches. The chance is small for crowding of the permanent dentition in the patient seen in Figure 4-13.

A. Development of primary occlusion

The primary teeth should be in normal alignment and occlusion should occur shortly after the age of 2 years, with all the roots fully formed by the time the child is 3 years old. With the growth of the jaws, the anterior teeth separate, beginning between 4 and 5 years of age. The primary occlusion is also supported and made more efficient by the emergence of the first permanent molars (sometimes referred to as *6-year molars*) immediately distal to the primary second molars, as illustrated in the development of occlusion shown in Figure 4-14, *A, B*. The sequence of eruption (in months) is depicted in Figure 4-14, *C*. The completion of the primary occlusion and developing permanent dentition is shown in Figure 4-14, *D*.

B. Development of permanent occlusion

The development of the permanent occlusion (Figure 4-15, *A*) begins with the emergence and contacts of the first permanent molars at about 6 years of age and, except for the third molar, is concluded at about 15 to 18 years of age. The emergence of the mandibular incisors (Figure 4-15, *B*) follows the 6-year molars at 6 to 7 years of age. The most favorable sequence of eruption/emergence of the permanent dentition for a normal occlusion is shown in Figure 4-15, *C*. The third molars emerge and come into occlusal contact later, usually by 25 years of age (Figure 4-15, *D*).

When the teeth are in ideal alignment so that proximal contacts and marginal ridges are in proper position (Figure 4-16), there is less of a chance of impaction of food into the interproximal areas, resulting in loss of periodontal attachment.

C. Tooth size, arch form, and arch dimensions

Room for the development, eruption, and emergence of the permanent teeth during the mixed dentition period is influenced by the forward rotation of the maxillomandibular complex. An important part in the development of the occlusion of the permanent dentition is the premolar segment where the erupting premolars are significantly smaller in the mesiodistal diameter than the primary molars, which they replace (i.e., the mesiodistal diameters of the mandibular primary molars are greater than the mesiodistal diameter of the replacing premolars). This gain in space between the primary and permanent dentition in the dental arch is referred to as the *leeway space*. It has importance for the alignment of the mandibular incisors and for mandibular molar movement to correct for the end-to-end molar relationship in the mixed dentition period into a normal molar relationship in the permanent dentition (e.g., mesiobuccal cusp of the

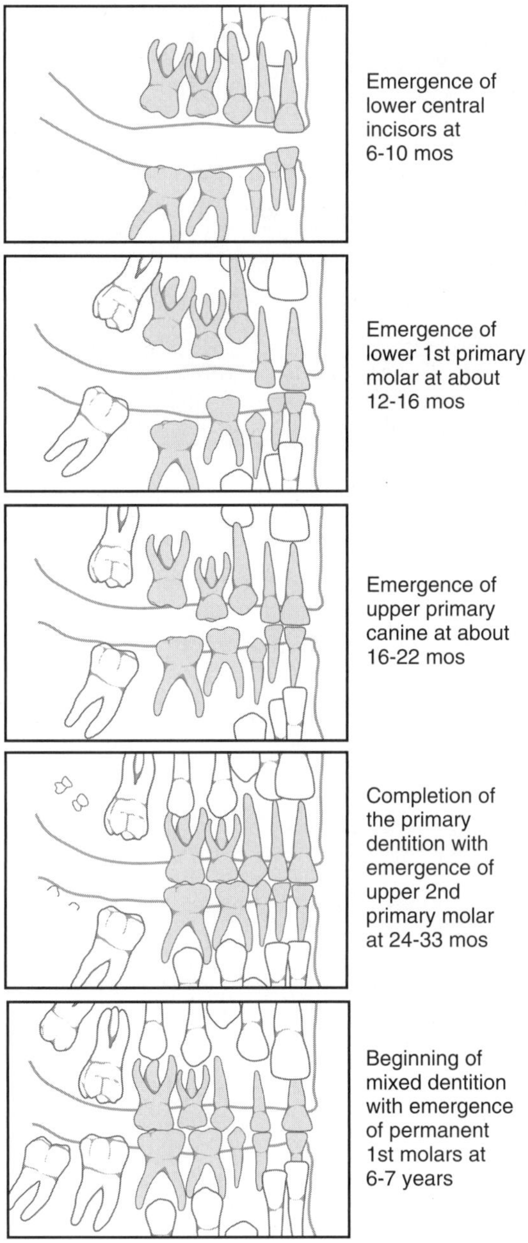

A

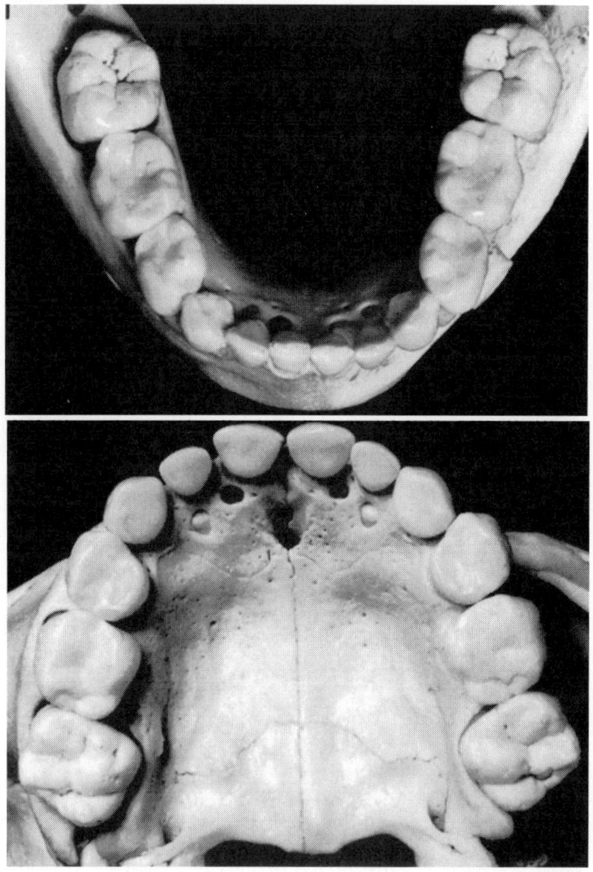

B

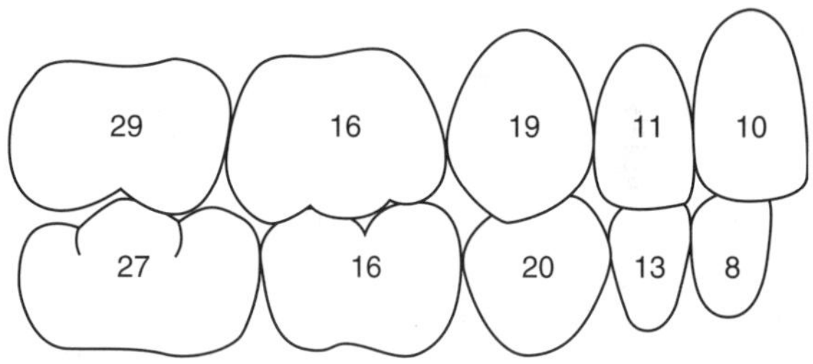

C

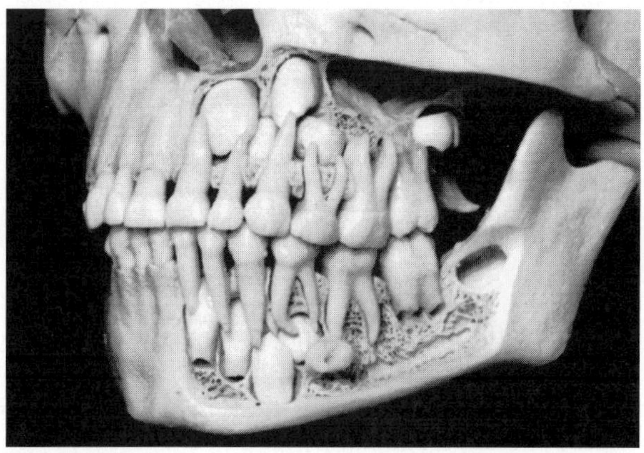

D

Figure 4–14. Development of primary occlusion. A, Birth to mixed dentition. (From Schour L, Massler M: Studies in tooth development: the growth pattern of human teeth. Part II. *J Am Dent Assoc* 27:1918, 1940.) **B**, Mixed dentition with first permanent molar in position. **C**, Mean age of emergence (in months) primary teeth. **D**, Anterior-lateral view of mixed dentition with first permanent molars in position and developing permanent dentition (empty crypt is a preparation artifact). (From Ash MM, Ramfjord SP: Occlusion. Philadelphia: WB Saunders, 1995.)

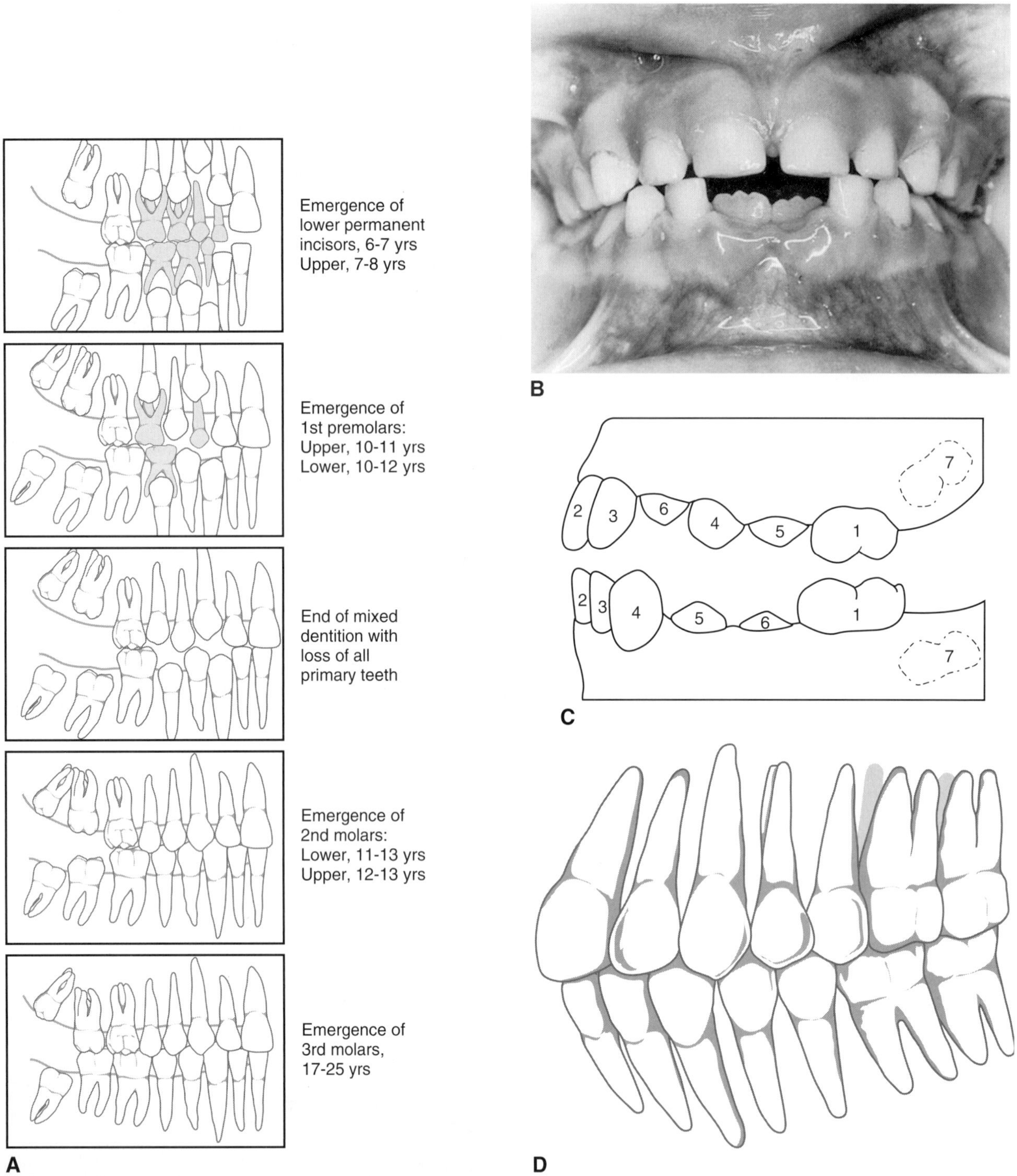

Figure 4–15. Development of the permanent occlusion. **A,** Schematic representation of developing occlusion. (From Schour L, Massler M: The development of the human dentition. *J Am Dent Assoc* 28:1153, 1941.) **B,** Emergence of the mandibular central incisors. **C,** Sequence of eruption of the permanent teeth. **D,** Permanent dentition of 28 teeth at about 14 to 16 years of age.

maxillary first molar occluding in the mesiobuccal developmental groove of the mandibular first molar, as shown in Figure 4-17, *A*, which is an angle class I molar relationship).

The arch form and width of the primary dentition is established generally for both the primary and permanent dentitions by the age of 9 months. What does change is the increase in anterior-posterior dimensions of the jaws, which is necessary for the incorporation of the molars into the occlusion. The supporting alveolar bone and basal bone determine the shape of the dental arches.

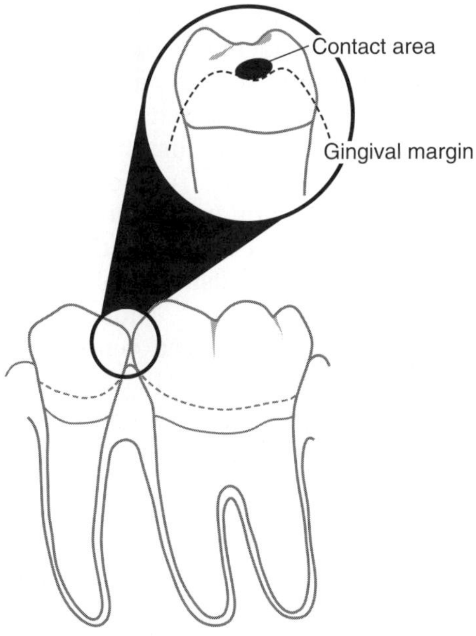

Figure 4-16. Schematic illustration of proximal contact areas and relationship to gingival margin.

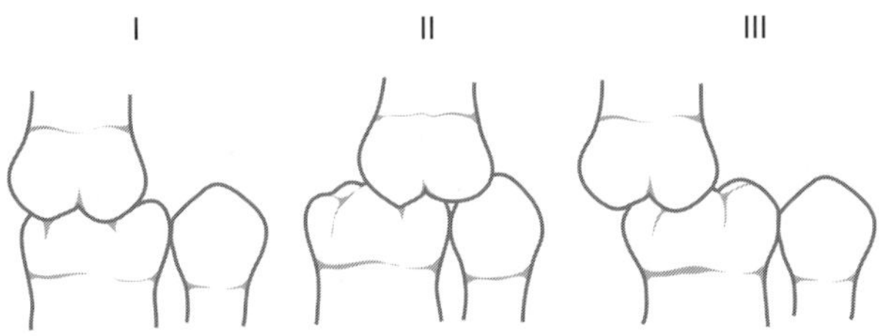

Figure 4–17. Molar relationships of the permanent dentition used in angle classification. A, Class I (normal). **B,** Class II (retrognathism). **C,** Class III (prognathism).

There is a general relationship between the size of the teeth and the size of the dental arches; however, when a discrepancy is evident between the aggregate mesiodistal diameters of the crowns of the teeth and the size of the bony supporting arches, crowding or protrusion can occur. Arch width and perimeter dimensions can relate to differences between crowded and uncrowded dentitions.

In cases of restorative dentistry, the dimensions of the replacement teeth must be related to the size of the existing teeth and arch dimensions. For example, for a maxillary arch length of 128 mm and a mandibular arch length of 126 mm, the sum of the mesiodistal diameter of all the mandibular teeth would have to be 126 mm, and the sum of the mesiodistal diameter of all the maxillary teeth would have to be 128 mm. Arch dimensions and tooth size vary considerably, and there is no template for any patient. The aesthetics of tooth form, size, and color are important considerations in restoring teeth.

8.0 OCCLUSAL CONTACT RELATIONS AND MANDIBULAR MOVEMENTS

The restorative dentist must preserve comfort and health throughout the functional (chewing) and parafunctional range of the patient's mandibular movements. Concepts of occlusion that incorporate principles of mandibular movement require a basic understanding of occlusal relations and potential influences upon dental anatomy as a foundation. This section will introduce occlusal contact relations that occur in maximum intercuspation of the teeth (centric positions) and the basic relations associated with mandibular movement (eccentric positions).

A. Static occlusal relationships

In the generally accepted definition of normal occlusion, each mandibular tooth is positioned lingual to the maxillary counterpart. It may also be helpful to note that the mandibular teeth are positioned about one half of a tooth anterior to the maxillary counterpart, excluding the central incisors (Figure 4-18). In this position, occlusal contacts may follow two primary forms. (Figure 4-19). It should be noted that the following descriptions relate to so-called idealized contact relations—a concept that can be used as a basis for discussion, as well as for developing occlusal contact relations in restorative dentistry and orthodontics. Individuals may often show variations from the patterns as presented *without* having occlusal dysfunction.

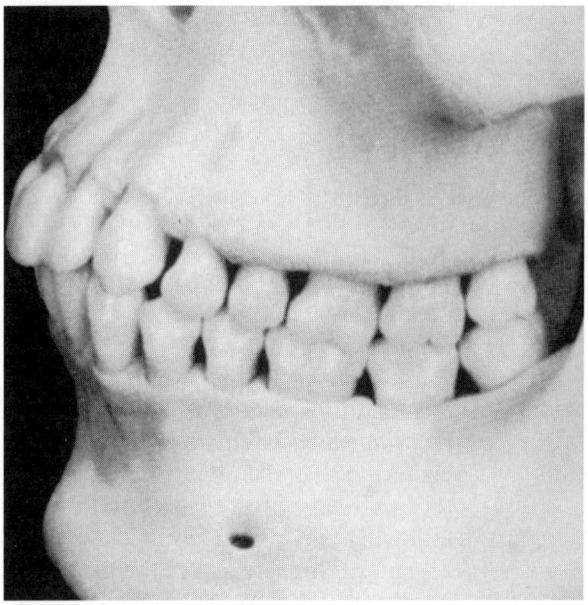

Figure 4–18. View of the step relationship of maxillary and mandibular teeth.

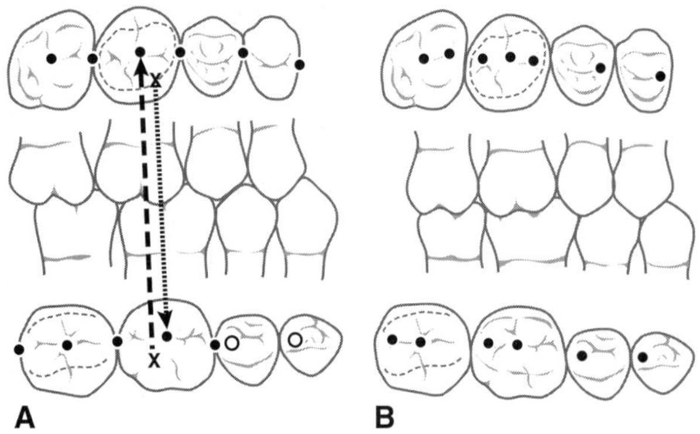

Figure 4–19. A, Cusp/embrasure contact relationship. B, Cusp/fossa contact relationship.

1. Posterior cusp-fossa/cusp-embrasure occlusion, from an occlusal view (Figure 4-19, *A*). The mandibular buccal cusps (mandibular supporting cusps) will occlude as follows:
   a. The first premolar cusp contacts the marginal ridges between the maxillary canine and first premolar.
   b. The second premolar contacts marginal ridges between the first maxillary premolar and second maxillary premolar.
   c. The mesiobuccal cusp of the first molar contacts the marginal ridges between the second maxillary premolar and first molar.
   d. The distobuccal cusp of the first molar contacts the central fossa of the maxillary first molar (this is a key contact relationship to remember).
   e. The distal cusp of the first molar contacts the distal fossa of the maxillary first molar.
   f. The mesiobuccal cusp of the second molar contacts the marginal ridges between the first and second maxillary molars.
   g. The distobuccal cusp of the second molar contacts the central fossa of the maxillary second molar.

   Again, from Figure 4-19, *A*, the contact relations occurring with the *maxillary lingual cusps* (maxillary supporting cusps) follow a similar embrasure contact pattern, with the exception of the following two cusps:

   h. The mesiolingual cusp of the first molar contacts the central fossa of the mandibular first molar (this is a key contact relationship to remember).
   i. The mesiolingual cusp of the second molar contacts the central fossa of the mandibular second molar.
2. Posterior cusp-fossa/cusp-fossa occlusion

   The cusp-fossa/cusp-fossa occlusion shares the same relationship as the embrasure form when considering the mesiolingual cusps of the maxillary molars and the distobuccal cusps of the mandibular molars. Those supporting cusps will contact the central fossae of the opposing counterparts in maximum intercuspation. The contact relations for the right mandibular supporting cusps and incisors are indicated in Figure 4-19, *B*. The mandibular cusp pattern results in a fossa contact for each supporting cusp and results in a "one tooth contacting one tooth" relationship, as opposed to the mandibular teeth contacting the maxillary counterpart and the mesially occurring tooth as described for the cusp-embrasure occlusion (Figure 4-19, *A*). The *mandibular supporting cusp* relations will occur (Figure 4-19, *B*) as follows:
   a. The first premolar contacts the mesial triangular fossa of the maxillary first premolar.
   b. The second premolar contacts the mesial triangular fossa of the maxillary second premolar.
   c. The mesiobuccal cusp of the first molar contacts the mesial triangular fossa of the maxillary first molar.
   d. The distobuccal cusp of the first molar contacts the central fossa of the maxillary first molar.
   e. The distal cusp of the first molar contacts the distal triangular fossa of the maxillary first molar.
   f. The mesiobuccal cusp of the second molar contacts the mesial triangular fossa of the maxillary second molar.
   g. The distobuccal cusp of the second molar contacts the central fossa of the maxillary second molar.

   As shown in Figure 4-19, *B*, the maxillary supporting cusp relationships follow a similar contact relationship with the mandibular counterparts. Note that with the exception of the mesiolingual cusps of the maxillary molars, the remaining contacts in maximum intercuspation occur in the distal fossa of the mandibular counterparts.

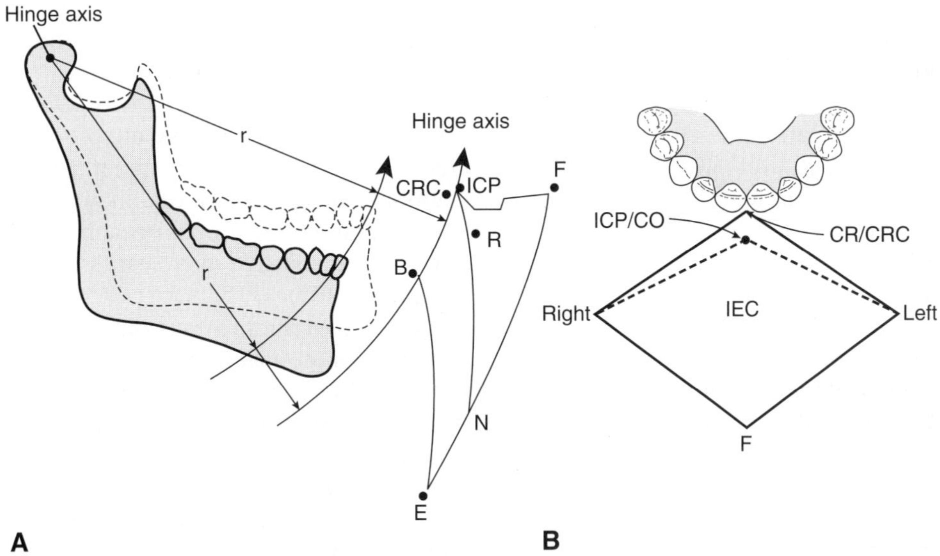

Figure 4–20. Border movements of the mandible. A, Sagittal plane. *F,* maximum protrusive; *ICP,* intercuspal position/centric occlusion (maximum intercuspation); *CRC,* retruded contact position in centric relation; *B* to *CRC,* hinge axis movement; *E,* point of maximum opening; *ICP* to *N,* normal range of opening/closing movements; *IEC,* incisal edge contacts. **B,** Horizontal plane. Maximum right, left, and protrusive movements.

B. Border movements of the mandible

Primary movements of the temporomandibular joint (TMJ) involve some degree of rotation (hinge movement) and translation (sliding movements) of both joints. Although the TMJ will be discussed separately, basic mandibular movements may be better understood by studying the border movements of the mandible. Border movements are the limits to which the mandible can move, whereas the functional movements generally occur within the border positions. Plane diagrams may be helpful to visualize the various positions and movements. Sagittal and horizontal plane diagrams of border movements are shown in Figure 4-20. Unassisted maximum opening for a normal person is considered to be about 40+ mm. Unassisted normal maximum lateral movements are considered to be about 10 to 12 mm. Maximum protrusion from incisal edge contact (IEC) is normally about 4 to 5+ mm. Chewing function takes place usually within a few millimeters of the intercuspal position (ICP) or centric occlusion (CO), which are terms used to define maximum intercuspation of the teeth.

1. Mandibular movements viewed from the frontal/coronal plane

   Healthy individuals are able to move their mandibles laterally to both the left and right. Chewing generally occurs on the side to which the mandible moves, as shown in Figure 4-21.

   When the mandible moves to the right, the right side movement is termed *laterotrusive movement* (right working movement). The left side would then move medially and protrusively to result in a mediotrusive movement (balancing or nonworking movement) (Figure 4-22). It

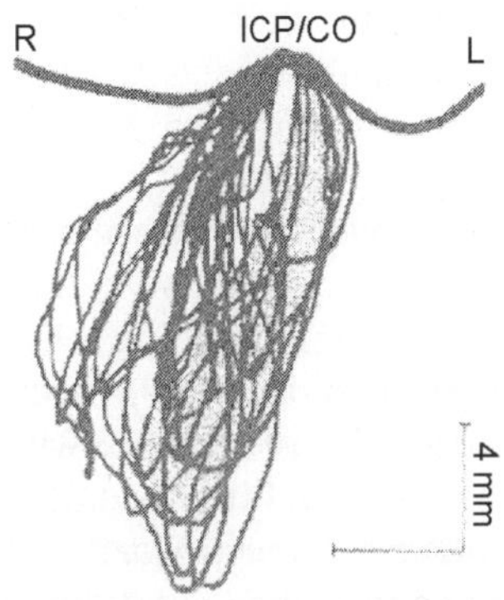

Figure 4–21 Mandibular movements during the process of chewing naturally. Incisor point movement seen in the frontal plane. *R,* right; *L,* left; *ICP/CO,* intercuspal position/centric occlusion. (Modified from Ash MM, Nelson SJ: Wheeler's Dental Anatomy, Physiology and Occlusion [8th edition]. Philadelphia: WB Saunders, 2003.)

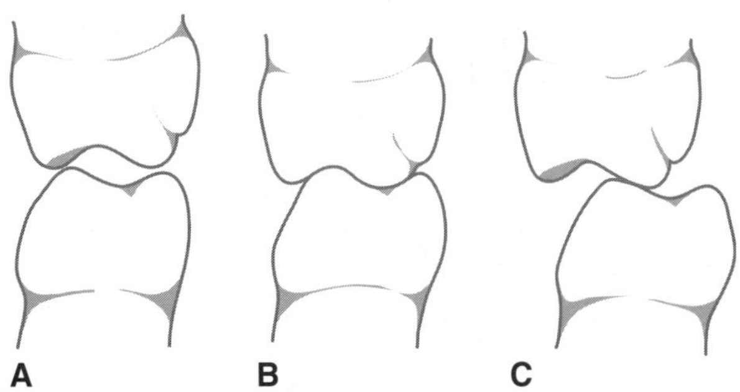

Figure 4–22. Mandibular movement contact relations seen from the coronal plane; contact relations of maxillary and mandibular molars. A, Right laterotrusive (working side). **B,** Intercuspal; position (centric occlusion). **C,** Mediotrusive (nonworking side/balancing) left side.

follows, then, that the laterotrusive movements and mediotrusive movements reverse sides when the mandible moves to the left.

From the basic contact relations occurring in maximum intercuspation (ICP), potential tooth contacts occurring when the mandible moves laterally and protrusively can be described.

2. Mandibular movements viewed from the horizontal plane

   When viewed in the horizontal plane, the paths for the mesiolingual cusp of the maxillary first molar and the distobuccal cusp of the mandibular first molar are shown in Figure 4-23.

   a. In a normal alignment of the dentition, the mesiolingual cusp of the maxillary first molar opposes the central fossa of the mandibular first molar.
   b. From this position, the cusp will pass through the lingual groove when a laterotrusive (working) movement occurs.
   c. During a mediotrusive movement (nonworking or balancing), the same cusp will oppose the distobuccal groove.
   d. Mandibular protrusion will result in the mesiolingual cusp passing through the central groove toward the distal marginal ridge of the mandibular molar.
   e. Retrusive movement of the mandible will result in the potential for contacts mesial to the intercuspal contacts on mandibular posterior teeth.

3. A similar pattern exists for mandibular movements as related to the anatomy of maxillary posterior teeth.

   a. The distobuccal cusps of the mandibular first molars oppose the central fossa of the maxillary first molars.
   b. During a laterotrusive movement, that cusp will pass through the buccal groove of the maxillary molar.
   c. A mediotrusive movement will oppose the maxillary mesiolingual cusp.
   d. It should be apparent that the maxillary supporting cusps and the mandibular supporting cusps oppose each other during mediotrusive movements (Figure 4-22).
   e. Protrusive movements result in the mandibular distobuccal cusp passing through the maxillary central groove toward the mesial marginal ridge.
   f. Occlusal contacts occurring during retrusive movements will occur distal to the contacts in maximal intercuspation on maxillary teeth.

   What has just been described uses the first molars only; however, a similar pattern is generated for each supporting cusp.

   Examining eccentric occlusal contact relations again from the frontal view, it is apparent that occlusal contact is possible along three primary anatomical areas of the posterior teeth.

   g. During a right working movement, the right side molar teeth may contact along the lingual inclines of the maxillary buccal cusps and the buccal inclines of the mandibular buccal cusps (Figure 4-22). Likewise, the lingual inclines of the maxillary lingual cusps may contact the buccal inclines of the mandibular lingual cusps. This relationship is sometimes called a *cross-tooth balance.*
   h. When examining the mediotrusive side (left side nonworking), contact is also possible along the buccal inclines of the left maxillary lingual cusps and the lingual inclines of the left mandibular buccal cusps. Note: this relationship of bilateral occlusal contact during lateral excursions is sometimes referred to as a *balanced* or *cross-arch-balanced relationship.*

   The description above has been based upon a right side working and left side nonworking movement. A left working movement would produce a similar but reversed contact relationship between the right and left sides.

   Three occlusal relationships for working movements considered acceptable

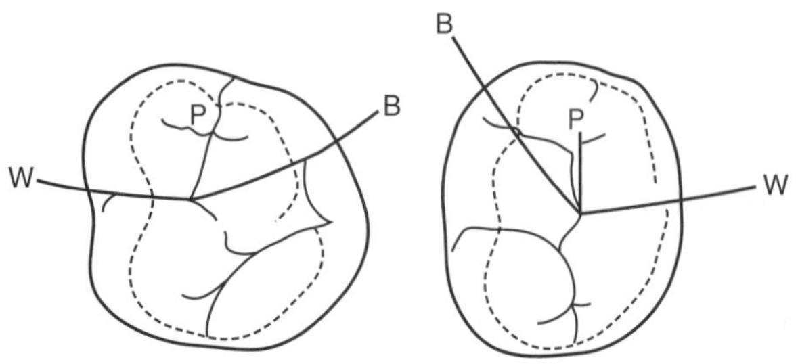

Figure 4–23. Movement paths in horizontal plane made by supporting cusp on right maxillary first molar and on right mandibular first molar.
W, Laterotrusive; *B,* mediotrusive; *P,* protrusive.

restorative concepts for the natural dentition are described as follows:

i. If contact occurs only on the cuspid teeth during working movements, the relationship is sometimes referred to as a *canine-guided, canine rise,* or *cuspid-protected occlusion*. In this relationship, contact of the maxillary and mandibular canine teeth will occur to the extent that all posterior teeth are separated on the working and nonworking sides.

j. If the canine and the buccal cusps of the posterior teeth contact simultaneously during the working movement, to the extent that the nonworking side teeth are separated, the relationship may be referred to as a *group function occlusion*.

k. As the mandible slides into a protrusive position, contact will generally occur along the lingual surface of the maxillary anterior teeth and the facial surface or incisal edge of the mandibular anterior teeth. Most restorative concepts of occlusion for the natural dentition recommend that anterior contacts separate the posterior teeth during protrusive movement. This relationship is referred to as *anterior guidance* or *incisal guidance*. Although these descriptions may be generally accepted, it should be recognized that posterior tooth contact in protrusive movement does occur naturally, as well as posterior contact on the nonworking side. For example, the dentist may choose to apply these contact relationships during certain prosthodontics procedures.

9.0 ANATOMY, PHYSIOLOGY, AND FUNCTION OF THE TEMPOROMANDIBULAR JOINT

The TMJ is a complex joint that allows a wide degree of freedom for many possible movements. Actions of the joints may have a profound effect on restorative dentistry and a person's ability to function normally. Understanding the anatomy of the TMJ and functional movements is a prerequisite to comprehensive diagnosis and treatment in the dental clinic.

A. TMJ anatomy

The primary anatomical features of the TMJ are reviewed in the following diagrams showing a sagittal view of the joint, capsule, TMJ ligament, oblique band, and the TMJ horizontal band (Figure 4-24). The disc is attached to the medial and lateral poles of the condyle by discal ligaments. These ligaments limit movement within the lower joint space to rotation. The glenoid fossa and the condyle are covered by dense fibrous connective tissue (Figure 4-25). The articular meniscus (disc) is a biconcave structure composed of dense collagenous (hyaline) connective

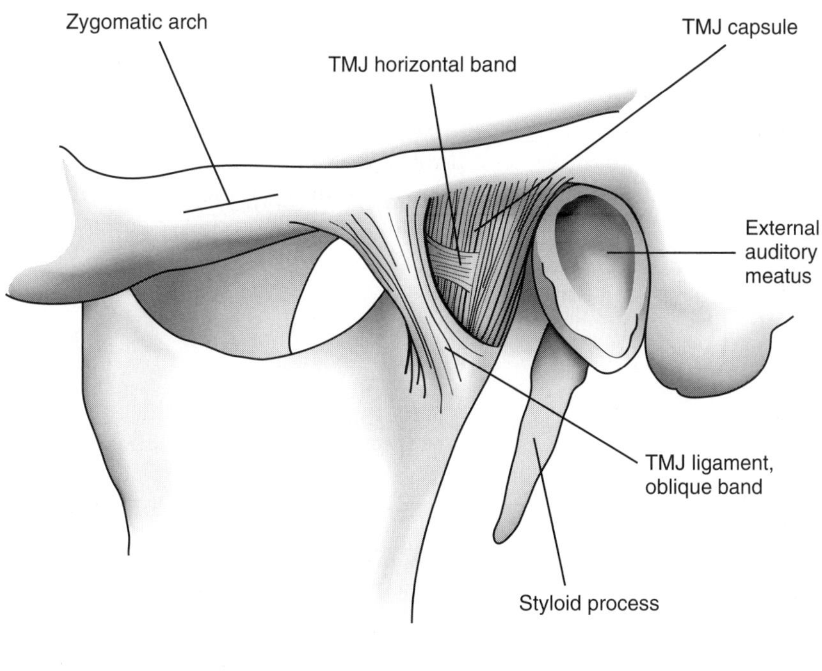

Figure 4–24. TMJ capsule and TMJ ligaments.

tissue. The central areas are primarily avascular and noninnervated in the adult. The anterior band aspect of the meniscus (disc/meniscus) inserts into the superior belly of the lateral pterygoid muscle (Figure 4-25). These areas are innervated and vascular. The posterior discal attachment is called the *bilaminar zone* or *retrodiscal lamina* (Figure 4-26). This area is both vascularized and innervated. Elastic fibers are found in the superior lamina and collagen fibers inferiorly.

B. TMJ innervation

The sensory innervation (not shown) for the TMJ is provided primarily by the auriculotemporal nerve (posterior and lateral TMJ). Anterior innervation occurs through a branch from the deep temporal nerve.

C. Ligaments

Three primary ligaments and two accessory ligaments support the TMJ. Primary ligaments include the lateral and medial capsular ligament, the discal ligaments, and a very strong temporomandibular ligament (see Figure 4-24). The TMJ ligament consists of an inner layer of horizontal fibers and an outer portion of oblique fibers. The stylomandibular and sphenomandibular ligaments (Figure 4-27) make up the accessory ligaments,

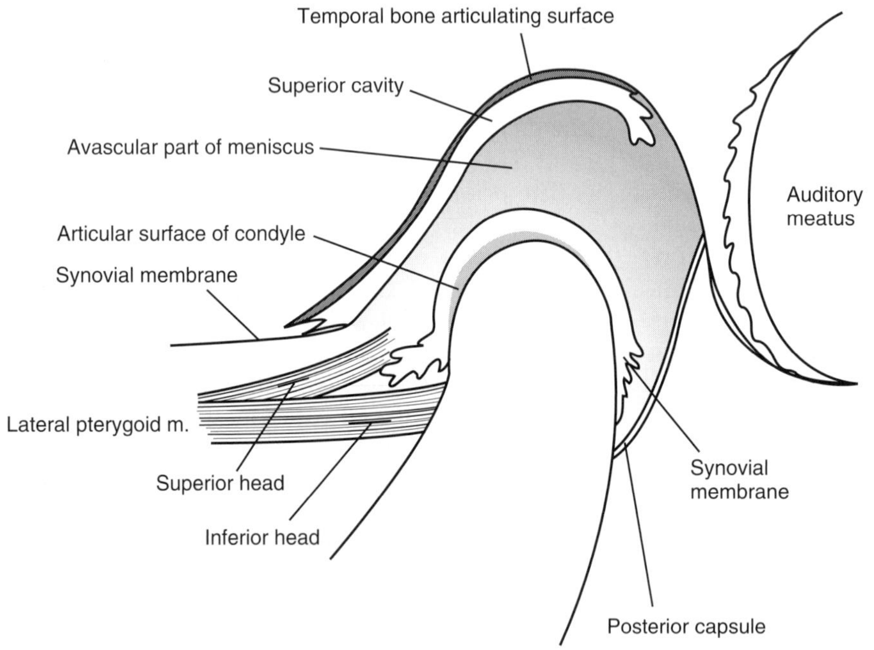

Figure 4–25. Schematic representation of the TMJ.

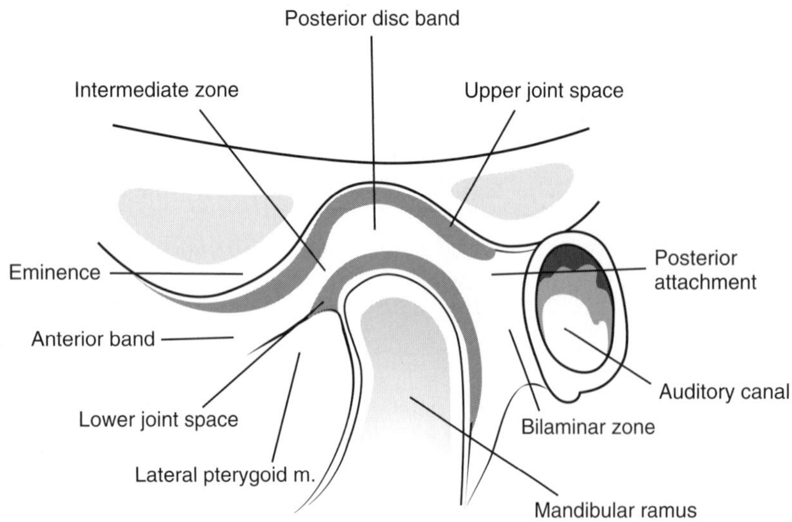

Figure 4–26. Articular disc of the TMJ. (From Ash MM, Ramfjord SP: Occlusion. Philadelphia: WB Saunders, 1995; redrawn from Dolwick MF, Sanders B: Internal Derangement and Arthrosis. St. Louis: Mosby, 1985.)

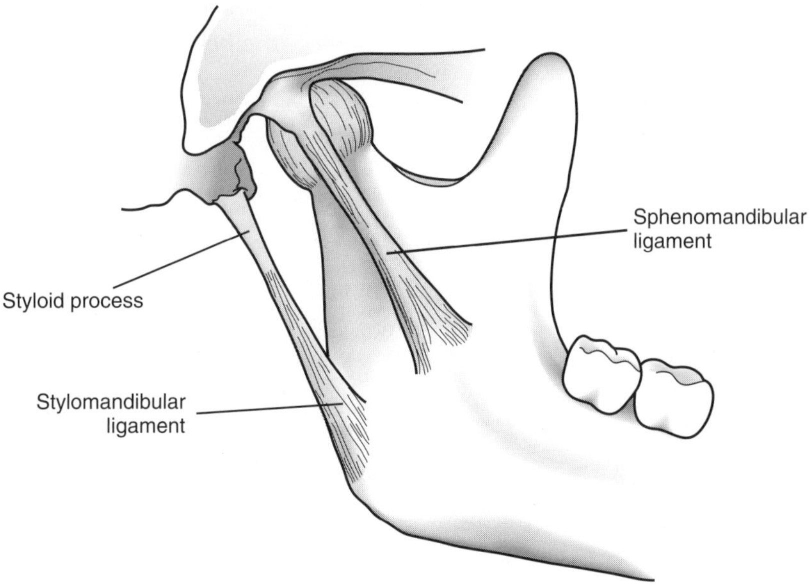

Figure 4–27. Accessory ligaments of the TMJ.

which function with the primary ligaments to limit excessive movement of the joint. The dense collagenous connective tissue in these ligaments does not stretch; however, it should be recognized that the ligaments and masticatory muscles act like a hammock to suspend the condyle within the joint. This arrangement of structures enables complex movements, such as chewing.

D. Synovial joint

The TMJ is a synovial joint in that the upper and lower joint spaces are lined by synovial cells (see Figure 4-25). Synovial fluid moistens these surfaces and provides lubrication and perhaps nutritional or metabolic functions.

E. Joint actions

The TMJ is often referred to as a *ginglymoarthrodial joint,* meaning hinge and glide. The TMJ is also somewhat capable of free movement or diarthrosis. As the mandible articulates with both left and right TMJs, mandibular movement results in actions of both joints simultaneously. Hinge (rotation) occurs in the lower joint space. Glide (translation) occurs in the upper joint space. Each TMJ is able to rotate in three separate planes or axes.

It should be recognized that an action or rotation that occurs in one joint may produce a different action at the other (i.e., while the working condyle rotates in the frontal [vertical] axis, the nonworking condyle translates). In any event, maximum opening equals the maximum rotation and maximum translation of both condyles.

10.0 MASTICATORY MUSCLES

This section deals with the basic musculature involved with mastication. As in previous sections, the reader is directed to more detailed anatomical works for further study. This section serves only as a basic review. At a minimum, the reader should be knowledgeable about the origin, insertion, innervation, and action of the basic muscles of mastication as related to the basic mandibular movements.

A. Masseter muscles (Figure 4-28)
   1. Superficial layer of masseter muscle
      a. Origin: lower border of the zygomatic arch, the lateral surface of the ascending ramus, and body of the mandible.
      b. Insertion: mandibular angle extending from the lateral surface of the mandible near the second molar to the posterior lateral surface of the ramus.
      c. Innervation: V_3 fifth nerve (masseter nerve branch).
      d. Function: it is a powerful mandibular elevator muscle.
   2. Deep layer masseter muscle/zygomaticomandibular muscle
      a. Origin: the tendinous attachment of this muscle originates on the lower lateral border of the zygomatic arch and lateral surface of the mandibular ramus.
      b. Insertion: its insertion is concurrent with the superficial layer at the level of the mandibular angle.

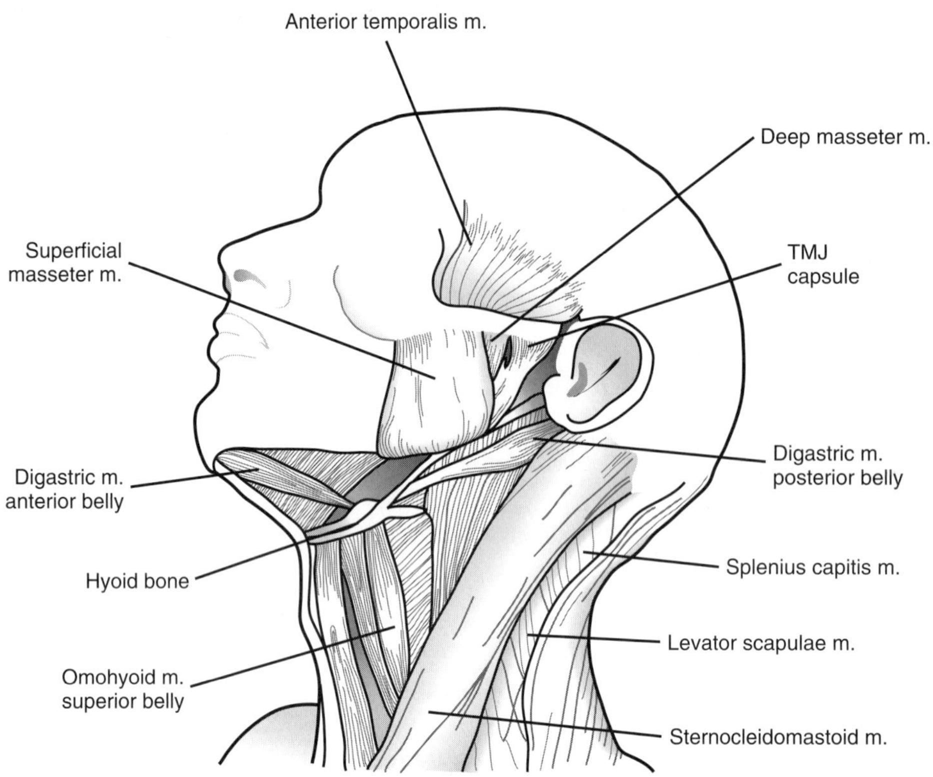

Figure 4–28. Muscles of the head and neck.

c. Function: aids in retrusive mandibular movements.

B. Temporalis muscle (Figure 4-28)
   1. Fan-shaped muscle located on the lateral side of the skull
      a. Origin: the temporal fossa and fascia.
      b. Insertion: a tendinous attachment to the anterior border and mesial surface of the coronoid process and ascending mandibular ramus.
      c. Innervation: temporal branches of the mandibular division, fifth nerve.
      d. Function: the anterior and intermediate bundles of this muscle assist in mandibular elevation. The posterior bundle, due to its horizontal orientation, retrudes the mandible.

C. Pterygoid muscles (Figure 4-29)
   1. Medial pterygoid muscle: an intraoral muscle located medial to the ascending ramus of the mandible. The medial pterygoid is orientated almost parallel to the masseter muscle.
      a. Origin: medial surface of the lateral pterygoid plate, pyramidal process of the palatine bone.
      b. Insertion: its insertion is on the internal surface of the mandibular ramus and angle of the mandible.
      c. Innervation: branch from the mandibular division of the fifth nerve.
      d. Function: mandibular elevation and lateral positioning.
   2. Lateral pterygoid muscle: superior (SHLP) and inferior heads (IHLP)
      a. Origin: superior head origin is the greater sphenoid wing. The origin occurs on the lateral surface of the pterygoid plate.
      b. Insertion: the insertion of the tendinous process of the superior head is part of the anterior border of the condyle, articular disc, and joint capsule. The insertion of the lower head is to the condylar capsule and pterygoid fovea on the anterior surface of the neck of the condyle.
      c. Innervation: fifth cranial nerve.
      d. Function: although reports vary, the SHLP is thought to be responsible for the stabilization of the condylar head and disc against the articular eminence during closing or clenching.

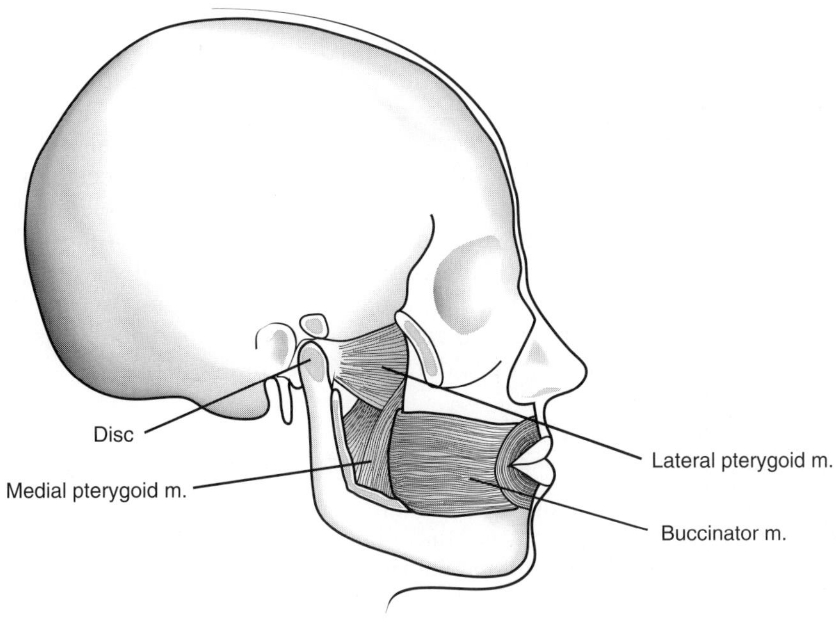

Figure 4–29. Lateral and medial pterygoid muscles (cutaway sections).

Hypothetically, both the SHLP and IHLP can be regarded as parts of one muscle, with distribution of activities shaded according to the biomechanical demands of the task. The IHLP plays a major role in the generation and fine control of horizontal forces, especially in the contralateral direction, which is required in masticatory and parafunctional activities.

3. Digastric muscle: anterior and posterior parts (Figure 4-28)
   a. Attachments (anterior belly): the attachment of this muscle is at the digastric fossa on the inner surface of the mandibular body near the midline. From this attachment, the muscle moves in a lateral, posterior, and inferior direction where it joins with the tendinous insertion of the posterior belly of the digastric muscle on the same side of the head. Both tendons pass through a fibrous loop of the hyoid bone.
   b. Attachments (posterior belly): the origin of this muscle is at the mastoid notch of the temporal bone. From this origin, the muscle is oriented in a forward, medial, and inferior direction to join with the tendon of the anterior belly.
   c. Innervation: anterior part is a branch from the nerve to the mylohyoid, mandibular division of the fifth nerve. The posterior part is innervated by the digastric branch of the facial nerve.
   d. Function: this pair of muscles is an important depressor of the mandible.

11.0 MASTICATORY SYSTEM AND ROLE OF OCCLUSION

Occlusion relates to the study of oral motor function and behavior. This beautifully complex system involves the peripheral and central nervous systems, head and neck musculature, TMJs, periodontal tissues, and the teeth. These individual components all act together during the performance of daily functional activities such as chewing, sucking, swallowing, speech, respiration, and (perhaps a daily activity) kissing. In addition, these systems are involved in activities not routinely recognized as functional. Aggressive clenching or grinding of the teeth (bruxism) and habits such as biting fingernails are generally considered parafunctional.

As an introductory study of a masticatory action, the process will be simplified into three basic phases. The masticatory activity is first initiated with actions that are responses to need, including hunger or thirst. Thus, a person may make a conscious decision to eat or drink something, initiating an action. The second phase is very complex and involves neuromuscular programming before actually performing the task. An example of this would be opening one's mouth large enough to insert a candy bar and then knowing how hard to bite on the candy bar to incise or chew it. Actually, the programming phase involves many things, such as one's previous experience with the food type, hardness, and so forth, as well as input from sensory receptors of the periodontal tissues and oral soft tissues (e.g., lips and tongue). The third and final phase of process is to execute the action. Current belief is that cyclical actions such as chewing probably involve neural activity of a so-called brainstem pattern generator. This pattern generator allows complex coordinated movement without much conscious input from the higher brain centers. However, these preprogrammed actions can be stopped at any time from any part of the system providing sensory feedback. Remember how quickly chewing is stopped when one unexpectedly bites the cheek or tongue, and perhaps how hard it is to swallow an unwanted raw fish delicacy.

Basically, the masticatory system is remarkably adaptable, which is why we can perform clinical dentistry with such high success. The masticatory system tends to reach a state of homeostasis (stability). This is achieved when forces exerted by the lips and cheeks, tongue, occlusal forces, and the support provided by the periodontal tissues work together to maintain tooth position within the dental arches. Obviously, the health of the masticatory muscles and TMJs also influences the homeostasis or stability by influencing jaw position and occlusal forces.

As age, wear, and disease affect the masticatory system, a process of adaptation will generally occur. Functional adaptation occurs when jaw position changes due to pain, drifted teeth, or high restorations. If a high restoration prevents intercuspation in the normal jaw position, a patient may search to find a new position for the teeth. Adaptation may also occur structurally. In structural adaptation, changes occur to anatomic structures such as tooth attrition, resorption, mobility, or migration. Structural adaptation may occur with hyper or excessive force or function resulting in resorption or deposition of bone as a structural adaptation. A third adaptive process may also occur. Humans may respond or adapt by changing their behavior. The adage "If it hurts, don't do it" is an example of behavioral adaptation. Behavioral adaptation also relates to patients' perceptions of suffering. This is an emotional condition relating to how pleasant or unpleasant the adaptation is to the patient. This is sometimes referred to as a person's *affect.*

All of these factors influence function of the masticatory system. The system tends to balance the effects of disease, aging, and restorative treatment through adaptive processes. Since there is no way to predict how well an individual will be able to adapt to disease or influences from restorative treatment, the dentist's challenge is to prevent disease and provide treatment that minimizes a patient's need to adapt. In other words, a dentist telling a patient "You will get used to it" may be correct given enough time, but this is never considered sound dental practice.

References

American Dental Association, Committee on Nomenclature: Committee adopts official method for the symbolic designation of teeth. *J Am Dent Assoc* 34:647, 1947.

American Dental Association, Committee on Dental Education and Hospitals: Tooth numbering and radiographic mounting. *Am Dent Assoc Trans* 109:25, 109:247, 1968.

Arulmozhi DK et al.: Migraine: current concepts and emerging therapies. *Vascul Pharmacol* 43:176, 2005.

Ash MM, Nelson SJ: *Wheeler's Dental Anatomy, Physiology and Occlusion* (8th edition). Philadelphia: WB Saunders, 2003.

Ash MM, Ramfjord SP: *Occlusion* (4th edition). Philadelphia: WB Saunders, 1995.

Ash MM, Ramfjord SP: *An Introduction to Functional Occlusion*. Philadelphia: WB Saunders, 1982.

Bader G, Lavigne G: Sleep bruxism: an overview of an oromandibular sleep movement disorder. *Sleep Medicine Reviews* 4:27, 2000.

Black GV: *Descriptive Anatomy of the Human Teeth* (4th edition). Philadelphia: SS White Dental Manufacturing, 1897.

Carlsen O: *Dental Morphology*. Copenhagen: Munksgaard, 1987.

Charlick RE et al.: *Dental Anatomy*. Ann Arbor, MI: University of Michigan, 1974.

De Moor RJG et al.: The radix entomolaris in mandibular first molars: an endodontic challenge. *Int Endodontic J* 37:789, 2004.

Devlin TM (ed): *Textbook of Biochemistry with Clinical Correlations* (5th edition). New York: John Wiley (Wiley-Liss), 2002.

Dolwick MF, Sanders B: *Internal Derangement and Arthrosis*. St. Louis: Mosby, 1985.

dos Santos J: *Occlusion: Principles and Concepts*. St. Louis: Ishiyaki EuroAmerica, 1985.

Ellison JA, Stanziani P: SSRI-associated bruxism in four patients. *J Clin Psychiatry* 54:432, 1993.

Fédéeration Dentaire Internationale: Two-digit system of designating teeth. *Int Dent J* 21:104, 1971.

Fuller JL, Denehy GE: *Concise Dental Anatomy and Morphology* (2nd edition). Chicago: Year Book, 1984.

Gay T, Piecuch JF: An electromyographic analysis of jaw movements. *Electromyogr Clin Neurophysiol* 26:365, 1986.

Gear RW: Neural control of oral behavior and its impact on occlusion. In: McNeill C (ed): *Science and Practice* of Occlusion. Chicago: Quintessence, 1997.

Gerber PB, Lynd LD: Selective serotonin-reuptake inhibitor-induced movement disorders. *Ann Pharm* 32:692, 1998.

Goadsby PJ et al.: Migraine: current understanding and treatment. *N Engl J Med* 346:257, 2002.

Goodman P: A universal system for identifying permanent and primary teeth. *J Dent Child* 34:312, 1987.

Gülekon N et al.: Variations in the anatomy of the auriculotemporal nerve. *Clin Anat* 18:15, 2005.

Haderup V: Dental nomenklatur og stenograft. *Dansk Tandl Tidskr* 3:3, 1891.

Hannam AG: Jaw muscle structure and function. In: McNeill C (ed): *Science and Practice of Occlusion*. Chicago: Quintessence, 1997.

Hannam AG, McMillan AS: Internal organization in the human jaw muscles. *Crit Rev Oral Biol Med* 5:55, 1994.

Hirsh J et al.: Oral anticoagulants: mechanism of action, clinical effectiveness, and optimal therapeutic range. *Chest* 108:231, 1995.

Ismail AI, Bandekar RR: Fluoride supplements and fluorosis: a meta-analysis. *Community Dent Oral Epidemiol* 27:48, 1999.

Kato T et al.: Topical review: sleep bruxism and the role of periphery sensory influences. *J Orofac Pain* 17:191, 2003.

Knott J, Meredith HV: Statistics on the eruption of the permanent dentition from serial data from North American white children. *Angle Orthod* 36:68, 1966.

Kraus BS, Jordon RE: *The Human Dentition Before Birth*. Philadelphia: Lea & Febiger, 1965.

Kraus BS et al.: *Dental Anatomy and Occlusion*. Baltimore: Williams & Wilkins, 1969.

Kronfeld R, Scour I: Neonatal dental hypoplasia. *J Am Dent Assoc* 26:18, 1939.

Lavigne GJ et al.: Neurobiological mechanisms involved in sleep bruxism. *Crit Rev Oral Biol Med* 14:30, 2003.

Lobbezoo F, Naeije M: Bruxism is mainly regulated centrally, not peripherally. *J Oral Rehabil* 8:1085, 2001.

Logan WHG, Kronfeld R: Development of the human jaws and surrounding structures from birth to age fifteen. *J Am Dent Assoc* 20:379, 1933.

Lunt RC, Law DB: A review of the chronology of deciduous teeth. *J Am Dent Assoc* 89:87, 1974.

Lyons H: Committee adopts official method for the symbolic designation of teeth. *J Am Dent Assoc* 34:647, 1947.

Lysell L et al.: Time and order of eruption of the primary teeth: a longitudinal study. *Odont Rev* 13:21, 1962.

Masters DH, Hoskins SW: Projection of cervical enamel into molar furcations. *J Periodontol* 35:49, 1964.

McCauley HB: *Dent Radiogr Photogr* 18:1, 1945.

Mignogna MD et al.: Oral tuberculosis: a clinical evaluation of 42 cases. *Oral Dis* 6:25, 2000.

Milosevic A et al.: The occurrence of tooth wear in users of Ecstasy (3,4-methylenedioxymethamphetamine). *Community Dent Oral Epidemiol* 27:283, 1999.

Montgomery R et al.: *Biochemistry. A Case-Orientated Approach* (6th edition). St. Louis: Mosby, 1996.

Nomata N: A chronological study on the crown formation of the human deciduous dentition. *Bull Tokyo Med Dent Univ* 11:55, 1964.

Okeson JP: *Management of Temporomandibular Disorders and Occlusion* (3rd edition). St. Louis: Mosby, 1993.

Orban B: *Oral Histology and Embryology* (2nd edition). St. Louis: Mosby, 1944.

Palmer C: Palmer's dental notation. *Dental Cosmos* 33:194, 1981.

Peck S, Peck L: A time for change of tooth numbering systems. *J Dent Educ* 57:643, 1993.

Pelletier CE: *Pharmacology*. New York: Lange Medical Books, 2003.

Pindborg JJ: *Pathology of the Dental Hard Tissue*. Philadelphia: WB Saunders, 1970.

Rees LA: The structure and function of the temporomandibular joint. *Brit Dent J* 96:125, 1954.

Regezi JA, Sciubba JJ: *Oral Pathology. Clinical Pathological Correlations* (3rd edition). Philadelphia: WB Saunders, 1999.

Richardson AS, Castaldi CR: Dental development during the first two years of life. *J Can Dent Assoc* 33:418, 1967.

Romanelli F et al.: Possible paroxetine-induced bruxism. *Ann Pharmacother* 30:1246, 1996.

Ruangsri S et al.: Functional activity of superior head of human lateral pterygoid muscle during isometric force. *J Dent Res* 84:548, 2005.

Samaranayake LP: *Essential Microbiology for Dentistry*. New York: Churchill Livingstone, 1996.

Scapino RP: Morphology and mechanism of the jaw joint. In: McNeill C (ed): *Science and Practice of Occlusion*. Chicago: Quintessence, 1997.

Schour L, Massler M: Studies in tooth development: the growth pattern of human teeth. Part II. *J Am Dent Assoc* 27:1918, 1940.

Schour L, Massler M: The development of the human dentition. *J Am Dent Assoc* 28:1153, 1941.

Shafer WG et al.: *A Textbook of Oral Pathology*. Philadelphia: WB Saunders, 1983.

Sowter JW (ed): *Dental Laboratory Technology: Dental Anatomy*. Chapel Hill, NC: University of North Carolina, 1972.

Su WJ: Recent advances in molecular diagnosis of tuberculosis. *J Microbiol Immunol Infect* 35:209, 2002.

Tortora GJ: *Atlas of the Human Skeleton*. New York: John Wiley & Sons, 2000.

Turner II CG, Nichol CR, Scott GR: Scoring procedures for key morphological traits of the permanent dentition: The Arizona State University Dental Anthropology System. In: Kelley MA, Larsen CS, (eds): *Advances in Dental Anthropology*, New York: Wiley-Liss, 1991.

Widmalm S, Lillie J, Ash M: Anatomical and electromyographic studies of the lateral pterygoid muscle. *J Oral Rehabil* 14:429, 1987.

Woelfel JB, Scheid RC: *Dental Anatomy: Its Relevance to Dentistry.* Philadelphia: Lippincott Williams & Wilkins, 2002.

World Health Organization: *Oral Health Surveys: Basic Methods* (3rd edition). Geneva: The World Health Organization, 1987.

Zsigmondy A: Ghrundzüge einer praktischen Methode zur raschen und genauen, Vonnerkung der zahnartzlichen Beobachtungen' und Operationen. *Dtsch Vjschr Zahnhk* 1:209, 1861.

Zsigmondy A: A practical method for rapidly noting dental observations and operations. *Br J Dent Science* 17:580, 1874.

SAMPLE QUESTIONS

1. ***There are several tooth numbering systems, some used more than others, and some used by dental specialties or by special organizations. The so-called universal system consists of:***
   A. Two-digit sets of numbers for each tooth in each arch quadrant (e.g., 18 to 11).
   B. Single sequential number for teeth repeated in each quadrant (e.g., 8 to 1).
   C. A sequential alphabet letter for each tooth in an entire dentition (e.g., A to T).
   D. Different symbols for each numbered tooth in each quadrant (e.g., $\underline{8}|$ to $\underline{1}|$).
2. ***From the occlusal perspective, which tooth in the primary dentition varies the most in form of which tooth in the permanent dentition varies the most?***
   A. Maxillary first primary molar.
   B. Maxillary second primary molar.
   C. Mandibular first primary molar.
   D. Mandibular second primary molar.
3. ***The primary* maxillary first molar *has which of the following characteristics?***
   A. It is larger in all dimensions than the primary maxillary second molar.
   B. All three roots can be seen from mesial perspective.
   C. Bifurcation of roots begins almost immediately at the site of the cervical line (CEJ).
   D. The mesial root is considerably shorter than the distal one.
4. ***From a mesial perspective, the crown of the primary* maxillary first molar *has which of the following characteristics?***
   A. Pronounced convexity on the buccal outline of the cervical third.
   B. The cervical line mesially shows some curvature in an apical direction.
   C. The dimension at the occlusal third is the same as at the cervical third.
   D. The mesiobuccal cusp is longer and sharper than the mesiolingual cusp.
5. ***From the lingual perspective, the crown of the primary* maxillary second molar *shows which of the following?***
   A. Small, well-developed mesiolingual cusp.
   B. Distolingual (DL) cusp smaller than the maxillary primary first molar DL cusp.
   C. There is no supplemental cusp apical to the mesiolingual cusp.
   D. Developmental groove separating the mesiolingual and distolingual cusps.
6. ***The primary* mandibular first molar *has which of the following characteristics?***
   A. Resembles other primary and permanent teeth.
   B. From the occlusal perspective, has a heart-shaped outline.
   C. The mesiobuccal cusp is smaller than the distobuccal cusp.
   D. No developmental groove is evident between the buccal cusps.
7. ***A comparison occlusally between the primary mandibular second molar and the permanent mandibular first molar shows which of the following differences?***
   A. The mesio-, distobuccal, and distal cusps of the primary molar are almost equal in size; the distal cusp of the permanent molar is smaller than the other two cusps.
   B. The primary molar crown is wider buccolingually (in comparison with its mesiodistal measurement) than is the permanent molar.
   C. The primary molar outline is somewhat hexagonal; the permanent molar is rhomboidal.
   D. The ratio of the crown/root length of both molars is the same.
8. ***In comparing permanent and primary teeth, which of the following differences are noted?***
   A. Crowns of anterior primary teeth are narrower mesiodistally (in comparison to their crown length) than the permanent teeth.
   B. Comparatively, the roots of primary anterior teeth are narrower and longer.
   C. Cervical ridges of enamel of the primary anterior teeth are less prominent.
   D. Buccal and lingual surfaces of primary molars are less flat above the cervical curvature than those of permanent molars
9. ***The overall length of the primary teeth that are given here are the average range of dimensions with one exception. Which range for what tooth is* not *correct?***
   A. Maxillary central incisor, 16 to 17 mm.
   B. Mandibular central incisor, 16 to 17 mm.
   C. Maxillary lateral incisor, 16 to 17 mm.
   D. Mandibular lateral incisor, 15 to 17 mm.
10. ***For each type of tooth, the primary teeth consistently show which of the following characteristics?***
   A. Greater mesiodistal diameter relative to crown height than permanent teeth.
   B. An elongated appearance of the primary crowns and roots.
   C. Crowns that are translucent white in color.
   D. Root trunk length is one-half of the crown height.

11. ***Which primary tooth is generally accepted as the first to erupt, and at about what mean age?***
    A. Maxillary central incisor, 8 to 12 months.
    B. Maxillary central incisor, 7 to 9 months.
    C. Mandibular central incisor, 6 to 10 months.
    D. Mandibular central incisor, 8 to 10 months.
12. ***A most favorable sequence of eruption for the permanent dentition is which of the following (right side)? (Eruption sequence given by numbers in parentheses.)***
    A. (1) 3, 30; (2) 8, 25; (3) 7, 26; (4) 27, 5; (5) 28, 4; (6) 29, 6; (7) 31, 2.
    B. (1) 3, 30; (2) 8, 25; (3) 26, 7; (4) 27, 6; (5) 28, 5; (6) 29, 4; (7) 31, 2.
    C. (1) 30, 3; (2) 25, 8; (3) 26, 7; (4) 27, 5; (5) 28, 4; (6) 29, 6; (7) 31, 2.
    D. (1) 30, 3; (2) 25, 8; (3) 26, 7; (4) 27, 6; (5) 28, 5; (6) 29, 4; (7) 2, 31.
13. ***Which primary tooth generally erupts last?***
    A. Mandibular second molar.
    B. Maxillary second molar.
    C. Maxillary canine.
    D. Mandibular canine.
14. ***Comparing the overall length of primary central incisors (E|F) with permanent maxillary central incisors (8|9), which is the correct ratio expressed as a percentage?***
    A. About 50%.
    B. About 60%.
    C. About 70%.
    D. About 80%.
15. ***At what time is the crown completed for the tooth indicated?***
    A. Primary maxillary central incisor, 3 weeks.
    B. Permanent maxillary central incisor, 2 to 3 years.
    C. Primary maxillary lateral incisor, 2 to 3 months.
    D. Permanent maxillary lateral incisor, 2 to 3 years.
16. ***When are the crowns of the primary maxillary second molars completed?***
    A. 11 months.
    B. 10 months.
    C. 9 months.
    D. 8 months.
17. ***Which of the following is* not *a type trait of the permanent maxillary second premolar?***
    A. Buccal view: narrow shoulders (margins of crown; mesio- and disto-occlusal angles).
    B. Occlusal table outline: ovoid.
    C. Mesiomarginal groove interrupts mesial marginal ridge.
    D. Lingual view: buccal profile is not visible.
18. ***Which of the following are* not *type traits of permanent maxillary molars?***

	First Molar	Second Molar	Third Molar
A. Buccal view:	Widest molar	Intermediate width	Smallest molar
B. DL cusp:	Same size as M_2	Same size as M_1	Smallest size
C. Occlusal view:	Square/ rhomboid	More rhomboidal	Triangle- or heart-shaped
D. MB root apex:	In line with cusp tip	In line with crown center	Roots dis-placed

19. ***Which of the following is* not *an arch trait of the maxillary canine?***
    A. In the same dentition, the crown is larger than the mandibular canine.
    B. The incisal margin of the crown occupies at least one third to one half of crown height.
    C. Labial aspect: mesial and distal marginal ridges converge toward cervix.
    D. Marked symmetry of mesial/distal halves when viewed from incisal.
20. ***Which one of the following morphological characteristic is representative of* all *posterior maxillary teeth?***
    A. Marked mesial concavity on crowns and roots.
    B. Tips of cusps are well within the confines of the root trunks.
    C. From mesial/distal aspect, crowns are rhomboidal in shape.
    D. From mesial/distal aspect, all maxillary posterior crowns are trapezoidal with shortest uneven side toward occlusal surface.
21. ***In terms of vertical dimension, where is the mental foramen found most frequently?***
    A. At the apices of the premolars.
    B. Coronal to the apices.
    C. Below the apices.
    D. No particular location predominates.
22. ***A major anatomical variant of the two-rooted mandibular molar is a tooth with an additional distolingual and third root. What is the prevalence of these three-rooted mandibular first molars?***
    A. May exceed 10% in Caucasians.
    B. Less than 1% in Eurasian and Asian populations.
    C. Greater than 5% (even up to 40%) in populations with Mongolian traits.
    D. Greater than 8% in African populations.
23. ***Which jaw activity does* not *involve one of the following muscles?***
    A. Clenching, superior heads of lateral pterygoid muscles (LPM).
    B. Clenching, inferior heads of LPM.
    C. Ipsilateral jaw movements, inferior heads of LPM.
    D. Simple jaw opening, deep masseter muscle.

24. ***If jaw opening is divided into phases, and it is assumed that the surfaces of the articulating bones and disc are associated throughout jaw opening, what is the relationship of the disc and condyle in the following phases?***

A. In the very earliest phase, the condyle moves forward before the disc.
B. In the early phase, the disc and condyle move anteriorly in concert.
C. In an intermediate phase, the condyle moves forward at a slower rate.
D. In the final phase, the disc moves forward at a faster rate.

25. ***Occlusal interferences can be defined by* all *of the following* except:**

A. Occlusal contact relations that interfere with function.
B. Interference to jaw closure into the intercuspal position.
C. Interferences to laterotrusive movements.
D. Interferences to jaw opening.

26. ***If posterior teeth on the* left side *contact occlusally during a right lateral excursion of the mandible, the left side occlusal contact would be referred to as:***

A. Laterotrusive contact.
B. Protrusive contact.
C. Mediotrusive contact.
D. Centric relation.

27. ***Which one of the following is considered a primary ligament of the TMJ?***

A. Stylomandibular.
B. Sphenomandibular.
C. Stylohyoid.
D. Temporomandibular.

28. ***Mandibular movement resulting from occlusal contacts of the teeth from retruded contact position (CRC) to intercuspal position (slide in centric) may show all* except *one of the following directional components when viewed only in the horizontal plane. Which is the* exception?**

A. Vertical component.
B. Horizontal component.
C. Lateral component.
D. Protrusive component.

29. ***Where is the height of contour located relative to the following teeth (viewed from the mesial)?***

A. Facial surfaces of all molars, middle third.
B. Lingual surfaces of all premolars and molars, cervical third.
C. Lingual surfaces of molars and premolars, cervical or middle third.
D. Anterior teeth, cervical or middle third.

30. ***The occlusal surface of a primary mandibular first molar often has a prominent faciolingual ridge. This* transverse ridge *connects which two cusps?***

A. Buccal and distolingual.
B. Mesiolingual and distobuccal.
C. Mesiobuccal and mesiolingual.
D. Distobuccal and distolingual.

31. ***Which premolar would be the* most *likely to have a single pulp horn?***

A. Maxillary first.
B. Mandibular first.
C. Mandibular second.
D. Maxillary second.

32. ***Which one of the following is* not *a normal anatomical feature of mandibular incisors?***

A. Bifurcated roots.
B. Inconspicuous cingula.
C. Four developmental lobes.
D. Incisal edges placed slightly lingually.

33. ***The heights of contour of the* distal *surfaces of permanent mandibular central incisors are located in which coronal third?***

A. Middle.
B. Cervical.
C. Occlusal.
D. Incisal.

34. ***On average, approximately what is the dimension of the permanent* maxillary canine *at the widest mesiodistal diameter of the crown?***

A. 5.5 mm.
B. 6.5 mm.
C. 7.5 mm.
D. 8.5 mm.

35. ***Which one of the following is found on the crown of permanent mandibular first molars but is* not *found on the crowns of mandibular second molars?***

A. MB cusp.
B. Distobuccal groove.
C. Lingual groove.
D. DB cusp.

36. ***The Y-shaped central developmental groove is most likely found on which of the following premolars?***

A. Maxillary first.
B. Mandibular first.
C. Maxillary second.
D. Mandibular second.

37. ***In a cusp–embrasure relationship, the maxillary first premolar is most likely to articulate with which of the following mandibular teeth?***

A. First premolar only.
B. First molar only.
C. Canine and first premolar.
D. First and second premolars.

38. ***Equal contracture of the lateral pterygoid muscle bilaterally produces which of the following mandibular movements?***
   A. Retrusive.
   B. Elevation.
   C. Protrusive.
   D. Lateral.

Test items 39–51 relate to the following case presentation.

A 35-year-old woman presents with a painful limitation of jaw opening (28 mm), a painful tooth on the right side, and swelling at the angle of the jaw. She has a history of temporomandibular disease (TMD) and conservative treatment. Medical history reveals that the patient is being treated for tuberculosis with combination antituberculosis drugs including rifampin (Rifadin). She is also being treated with an anticoagulant, warfarin (Coumadin), a low level of aspirin, and paroxetine (Paxil) for depression. The intraoral examination shows extensive teeth wear from bruxism, diagnosed by a sleep specialist as sleep bruxism. Tooth 32 has a deep carious lesion and, on radiographic examination, a periapical radiolucency.

39. ***The incidence of tuberculosis is increasing as a result of an association with AIDS. Oral infections of tuberculosis (TBC) do occur but are uncommon. Diagnosis of oral lesions may present several challenges, as set forth in all of the following statements* except one. *Which one of the following statements is false?***
   A. Lesions secondary to HIV may be present.
   B. Isolation of *M. tuberculosis* by culture requires 4 to 6 weeks or longer.
   C. Mycobacteria can be demonstrated by special stains in only 27% to 60% of cases.
   D. Molecular tests (e.g., polymerase chain reaction) show slow turnaround times.
40. ***All the following side effects have been reported to be related to the use of rifampin* except one. *Which is the* exception?**
   A. Green bodily fluids—sweat, tears, urine.
   B. Hepatotoxicity.
   C. Thrombocytopenia.
   D. Rashes.
41. ***Which of the following modes of action* does not *relate to rifampin?***
   A. Inhibits RNA synthesis.
   B. Binds tightly to eukaryotic RNA polymerase.
   C. Tuberculocidal to intracellular and extracellular organisms.
   D. Reduces activity of hepatic mixed-function oxidases.
42. ***Exacerbation of bruxism has been reported to occur with all the following agents* except one? *Which is the* exception?**
   A. Paroxetine (Paxil).
   B. Selective serotonin reuptake inhibitors.
   C. Naproxen (Naprosyn).
   D. Amphetamine derivative (“Ecstasy”).
43. ***Migraine is a form of headache that is currently thought to be best understood on the basis of all the following with one exception. The* exception *is which of the following?***
   A. As a dysfunction of brainstem pathways or diencephalic nuclei.
   B. As a primary disorder of the brain.
   C. As similar in mechanism to tension headaches.
   D. As a neurovascular headache.
44. ***Three key factors in the pathogenesis of pain in migraine are usually considered. Which of the following is* not *considered to be a key factor?***
   A. Cranial blood vessels.
   B. β-amyloid-containing plaques in the brain.
   C. Trigeminal innervation of the vessels.
   D. Reflex connection of trigeminal system with cranial parasympathetic outflow.
45. ***The treatment of the patient with low levels of aspirin is done for which of the following reasons?***
   A. To reduce the likelihood of platelet aggregation.
   B. To stimulate cyclo-oxygenase in the platelets.
   C. To increase the formation of thromboxane.
   D. To cause platelets to regenerate cyclo-oxygenase.
46. ***When there is a pulpal-periodontal infection of a mandibular third molar, which of the following listed facial and cervical spaces is* most *likely to have become infected when there is swelling at the angle of the jaw?***
   A. Retromolar space.
   B. Submaxillary space.
   C. Submasseteric space.
   D. Parotid space.
47. ***Lymphatic drainage from tooth 32 will first involve which of the following node groups?***
   A. Lateral upper deep cervical node.
   B. Medial upper deep cervical node.
   C. Lateral lower deep cervical node.
   D. Submaxillary node.
48. ***All but one the following are considerations relevant to the diagnosis and treatment of tuberculosis. Which of the following statements is* not *true?***
   A. Increase in the prevalence of TB.
   B. Oral TB lesions occur most frequently on the gingival.
   C. Emergence of multidrug-resistant strains.
   D. High risk of *M. tuberculosis* infection in patients infected with human immunodeficiency virus (HIV).

49. Extraction of tooth 32 revealed attached soft tissue. Which of the following is* most important *for a presumptive diagnosis of tuberculosis?
A. Caseous necrotic areas.
B. Acid-fast bacilli.
C. Epithelioid histiocytes.
D. Langerhans giant cells.

50. Which one of the following disorders is the* least *likely to be a differential diagnostic factor in the patient's limited jaw opening?
A. Exacerbation of TMJ and TMD.
B. Trismus secondary to TMJ pain.
C. Myalgia secondary to TMD.
D. Myositis secondary to bruxing.

51. The patient is on an anticoagulant drug (e.g., warfarin [Coumadin]) as well as rifampin. What is the effect of rifampin on the anticoagulation effect of warfarin (Coumadin)?
A. Increases the anticoagulant effect of warfarin.
B. Increases the cyclic conversion of vitamin K epoxide reductase.
C. Anticoagulation effect is inhibited.
D. Decreases its metabolic clearance by inducing activity of hepatic oxidases.

52. A transverse ridge is:
A. The combination name for joining oblique and triangular ridges
B. A combination name for joining buccal and lingual cusp triangular ridges
C. Characteristically found on all primary and permanent molars
D. Found occasionally on maxillary primary first molar

53. From the occlusal aspect, the primary* maxillary first molar *has which of the following characteristics?
A. Crown outline diverges lingually and distally.
B. Small traverse ridge frequently present called an oblique ridge.
C. Four cusps are present.
D. Mesial marginal ridge is thin and poorly developed.

54. From the lingual perspective the primary* maxillary first molar *has which of the following characteristics?
A. Distolingual cusp is the most prominent cusp.
B. Mesiolingual cusp poorly defined.
C. Distobuccal cusp cannot be seen from lingual aspect.
D. Crown converges considerably in a lingual direction.

55. The primary* maxillary second molar *has what characteristics?
A. Does not have a well-defined mesial triangular fossa.
B. Oblique ridge absent or not well developed.
C. Development (central) groove is well defined.
D. A tubercle of Carabelli (Supplementary cusp) is well developed.

56. From the occlusal aspect the primary* maxillary second molar *has which of the following characteristics?
A. Somewhat rhomboidal in form.
B. Three well developed cusps.
C. Two supplemental cusps, including tubercle of Carabelli.
D. Poorly defined mesial triangular fossa.

57. From the occlusal aspect, the primary* mandibular second molar *has which of the following characteristics?
A. Somewhat rectangular in form.
B. The outline of the crown converges mesially.
C. Three buccal cusps are dissimilar in size.
D. Cusps do not have well defined triangular ridges.

58. A comparison of the pulp chambers and root canals of maxillary primary and permanent second molars shows which of the following?
A. Enamel cap of primary tooth is relatively thick but less consistent in depth.
B. Comparatively less thickness of dentin at the occlusal fossa of primary molars.
C. Pulp chambers are proportionally larger in primary molars.
D. Pulp horns are lower in primary molars, especially distal horns.

59. In a comparison of maxillary, primary and permanent second molars, which of the following differences are noted?
A. Enamel rods at the cervix slope gingivally in the primary molar.
B. Enamel rods at the cervix slope occlusally in the permanent molar.
C. Buccal cervical ridges are less pronounced in the primary molar.
D. Roots of primary teeth are longer and more slender in comparison with crown size than those of permanent teeth.

60. Based on average MD diameters of the crowns of primary teeth, the range for average overall length of the primary maxillary arch is about what dimension?
A. 60–68 mm.
B. 68–76 mm.
C. 76–84 mm.
D. 84–92 mm.

61. What is the average height of curvature of the cervical line (CEJ) on the mesial and distal of the permanent maxillary and mandibular incisors?
A. About 3.5 mm on the mesial of the maxillary central incisor.
B. About 1.5 mm on the distal of the maxillary central incisor.
C. About 2.0 mm on the mesial of the mandibular central incisor.
D. About 1.0 mm on the distal of the mandibular central incisor.

62. ***Considering the period of 2½ months to about 6 years of age which of the following is true?***
   A. Not all the primary teeth have attained their occlusal level.
   B. Parts of both jaws containing primary teeth change noticeably in size.
   C. A significant increase in intercanine width occurs shortly before and during the time the primary teeth are lost and the permanent teeth emerge.
   D. Dental arch form is more or less constant and practically no dimensional changes take place in depth or width after 9 months of age.

63. ***Which sequence of eruption of permanent teeth occurs most often? (8-7-6-5-4-3-2-1 = M_3-M_2-M_1-P_2-P_1-C-LI-CI). First #, #'s in each series is considered to be the first to erupt.***
   A. 6-1-2-4-3-5-7-8 (Maxilla).
   B. 6-1-2-3-4-5-7-8 (Maxilla).
   C. (6-1)-2-4-3-5-7-8 (Mandible).
   D. 1-6-2-4-5-3-7-8 (Mandible).

64. ***The first evidence of calcification (weeks in utero) in the primary dentition occurs in which of the following teeth at about what age?***
   A. Maxillary central incisor—14 (13–16) weeks.
   B. Mandibular central incisor—12 (10–13) weeks.
   C. Maxillary lateral incisor—14 (13–16) weeks.
   D. Mandibular lateral incisor—14 (13–15) weeks.

65. ***A most characteristic feature of the* primary maxillary central incisor *is which of the following?***
   A. Faciolingual breadth of the crown.
   B. Mesiodistal width of the crown.
   C. Mesial and distal margin outlines in line with profiles of root.
   D. Root/crown ratio.

66. ***When is the crown of the permanent mandibular second molar completed?***
   A. About 7–8 years.
   B. About 8–9 years.
   C. About 9–10 years.
   D. About 10–11 years.

67. ***Which of the following is NOT a type trait of the permanent maxillary first premolar?***
   A. Occlusal table outline, trapezoidal.
   B. Generally two roots – mesial and distal.
   C. Central groove is long.
   D. Supplementary grooves are rare.

68. ***Which of the following are NOT type traits of permanent mandibular first and second premolars?***

	First Premolar	Second Premolar
A. Buccal view:	Crown bilaterally Asymmetrical	Bilaterally symmetrical
B. Lingual aspect:	Entire buccal profile visible	Buccal profile not seen
C. Lingual aspect:	Most of occlusal surface visible	Little, if any seen
D. Lingual aspect:	Contour height: Middle third	Cervical third

69. ***Which of the following are NOT arch traits of the canines?***

	Maxillary Canine (6)	Mandibular Canine (27)
A. Crown size	Larger (same dentition)	Smaller (same dentition)
B. Lingual pits/grooves	Common	None
C. Labiolingual diameter	Near cervix same as 27	Near cervix same as 6
D. Incisal view, M/D halves	Symmetrical	Marked asymmetry

70. ***Which of the following are NOT type traits of the permanent maxillary central and lateral incisors?***

	Central Incisor	Lateral Incisor
A. Labial view: Mesial Contact	Incisal 3rd	Jnct. incisal/ mid 3rd
B. Labial view: Distal Contact	Jnct. incisal/ mid 3rd	Middle third
C. Mesial view: contacts	Within incisal third	Jnct. incisal/ mid 3rd
D. Labial: mesioincisal angle	Slightly rounded	Sharp rt.angle

71. ***Which position of the mental foramen relative to the mandibular premolars and first molar occurs most frequently?***
   A. Between the first and second premolars.
   B. In line with the second premolar.
   C. Distal to the second premolar.
   D. In line with the mesial root of the first molar.

72. ***The maxillary sinus overlies the alveolar processes in particular what teeth?***
   A. First and second maxillary molars.
   B. All maxillary molars.
   C. First and second premolars.
   D. First and second premolars and first and second molars.

73. ***The masseter muscle, which has a complex of internal components, includes all the following EXCEPT?***
   A. Pennation.
   B. Structural composition permitting regional activation.
   C. Multiple internal aponeuroses.
   D. Internal aponeuroses that do not move or deform.

74. ***Sleep bruxism can be characterized by which of the following?***
   A. Episodes of massive, bilateral clenching.
   B. Tooth grinding that may last for up to 20 minutes.
   C. Often coincides with passage from lighter to deeper sleep.
   D. Occurs approximately every 20 minutes in the sleep cycle.

75. *Recent focus on causative factors in bruxism include ALL of the following Except?*
A. Occlusal interferences.
B. Part of a sleep arousal response.
C. Pathophysiological factors.
D. Neurotransmitters in the central nervous system.

76. *ALL of the following are supporting cusps EXCEPT?*
A. Buccal cusp of Tooth #29.
B. Lingual cusp of tooth # 4.
C. ML cusp of tooth #3.
D. ML cusp of tooth # 19.

77. *Measurement of* horizontal overlap *(over jet) of the teeth is easily done by which of the following methods?*
A. Measure from the facial surface of a mandibular incisor to the facial surface of a maxillary incisor with the subject in intercuspal position.
B. With the subject intercuspal position, mark the position of the maxillary incisal edge on the facial surface of the mandibular incisor with a pencil.
Then have the subject open the mouth and measure from the mark that you made to the incisal edge of the mandibular incisor.
C. Measure from the midline between the maxillary central incisors to the midline of the mandibular central incisors.
D. Measure from the incisal edge of a maxillary incisor to the incisal edge of a mandibular incisor with the mandible in the maximum open position.

78. *In a cusp-fossa occlusal relationship, the maxillary second premolar is most likely to articulate with which of the following mandibular teeth?*
A. First premolar only.
B. Second premolar only.
C. Canine and first premolar.
D. First and second premolars.

79. *Which of the following contributes primary sensory innervation to the temporomandibular joint?*
A. Auriculotemporal nerve.
B. Infraorbital nerve.
C. Branch of the lingual nerve.
D. Facial nerve.

80. *The smallest cusp on the crown of a 5 lobed mandibular second premolar is the:*
A. Buccal cusp.
B. Distobuccal cusp.
C. Distal cusp.
D. Distolingual cusp.

81. *A typical primary mandibular first molar has how many pulp horns?*
A. 1.
B. 2.
C. 3.
D. 4.

82. *Rest position (RP) is defined:*
A. As any position of the mandible that lacks contact of the teeth.
B. As the centric relation position of the condyles with the teeth apart.
C. As a mandibular position with masticatory muscles at complete rest.
D. As a clinical mandibular position in relation to the interocclusal space.

83. *Name the point angle which represents the junction of the cutting edge of an incisor with the surface that is toward the tongue and the surface that is away from the midline.*
A. Distoproximoincisal.
B. Distolabioincisal.
C. Distolinguoincisal.
D. Labioincisolinguo.

84. *Root bifurcation would be a more likely finding in which of the following permanent teeth?*
A. Maxillary canine.
B. Mandibular canine.
C. Maxillary central incisor.
D. Mandibular lateral incisor.

85. *What is the correct schematic outline of the following teeth?*
A. Mandibular premolars, viewed from occlusal, rhomboidal.
B. Maxillary central incisors, viewed from facial, triangles.
C. Maxillary lateral incisors, viewed from mesial, trapezoidal.
D. All mandibular posterior teeth, distal aspect, rhomboidal.

86. *A distinct central developmental groove, prominent buccal triangular ridge, two cusps and distinct mesial and distal occlusal pits would be most characteristic of:*
A. Mandibular first premolars.
B. Primary mandibular first molars.
C. Primary mandibular second molars.
D. Mandibular second premolars.

87. *From the incisal view, a greater mesiodistal measurement than faciolingual measurement can be seen in which of the following permanent anterior crowns?*
A. Maxillary central incisor.
B. Maxillary canine.
C. Mandibular canine.
D. Mandibular central incisor.

88. *Maximum rotation and translation of both condyles takes place at:*
A. Maximum opening.
B. Maximum protrusive.
C. Right and left lateral excursive movements.
D. Hinge movement.

Questions 89–100 relate to the following history and examination

A mother brings her 12-year-old boy to the dentist to ask about her son grinding his teeth and about some white "spots" located on the smooth-surfaced enamel of several of his anterior teeth and premolars. Among other questions about the cause of the defects, the mother then asks when a systemic disturbance occurred that may have caused the "spots." The patient has excessive tooth wear from bruxing and clenching. The dentist measures the cervical-incisal length of the permanent maxillary central incisor (10.5 mm). Also measured is the distance from the CEJ to the midpoint of the defect (5.5 mm). Given that the crown is completed over a period of 4 to 5 years it is possible to estimate the age at which the hypoplasia occurred using 6 months or yearly periods in the following formula:

ADF = ACF – (yrs. of formation/crown height × distance of defect from CEJ)

89. ***Using an average age of crown formation (ACF) of both 4 and 5 years, the age of defect formation (ADF) is estimated to be about what time?***
   A. 7–9 months in utero.
   B. 0–1 years of age.
   C. 1–2 years.
   D. 2–3 years.
90. ***The increase of fluorosis of permanent teeth in both nonfluoridated and optimally fluoridated populations points to the need for dentists to caution parents with children about potential causes of fluorosis in children. Which of the following cautions about fluoride is correct, but the age or implied age is NOT Correct?***
   A. Excess (> 1 ppm) fluoride in the drinking water during enamel formation.
   B. Excessive (> pea-sized amount) use of fluoride toothpaste under 6 years of age.
   C. Use of fluoride toothpaste for children under 4 years of age.
   D. Use of a 1.1% sodium fluoride toothpaste or gel by pediatric patients only when 6 years of age and older.
91. ***Systemic etiologic factors that are said to be associated with enamel defects such as hypoplasia occur generally in what period of time?***
   A. Before birth.
   B. Generally after birth and before the age of 6 years.
   C. During the first year postpartum for Hutchinson's incisors.
   D. During birth.
92. ***The differential diagnosis of white "spots" of the enamel of primary and permanent teeth should include disorders that have a substantiated cause. Which of the following DO NOT have an evidence-based causal relationship with enamel hypoplasia?***
   A. Rickets.
   B. Congenital syphilis.
   C. Measles.
   D. Fluorosis.
93. ***Clenching and grinding of teeth involves contraction of skeletal type muscles. Several types of myofilaments are present in the contractile elements of skeletal muscles. Which statement about muscle filaments IS NOT true?***
   A. Myosin forms the thick filament of muscle.
   B. Actin is a major protein of thin filaments.
   C. Titin is a protein of elastic filament.
   D. Connectin is a protein of intermediate filament.
94. ***The clinical examination of the patient reveals extensive wear of the right canines, and somewhat less wear of the lateral incisors. Also there is tenderness of the jaw closing muscles, particularly on the right side. The muscle(s) that would be involved primarily in providing most of the force for anterior tooth clenching include which of the following masticatory muscles?***
   A. Inferior lateral pterygoid muscle.
   B. Superior lateral pterygoid muscle.
   C. Anterior temporalis muscle.
   D. Masseter muscle.
95. ***Sleep bruxism (SB) is defined by many but not all of the following characteristics. Which is the EXCEPTION?***
   A. Stereotypical movement disorder.
   B. Grinding and clenching of the teeth during sleep.
   C. More frequent in the younger generation.
   D. Individuals who brux during the daytime inevitably brux at night.
96. ***Recent physiologic evidence suggests that central and/or autonomic nervous systems rather than peripheral sensory factors play a dominant role in the genesis of sleep bruxism (SB). Which statement about the central genesis of SB is NOT true?***
   A. During sleep the mouth is usually open due to motor repression.
   B. Tooth contact most likely occurs in association with sleep arousal.
   C. Some peripheral sensory factors may exert an influence on SB through their interaction with sleep-awake mechanisms.
   D. Sequential change from autonomic (cardiac)/brain cortical activities follows SB-related jaw motor activity.

97. ***Aggravation of bruxism has been suggested to occur secondarily to all of the following occlusal relationships except one. Which one is the EXCEPTION?***

A. Occlusal interferences in centric relation.
B. Occlusal interferences in the intercuspal position.
C. Iatrogenic occlusal relations that *interfere* with bruxism.
D. Angle Class III malocclusion (prognathism).

98. ***The differential diagnosis of enamel hypoplasia should take into account suggested differences between non-fluoride and fluoride opacities. Which of the following statements does not suggest a basis for a diagnosis of non-fluoride (NF) enamel hypoplasia?***

A. Levels of F in drinking water that range from 0.2 to 0.34 ppm have been reported to be associated with prevalences of NF enamel opacities ranging from 22% to 35 %.
B. At a level of 1 to 1.5 ppm of F in drinking water, only few F opacities occur.
C. Most NF enamel opacities appear as white, opaque spots in smooth surface enamel; areas of mild dental fluorosis are lusterless, opaque white patches.
D. Fluorosis and NF opacities are clinically significantly different.

99. ***During muscle contraction what physical change DOES NOT occur relative to muscle fiber contraction?***

A. Sarcomeres—shorten.
B. Thick and thin filaments—shorten.
C. I Band—shortens.
D. H zone—shortens.

100. ***Regarding the superior and inferior heads of the lateral pterygoid muscle (SHLP and IHLP), which of the following statements is NOT TRUE?***

A. Hypothetically, SHLP and IHLP can be considered to be parts of one muscle.
B. Distributions of SHLP and IHLP activities are shaded according to biochemical demands of tasks.
C. SHLP stabilizes the condyle and disk against the articular eminence in a wide range of jaw movements and forces.
D. IHLP plays a major role in the generation and fine control of horizontal forces.

Sample Exam

1. ***ALL of the following are supporting cusps EXCEPT?***
   A. Buccal cusp of Tooth #29.
   B. Lingual cusp of tooth #4.
   C. ML cusp of tooth #3.
   D. ML cusp of tooth #19.
2. ***The lateral pterygoid muscle attaches to which of the following?***
   A. Lateral surface of the lateral pterygoid plate.
   B. Medial surface of the lateral pterygoid plate.
   C. Lateral surface of the medial pterygoid plate.
   D. Medial surface of the medial pterygoid plate.
   E. Pyramidal process of palatine bone.
3. ***A transverse ridge is:***
   A. The combination name for joining oblique and triangular ridges
   B. A combination name for joining buccal and lingual cusp triangular ridges
   C. Characteristically found on all primary and permanent molars
   D. Found occasionally on maxillary primary first molar
4. ***Bronchogenic carcinoma is a complication most characteristic of which of the following conditions?***
   A. Silicosis.
   B. Asbestosis.
   C. Anthracosis.
   D. Sarcoidosis.
   E. Bronchiectasis.
5. ***Which of the following statements regarding tubular reabsorption is true?***
   A. Most calcium filtered is passively reabsorbed and not regulated under any conditions.
   B. Most urea is reabsorbed passively and is unaffected by regulatory mechanisms.
   C. Glucose is reabsorbed by secondary active transport and facilitated diffusion.
   D. Most filtered phosphate is reabsorbed in the collecting ducts and is unaffected by regulatory mechanisms.
6. ***The class of antibodies that plays an important role in type I hypersensitivity reactions is _____.***
   A. IgA
   B. IgD
   C. IgE
   D. IgG
   E. IgM
7. ***The amount of cytosine will be equal to the amount of guanine in which of the following molecules?***
   A. DNA.
   B. RNA.
   C. DNA and RNA.
   D. mRNA.
8. ***The branchial arches disappear when the _____ branchial arch grows down to contact the _____.***
   A. second; third branchial arch
   B. second; fifth branchial arch
   C. third; fifth branchial arch
   D. first; first branchial groove
   E. first; sixth branchial groove

9. ***Glucagon will decrease which of the following?***
   A. Glycogenolysis.
   B. Gluconeogenesis.
   C. Glycogenesis.
   D. Blood glucose.
10. ***When an enzyme is competitively inhibited, which of the following changes occur?***
   A. The apparent Km is unchanged.
   B. The apparent Km is decreased.
   C. Vmax is decreased.
   D. Vmax is unchanged.
11. ***A typical primary mandibular first molar has how many pulp horns?***
   A. 1.
   B. 2.
   C. 3.
   D. 4.

Test items 12–14 refer to the following testlet.

A 3-year-old African girl presents in the emergency room with a palpable mass in her lower right mandible. She is currently in the United States visiting relatives with her parents. Her mom claims that a few days ago she noticed a growing mass in her daughter's jaw. There appears to be slight swelling around the area, although it is painless and not tender to the touch. After further examination, a biopsy was taken, and the diagnosis of Burkitt's lymphoma was made.

12. ***Burkitt's lymphoma is a malignancy that affects which of the following cells?***
   A. Macrophages.
   B. T lymphocytes.
   C. B lymphocytes.
   D. Neutrophils.
   E. Keratinocytes.
13. ***The pathology report reveals a characteristic pattern of tumor cells that is classically associated with Burkitt's lymphoma. Which of the following describes this histopathologic pattern?***
   A. Honeycomb.
   B. Cobweb.
   C. Cotton wool.
   D. Sun ray.
   E. Starry sky.
14. ***The African form of Burkitt's lymphoma has been linked to the Epstein-Barr virus. This virus is also responsible for which of the following diseases?***
   A. Mononucleosis.
   B. Shingles.
   C. Chicken pox.
   D. Kaposi's sarcoma.
   E. Herpangina.
15. ***Measurement of horizontal overlap (over jet) of the teeth is easily done by which of the following methods?***
   A. Measure from the facial surface of a mandibular incisor to the facial surface of a maxillary incisor with the subject in intercuspal position.
   B. With the subject intercuspal position, mark the position of the maxillary incisal edge on the facial surface of the mandibular incisor with a pencil. Then have the subject open the mouth and measure from the mark that you made to the incisal edge of the mandibular incisor.
   C. Measure from the midline between the maxillary central incisors to the midline of the mandibular central incisors.
   D. Measure from the incisal edge of a maxillary incisor to the incisal edge of a mandibular incisor with the mandible in the maximum open position.
16. ***Increasing the radius of arterioles will increase which of the following?***
   A. Systolic blood pressure.
   B. Diastolic blood pressure.
   C. Viscosity of the blood.
   D. Capillary blood flow.
17. ***Which of the following nerves supplies taste sensation to the anterior two-thirds of the tongue?***
   A. Hypoglossal.
   B. Glossopharyngeal.
   C. Lingual.
   D. Facial.
   E. Mental.
18. ***Which of the following are NOT arch traits of the canines?***

	Maxillary Canine (6)	**Mandibular Canine (27)**
A. Crown size	Larger (same dentition)	Smaller (same dentition)
B. Lingual pits/grooves	Common	None
C. Labiolingual diameter	Near cervix same as 27	Near cervix same as 6
D. Incisal view, M/D halves	Symmetrical	Marked asymmetry

19. ***Which of the following statements regarding the regulation of gastrointestinal motility is true?***
   A. Sympathetic stimulation inhibits motility.
   B. Parasympathetic stimulation inhibits motility.
   C. Gastrointestinal motility is not influenced by the central nervous system (CNS).
   D. Gastrointestinal motility is not influenced by hormones.

20. Which of the following structures is the most common site for oral cancer?
A. Soft palate.
B. Lateral border of the tongue.
C. Lower lip.
D. Floor of mouth.
E. Buccal mucosa.

21. Mandibular movement resulting from occlusal contacts of the teeth from retruded contact position (CRC) to intercuspal position (slide in centric) may show all except one of the following directional components when viewed only in the horizontal plane. Which is the exception?
A. Vertical component.
B. Horizontal component.
C. Lateral component.
D. Protrusive component.

22. Which of the following muscles is responsible for the formation of the posterior tonsillar pillar?
A. Stylopharyngeus.
B. Tensor veli palatine.
C. Palatoglossus.
D. Palatopharyngeus.
E. Levator veli palatine.

23. Which of the following does not occur to compensate for a fall in blood pressure below normal values?
A. Increased cardiac output.
B. Increased stroke volume.
C. Increased heart rate.
D. Decreased total peripheral resistance.

24. Relative or absolute lack of insulin in humans would result in which one of the following reactions in the liver?
A. Increased glycogen synthesis.
B. Increased gluconeogenesis.
C. Decreased glycogen breakdown.
D. Increased amino acid uptake.

25. In 2% glutaraldehyde, which of the following times is minimally sufficient for achieving sterilization?
A. 15 minutes.
B. 1–2 hours.
C. 6 hours.
D. 12 hours.

26. Which of the following bones is part of the superior wall (roof) of the orbit?
A. Zygomatic.
B. Lacrimal.
C. Sphenoid.
D. Maxilla.
E. Ethmoid.

27. On average, approximately what is the dimension of the permanent maxillary canine at the widest mesiodistal diameter of the crown?
A. 5.5 mm.
B. 6.5 mm.
C. 7.5 mm.
D. 8.5 mm.

28. Both active transport and facilitated diffusion are characterized by which of the following?
A. Transport in one direction only.
B. Hydrolysis of ATP.
C. Transport against a concentration gradient.
D. Competitive inhibition.

29. Which of the following bacteria would be expected to first colonize onto plaque?
A. *Streptococci.*
B. *Bacteroides.*
C. *Fusobacterium.*
D. *Actinomyces.*
E. *Prevotella.*

30. Cell membrane typically contain the following compounds except:
A. Phospholipids
B. Proteins
C. Cholesterols
D. Triacylglycerols
E. Sphingolipids

31. Which of the following muscles adducts the vocal cords?
A. Lateral cricoarytenoid.
B. Posterior cricoarytenoid.
C. Cricothyroid.
D. Vocalis.
E. Tensor veli palatine.

32. Which of the following best describes anaplastic cells that have not invaded the basement membrane and are confined within their epithelium of origin?
A. Dysplasia.
B. Hyperplasia.
C. Metaplasia.
D. Sarcoma.
E. Carcinoma in situ.

33. Which muscle of the anterolateral abdominal wall is described as being belt- or strap-like?
A. External oblique muscle.
B. Internal oblique muscle.
C. Transversus abdominis muscle.
D. Rectus abdominis muscle.
E. Quadratus lumborum muscle.

34. In a comparison of maxillary, primary and permanent second molars, which of the following differences are noted?
A. Enamel rods at the cervix slope gingivally in the primary molar.
B. Enamel rods at the cervix slope occlusally in the permanent molar.
C. Buccal cervical ridges are less pronounced in the primary molar.
D. Roots of primary teeth are longer and more slender in comparison with crown size than those of permanent teeth.

Test items 35–37 refer to the following testlet.

A mother brings her 6-year-old daughter in for an examination because she noticed brown macules on her daughter's leg. The macules have jagged edges but do not appear raised. The mother is worried that her daughter may have a malignancy. After further evaluation and tests, the macules are identified as café au lait spots.

35. ***Café au lait spots are seen in conjunction with polyostotic fibrous dysplasia and endocrine abnormalities in which of the following disorders?***
    A. McCune-Albright's syndrome.
    B. Stevens-Johnson syndrome.
    C. Marfan's syndrome.
    D. Gorlin-Goltz syndrome.
    E. Peutz-Jeghers syndrome.
36. ***The patient's radiographs could be described as having what type of characteristic appearance?***
    A. Cotton wool.
    B. Ground glass.
    C. Cobweb.
    D. Soap bubble.
    E. Starry sky.
37. ***A bone biopsy was taken from the patient. Which of the following would most likely be observed under the microscope?***
    A. A dense inflammatory infiltrate.
    B. Fibrous tissue.
    C. Pleomorphic cells.
    D. Metastatic calcifications.
    E. Giant cells.
38. ***The overall length of the primary teeth that are given here are the average range of dimensions with one exception. Which one is the exception?***
    A. Maxillary central incisor, 16 to 17 mm.
    B. Mandibular central incisor, 16 to 17 mm.
    C. Maxillary lateral incisor, 16 to 17 mm.
    D. Mandibular lateral incisor, 15 to 17 mm.
39. ***Fibrotic and thickened heart valves that result in a reduction of blood flow through the valve characterize which of the following?***
    A. Stenosis.
    B. Regurgitation.
    C. Insufficiency.
    D. Prolapse.
    E. Ischemia.
40. ***From the occlusal aspect the primary maxillary second molar has which of the following characteristics?***
    A. Somewhat rhomboidal in form.
    B. Three well developed cusps.
    C. Two supplemental cusps, including tubercle of Carabelli.
    D. Poorly defined mesial triangular fossa.
41. ***All of the following local chemical factors will cause vasodilatation of the arterioles, except:***
    A. Decreased K
    B. Increased CO_2
    C. Nitric oxide
    D. Decreased O_2
    E. Histamine release
42. ***The inferior aspect of the diaphragm is supplied with blood by which of the following arteries?***
    A. Median sacral artery.
    B. Lumbar arteries.
    C. Inferior phrenic arteries.
    D. Celiac trunk.
    E. Superior mesenteric artery.
43. ***The coenzyme essential for normal amino acid metabolism is _____.***
    A. Biotin
    B. Tetrahydrofolate
    C. Pyridoxal phosphate
    D. Niacin
44. ***Equal contracture of the lateral pterygoid muscle bilaterally produces which of the following mandibular movements?***
    A. Retrusive.
    B. Elevation.
    C. Protrusive.
    D. Lateral.
45. ***Which of the following cells forms the myelin sheath around myelinated nerves in the central nervous system?***
    A. Schwann cells.
    B. Astrocytes.
    C. Microglia.
    D. Oligodendrocytes.
    E. Amphicytes.
46. ***Which of the following mineralized tissues have the greatest percentage of inorganic material?***
    A. Enamel.
    B. Dentin.
    C. Bone.
    D. Calculus.
47. ***Which of the following is not a feature of poststreptococcal glomerulonephritis?***
    A. Hematuria.
    B. Hypertension.
    C. Edema.
    D. Polyuria.
48. ***In a cusp–embrasure relationship, the maxillary first premolar is most likely to articulate with which of the following mandibular teeth?***
    A. First premolar only.
    B. First molar only.
    C. Canine and first premolar.
    D. First and second premolars.

49. ***There are several tooth numbering systems, some used more than others, and some used by dental specialties or by special organizations. The so-called universal system consists of:***
   A. Two-digit sets of numbers for each tooth in each arch quadrant (e.g., 18 to 11).
   B. Single sequential number for teeth repeated in each quadrant (e.g., 8 to 1).
   C. A sequential alphabet letter for each tooth in an entire dentition (e.g., A to T).
   D. Different symbols for each numbered tooth in each quadrant (e.g., $\underline{8}|$ to $\underline{1}|$).

Test items 50–55 refer to the following testlet.

A 24-year-old man presents to your office for an emergency visit, after being hit on the left side of his face with a soccer ball. He complains that his "tooth got knocked out" and that his jaw feels "out of place." He has no other medical conditions.

50. ***During intraoral examination, you find that the patient's lower second premolar is missing. Which type of alveolodental fibers was least involved in resisting the force that pulled this patient's tooth out of its socket?***
   A. Apical.
   B. Oblique.
   C. Alveolar crest.
   D. Interradicular.
51. ***You also notice that a cusp of his mandibular second molar has fractured off and that dentin is exposed. If this patient were to drink something cold, what will he sense?***
   A. Pain.
   B. Pressure.
   C. Vibration.
   D. Temperature.
52. ***You decide to take a radiograph of the fractured tooth. On the first film you miss the apex of the tooth, so you decide to take another radiograph. Relaxation of which of the patient's muscles would help you in taking the second film?***
   A. Geniohyoid.
   B. Stylohyoid.
   C. Mylohyoid.
   D. Levator veli palatine.
   E. Palatopharyngeus.
53. ***On further examination, you determine that the articular disc of the patient's temporomandibular joint has been displaced. If the patient contracts his lateral pterygoid muscle, the disc will move _____.***
   A. Posteriorly and medially
   B. Anteriorly and medially
   C. Posteriorly and laterally
   D. Anteriorly and laterally
54. ***During the examination, the patient observes that he cannot feel it when you touch part of his cheek and his upper lip. Which of the following nerves was probably damaged during the accident?***
   A. Lingual.
   B. Maxillary.
   C. Long buccal.
   D. Superior alveolar.
   E. Inferior alveolar.
55. ***You decide to restore the missing cusp on the patient's molar. During the administration of the inferior alveolar nerve block, which of the following ligaments is most likely damaged?***
   A. Sphenomandibular.
   B. Stylomandibular.
   C. Temporomandibular.
   D. Interdental.

56. ***Polycystic kidney disease is most commonly associated with _____.***
   A. Renal cell carcinoma
   B. Peripheral neuropathy
   C. Urolithiasis
   D. Berry aneurysm
   E. Non-Hodgkin's lymphoma
57. ***Which of the following types of epithelium lines the oropharynx?***
   A. Simple squamous.
   B. Stratified squamous.
   C. Simple cuboidal.
   D. Simple columnar.
   E. Pseudostratified columnar.
58. ***A scientist has discovered a new peptide hormone. He thinks it acts through the second messenger system, which utilizes cAMP. If this is true, which of the following substances should decrease the response of this new peptide hormone in cells?***
   A. Adenylate cyclase.
   B. Monoamine oxidase inhibitors.
   C. Phosphodiesterase.
   D. Aspirin.
59. ***From the occlusal perspective, which tooth in the primary dentition varies the most in form from that of any tooth in the permanent dentition?***
   A. Maxillary first primary molar.
   B. Maxillary second primary molar.
   C. Mandibular first primary molar.
   D. Mandibular primary second molar.
60. ***The most common cause of osteomyelitis is _____.***
   A. *Streptococcus pyogenes*
   B. *Staphylococcus aureus*
   C. *Lactobacillus casei*
   D. *Pseudomonas aeruginosa*
   E. *Escherichia coli*

61. *The muscle that is found in the walls of the heart is characterized by _____.*
A. A peripherally placed nucleus
B. Multiple nuclei
C. Intercalated discs
D. Fibers with spindle-shaped cells

62. *The smallest cusp on the crown of a 5 lobed mandibular second premolar is the:*
A. Buccal cusp.
B. Distobuccal cusp.
C. Distal cusp.
D. Distolingual cusp.

63. *Which of the following is not involved in the process of mineralization?*
A. Matrix vesicles.
B. Amelogenins.
C. Fluoride.
D. Phosphoryns.

64. *T-cell lymphoma is most likely to occur in a patient with which of the following conditions?*
A. Chronic granulomatous disease.
B. Myasthenia gravis.
C. Osteochondroma.
D. Wilson's disease.
E. Celiac sprue.

65. *For which of the following substances would you expect the renal clearance to be the lowest, under normal conditions?*
A. Urea.
B. Creatinine.
C. Sodium.
D. Water.
E. Glucose.

66. *DiGeorge's syndrome is characterized by a deficiency of _____.*
A. B lymphocytes
B. T lymphocytes
C. Both B and T lymphocytes
D. Antibodies
E. Complement inhibitor

67. *Which of the following phrases best describes restriction enzymes?*
A. Site-specific endonucleases.
B. Enzymes that regulate RNA.
C. Nonspecific endonucleases.
D. Topoisomerases.

68. *The gallbladder arises from the _____.*
A. Common hepatic duct
B. Common bile duct
C. Left hepatic duct
D. Cystic duct
E. Bile canaliculi

69. *Which one of the following disorders is the least likely to be a differential diagnostic factor in the patient's limited jaw opening?*
A. Exacerbation of TMJ and TMD.
B. Trismus secondary to TMJ pain.
C. Myalgia secondary to TMD.
D. Myositis secondary to bruxing.

70. *The superior and inferior ophthalmic veins drain into the _____.*
A. Internal jugular vein
B. Pterygoid plexus
C. Frontal vein
D. Infraorbital vein
E. Facial vein

Test items 71–74 refer to the following testlet.

A 6-year-old boy presents with a history of severe epistaxis. For the past 3 years the patient has experienced these nose bleeds, often without any apparent cause. The patient is otherwise in good health, but his mother has noticed that he "bruises easily." Laboratory tests are ordered.

71. *The laboratory test results show a normal PT but a prolonged PTT. A prolonged PTT test suggests that the patient has an abnormality affecting which component of the coagulation cascade?*
A. Activation of platelets.
B. Activation of thromboplastin.
C. Activation of plasminogen.
D. Intrinsic pathway.
E. Extrinsic pathway.

72. *The diagnosis of hemophilia A is made. This disease is caused by a deficiency of _____.*
A. Factor V.
B. Factor VII.
C. Factor VIII.
D. Factor IX.
E. Factor X.

73. *Which of the following describes the hereditary transmission of this disease?*
A. Autosomal dominant.
B. Autosomal recessive.
C. X-linked.
D. It is not genetically transmitted.

74. *The clinical presentation of hemophilia B is indistinguishable from hemophilia A. Which of the following best describes the laboratory method needed to distinguish these two conditions?*
A. Bleeding time.
B. Assay of coagulation factor levels.
C. Assay of von Willebrand's factor.
D. Blood smear.
E. Platelet count.

75. *Hydrolysis of which of the following compounds yields urea?*
A. Ornithine.
B. Argininosuccinate.
C. Aspartate.
D. Citrulline.

76. ***The median pharyngeal raphe serves as the attachment site for which of the following muscles?***
   A. Lateral pterygoid muscle
   B. Palatopharyngeus muscle
   C. Levator veli palatine muscle
   D. Salpingopharyngeus
   E. Superior constrictor muscle
77. ***A most favorable sequence of eruption for the permanent dentition is which of the following (right side)? (Eruption sequence given by numbers in parentheses.)***
   A. (1) 3, 30; (2) 8, 25; (3) 7, 26; (4) 27, 5; (5) 28, 4; (6) 29, 6; (7) 31, 2.
   B. (1) 3, 30; (2) 8, 25; (3) 26, 7; (4) 27, 6; (5) 28, 5; (6) 29, 4; (7) 31, 2.
   C. (1) 30, 3; (2) 25, 8; (3) 26, 7; (4) 27, 5; (5) 28, 4; (6) 29, 6; (7) 31, 2.
   D. (1) 30, 3; (2) 25, 8; (3) 26, 7; (4) 27, 6; (5) 28, 5; (6) 29, 4; (7) 2, 31.
78. ***Which of the following metabolic activities is increased 1 hour after a meal (during the absorptive state)?***
   A. Glycogenolysis.
   B. Oxidation of free fatty acids.
   C. Glucagon release.
   D. Glycolysis.
79. ***The most prominent mechanism of spread of the hepatitis A virus is by which of the following routes?***
   A. Oral-anal.
   B. Respiratory.
   C. Sexual contact.
   D. Perinatal.
   E. Insect vectors.
80. ***If the molar percentage of guanine in a human DNA is 30%, what is the molar percentage of adenine in that molecule?***
   A. 10%.
   B. 20%.
   C. 30%.
   D. 40%.
   E. 50%.
81. ***The muscularis externa has a third layer in the _____.***
   A. Esophagus
   B. Stomach
   C. Liver
   D. Small intestine
   E. Large intestine
82. ***An infection by which of the following bacteria may result in the formation of gummas?***
   A. *Mycobacterium tuberculosis.*
   B. *Neisseria gonorrhoeae.*
   C. *Treponema pallidum.*
   D. *Bordetella pertussis.*
   E. *Streptococcus pyogenes.*
83. ***Hassall's corpuscles are found in the medulla of which of the following glands?***
   A. Thymus.
   B. Thyroid.
   C. Parathyroid.
   D. Pineal.
   E. Suprarenal.
84. ***The masseter originates from the _____.***
   A. Condyle of the mandible.
   B. Infratemporal crest of the sphenoid bone.
   C. Inferior border of the zygomatic arch.
   D. Pyramidal process of the palatine bone.
   E. Mastoid process of temporal bone.
85. ***Considering the period of $2\frac{1}{2}$ months to about 6 years of age which of the following is true?***
   A. Not all the primary teeth have attained their occlusal level.
   B. Parts of both jaws containing primary teeth change noticeably in size.
   C. A significant increase in intercanine width occurs shortly before and during the time the primary teeth are lost and the permanent teeth emerge.
   D. Dental arch form is more or less constant and practically no dimensional changes take place in depth or width after 9 months of age.
86. ***The primary factor determining the percent of hemoglobin saturation is:***
   A. Blood PO_2.
   B. Blood PCO_2.
   C. Diphosphoglycerate concentration.
   D. The temperature of the blood.
   E. The acidity of the blood.
87. ***What is the average height of curvature of the cervical line (CEJ) on the mesial and distal of the permanent maxillary and mandibular incisors?***
   A. About 3.5 mm on the mesial of the maxillary central incisor.
   B. About 1.5 mm on the distal of the maxillary central incisor.
   C. About 2.0 mm on the mesial of the mandibular central incisor.
   D. About 1.0 mm on the distal of the mandibular central incisor.
88. ***Which of the following describes cells that are abnormal in appearance and may become premalignant?***
   A. Aplasia.
   B. Dysplasia.
   C. Karyomegaly.
   D. Pleomorphism.
   E. Metaplasia.
89. ***Which jaw activity does not involve one of the following muscles?***
   A. Clenching, superior heads of lateral pterygoid muscles (LPM).
   B. Clenching, inferior heads of LPM.
   C. Ipsilateral jaw movements, inferior heads of LPM.
   D. Simple jaw opening, deep masseter muscle.

90. *Hemorrhagic infarction and tissue necrosis suggest which of the following?*
A. Aspergillosis.
B. Blastomycosis.
C. Histoplasmosis.
D. Mucormycosis.
E. Toxoplasmosis.

91. *Which of the following ribs cannot be palpated?*
A. First
B. Second
C. Third
D. A and B

92. *Which of the following is released by mast cells after antigen binding?*
A. IgE.
B. Lysozyme.
C. IL-4.
D. Leukotriene.
E. Interferon.

93. *Where are the temperature control centers located?*
A. Cerebellum.
B. Hypothalamus.
C. Medulla.
D. Cerebral cortex.

94. *Which of the following is a major complication of chronic bronchitis?*
A. Myxedema.
B. Pneumothorax.
C. Emphysema.
D. Pernicious anemia.
E. Malignant transformation.

95. *A comparison occlusally between the primary mandibular second molar and the permanent mandibular first molar shows which of the following differences?*
A. The mesio-, distobuccal, and distal cusps of the primary molar are almost equal in size; the distal cusp of the permanent molar is smaller than the other two cusps.
B. The primary molar crown is wider buccolingually (in comparison with its mesiodistal measurement) than is the permanent molar.
C. The primary molar outline is somewhat hexagonal; the permanent molar is rhomboidal.
D. The ratio of the crown/root length of both molars is the same.

96. *Calcium binds to which of the following for contraction in smooth muscle?*
A. Troponin C.
B. Calmodulin.
C. Myosin.
D. Actin.
E. Desmosomes.

97. *The effects of which one of the following hormones are not mediated through cAMP?*
A. Estrogen.
B. Glucagon.
C. Epinephrine.
D. Norepinephrine.

Test items 98–102 refer to the following testlet.

A 43-year-old man presents for an emergency dental appointment complaining of a burning sensation in his mouth. Upon examination, white plaques are observed along the oral mucosa. The patient otherwise appears healthy. There is no history of systemic illness, but the patient did state that he had a blood transfusion more than 10 years ago following a car accident. The doctor referred the patient to emergency room for further tests.

98. *Upon further evaluation, the doctor requests an HIV and hepatitis test. The laboratory performed both an ELISA test and Western blot, revealing that the patient is HIV-positive. The Western blot is used to identify which of the following?*
A. Antibodies.
B. DNA.
C. RNA.
D. Proteins.
E. Plaque-forming units.

99. *Given the patient's history, if the patient was later diagnosed with active hepatitis, which of the following would most likely be the causative agent?*
A. Hepatitis A.
B. Hepatitis B.
C. Hepatitis C.
D. Hepatitis D.
E. Hepatitis E.

100. *Which of the following would the doctor likely prescribe for the patient's intraoral infection?*
A. Amoxicillin.
B. Vancomycin.
C. Ciprofloxacin.
D. Nystatin.
E. Chlorhexidine.

101. *All of the following molecules may be found within the nucleocapsid of an HIV virus except one. Which one is the exception?*
A. Reverse transcriptase.
B. Integrase.
C. Neuraminidase.
D. Protease.
E. Ribonucleic acid.

102. The patient is referred to an infectious disease specialist and placed on "triple therapy." Two years later, the patient is admitted to the emergency room with a dry cough and shortness of breath. His temperature is 101° F. The most likely cause of the patient's pneumonia is _____.

A. *Staphylococcus aureus*
B. *Haemophilus influenzae*
C. *Pneumocystis jiroveci (carinii)*
D. *Klebsiella pneumoniae*
E. *Streptococcus pneumoniae*

103. The primary maxillary first molar has which of the following characteristics?

A. It is larger in all dimensions than the primary maxillary second molar.
B. All three roots can be seen from mesial perspective.
C. Bifurcation of roots begins almost immediately at the site of the cervical line (CEJ).
D. The mesial root is considerably shorter than the distal one.

104. Which of the following is the end product of purine degradation in humans?

A. Urea.
B. Uric acid.
C. Adenosine.
D. Xanthine.

105. Which of the following is an essential amino acid?

A. Tyrosine.
B. Tryptophan.
C. Proline.
D. Serine.
E. Alanine.

106. Which of the following are the most abundant in the fovea centralis of the eyeball?

A. Rod cells.
B. Cone cells.
C. Rod and cone cells.
D. Amacrine cells.

107. The middle trunk of the brachial plexus of nerves arises from:

A. C5
B. C6
C. C7
D. C8

108. Tinea pedis, which is commonly known as athlete's foot, is a fungal infection that is caused by the following dermatophyte(s):

A. *Microsporum*
B. *Trichophyton*
C. *Epidermophyton*
D. Both A and B
E. Both B and C

109. In comparing permanent and primary teeth, which of the following differences are noted?

A. Crowns of anterior primary teeth are narrower mesiodistally (in comparison to their crown length) than the permanent teeth.
B. Comparatively, the roots of primary anterior teeth are narrower and longer.
C. Cervical ridges of enamel of the primary anterior teeth are less prominent.
D. Buccal and lingual surfaces of primary molars are less flat above the cervical curvature than those of permanent molars

110. Cystic fibrosis is a hereditary disorder that results from defective _____.

A. Collagen
B. Lysosomal enzymes
C. Chloride channels
D. Fibrillin
E. Myelin

111. Which of the following strata of oral epithelium is engaged in mitosis?

A. Basale.
B. Granulosum.
C. Corneum.
D. Spinosum.

112. The class of antibodies that plays an important role in mucosal immunity is _____.

A. IgA
B. IgD
C. IgE
D. IgG
E. IgM

113. Which of the following cells are defective in chronic granulomatous disease?

A. Neutrophils.
B. Lymphocytes.
C. Plasma cells.
D. Killer T cells.
E. Macrophages.

114. The coenzyme that serves as an intermediate carrier of one-carbon units in the synthesis of nucleic acids is which of the following?

A. Ascorbic acid.
B. Tetrahydrofolic acid.
C. Biotin.
D. Pyridoxine.

115. Which of the following genetic diseases that results from a deficiency in the liver enzyme that converts phenylalanine to tyrosine?

A. Albinism.
B. Homocystinuria.
C. Porphyria.
D. Phenylketonuria.

Test items 116–127 relate to the following case presentation.

A 35-year-old woman presents with a painful limitation of jaw opening (28 mm), a painful tooth on the right side, and swelling at the angle of the jaw. She has a history of temporomandibular disease (TMD) and conservative treatment. Medical history reveals that the patient is being treated for tuberculosis with combination antituberculosis drugs including rifampin (Rifadin). She is also being treated with an anticoagulant, warfarin (Coumadin), a low level of aspirin, and paroxetine (Paxil) for depression. The intraoral examination shows extensive teeth wear from bruxism, diagnosed by a sleep specialist as sleep bruxism. Tooth 32 has a deep carious lesion and, on radiographic examination, a periapical radiolucency.

116. The incidence of tuberculosis is increasing as a result of an association with AIDS. Oral infections of tuberculosis (TBC) do occur but are uncommon. Diagnosis of oral lesions may present several challenges, as set forth in all of the following statements except one. Which one of the following statements is false?

A. Lesions secondary to HIV may be present.
B. Isolation of *M. tuberculosis* by culture requires 4 to 6 weeks or longer.
C. Mycobacteria can be demonstrated by special stains in only 27% to 60% of cases.
D. Molecular tests (e.g., polymerase chain reaction) show slow turnaround times.

117. All the following side effects have been reported to be related to the use of rifampin except one. Which is the exception?

A. Green bodily fluids—sweat, tears, urine.
B. Hepatitis.
C. Leucopenia.
D. Nephrotoxicity.

118. Which of the following modes of action does not relate to rifampin?

A. Inhibits RNA synthesis.
B. Binds tightly to eukaryotic RNA polymerase.
C. Tuberculocidal to intracellular and extracellular organisms.
D. Reduces activity of hepatic mixed-function oxidases.

119. Exacerbation of bruxism has been reported to occur with all the following agents except one? Which is the exception?

A. Paroxetine (Paxil).
B. Selective serotonin reuptake inhibitors.
C. Naproxen (Naprosyn).
D. Amphetamine derivative ("Ecstasy").

120. Migraine is a form of headache that is currently thought to be best understood on the basis of all the following with one exception. The exception is which of the following?

A. As a dysfunction of brainstem pathways or diencephalic nuclei.
B. As a primary disorder of the brain.
C. As similar in mechanism to tension headaches.
D. As a neurovascular headache.

121. Three key factors in the pathogenesis of pain in migraine are usually considered. Which of the following is not considered to be a key factor?

A. Cranial blood vessels.
B. β-amyloid–containing plaques in the brain.
C. Trigeminal innervation of the vessels.
D. Reflex connection of trigeminal system with cranial parasympathetic outflow.

122. The treatment of the patient with low levels of aspirin is done for which of the following reasons?

A. To reduce the likelihood of platelet aggregation.
B. To stimulate cyclo-oxygenase in the platelets.
C. To increase the formation of thromboxane.
D. To cause platelets to regenerate cyclooxygenase.

123. When there is a pulpal-periodontal infection of a mandibular third molar, which of the following listed facial and cervical spaces is most likely to have become infected when there is swelling at the angle of the jaw?

A. Retromolar space.
B. Submaxillary space.
C. Submasseteric space.
D. Parotid space.

124. Lymphatic drainage from tooth 32 will first involve which of the following node groups?

A. Lateral upper deep cervical node.
B. Medial upper deep cervical node.
C. Lateral lower deep cervical node.
D. Submaxillary node.

125. All but one the following are considerations relevant to the diagnosis and treatment of tuberculosis. Which of the following statements is not true?

A. Increase in the prevalence of TB.
B. Oral TB lesions occur most frequently on the gingival.
C. Emergence of multidrug-resistant strains.
D. High risk of *M. tuberculosis* infection in patients infected with human immunodeficiency virus (HIV).

126. *Extraction of tooth 32 revealed attached soft tissue. Which of the following is most important for a presumptive diagnosis of tuberculosis?*
A. Caseous necrotic areas.
B. Acid-fast bacilli.
C. Epithelioid histiocytes.
D. Langerhans giant cells.

127. *The patient is on an anticoagulant drug (e.g., warfarin [Coumadin]) as well as rifampin. What is the effect of rifampin on the anticoagulation effect of warfarin (Coumadin)?*
A. Increases the anticoagulant effect of warfarin.
B. Increases the cyclic conversion of vitamin K epoxide reductase.
C. Anticoagulation effect is inhibited.
D. Decreases its metabolic clearance by inducing activity of hepatic oxidases.

128. *Gut-associated lymphoid tissue (GALT) produces secretory _____.*
A. IgA
B. IgD
C. IgE
D. IgG
E. IgM

129. *Antinuclear antibodies are seen in the serum samples from patients with _____.*
A. Hypogammaglobulinemia
B. Chronic granulomatous disease
C. Systemic lupus erythematosus
D. Multiple myeloma
E. Pheochromocytoma

130. *What is the correct general structure of the backbone of DNA and RNA?*
A. Sugar-base–sugar.
B. Bases linked through phosphodiester linkages.
C. Bases linked through hydrogen bonds.
D. Sugars linked through phosphodiester linkages.

131. *All of the following are found in the posterior triangle of the neck except one. Which one is the exception?*
A. External jugular vein.
B. Subclavian vein.
C. Hypoglossal nerve.
D. Phrenic nerve.
E. Brachial plexus.

132. *Which of the following amino acids is positioned at every third residue in the primary structure of the helical portion of the collagen-α chains?*
A. Glycine.
B. Glutamate.
C. Proline.
D. Lysine.
E. Hydroxyproline.

133. *Which of the following factors would result in decreased glomerular filtration rate?*
A. A fall in plasma protein concentration.
B. An obstruction of the tubular system which would increase capsular hydrostatic pressure.
C. Vasodilation of the afferent arterioles.
D. Inulin administration.

134. *The most common form of breast cancer is _____.*
A. Adenocarcinoma
B. Teratoma
C. Follicular lymphoma
D. Sarcoma
E. Carcinoma

135. *Which of the following are NOT type traits of the permanent maxillary central and lateral incisors?*

		Central Incisor	Lateral Incisor
A.	Labial view: Mesial Contact	Incisal 3rd	Jnct. incisal/mid 3rd
B.	Labial view: Distal Contact	Jnct. incisal/mid 3rd	Middle third
C.	Mesial view: contacts	Within incisal third	Jnct. incisal/mid 3rd
D.	Labial: mesioincisal angle	Slightly rounded	Sharp rt. angle

136. *The apex of a medullary pyramid in the kidney is called the _____.*
A. Cortex
B. Medulla
C. Renal papilla
D. Major calyx
E. Minor calyx

137. *All of the following conditions are commonly associated with a group A, β-hemolytic streptococci infection except one. Which one is the exception?*
A. Scarlet fever.
B. Toxic shock syndrome.
C. Pharyngitis.
D. Endocarditis.
E. Impetigo.

138. *The auriculotemporal nerve encircles which of the following vessels?*
A. Maxillary artery.
B. Superficial temporal artery.
C. Deep auricular artery.
D. Middle meningeal artery.
E. Anterior tympanic artery.

Test items 139–143 refer to the following testlet.

A 55-year-old man presents with malaise and dyspnea. He has a low-grade fever and reports that his shortness of breath has increased steadily over the past week and a half. He has a history of rheumatic fever and denies ever using recreational drugs. He is currently being treated by a dentist for full mouth reconstruction.

139. ***Upon further examination, a heart murmur was detected. Given the patient's past medical history, which heart valve is most likely affected?***
A. Mitral valve.
B. Tricuspid valve.
C. Aortic valve.
D. Pulmonary valve.

140. ***Before the patient's development of rheumatic fever, he likely suffered from which of the following conditions?***
A. Cystitis.
B. Pharyngitis.
C. Food poisoning.
D. Thrombocytopenia.
E. Meninigitis.

141. ***After further evaluation and tests, the patient is diagnosed with subacute endocarditis. If the infecting microbe was cultured in the laboratory, the results would most likely show that this microbe is positive for ____.***
A. α-hemolysis
B. β-hemolysis
C. γ-hemolysis
D. Coagulase
E. Lecithinase

142. ***Which of the following is the most likely complication that may occur from the vegetations forming on the patient's defective heart valve?***
A. Myocardial infarction.
B. Hemorrhage.
C. Petechiae.
D. Cor pulmonale.
E. Embolus.

143. ***After the diagnosis is made, the patient is immediately placed on high-dose, IV antibiotics. One of the antibiotics that is administered to the patient is streptomycin, an aminoglycoside. The antimicrobial effect of streptomycin is to inhibit the synthesis of ____.***
A. The bacterial cell wall
B. Folate
C. Proteins
D. Nucleic acids
E. β-lactamase

144. ***The conversion of information from DNA into mRNA is called which of the following?***
A. Translation.
B. Transcription.
C. Transduction.
D. Transformation.

145. ***Maximum rotation and translation of both condyles takes place at:***
A. Maximum opening.
B. Maximum protrusive.
C. Right and left lateral excursive movements.
D. Hinge movement.

146. ***The right subclavian artery arises from the ____ and the left subclavian artery arises from the ____.***
A. Axillary artery; aortic arch
B. Brachiocephalic artery; aortic arch
C. Aortic arch; brachiocephalic artery
D. Brachiocephalic artery; axillary artery
E. Axillary artery; brachial artery

147. ***Rest position (RP) is defined:***
A. As any position of the mandible that lacks contact of the teeth.
B. As the centric relation position of the condyles with the teeth apart.
C. As a mandibular position with masticatory muscles at complete rest.
D. As a clinical mandibular position in relation to the interocclusal space.

148. ***Which of the following ions has a higher intracellular concentration compared to the extracellular fluid?***
A. Na^+.
B. K^+.
C. Cl^-.
D. HCO_3^-
E. Ca^{2+}.

149. ***All of the following cells are associated with chronic inflammation except one. Which one is the exception?***
A. Macrophages.
B. Neutrophils.
C. T lymphocytes.
D. B lymphocytes.
E. Plasma cells.

150. ***When is the crown of the permanent mandibular second molar completed?***
A. About 7–8 years.
B. About 8–9 years.
C. About 9–10 years.
D. About 10–11 years.

151. ***Which of the following proteoglycans is present in extracellular space?***
A. Hyaluronic acid.
B. Keratan sulfate.
C. Chondroitin sulfate.
D. Dermatan sulfate.
E. Heparin.

152. *The pancreas is enveloped at its head by the _____.*
A. First part of the duodenum
B. Second part of the duodenum
C. Third part of the duodenum
D. Fourth part of the duodenum
E. First part of the jejunum

153. *Mucopolysaccharidoses are hereditary disorders that are characterized by the accumulation of glycosaminoglycans in various tissues due to which of the following?*
A. Overproduction (synthesis) of proteoglycans.
B. Deficiency of one of the lysosomal, hydrolytic enzymes normally involved in the degradation of one or more of the glycosaminoglycans.
C. The synthesis of abnormal proteoglycans.
D. The synthesis of highly branched glycosaminoglycan chains.
E. Arginine.

154. *A hormone acts to stimulate its neighboring cell to divide. This hormone would best be described as belonging to which category of hormones?*
A. Paracrine.
B. Autocrine.
C. Endocrine.

155. *The most common cause of pyelonephritis is _____.*
A. *Staphylococcus aureus*
B. *Vibrio cholerae*
C. *Escherichia coli*
D. *Helicobacter pylori*
E. *Bordetella pertussis*

156. *Which of the following types of epithelium acimar units of lines salivary glands?*
A. Simple squamous.
B. Stratified squamous.
C. Simple cuboidal.
D. Simple columnar.
E. Pseudostratified columnar.

157. *The _____ is a component of the juxtaglomerular apparatus which functions in regulation of blood pressure.*
A. Proximal convoluted tubule
B. Distal convoluted tubule
C. Bowman's capsule
D. Glomerulus
E. Macula densa

158. *The masseter muscle, which has a complex of internal components, includes all the following EXCEPT?*
A. Pennation.
B. Structural composition permitting regional activation.
C. Multiple internal aponeuroses.
D. Internal aponeuroses that do not move or deform.

159. *The cricopharyngeus muscle of the esophagus _____.*
A. Is a parasympathetic stimulator of peristalsis
B. Is a sympathetic inhibitor of peristalsis
C. Prevents swallowing air at the pharyngeal end
D. Prevents regurgitation of stomach contents at the abdominal end
E. Controls the gag reflex

160. *The most common cause of bacterial meningitis in newborns is _____.*
A. *Staphylococcus aureus*
B. *Streptococcus pneumoniae*
C. *Escherichia coli*
D. *Haemophilus influenzae*
E. *Listeria monocytogenes*

161. *In which one of the following tissues is glucose transport into the cell unaffected by insulin?*
A. Skeletal muscle.
B. Liver.
C. Adipose tissue.
D. Smooth muscle.

162. *Deoxygenated blood from the transverse sinus drains into the _____.*
A. Inferior sagittal sinus
B. Confluence of sinuses
C. Sigmoid sinus
D. Straight sinus
E. Internal jugular vein

163. *The primary maxillary second molar has what characteristics?*
A. Does not have a well-defined mesial triangular fossa.
B. Oblique ridge absent or not well developed.
C. Development (central) groove is well defined.
D. A tubercle of Carabelli (Supplementary cusp) is well developed.

164. *Facial nerves are derived from the ____ branchial arch.*
A. First
B. Second
C. Third
D. Fourth
E. Fifth and sixth

165. *Analysis of DNA fragments (probing) is possibly due to which of the following properties of DNA?*
A. Phosphodiester bonds.
B. Complimentary strands.
C. Protein binding.
D. Western blotting.

166. *From the occlusal aspect, the primary mandibular second molar has which of the following characteristics?*
A. Somewhat rectangular in form.
B. The outline of the crown converges mesially.
C. Three buccal cusps are dissimilar in size.
D. Cusps do not have well defined triangular ridges.

167. Which of the following are not type traits of permanent maxillary molars?

	First Molar	*Second Molar*	*Third Molar*
A. Buccal view:	Widest molar	Intermediate width	Smallest molar
B. DL cusp:	Same size as M_2	Same size as M_1	Smallest size
C. Occlusal view:	Square/rhomboid	More rhomboidal	Triangle or heart-shaped
D. MB root apex:	In line with cusp tip	In line with crown center	Roots displaced

168. A cotton wool appearance may be used to describe the radiograph of a patient with _____.

A. Osteopetrosis
B. Osteitis deformans
C. Peutz-Jeghers syndrome
D. Seborrheic keratosis
E. Osteogenesis imperfecta

169. The energy for skeletal muscle contraction is derived from which of the following processes?

A. Calcium release from sarcoplasmic membranes and binding to troponin.
B. Cleavage of ATP by the myosin head.
C. Membrane sodium-potassium ATPase pump.
D. Sodium influx during the action potential.

170. Which of the following is a property of C fibers?

A. Have the slowest conduction velocity of any nerve fiber type.
B. Have the largest diameter of any nerve fiber type.
C. Are afferent nerves from muscle spindles.
D. Are afferent nerves from Golgi tendon organs.
E. Are preganglionic autonomic fibers.

171. To which of the following bones is the tensor tympani attached?

A. Incus.
B. Malleus.
C. Stapes.
D. Hyoid.
E. Mandible.

172. An increase in alkaline phosphatase may be seen in all of the following conditions except one. Which one is the exception?

A. Hyperparathyroidism.
B. Osteoporosis.
C. Osteitis deformans.
D. Adenocarcinoma of the prostate.
E. Multiple myeloma.

173. The hereditary transmission of Peutz-Jeghers syndrome is _____.

A. Autosomal dominant
B. Autosomal recessive
C. Sex-linked dominant
D. Sex-linked recessive
E. Not genetically transmitted

174. Which one of the following is considered a primary ligament of the TMJ?

A. Stylomandibular.
B. Sphenomandibular.
C. Stylohyoid.
D. Temporomandibular.

Test items 175–180 refer to the following testlet.

A 60-year-old homeless man who lives in a community shelter presents with history of coughing for the past 6 months. He has a slight fever, hemoptysis, and productive cough with a yellowish sputum discharge. After further examination and tests, the patient is diagnosed with active tuberculosis.

175. When the sputum samples were taken to the laboratory, what test did the doctor order to be performed to help make the diagnosis?

A. Gram stain.
B. Acid-fast stain.
C. Spore stain.
D. PPD test (tuberculin test).
E. Voges-Proskauer test.

176. After 2 weeks, the bacterial cultures came back from the lab confirming the initial diagnosis, positively identifying the organism Mycobacterium tuberculosis. M. tuberculosis is known to infect which of the following cells?

A. Fibroblasts.
B. Basal cells.
C. Type I pneumocytes.
D. Macrophages.
E. Erythrocytes.

177. Which of the following is a glycolipid found on the surface of M. tuberculosis that plays a role in its pathogenesis?

A. Cord factor.
B. O antigen.
C. Protein A.
D. Exotoxin A.
E. Lecithinase.

178. Since the patient was living in a homeless shelter, the tuberculin test was administered to all of the staff and residents living at the shelter. This test is based on a delayed type hypersensitivity reaction that is mediated by _____.

A. Only IgG
B. IgG and IgM
C. IgE
D. T cells and macrophages
E. Mast cells and basophils

179. Which of the following is the most appropriate drug used in combination therapy for tuberculosis to treat the patient?
A. Amoxicillin.
B. Clindamycin.
C. Cephalosporin.
D. Tetracycline.
E. Rifampin.

180. After 3 weeks, the patient was feeling "much better" and was discharged from the hospital, although he remained on his drug therapy for another 6 months. Which of the following best describes the calcified scar that later formed in the affected lung parenchyma and hilar lymph node?
A. Gumma.
B. Chancre.
C. Metastatic calcifications.
D. Tubercle.
E. Ghon complex

181. An infection in a mandibular incisor with an apex below the mylohyoid muscle drains into which of the following spaces?
A. Sublingual space
B. Submental space
C. Submandibular space
D. Parapharyngeal space

182. Phospholipase C is an enzyme that plays an important role in the production of second messengers, which produce intracellular responses. Which two second messengers are produced through the action of this enzyme?
A. cAMP and tyrosine kinase.
B. Acetylcholine and histidine.
C. Adenylate cyclase and protein kinase.
D. 1,2-diacylglycerol and inositol 1,4,5-triphosphate.

183. Which of the following cytokines stimulate B lymphocytes to differentiate into plasma cells?
A. IL-1.
B. IL-2.
C. IL-3.
D. IL-4.
E. IL-5.

184. Which of the following statements regarding the parasympathetic nervous system is true?
A. The third cranial nerve (the oculomotor nerve) carries sympathetic fibers to the smooth muscles of the eye.
B. The facial and the glossopharyngeal cranial nerves carry the parasympathetic preganglionic fibers for the autonomic innervation to the salivary glands.
C. The parasympathetic nervous system innervates primarily striated muscle in the body.
D. The parasympathetic nervous system is organized for diffuse activation and responses.

185. From the incisal view, a greater mesiodistal measurement than faciolingual measurement can be seen in which of the following permanent anterior crowns?
A. Maxillary central incisor.
B. Maxillary canine.
C. Mandibular canine.
D. Mandibular central incisor.

186. The vestigial cleft of Rathke's pouch in the hypophysis is located between the _____.
A. Anterior and posterior lobes
B. Anterior lobe and hypothalamus
C. Posterior lobe and hypothalamus
D. Median eminence and the optic chiasm

187. A comparison of the pulp chambers and root canals of maxillary primary and permanent second molars shows which of the following?
A. Enamel cap of primary tooth is relatively thick but less consistent in depth.
B. Comparatively less thickness of dentin at the occlusal fossa of primary molars.
C. Pulp chambers are proportionally larger in primary molars.
D. Pulp horns are lower in primary molars, especially distal horns.

188. The center that provides output to the respiratory muscles is located in the _____.
A. Pons
B. Medulla
C. Cerebral cortex
D. Cerebellum
E. Hypothalamus

189. The brachial plexus of nerves arises from which of the following roots of the anterior primary rami of spinal nerves?
A. All cervical roots (C1–C8).
B. All thoracic roots (T1–T12).
C. C 8 and T1.
D. C5 through C8 and T1.
E. C5 through C8 and T1 through T4.

190. Aschoff bodies are observed in which of the following conditions?
A. Acute myelogenous leukemia.
B. Pheochromocytoma.
C. Osteopetrosis.
D. Rheumatic fever.
E. Scleroderma.

191. Nonsteroidal anti-inflammatory agents are painrelieving and anti-inflammatory. They are effective since they act to inhibit prostaglandin synthesis by:
A. Inhibiting fatty acid lipo-oxygenase activity.
B. Inhibiting fatty acid-specific cyclo-oxygenase activity.
C. Inhibiting fatty acid-specific hydroperoxidase activity.
D. Inhibiting phospholipase A2.

192. *Terminal bronchioles are characterized by _____ cells.*
A. Goblet
B. Ciliated cuboidal
C. Nonciliated cuboidal
D. Ciliated squamous
E. Nonciliated squamous

193. *A major anatomical variant of the two-rooted mandibular molar is a tooth with an additional distolingual and third root. What is the prevalence of these three-rooted mandibular first molars?*
A. May exceed 10% in Caucasians.
B. Less than 1% in Eurasian and Asian populations.
C. Greater than 5% (even up to 40%) in populations with Mongolian traits.
D. Greater than 8% in African populations.

194. *Which one of the following statements regarding the regulation of gastrointestinal function is true?*
A. The main sympathetic nerve supply to the digestive tract is the vagus.
B. In general, sympathetic stimulation is excitatory to digestive activity.
C. Salivary secretion is stimulated by both branches of the autonomic nervous system, although not to the same degree.
D. Parasympathetic stimulation of the salivary glands produces a saliva rich in mucus.

195. *The occlusal surface of a primary mandibular first molar often has a prominent faciolingual ridge. This transverse ridge connects which two cusps?*
A. Buccal and distolingual.
B. Mesiolingual and distobuccal.
C. Mesiobuccal and mesiolingual.
D. Distobuccal and distolingual.

196. *Which of the following disorders is least likely to be included in the differential diagnosis of a patient with jaundice?*
A. Hepatitis.
B. Hemolytic anemia.
C. Cholelithiasis.
D. Glomerulonephritis.
E. Carcinoma of the pancreas.

197. *Arteriovenous anastomoses in deeper skin are important in _____.*
A. Immunity
B. Thermoregulation
C. Controlling the arrector pili muscle
D. Pigmentation
E. Pain sensation

198. *Complications of Barrett's esophagus include all of the following except one. Which one is the exception?*
A. Varices.
B. Stricture.
C. Hemorrhage.
D. Adenocarcinoma.
E. Ulceration.

Test items 199–202 refer to the following testlet.

A 30-year-old woman comes to your office for a dental examination. She has not been to the dentist in 2 years. The patient has type I diabetes, which requires her to take insulin. She is otherwise in good health. On intraoral examination, you notice that the dorsum of her tongue has a thick, matted appearance and diagnose her with hairy tongue. You also find that the patient has deep caries in her upper second maxillary molar.

199. *Which type of papillae is affected that causes the hair-like appearance of her tongue?*
A. Foliate.
B. Circumvallate.
C. Fungiform.
D. Filiform.

200. *On the patient's radiograph, you notice that the pulp chamber in the carious molar appears smaller than the surrounding teeth. This is most likely due to the deposition of which type of dentin?*
A. Secondary.
B. Tertiary.
C. Mantle.
D. Sclerotic.

201. *You decide to remove the caries and prepare the patient for anesthesia. Which nerve must you anesthetize to ensure adequate anesthesia for the patient?*
A. Nasopalatine nerve.
B. Greater palatine nerve.
C. Anterior superior alveolar nerve.
D. Middle superior alveolar nerve.
E. Posterior superior alveolar nerve.

202. *After administering the anesthetic, the patient complains that her "heart feels like it's racing." You explain to her that it may be from the epinephrine in the anesthesia. Which of the following glands could most likely cause the same symptoms in the patient?*
A. Hypophysis.
B. Thyroid.
C. Pineal.
D. Suprarenal.

203. *Which of the following microbes is the most common cause of gastroenteritis in children?*
A. Reoviruses.
B. Picornaviruses.
C. Togaviruses.
D. Paramyxoviruses.

204. *Name the point angle which represents the junction of the cutting edge of an incisor with the surface that is toward the tongue and the surface that is away from the midline.*
A. Distoproximoincisal.
B. Distolabioincisal.
C. Distolinguoincisal.
D. Labioincisolinguo.

205. Ureters travel inferiorly just _____ the parietal peritoneum of the posterior body wall. They pass _____ to the common iliac arteries as they enter the pelvis.
A. Above; posterior
B. Above; anterior
C. Below; posterior
D. Below; anterior
E. Above; superior

206. Aspartame contains aspartic acid and which of the following amino acids?
A. Phenylalanine.
B. Leucine.
C. Isoleucine.
D. Lysine.
E. Proline.

207. Injury to which of the following nerves would affect abduction of the eyeball?
A. Optic nerve.
B. Oculomotor.
C. Trochlear.
D. Trigeminal.
E. Abducens.

208. Which of the following statements regarding tubular secretion in the kidney is true?
A. The secretion of K^+ increases when a person is in acidosis.
B. The secretion of H^+ increases when a person is in alkalosis.
C. It is a process that transports substances from the filtrate to the capillary blood.
D. It accounts for most of the K^+ in the urine.

209. _____ marks the end of growth in length of long bones.
A. Diaphyseal closure
B. Epiphyseal closure
C. Ossification
D. Formation of periosteum
E. Cessation of bone remodeling

210. The presence of M-protein antibodies suggests immunity to infection by which type of bacteria?
A. *Streptococcus pyogenes.*
B. *Streptococcus viridans.*
C. *Streptococcus sanguis.*
D. *Staphylococcus aureus.*
E. *Lactobacillus casei.*

211. The synthesis of all steroid hormones involves which of the following compounds?
A. Pregnenolone.
B. Progesterone.
C. Aldosterone.
D. Cortisone.
E. Testosterone.

Questions 212–223 relate to the following history and examination

A mother brings her 12-year-old boy to the dentist to ask about her son grinding his teeth and about some white "spots" located on the smooth-surfaced enamel of several of his anterior teeth and premolars. Among other questions about the cause of the defects, the mother then asks when a systemic disturbance occurred that may have caused the "spots". The patient has excessive tooth wear from bruxing and clenching. The dentist measures the cervical-incisal length of the permanent maxillary central incisor (10.5 mm). Also measured is the distance from the CEJ to the midpoint of the defect (5.5 mm). Given that the crown is completed over a period of 4 to 5 years it is possible to estimate the age at which the hypoplasia occurred using 6 months or yearly periods in the following formula:

$$\text{ADF} = \text{ACF} - (\text{yrs. of formation/crown height} \times \text{distance of defect from CEJ}).$$

212. Using an average age of crown formation (ACF) of both 4 and 5 years, the age of defect formation (ADF) is estimated to be about what time?
A. 7–9 months in utero.
B. 0–1 years of age.
C. 1–2 years.
D. 2–3 years.

213. The increase of fluorosis of permanent teeth in both nonfluoridated and optimally fluoridated populations points to the need for dentists to caution parents with children about potential causes of fluorosis in children. Which of the following cautions about fluoride is correct, but the age or implied age is NOT Correct?
A. Excess (> 1 ppm) fluoride in the drinking water during enamel formation.
B. Excessive (> pea-sized amount) use of fluoride toothpaste under 6 years of age.
C. Use of fluoride toothpaste only for children under 4 years of age.
D. Use of a 1.1% sodium fluoride toothpaste or gel by pediatric patients only when 6 years of age and older.

214. Systemic etiologic factors that are said to be associated with enamel defects such as hypoplasia occur generally in what period of time?
A. Before birth.
B. Generally after birth and before the age of 6 years.
C. During the first year postpartum for Hutchinson's incisors.
D. During birth.

215. *The differential diagnosis of white "spots" of the enamel of primary and permanent teeth should include disorders that have a substantiated cause. Which of the following DO NOT have an evidence-based causal relationship with enamel hypoplasia?*
A. Rickets.
B. Congenital syphilis.
C. Measles.
D. Fluorosis.

216. *Clenching and grinding of teeth involves contraction of skeletal type muscles. Several types of myofilaments are present in the contractile elements of skeletal muscles. Which statement about muscle filaments IS NOT true?*
A. Myosin forms the thick filament of muscle.
B. Actin is a major protein of thin filaments.
C. Titin is a protein of elastic filament.
D. Connectin is a protein of intermediate filament.

217. *The clinical examination of the patient reveals extensive wear of the right canines, and somewhat less wear of the lateral incisors. Also there is tenderness of the jaw closing muscles, particularly on the right side. The muscle(s) that would be involved primarily in providing most of the force for anterior tooth clenching include which of the following masticatory muscles?*
A. Inferior lateral pterygoid muscle.
B. Superior lateral pterygoid muscle.
C. Anterior temporalis muscle.
D. Masseter muscle.

218. *Sleep bruxism (SB) is defined by many but not all of the following characteristics. Which is the EXCEPTION?*
A. Stereotypical movement disorder.
B. Grinding and clenching of the teeth during sleep.
C. More frequent in the younger generation.
D. Individuals who brux during the daytime inevitably brux at night.

219. *Recent physiologic evidence suggests that central and/or autonomic nervous systems rather than peripheral sensory factors play a dominant role in the genesis of sleep bruxism (SB). Which statement about the central genesis of SB is NOT true?*
A. During sleep the mouth is usually open due to motor repression.
B. Tooth contact most likely occurs in association with sleep arousal.
C. Some peripheral sensory factors may exert an influence on SB through their interaction with sleep-awake mechanisms.
D. Sequential change from autonomic (cardiac)/brain cortical activities follows SB-related jaw motor activity.

220. *Aggravation of bruxism has been suggested to occur secondarily to all of the following occlusal relationships except one. Which one is the EXCEPTION?*
A. Occlusal interferences in centric relation.
B. Occlusal interferences in the intercuspal position.
C. Iatrogenic occlusal relations that *interfere* with bruxism.
D. Angle Class III malocclusion (prognathism).

221. *The differential diagnosis of enamel hypoplasia should take into account suggested differences between non-fluoride and fluoride opacities. Which of the following statements does not suggest a basis for a diagnosis of non-fluoride (NF) enamel hypoplasia?*
A. Levels of F in drinking water that range from 0.2 to 0.34 ppm have been reported to be associated with prevalences of NF enamel opacities ranging from 22% to 35%.
B. At a level of 1 to 1.5 ppm of F in drinking water, only few F opacities occur.
C. Most NF enamel opacities appear as white, opaque spots in smooth surface enamel; areas of mild dental fluorosis are lusterless, opaque white patches.
D. Fluorosis and NF opacities are clinically significantly different.

222. *During muscle contraction what physical change DOES NOT occur relative to muscle fiber contraction?*
A. Sarcomeres—shorten.
B. Thick and thin filaments—shorten.
C. I Band—shortens.
D. H zone—shortens.

223. *Regarding the superior and inferior heads of the lateral pterygoid muscle (SHLP and IHLP), which of the following statements is NOT TRUE?*
A. Hypothetically, SHLP and IHLP can be considered to be parts of one muscle.
B. Distributions of SHLP and IHLP activities are shaded according to biochemical demands of tasks.
C. SHLP stabilizes the condyle and disk against the articular eminence in a wide range of jaw movements and forces.
D. IHLP plays a major role in the generation and fine control of horizontal forces.

224. *The process of active sodium transport in the ascending limb of the loop of Henle is absolutely essential for which of the following processes?*
A. Regulation of chloride excretion.
B. Regulation of pH in extracellular fluid.
C. Regulation of aldosterone excretion.
D. Regulation of water excretion.

225. *Hypertension (long-term) will be compensated by which of the following renal mechanisms?*
A. Increased circulating ADH (vasopressin).
B. Increased sympathetic activity.
C. Decreased circulating aldosterone.
D. Increased circulating angiotensin II.

226. *The most superficial layer of the epidermis is the stratum _____.*
A. Spinosum
B. Basale
C. Granulosum
D. Lucidum
E. Corneum

227. *Where are the cells that produce calcitonin located?*
A. Red marrow.
B. Adrenal gland.
C. Parathyroid gland.
D. Thyroid gland.
E. Spleen.

228. *In mature dentin, the ratio of inorganic to organic matter is approximately _____.*
A. 94:6
B. 50:50
C. 70:30
D. 80:20
E. 60:40

229. *All of the following symptoms are mediated by antibodies except one. Which one is the exception?*
A. Arthus reaction.
B. Tuberculin reaction.
C. Asthma.
D. Erythroblastosis fetalis.
E. Serum sickness.

230. *The pancreas produces enzymes that are responsible for the digestion of dietary compounds. Which of the following foods would not be digested by enzymes synthesized and secreted by the pancreas?*
A. Carbohydrates.
B. Lipids.
C. Vitamins.
D. Protein.

231. *The primary sensory neurons' nucleus of termination involved in the jaw jerk reflex is the _____.*
A. Facial nucleus
B. Trochlear nucleus
C. Mesencephalic nucleus
D. Spinal trigeminal nucleus
E. Nucleus of solitary tract

232. *Aldosterone _____.*
A. Stimulates N reabsorption in the distal and collecting ducts
B. Is secreted by the juxtaglomerular apparatus
C. Stimulates K absorption in the distal tubule
D. Stimulates bicarbonate reabsorption in the proximal tubule

233. *The first evidence of calcification (weeks in utero) in the primary dentition occurs in which of the following teeth at about what age?*
A. Maxillary central incisor—14 (13–16) weeks.
B. Mandibular central incisor—12 (10–13) weeks.
C. Maxillary lateral incisor—14 (13–16) weeks.
D. Mandibular lateral incisor—14 (13–15) weeks.

234. *From the lingual perspective, the crown of the primary maxillary second molar shows which of the following?*
A. Small, well-developed mesiolingual cusp.
B. Distolingual (DL) cusp smaller than the maxillary primary first molar DL cusp.
C. There is no supplemental cusp apical to the mesiolingual cusp.
D. Developmental groove separating the mesiolingual and distolingual cusps.

235. *An 8-year-old boy presents with macroglossia and delayed eruption of his primary teeth. Of the following choices, which one is most likely?*
A. Plummer's disease.
B. Osteochondroses.
C. Cretinism.
D. Wilson's disease.
E. Mallory-Weiss syndrome.

236. *A major function of surfactant is to increase which of the following?*
A. Pulmonary compliance.
B. Alveolar surface tension.
C. The work of breathing.
D. The tendency of the lungs to collapse.

237. *Red pulp in the spleen consists of _____.*
A. Fibroblasts
B. T lymphocytes
C. B lymphocytes
D. Macrophages
E. Chromaffin cells

238. *The velocity of blood flow _____.*
A. Is higher in the capillaries than the arterioles
B. Is higher in the veins than in the venules
C. Is higher in the veins than in the arteries
D. Falls to zero in the descending aorta during diastole

239. *Neuraminidase is produced by _____.*
A. Influenza virus
B. Hepatitis C viruses
C. Human immunodeficiency virus
D. Measles virus
E. Rubella virus

240. *Which sequence of eruption of permanent teeth occurs most often? (8-7-6-5-4-3-2-1 = M3-M2-M1-P2-P1-C-LI-CI). First #, #'s in each series is considered to be the first to erupt.*
A. 6-1-2-4-3-5-7-8 (Maxilla).
B. 6-1-2-3-4-5-7-8 (Maxilla).
C. (6-1)-2-4-3-5-7-8 (Mandible).
D. 1-6-2-4-5-3-7-8 (Mandible).

241. *All of the following are histopathologic features of malignant cells except one. Which one is the exception?*
A. Anaplasia.
B. Pleomorphism.
C. Aneuploidy.
D. Large nuclei.
E. Low nuclear-cytoplasmic ratio.

242. *The vertebral artery meets with the basilar artery at the lower border of the _____.*
A. Midbrain
B. Pons
C. Medulla
D. Temporal lobe
E. C1

243. *Which of the following is not involved in the process of gene cloning?*
A. DNA polymerase.
B. RNA ligase.
C. RNA polymerase.
D. Restriction endonuclease.

244. *Which of the following is the most significant stimulant of the respiratory center?*
A. Decreased blood oxygen tension.
B. Increased blood hydrogen ion concentration.
C. Decreased blood hydrogen ion concentration.
D. Increased blood carbon dioxide tension.

245. *The infraorbital nerve is a branch of the _____.*
A. Optic nerve
B. Oculomotor nerve
C. Ophthalmic nerve
D. Maxillary nerve
E. Mandibular nerve

246. *Root bifurcation would be a more likely finding in which of the following permanent teeth?*
A. Maxillary canine.
B. Mandibular canine.
C. Maxillary central incisor.
D. Mandibular lateral incisor.

247. *Which one of the following carbohydrates is a ketose sugar?*
A. Galactose.
B. Fructose.
C. Glucose.
D. Mannose.
E. Glyceraldehydes.

248. *Which of the following antimicrobials is bacteriostatic and inhibits protein synthesis in bacteria?*
A. Streptomycin.
B. Penicillin V.
C. Ciprofloxacin.
D. Cephalexin.
E. Tetracycline.

249. *The auricular hillocks are derived from the _____.*
A. First branchial arch
B. Second branchial arch
C. First and second branchial arch
D. Lateral nasal process
E. Medial nasal process

250. *Comparing the overall length of primary central incisors (E|F) with permanent maxillary central incisors (8|9), which is the correct ratio expressed as a percentage?*
A. About 50%.
B. About 60%.
C. About 70%.
D. About 80%.

251. *Ehlers-Danlos syndrome is a disease affecting _____.*
A. Bone
B. Connective tissue
C. Muscle
D. Joints
E. Glycogen synthesis

252. *Which of the following participate in both fatty acid biosynthesis and b-oxidation of fatty acids?*
A. Malonyl CoA.
B. FAD.
C. Acetyl CoA.
D. NAD.

253. *Insulin produces which of the following changes in mammalian cells?*
A. Increase in liver glycogen production.
B. Increase in blood glucose concentration.
C. Decrease in the transport of glucose into muscle.
D. Increase in the transport of glucose into the brain.

254. *Osteocytes are found in _____ in mature bone.*
A. Trabeculae
B. Lacunae
C. The central canal
D. Canaliculi
E. Spicules

255. *Which one of the following morphological characteristic is representative of all posterior maxillary teeth?*
A. Marked mesial concavity on crowns and roots.
B. Tips of cusps are well within the confines of the root trunks.
C. From mesial/distal aspect, crowns are rhomboidal in shape.
D. From mesial/distal aspect, all maxillary posterior crowns are trapezoidal with shortest uneven side toward occlusal surface.

256. *Nephrolithiasis is most likely to be associated with which of the following conditions?*
A. Hyperparathyroidism.
B. Myxedema.
C. Pyelonephritis.
D. Wilson's disease.
E. Thrombocytopenia.

257. *The rate-limiting enzyme in glycolysis is which of the following?*
A. Fructose bisphosphatase.
B. Phosphofructokinase.
C. Phosphoglucose isomerase.
D. Glucokinase.

258. *The type of collagen characteristically found in cartilage is which of the following?*
A. Type I.
B. Type II.
C. Type III.
D. Type IV.

259. *A most characteristic feature of the primary maxillary central incisor is which of the following?*
A. Faciolingual breadth of the crown.
B. Mesiodistal width of the crown.
C. Mesial and distal margin outlines in line with profiles of root.
D. Root/crown ratio.

260. *The spread of an odontogenic infection to which of the following spaces would MOST likely be considered life-threatening?*
A. Submandibular space
B. Sublingual space
C. Parapharyngeal space
D. Retropharyngeal space
E. Pterygomandibular space

261. *The most common mutation accounting for the pathogenesis of trisomy 21 is _____.*
A. Chromosome translocation
B. Meiotic nondisjunction
C. Mitotic nondisjunction
D. Single deletion
E. X-linked inheritance

262. *What type of collagen is found in cementum?*
A. Type I collagen.
B. Type II collagen.
C. Type III collagen.
D. Type IV collagen.
E. Type V collagen.

263. *What happens to net filtration in the glomerulus when plasma protein concentration is decreased?*
A. Net filtration (ultrafiltration) increases.
B. Net filtration (ultrafiltration) decreases.
C. Net filtration remains unchanged.
D. Net filtration ceases.

264. *The presence of Auer rods in a peripheral blood smear suggests which of the following conditions?*
A. Acute lymphocytic leukemia.
B. Acute lymphoblastic leukemia.
C. Acute myelogenous leukemia.
D. Chronic lymphocytic leukemia.
E. Hodgkin's lymphoma.

265. *Hormones secreted by the posterior pituitary gland include which of the following?*
A. Prolactin.
B. Follicle-stimulating hormone.
C. Luteinizing hormone.
D. Vasopressin.

266. *Which of the following is the predominant immunoglobulin in whole saliva?*
A. Secretory IgA.
B. Secretory IgG.
C. Secretory IgM.
D. Secretory IgB.

267. *Which of the following is not an arch trait of the maxillary canine?*
A. In the same dentition, the crown is larger than the mandibular canine.
B. The incisal margin of the crown occupies at least one third to one half of crown height.
C. Labial aspect: mesial and distal marginal ridges converge toward cervix.
D. Marked symmetry of mesial/distal halves when viewed from incisal.

268. *During exercise, which of the following is decreased?*
A. Oxidation of fatty acids.
B. Glucagon release.
C. Glycogenolysis.
D. Lipogenesis.

269. *Involution of the thymus would occur following which year in a healthy individual?*
A. 0 years (at birth).
B. 12th year.
C. 20th year.
D. 60th year.

270. *Monoamine oxidase (MAO) _____.*
A. Inactivates reduced steroid derivatives
B. Is activated by MAO inhibitors
C. Inactivates catecholamines by oxidative deamination
D. Is located in the synapse where it inactivates the neurotransmitter acetylcholine

271. *Sleep bruxism can be characterized by which of the following?*
A. Episodes of massive, bilateral clenching.
B. Tooth grinding that may last for up to 20 minutes.
C. Often coincides with passage from lighter to deeper sleep.
D. Occurs approximately every 20 minutes in the sleep cycle.

272. *An endocrine disorder that causes an early loss of primary teeth and the early eruption of secondary teeth is _____.*
A. Myxedema
B. Hashimoto's thyroiditis
C. DiGeorge's syndrome
D. Plummer's disease
E. Dwarfism

273. *Which of the following factors will not influence the rate at which a meal will leave the stomach?*
A. Acidification of the duodenum.
B. Increasing the tonicity of the intestine.
C. Saline in the duodenum.
D. Lipid in the intestine.

274. *Occlusal interferences can be defined by all of the following except:*
A. Occlusal contact relations that interfere with function.
B. Interference to jaw closure into the intercuspal position.
C. Interferences to laterotrusive movements.
D. Interferences to jaw opening.

275. *The olecranon fossa is located on the _____ surface of the _____.*
A. Superior; radius
B. Anterior; humerus
C. Posterior; humerus
D. Anterior; radius

276. *Which of the following is usually least malignant?*
A. Acute lymphoblastic leukemia.
B. Acute lymphocytic leukemia.
C. Acute myelogenous leukemia.
D. Chronic lymphocytic leukemia.
E. Chronic myelogenous leukemia.

277. *Each of the following describes collagen except one. Which is the exception?*
A. Most abundant protein in the body.
B. Modifications to procollagen occur in the extracellular matrix.
C. Incorporates hydroxyproline into the molecule by Trna.
D. Hydroxylation of proline requires vitamin C and molecular oxygen.

278. *Which position of the mental foramen relative to the mandibular premolars and first molar occurs most frequently?*
A. Between the first and second premolars.
B. In line with the second premolar.
C. Distal to the second premolar.
D. In line with the mesial root of the first molar.

279. *From the lingual perspective the primary maxillary first molar has which of the following characteristics?*
A. Distolingual cusp is the most prominent cusp.
B. Mesiolingual cusp poorly defined.
C. Distobuccal cusp cannot be seen from lingual aspect.
D. Crown converges considerably in a lingual direction.

280. *In addition to the esophagus itself, which of the following structures also passes through the diaphragm through the esophageal opening?*
A. The aorta.
B. The inferior vena cava.
C. The azygos vein.
D. The posterior and anterior vagal trunks.
E. The splanchnic nerves.

281. *Which one of the following does not release acetylcholine?*
A. Sympathetic preganglionic fibers.
B. Sympathetic postganglionic fibers that innervate the heart.
C. Parasympathetic postganglionic fibers to effector organs.
D. Parasympathetic preganglionic fibers.

282. *An infant diagnosed with osteopetrosis has dysfunctional _____.*
A. Chondrocytes
B. Osteoblasts
C. Osteoclasts
D. Fibroblasts
E. Lymphocytes

283. *Langerhans' cells are located primarily in stratum _____.*
A. Corneum
B. Lucidum
C. Granulosum
D. Spinosum
E. Basale

284. *Which of the following would be expected to raise blood pressure?*
A. A drug that inhibits the angiotensin IIconverting enzyme and thus the production of angiotensin II (ACE inhibitors).
B. A drug that inhibits the synthesis of nitric oxide.
C. A drug that blocks vasopressin receptors.
D. Increased stimulation of the carotid baroreceptor.

285. *When are the crowns of the primary maxillary second molars completed?*
A. 11 months.
B. 10 months.
C. 9 months.
D. 8 months.

286. *Which of the following processes is not a true component of swallowing?*
A. Closure of the glottis.
B. Involuntary relaxation of the upper esophageal sphincter.
C. Involuntary movements of the tongue against the palate.
D. Esophageal peristalsis.

287. *Which of the following receptors are recognized by CD8 lymphocytes?*
A. Class I MHC molecules.
B. Class II MHC molecules.
C. Surface IgE.
D. Surface IgM.
E. Histamine receptor.

288. *Which one of the following is not a normal anatomical feature of mandibular incisors?*
A. Bifurcated roots.
B. Inconspicuous cingula.
C. Four developmental lobes.
D. Incisal edges placed slightly lingually.

289. *The _____ differentiates into ameloblasts.*
A. Stellate reticulum
B. Inner enamel epithelium in the cap stage
C. Inner enamel epithelium in the bell stage
D. Outer enamel epithelium in the cap stage
E. Outer enamel epithelium in the bell stage

290. *Which of the following statements is true of the histology of the trachea?*
A. The mucosa is covered with oral epithelium.
B. Elastic cartilage rings lie deep to the submucosa.
C. The cartilage is ring-shaped; the open end of the ring faces anterior.
D. The cartilage is covered by a perichondrium.
E. Skeletal muscle extends across the open end of each cartilage.

291. *In pemphigus, autoantibodies are directed against which of the following structures?*
A. Acetylcholine receptor.
B. Sarcomere.
C. Epidermis.
D. Thyroid follicle.
E. Lysosomes.

292. *Which one of the following is elevated in plasma during the absorptive period (compared to the postabsorptive state)?*
A. Chylomicrons.
B. Acetoacetate.
C. Lactate.
D. Glucagon.

293. *Recent focus on causative factors in bruxism include ALL of the following Except?*
A. Occlusal interferences.
B. Part of a sleep arousal response.
C. Pathophysiological factors.
D. Neurotransmitters in the central nervous system.

294. *A distinct central developmental groove, prominent buccal triangular ridge, two cusps and distinct mesial and distal occlusal pits would be most characteristic of:*
A. Mandibular first premolars.
B. Primary mandibular first molars.
C. Primary mandibular second molars.
D. Mandibular second premolars.

295. *An autoclave sterilizes dental instruments by causing which of the following?*
A. Coagulation of proteins.
B. Denaturing of proteins.
C. Precipitation of nucleic acids.
D. Disruption of cell membranes.
E. Dissolution of lipids.

296. *Porphyrins use which amino acid in their synthesis?*
A. Alanine.
B. Phenylalanine.
C. Cysteine.
D. Glycine.

297. *The dental lamina arises from _____.*
A. Somites
B. Neural crest cells
C. The first branchial arch
D. The second branchial arch
E. The buccopharyngeal membrane

298. *Karyotyping can be used to diagnose which of the following diseases?*
A. Klinefelter's syndrome.
B. Multiple myeloma.
C. Niemann-Pick disease.
D. Pemphigus.
E. Peutz-Jeghers syndrome.

299. *Muscle spindle stretching when the patellar tendon is tapped produces which of the following responses?*
A. Muscle contraction within muscle where the spindles are located.
B. Increased sympathetic stimulation of the spindles.
C. A reduction in the number of afferent impulses entering the spinal cord.
D. An inhibition of the stretch reflex.

300. *In terms of vertical dimension, where is the mental foramen found most frequently?*
A. At the apices of the premolars.
B. Coronal to the apices.
C. Below the apices.
D. No particular location predominates.

301. *Urinary filtrate is most hypotonic in the _____.*
A. Proximal convoluted tubule
B. Descending limb of Henle's loop
C. Thin segment of Henle's loop
D. Thick ascending segment of Henle's loop
E. Distal convoluted tubule

302. *There are _____ pairs of true ribs.*
A. Four
B. Five
C. Seven
D. Eleven
E. Twelve

303. *Based on average MD diameters of the crowns of primary teeth, the range for average overall length of the primary maxillary arch is about what dimension?*
A. 60–68 mm.
B. 68–76 mm.
C. 76–84 mm.
D. 84–92 mm.

304. *Symptoms of a myocardial infarction include all of the following except one. Which one is the exception?*
A. Angina.
B. Diaphoresis.
C. Fever.
D. Vomiting.
E. Dyspnea.

305. *Which process transports amino acids across the luminal surface of the epithelia that lines the small intestine?*
A. Simple diffusion.
B. Primary active transport.
C. Cotransport with sodium ion.
D. Cotransport with chloride ion.

306. *Which of the following cells are capable of mitosis?*
A. Smooth muscle.
B. Skeletal muscle.
C. Cardiac muscle.
D. Type I pneumocytes.
E. Neurons.

307. *Vitamin K serves as a coenzyme for:*
A. The enzymatic hydroxylation of proline to 4-hydroxyproline.
B. The carboxylation of inactive prothrombin to form active prothrombin.
C. The synthesis of nucleic acids.
D. Protein synthesis.

308. *Squamous cell carcinoma is the most common oral cancer. It is a tumor of _____.*
A. Melanocytes
B. Basal cells
C. Fibroblasts
D. Keratinocytes
E. Macrophages

309. *Which of the following is NOT a type trait of the permanent maxillary first premolar?*
A. Occlusal table outline, trapezoidal.
B. Generally two roots—mesial and distal.
C. Central groove is long.
D. Supplementary grooves are rare.

310. *Which of the following skin lesions is most likely premalignant?*
A. Verruca vulgaris.
B. Keloids.
C. Seborrheic keratosis.
D. Actinic keratosis.
E. Compound nevus.

311. *Which of the following statements regarding the hormone secretin is true?*
A. It is responsible for activating chymotrypsinogen.
B. It stimulates the release of pancreatic secretion rich in bicarbonate.
C. It stimulates the release of pancreatic enzymes.
D. It stimulates the contraction of the gallbladder to release bile.

312. *Which primary tooth generally erupts last?*
A. Mandibular second molar.
B. Maxillary second molar.
C. Maxillary canine.
D. Mandibular canine.

313. *The latissimus dorsi muscle is supplied by the _____ nerve.*
A. Medial pectoral
B. Cranial nerve XI
C. Dorsal scapular
D. Thoracodorsal

314. *Which of the following responses is due to the stimulation of α-adrenergic receptors?*
A. Slowing of heart rate.
B. Constriction of blood vessels in skin.
C. Increased gastrointestinal motility.
D. Increased renal blood flow.

315. *Which of the following contributes primary sensory innervation to the temporomandibular joint?*
A. Auriculotemporal nerve.
B. Infraorbital nerve.
C. Branch of the lingual nerve.
D. Facial nerve.

316. *All of the following arteries are branches of the mandibular division of the maxillary artery except one. Which one is the exception?*
A. Incisive artery.
B. Submental artery.
C. Middle meningeal artery.
D. Mylohyoid artery.
E. Deep auricular artery.

317. *Rheumatoid arthritis is characterized by inflammation of the _____.*
A. Articular capsule
B. Articular cartilage
C. Cortical bone
D. Perichondrium
E. Synovium

318. *Which of the following are NOT type traits of permanent mandibular first and second premolars?*

	First Premolar	Second Premolar
A. Buccal view:	Crown bilaterally Asymmetrical	Bilaterally symmetrical
B. Lingual aspect:	Entire buccal profile visible	Buccal profile not seen
C. Lingual aspect:	Most of occlusal surface visible	Little, if any seen
D. Lingual aspect:	Contour height: Middle third	Cervical third

319. *Which of the following muscles of the back is supplied by the CN XI?*
A. Levator scapulae.
B. Latissimus dorsi.
C. Trapezius.
D. Major rhomboid.
E. Minor rhomboid.

320. A positive quelling reaction can be observed in bacteria with a _____.
A. Thick peptidoglycan layer
B. Capsule
C. Flagella
D. Cell wall that contains teichoic acid
E. Glycocalyx coating

321. In which of the following might arterial blood pressure be abnormally high?
A. Ventricular fibrillation.
B. Heart failure.
C. Anaphylactic shock.
D. Increased intracranial pressure.

322. All of the following can be found in the cell wall of a gram-negative bacterium except one. Which one is the exception?
A. Endotoxin.
B. A thin peptidoglycan layer.
C. Lipopolysaccharide.
D. Teichoic acid.
E. O antigen.

323. The articulating surfaces of the temporomandibular joint are covered with _____.
A. Fibrocartilage
B. Hyaline cartilage
C. Articular cartilage
D. Elastic cartilage
E. Perichondrium

324. The binding of epinephrine or glucagon to the corresponding membrane receptor has which of the following effects on glycogen metabolism?
A. The net synthesis of glycogen is increased.
B. Glycogen phosphorylase is activated while glycogen synthase is inactivated.
C. Glycogen phosphorylase is inactivated while glycogen synthase is activated.
D. Both glycogen synthase and phosphorylase are activated.
E. Both glycogen synthase and phosphorylase are inactivated.

325. If posterior teeth on the left side contact occlusally during a right lateral excursion of the mandible, the left side occlusal contact would be referred to as:
A. Laterotrusive contact.
B. Protrusive contact.
C. Mediotrusive contact.
D. Centric relation.

326. Blood from the internal carotid artery reaches the posterior cerebral artery by the _____.
A. Anterior cerebral artery
B. Anterior communicating artery
C. Posterior communicating artery
D. Posterior superior cerebellar artery
E. Basilar artery

327. ATP is utilized directly for each of the following processes except:
A. Accumulation of Ca^{2+} by the sarcoplasmic reticulum.
B. Transport of Na^{+} from intracellular to extracellular fluid.
C. Transport of K^{+} from extracellular to intracellular fluid.
D. Transport of H^{+} from parietal cells into the lumen of the stomach.
E. Transport of glucose into muscle cells.

328. All of the following microbes listed are associated with infections secondary to an HIV infection except one. Which one is the exception?
A. *Pneumocystis jiroveci (carinii).*
B. Epstein-Barr virus.
C. Coxsackievirus.
D. *Mycobacterium tuberculosis.*
E. *Candida albicans.*

329. Which of the following is not a type trait of the permanent maxillary second premolar?
A. Buccal view: narrow shoulders (margins of crown; mesio- and disto-occlusal angles).
B. Occlusal table outline: ovoid.
C. Mesiomarginal groove interrupts mesial marginal ridge.
D. Lingual view: buccal profile is not visible.

330. What is the correct schematic outline of the following teeth?
A. Mandibular premolars, viewed from occlusal, rhomboidal.
B. Maxillary central incisors, viewed from facial, triangles.
C. Maxillary lateral incisors, viewed from mesial, trapezoidal.
D. All mandibular posterior teeth, distal aspect, rhomboidal.

331. Which of the following consists of glucose molecules linked together that act as the structural component of plaque?
A. Fructose.
B. Sucrose.
C. Levans.
D. Dextrans.
E. Fructans.

332. Hydroxyapatite _____.
A. Is weakened if fluoride is substituted for some of the hydroxyl ions
B. Is a noncrystalline structure
C. If containing carbonate ion becomes more soluble
D. Is composed of calcium and phosphate in a 1:1 ratio

333. Tooth enamel is derived from _____.
A. Endoderm
B. Mesoderm
C. Ectoderm
D. Endoderm and mesoderm
E. Ectoderm and mesoderm

334. *Which portion of uriniferous tubules contains squamous epithelial cells?*
A. Proximal convoluted tubule.
B. Thick descending limb of Henle's loop.
C. Thin segment of Henle's loop.
D. Thick ascending segment of Henle's loop.
E. Distal convoluted tubule.

335. *Which of the following enzymes found in the liver is involved in gluconeogenesis during the postabsorptive state?*
A. Glucose 6-phosphate dehydrogenase.
B. 6-phosphogluconate dehydrogenase.
C. Glucose 6-phosphatase.
D. Glucokinase.

336. *The heights of contour of the distal surfaces of permanent mandibular central incisors are located in which coronal third?*
A. Middle.
B. Cervical.
C. Occlusal.
D. Incisal.

337. *Accumulation of fluid in the pericardium occurs most often with which of the following conditions?*
A. Unstable angina.
B. Cardiomyopathy.
C. Myocarditis.
D. Acute pericarditis.
E. Tamponade.

338. *The correct order of tooth formation is _____.*
A. Ameloblasts form, odontoblasts form, ameloblasts start to form enamel, odontoblasts start to form dentin
B. Ameloblasts form, odontoblasts form, odontoblasts start to form dentin, ameloblasts start to form enamel
C. Odontoblasts form, odontoblasts start to form dentin, ameloblasts form, ameloblasts start to form enamel
D. Ameloblasts form, ameloblasts start to form enamel, odontoblasts form, odontoblasts start to form dentin
E. Odontoblasts form, ameloblasts form, odontoblasts start to form dentin, ameloblasts start to form enamel

339. *Reduction division occurs during the _____.*
A. First stage of mitosis
B. Second stage of mitosis
C. First stage of meiosis
D. Second stage of meiosis
E. Third stage of meiosis

340. *All of the following factors play a role in the virulence of the microbe that causes whooping cough except one. Which one is the exception?*
A. IgA protease.
B. Hemagglutinin.
C. Exotoxin.
D. Capsule.
E. Pili.

341. *The minimum volume of air that remains in the lungs after a maximal expiration is termed the _____.*
A. Tidal volume
B. Functional residual capacity
C. Residual volume
D. Vital capacity

342. *From a mesial perspective, the primary maxillary first molar has which of the following characteristics?*
A. Pronounced convexity on the buccal outline of the cervical third.
B. The cervical line mesially shows some curvature in an apical direction.
C. The dimension at the occlusal third is the same as at the cervical third.
D. The mesiobuccal cusp is longer and sharper than the mesiolingual cusp.

343. *The embryo develops from the _____.*
A. The entire blastocyst
B. The entire trophoblast
C. The embryonic disc
D. The extraembryonic coelem
E. The morula

344. *Which primary tooth is generally accepted as the first to erupt, and at about what mean age?*
A. Maxillary central incisor, 8 to 12 months.
B. Maxillary central incisor, 7 to 9 months.
C. Mandibular central incisor, 6 to 10 months.
D. Mandibular central incisor, 8 to 10 months.

345. *Blood levels of progesterone are highest during _____.*
A. The follicular phase of the ovarian cycle
B. The luteal phase of the ovarian cycle
C. Ovulation
D. Menstruation

346. *The _____ of the heart is also known as the mitral valve.*
A. Right atrioventricular valve
B. Left atrioventricular valve
C. Pulmonary valve
D. Aortic valve
E. Tricuspid valve

347. *The most common cause of death in diabetic patients is _____.*
A. Peripheral neuropathy
B. Pancreatic cancer
C. Cardiovascular disease
D. Kidney failure
E. Opportunistic infections

348. *At what time is the crown completed for the tooth indicated?*
A. Primary maxillary central incisor, 3 weeks.
B. Permanent maxillary central incisor, 2 to 3 years.
C. Primary maxillary lateral incisor, 2 to 3 months.
D. Permanent maxillary lateral incisor, 2 to 3 years.

349. *The Y-shaped central developmental groove is most likely found on which of the following premolars?*
A. Maxillary first.
B. Mandibular first.
C. Maxillary second.
D. Mandibular second.

350. *The sternal angle between the manubrium and the sternum marks the position of the _____ rib.*
A. First
B. Second
C. Third
D. Fourth
E. Fifth

351. *Which compound is produced in the hexose monophosphate (pentose phosphate) pathway?*
A. ATP.
B. NADH.
C. NADPH.
D. Fructose 1,6-bisphosphate.
E. Phosphoenolpyruvate.

352. *Which of the following is the most common cause of subacute endocarditis?*
A. *Staphylococcus aureus.*
B. *Staphylococcus epidermidis.*
C. *Streptococcus viridans.*
D. *Streptococcus pyogenes.*
E. *Streptococcus pneumoniae.*

353. *From the occlusal aspect, the primary maxillary first molar has which of the following characteristics?*
A. Crown outline diverges lingually and distally.
B. Small traverse ridge frequently present called an oblique ridge.
C. Four cusps are present.
D. Mesial marginal ridge is thin and poorly developed.

354. *Lymph from the mandibular incisors drain chiefly into _____.*
A. Submandibular nodes
B. Submental nodes
C. Superficial parotid nodes
D. Deep cervical nodes
E. Occipital nodes

355. *Which of the following may be observed in a child diagnosed with rickets?*
A. Dark pigmentation on the oral mucosa.
B. Early eruption of teeth.
C. Hutchinson's incisors.
D. Abnormal dentin.
E. Macroglossia.

356. *Which of the following coenzymes are involved in the metabolism of pyruvate to acetyl CoA?*
A. Thiamin pyrophosphate, lipoic acid, FAD, NAD, and coenzyme A.
B. NAD, tetrahydrofolate, lipoic acid, FAD, and vitamin B_{12}.
C. Mg_2, FAD, nicotinamide adenine dinucleotide, and biotin.
D. Coenzyme A, niacin, FAD, and ascorbic acid.

357. *The primary mandibular first molar has which of the following characteristics?*
A. Resembles other primary and permanent teeth.
B. From the occlusal perspective, has a heartshaped outline.
C. The mesiobuccal cusp is smaller than the distobuccal cusp.
D. No developmental groove is evident between the buccal cusps.

358. *Which of the following muscle attaches to the anterior end of the articular disc of the temporomandibular joint?*
A. Superficial head of the medial pterygoid muscle.
B. Deep head of the medial pterygoid muscle.
C. Superior head of the lateral pterygoid muscle.
D. Inferior head of the lateral pterygoid muscle.

359. *In a cusp-fossa occlusal relationship, the maxillary second premolar is most likely to articulate with which of the following mandibular teeth?*
A. First premolar only.
B. Second premolar only.
C. Canine and first premolar.
D. First and second premolars.

360. *The presence of which of the following in a patient's serum indicates that the patient is a highly infectious hepatitis B carrier?*
A. HBsAg.
B. HBsAb.
C. HBcAg.
D. HBeAg.
E. HBeAb.

361. *Which of the following statements regarding salivary secretion is true?*
A. In general, saliva is more hypertonic than plasma.
B. As salivary flow increases, bicarbonate concentration decreases.
C. As salivary flow increases, ionic concentration increases.
D. Salivary secretion is regulated primarily by hormonal stimulation.

362. *The pulmonary vein of the lung carries:*
A. Unoxygenated blood from the lungs to the heart
B. Oxygenated blood from the lungs to the heart
C. Unoxygenated blood to the lungs from the heart
D. Oxygenated blood to the lungs from the heart
E. Oxygenated blood from the heart to the lungs

363. *_____ vertebrae are characterized by a heartshaped body.*
A. Cervical
B. Thoracic
C. Lumbar
D. Sacral
E. Coccygeal

364. *Lipid micelles are stabilized by which of the following?*
A. Hydrophobic interactions.
B. Hydrophilic interactions.
C. Interactions of lipid and water.
D. Interaction of hydrophobic lipid tails with hydrophobic domains of proteins.

365. *The HIV virus binds directly to the surface receptors of CD4 lymphocytes with _____.*
A. Reverse transcriptase
B. Integrase
C. Hemagglutinin
D. Glycoprotein 120
E. Protease

366. *The maxillary sinus overlies the alveolar processes in particular what teeth?*
A. First and second maxillary molars.
B. All maxillary molars.
C. First and second premolars.
D. First and second premolars and first and second molars.

367. *If jaw opening is divided into phases, and it is assumed that the surfaces of the articulating bones and disc are associated throughout jaw opening, what is the relationship of the disc and condyle in the following phases?*
A. In the very earliest phase, the condyle moves forward before the disc.
B. In the early phase, the disc and condyle move anteriorly in concert.
C. In an intermediate phase, the condyle moves forward at a slower rate.
D. In the final phase, the disc moves forward at a faster rate.

368. *Endotoxin consists of _____.*
A. Lipopolysaccharide
B. M protein
C. Hyaluronidase
D. Lactic acid
E. Coagulase

369. *The trochlea of the humerus bone articulates with the _____.*
A. Ulna of the forearm
B. Radius of the forearm
C. Coronoid process of the ulna of the forearm
D. Olecranon of the ulna of the forearm
E. Medial epicondyle

370. *Increased formation of ketone bodies during fasting is a result of which of the following?*
A. Increased oxidation of fatty acids as a source of fuel.
B. Decreased formation of acetyl CoA in the liver.
C. Decreased levels of glucagon.
D. Increased glycogenesis in muscle.

371. *Nucleus ambiguus contains the cell bodies of which of the following cranial nerves?*
A. III, IV, and V.
B. VII, IX ,and X.
C. VII, IX, and XI.
D. IX, X, and XI.
E. IX, X, and XII.

372. *The participation of calcium in the contraction of skeletal muscle is facilitated or associated with which of the following?*
A. Calcium release from sarcoplasmic reticulum.
B. Calcium binding to the myosin heads.
C. Active transport of calcium out of longitudinal tubules.
D. Uptake of calcium by T-tubules.

373. *What type of vaccine is used for Clostridium tetani?*
A. Capsular polysaccharides.
B. Toxoids.
C. Killed bacteria.
D. Immunoglobulins.
E. No vaccine is available.

374. *Where is the height of contour located relative to the following teeth (viewed from the mesial)?*
A. Facial surfaces of all molars, middle third.
B. Lingual surfaces of all premolars and molars, cervical third.
C. Lingual surfaces of molars and premolars, cervical or middle third.
D. Anterior teeth, cervical or middle third.

375. *The gamma motor neurons control which of the following?*
A. Muscle spindles.
B. Iris of the eye.
C. Voluntary muscle fibers.
D. Pyloric sphincter.

376. *Which of the following organelles is surrounded by a double membrane?*
A. Ribosome.
B. Golgi apparatus.
C. Lysosome.
D. Cytoplasmic inclusion.
E. Mitochondria.
F. Ganglion cells.

377. Calcium that enters the cell during smooth muscle excitation binds with which of the following?
A. Calmodulin.
B. Inactive myosin kinase.
C. Troponin.
D. Myosin.
E. Actin.

378. The lumen of the gastrointestinal tract is lined with _____.
A. Mucosa
B. Submucosa
C. Muscularis externa
D. Fibrosa
E. Adventitia

379. Which one of the following is found on the crown of permanent mandibular first molars but is not found on the crowns of mandibular second molars?
A. MB cusp.
B. Distobuccal groove.
C. Lingual groove.
D. DB cusp.

380. Which of the following mediators aid in the killing of intracellular bacteria?
A. Histamine.
B. Interleukin-2.
C. Catalase.
D. IgG.
E. Lysozyme.

381. Chromosomes line up at a cell's equator during which phase of mitosis?
A. Telophase.
B. Metaphase.
C. Interphase.
D. Anaphase.
E. Prophase.

382. Following the production of Okazaki fragments, which of the following is required to close the gap between the fragments?
A. DNA ligase.
B. DNA polymerase.
C. RNA polymerase.
D. Reverse transcriptase.

383. The maxillary nerve passes through which of the following?
A. Superior orbital fissure.
B. Internal acoustic meatus.
C. Foramen ovale.
D. Foramen rotundum.
E. Foramen spinosum.

384. A productive cough may be seen in all of the following conditions except one. Which one is the exception?
A. Pneumonia.
B. Lung abscess.
C. Bronchiectasis.
D. Asthma.
E. Bronchogenic carcinoma.

385. For each type of tooth, the primary teeth consistently show which of the following characteristics?
A. Greater mesiodistal diameter relative to crown height than permanent teeth.
B. An elongated appearance of the primary crowns and roots.
C. Crowns that are translucent white in color.
D. Root trunk one-half that of crown height.

386. All of the following are rotator cuff muscles except:
A. Supraspinatous muscle
B. Infraspinatous muscle
C. Teres minor muscle
D. Teres major muscle
E. Subscapularis muscle

387. Which of the following does not affect the muscle tension produced during contraction?
A. The extent of motor-unit recruitment.
B. The proportion of each single motor unit that is stimulated to contract.
C. The number of muscle fibers contracting.
D. The frequency of stimulation.

388. Cytochrome P450 enzymes may be found in which of the following cellular organelles?
A. Mitochondria.
B. Golgi apparatus.
C. Lysosome.
D. Ribosome.
E. Endoplasmic reticulum.

389. A patient has a heart rate of 70 bpm. Her EDV (end-diastolic volume) is 140 mL. Her ESV (endsystolic volume) is 30 mL. Calculate the CO (cardiac output) of this individual.
A. 9800 mL.
B. 2100 mL.
C. 7700 mL.
D. 15,400 mL

390. Which premolar would be the most likely to have a single pulp horn?
A. Maxillary first.
B. Mandibular first.
C. Mandibular second.
D. Maxillary second.

391. Which of the following groups of microorganisms produce dipicolinic acid?
A. *Actinomycetes*.
B. *Histoplasma*.
C. *Streptococcus*.
D. *Staphylococcus*.
E. *Clostridium*.

392. Which of the following describes the function of RNA polymerase?
A. Translates DNA into protein.
B. Terminates transcription.
C. Removes introns during transcription.
D. Synthesizes RNA 5′→3′.

393. *Which of the following bones is formed by intramembranous ossification?*
A. Humerus.
B. Lumbar vertebrae.
C. Frontal bone of the skull.
D. Ribs.
E. Clavicle.

394. *The pressure in a capillary in skeletal muscle is 37 mmHg at the arteriolar end and 16 mmHg at the venular end. The interstitial pressure is 0 mmHg. The colloid osmotic pressure is 26 mmHg in the capillary and 1 mmHg in the interstitial fluid. The net force producing fluid movement across the capillary wall is which of the following ?*
A. 1 mmHg out of the capillary.
B. 3 mmHg out of the capillary.
C. 12 mmHg out of the capillary.
D. 3 mmHg into the capillary.

395. *Which of the following forms of thyroid hormone is most readily found in the circulation?*
A. Tri-iodothyronine (T3).
B. Thyroxine (T4).
C. Thyroglobulin.
D. TSH.

396. *Dust cells can be found in the _____.*
A. Brain
B. Heart
C. Lungs
D. Liver
E. Spleen

397. *The lateral thoracic wall of the axilla is covered by which of the following muscles?*
A. Pectoralis major.
B. Pectoralis minor.
C. Serratus anterior.
D. Subscapularis.
E. Latissimus dorsi.

398. *CO_2 generated in the tissues is carried in venous blood primarily in which form?*
A. CO_2 in the plasma.
B. H_2CO_3 in the plasma.
C. HCO_3^- in the plasma.
D. CO_2 in the red blood cells.
E. Carboxyhemoglobin in the red blood cells.

399. *Oral epithelium is composed of _____ epithelium.*
A. Keratinized simple squamous
B. Keratinized stratified squamous
C. Nonkeratinized simple squamous
D. Nonkeratinized stratified squamous
E. Nonkeratinized stratified columnar

400. *Chondroitin sulfate is a major component of which of the following?*
A. Bacterial cell walls.
B. Mucin.
C. IgA.
D. Cartilage.
E. Hair.

Answer Key for Section 1

1. **A.** The inferior head of the lateral pterygoid muscle attaches to the lateral surface of the lateral pterygoid plate of sphenoid bone. Its superior head attaches to the infratemporal crest of the greater wing of sphenoid bone. The deep fibers of the medial pterygoid muscle attaches to the medial surface of the lateral pterygoid plate.
2. **D.** The palatopharyngeus forms the posterior tonsillar pillar. It also functions to close off the nasopharynx and larynx during swallowing. The anterior tonsillar pillar is formed by the palatoglossus.
3. **E.** The superior and inferior ophthalmic veins drain into the facial vein and cavernous sinus.
4. **C.** The masseter originates from the inferior border of the zygomatic arch; specifically, its superficial head and deep head originate from the anterior two thirds or posterior one third of the inferior border, respectively. Its superficial head inserts into the lateral surface of the angle of the mandible; its deep head inserts into the ramus and body of the mandible.
5. **A.** Lateral cricoarytenoid. The oblique and transverse arytenoids and thyroartenoid also adduct the vocal folds. The posterior cricoarytenoids abducts the vocal cords. The cricothyroid muscle raises the cricoid cartilage and tenses the vocal cords.
6. **A.** The site of cell division (mitosis) occurs in the stratum basale (basal layer, stratum germinativum) of oral epithelium.
7. **D.** After branching from the mandibular nerve (CN V_3), the auriculotemporal nerve travels posteriorly and encircles the middle meningeal artery, remaining posterior and medial to the condyle. It then continues up towards the TMJ, external ear, and temporal region, passing through the parotid gland and traveling with the superficial temporal artery and vein.
8. **C.** Intercalated discs are only found in cardiac muscle. Multiple, peripherally positioned nuclei are found in the fibers of skeletal muscle. Smooth muscle cells are spindle-shaped.
9. **C.** The hypoglossal (CN XII) nerve is not found in the posterior triangle; it is, however, present in the submandibular triangle. Contents of the posterior triangle include the external jugular and subclavian vein and their tributaries, the subclavian artery and its branches, branches of the cervical plexus, CN XI, nerves to the upper limb and muscles of the triangle floor, the phrenic nerve, and the brachial plexus.
10. **C.** Deoxygenated blood from the transverse sinus drains to the sigmoid sinus, which empties into the internal jugular veins. The transverse sinuses receive blood from the confluence of sinuses, which is located in the posterior cranium.
11. **A.** The vestigial cleft of Rathke's pouch is located between the anterior and posterior lobes—specifically, between the pars intermedia and anterior lobe. It consists of cyst-like spaces (Rathke's cysts) and represents the vestigial lumen of Rathke's pouch.
12. **B.** The thymus is active at birth and increases in size until puberty (around age 12), after which it gradually atrophies and is replaced by fatty tissue.
13. **C.** The internal carotid artery is joined to the posterior cerebral artery via the posterior communicating artery, which is part of the circle of Willis.
14. **D.** It is a branch of the maxillary (CN V_2) nerve. The maxillary nerve branches from the trigeminal ganglion and exits the skull through the foramen rotundum. When it reaches the pterygopalatine ganglion, it terminates as the infraorbital and zygomatic nerves.

15. **A.** Of the cell types listed, only smooth muscle cells are capable of cell division.
16. **C.** The acinar units of salivary glands are lined by simple cuboidal epithelium. This type of epithelium also lines the bronchioles, thyroid gland, and ovary capsule.
17. **B.** The tendon of the tensor tympani is attached to the handle of the malleus in the middle ear. Loud sounds cause the tensor tympani to contract, pulling the malleus and tympanic membrane inward to reduce vibrations and prevent damage.
18. **C.** The ratio of inorganic to organic matter in mature dentin is approximately 70:30. In enamel and cementum, it is approximately 96:4 and 50:50, respectively.
19. **D.** Oligodendrocytes produce the myelin sheath around myelinated axons in the central nervous system. Schwann cells make up the myelin sheath around myelinated axons in the autonomic nervous system.
20. **D.** The facial nerve supplies special sensory (taste) to the anterior two thirds of the tongue, via one of its branches, the chorda tympani (Fig. 1–25). The chorda tympani branches from the facial nerve, carrying both sensory fibers for taste and preganglionic parasympathetic fibers. It exits from of the temporal bone to join the lingual nerve (a branch of CN V_3), as it courses inferiorly toward the submandibular ganglion. Postganglionic parasympathetic fibers emerge from the ganglion and continue toward the sublingual and submandibular glands. Sensory fibers also branch from the nerve and provide taste sensation to the anterior two thirds of the tongue.
21. **B.** Oblique alveolodental fibers resist occlusal forces that occur along the long axis of the tooth. The rest of the alveolodental (PDL) fibers listed provide resistance against forces which pull the tooth in an occlusal direction (i.e., forces that try to pull the tooth from its socket).
22. **A.** When pulpal nerves are stimulated, they can only transmit one signal: pain.
23. **C.** The mylohyoid muscle forms the floor of the mouth. Relaxation of this muscle would help the dentist push the film down, to help ensure that the apical root is captured on the radiograph.
24. **B.** Fibers of the lateral pterygoid muscle are attached to the anterior end of the disc. Contraction of this muscle pulls the disc in an anterior and medial direction.
25. **B.** The sensory distribution for the maxillary nerve (CN V_2) includes the cheek and upper lip, and lower eyelid, upper lip, nasopharynx, tonsils, palate, and maxillary teeth. The sensory distribution for the long buccal also includes the (lower) cheek; however, it does not include the upper lip. The long buccal is a branch of the mandibular nerve (CN V_3) and provides sensory nerves to the cheek, buccal gingiva of the posterior mandibular teeth, and buccal mucosa.
26. **A.** The inferior alveolar nerve (IAN) courses between the sphenomandibular ligament and the ramus of the mandible before entering the mandibular foramen. The sphenomandibular ligament may therefore be damaged during the administration of an IAN block.
27. **C.** The lateral thoracic wall of the axilla is covered by the serratus anterior muscle. The anterior wall is covered by pectoralis major and pectoralis minor. Latissimus dorsi contributes to the inferior aspect of the posterior wall.
28. **A.** The trochlea of the humerus articulates with the ulna of the forearm. The capitulum of the humerus bone articulates with the radius of the forearm. The coronoid fossa, located just superior to the trochlea, fits the coronoid process of the ulna of the forearm. The olecranon fossa of the humerus fits the olecranon of the ulna of the forearm. The medial epicondyle is on the humerus itself and serves as an attachment site for muscles.
29. **C.** The trapezius muscle is supplied by CN XI. Latissimus dorsi is supplied by the thoracodorsal nerve, levator scapulae is supplied by the dorsal scapular nerve, and the major and minor rhomboid muscles are supplied by the dorsal scapular nerve.
30. **C.** There are seven pairs of true ribs, meaning they attach directly to the sternum via costal cartilages. The remaining five pairs are called false ribs because they attach indirectly to the sternum via costal cartilages. The last pair does not attach at all.
31. **B.** Thoracic vertebrae are characterized by a heart-shaped body.
32. **B.** The sternal angle between the manubrium and the sternum marks the position of the second rib. From this location ribs can be counted externally. This is important, because the first rib cannot be palpated.
33. **D.** The rectus abdominus muscle of the anterolateral abdominal wall is described as being belt- or strap-like. The remaining three muscles of the anterolateral abdominal wall (external oblique muscle, internal oblique muscle, and transverses abdominus muscle) are all described as sheet-like. The quadratus lumborum muscle is part of the posterior abdominal wall.
34. **D.** The posterior and anterior vagal trunks pass through the diaphragm through the esophageal opening. The aorta enters the diaphragm through the median arch, the inferior vena cava through its own opening in the central tendon, the azygos vein through the right crus, and the splanchnic nerves through the crura.
35. **C.** The inferior aspect of the diaphragm is supplied with blood by the inferior phrenic arteries. The median sacral artery supplies the anterior aspect of the sacral area, and the lumbar arteries supply

the lower abdominal wall. The celiac trunk and superior mesenteric arteries are both unpaired branches to the gut and associated glands.

36. **D.** Oral epithelium is composed of nonkeratinized, stratified, squamous epithelium.
37. **D.** The cartilage of the trachea is covered by a perichondrium. The mucosa is covered with respiratory epithelium. Hyaline cartilage rings lie deep to the submucosa. The open end of the cartilage faces the posterior. Smooth muscle extends across the open end of each cartilage.
38. **B.** Terminal bronchioles are characterized by ciliated cuboidal cells.
39. **E.** The most superficial layer of the epidermis is the stratum corneum. From deep to superficial, the layers are basale, spinosum, granulosum, lucidum, and corneum.
40. **D.** Langerhans cells are located primarily in stratum spinosum.
41. **B.** Arteriovenous anastomoses in deeper skin are important in thermoregulation.
42. **C.** The frontal bone of the skull is formed by intramembranous ossification. The humerus, vertebrae, ribs, and clavicle all are formed by endochondral ossification.
43. **B.** Osteocytes are found in lacunae in mature bone.
44. **B.** Epiphyseal closure marks the end of growth in length of long bones.
45. **B.** The branchial arches disappear when the second arch grows down to contact the fifth branchial arch.
46. **B.** Facial nerves are derived from the second branchial arch. The trigeminal nerve is derived from the first branchial arch.
47. **E.** In the liver, smooth endoplasmic reticulum is involved in glycogen metabolism and detoxification of various drugs and alcohols; it therefore, contains P450 enzymes, which are cytochromes that are important in the detoxification process.
48. **A.** Type I collagen is the predominant collagen found in cementum. Type III collagen may be present during the formation of cementum, but it is largely reduced during maturation.
49. **B.** In smooth muscle, the binding of calcium to calmodulin will activate the enzyme myosin light chain kinase. This enzyme phosphorylates myosin, allowing it to bind to actin, and the muscle contracts. For contraction in skeletal and cardiac muscle, calcium binds to troponin C.
50. **B.** The mandibular incisors, as well as the lower lip, floor of the mouth, tip of the tongue and chin, primarily drain into the submental nodes. The rest of the mandibular teeth (premolars and molars) mainly drain into the submandibular nodes.
51. **C.** Fibers of the superior head of the lateral pterygoid muscle attach to the anterior end of the disc, which helps to balance and stabilize the disc during mouth closure.
52. **B.** The submental artery is a branch of the facial artery. Branches of the mandibular division of the maxillary artery include the inferior alveolar, deep auricular, anterior tympanic, mylohyoid, incisive, mental and middle meningeal arteries.
53. **D.** The maxillary nerve (CN V_2) exits the skull through the foramen rotundum. It then passes through the pterygopalatine fossa, where it communicates with the pterygopalatine ganglion. Contents of the superior orbital fissure include CN III, IV, V_1 and VI and the ophthalmic veins. CN VII and VIII pass through the internal acoustic meatus and CN V_3 (the mandibular nerve) passes through the foramen ovale. The foramen spinosum is not associated with any cranial nerves; it contains the middle meningeal vessels.
54. **E.** The abducens nerve (CN VI) provides innervation to the lateral rectus muscle, which moves the eyeball laterally, i.e. abducts the eye. The medial rectus muscle, which is innervated by the oculomotor nerve (CN III), is responsible for adduction of the eyeball.
55. **D.** The nucleus ambiguus is found in the medulla of the brainstem. It contains the cell bodies of motor neurons for CN IX, X and XI. The cell bodies of CN VII, IX and X's sensory neurons are contained in the nucleus of the solitary tract.
56. **A.** The articulating surfaces of the TMJ are covered with fibrocartilage, directly overlying periosteum. The non-articulating surfaces of the TMJ are covered with periosteum. The articulating surfaces of diarthrodial joints are covered with hyaline cartilage.
57. **C.** The mesencephalic nucleus contain the nuclei of the trigeminal sensory nerves (CN V) involved in proprioception and the jaw jerk reflex, including periodontal ligament fibers involved in the reflex. It is located in the midbrain and pons.
58. **D.** The red pulp of the spleen consists of cords, containing numerous macrophages, and venous sinusoids. It is the site of blood filtration. The white pulp of the spleen contains numerous T and B lymphocytes.
59. **B.** The two vertebral arteries join together at the border of the pons to form the basilar artery. Branches of the basilar provide blood supply to the pons.
60. **D.** Calcitonin is secreted by parafollicular cells (clear cells) that are located at the periphery of thyroid follicles in the thyroid gland. Calcitonin plays an important role in the regulation of calcium and phosphates. It suppresses bone reabsorption, resulting in decreased calcium and phosphate release.
61. **B.** During metaphase, mitotic spindles form. Chromosomes attach to these spindles, with their centromeres aligned with the equator of the cell.

62. **B.** The oropharynx is lined by stratified squamous epithelium. This type of epithelium also lines the oral cavity, laryngopharynx, esophagus, vaginal canal and anal canal.
63. **E.** The mitochondria is surrounded by a double (inner and outer) membrane. The nuclear membrane (not listed), which surrounds the nucleus, also consists of a double (inner and outer) membrane.
64. **A.** The medulla of the thymus contains Hassall's corpuscles, which consist of epithelial cells with keratohyaline granules. The medulla is the lighter-staining (less dense) central area of the gland, where T cells maturation occurs.
65. **B.** The fovea centralis only contains cone cells. It is located approximately 2.5 mm lateral to the optic disc in an yellow-pigmented area (macula luna). Vision is most acute from this area.
66. **C.** The roof of the orbit consists of lesser wing of the sphenoid bone and the orbital plate of the frontal bone (not listed).
67. **D.** The elongation and overgrowth of filiform papillae results in hairy tongue. Filiform papillae are thin, pointy projections that make up the most numerous papillae and gives the tongue's dorsal surface its characteristic rough texture. Note: a loss of filiform papillae results in glossitus.
68. **B.** Tertiary dentin, or reactive/reparative dentin, is dentin that is formed in localized areas in response to trauma or other stimuli, such as caries, tooth wear or dental work. Histologically, its consistency and organization varies; it has no defined dentinal tubule pattern.
69. **E.** Innervation to the maxillary second molar, as well as the palatal and distobuccal root of the maxillary first molar and the maxillary sinus, is provided by the Posterior superior alveolar nerve. The nerve is a branch of the maxillary nerve (CN V_2).
70. **D.** The suprarenal glands secrete epinephrine. Specifically, chromaffin cells of the the adrenal medulla, which act as modified postganglionic sympathetic neurons that synthesize, store and secrete catecholamines, produce epinephrine. It also produces norepinephrine.
71. **D.** The teres major muscle is a shoulder muscle, however, it is not a rotator muscle. All of the other four listed in this question are rotator cuff muscles.
72. **D.** The brachial plexus of nerves arises from five roots from the anterior primary rami of spinal nerves C5 through C8 and T1.
73. **B.** The right subclavian artery arises from the brachiocephalic artery, and the left subclavian artery arises from the aortic arch. The subclavian artery becomes the axillary artery upon crossing the first rib. The axillary artery becomes the brachial artery when it leaves the axilla.
74. **B.** The pulmonary vein of the lung carries oxygenated blood from the lungs to the left atrium of the heart. The pulmonary artery carries unoxygenated blood from the right ventricle of the heart to the lungs.
75. **B.** The left atrioventricular valve of the heart is also known as the mitral valve. The right atrioventricular valve of the heart is also known as the tricuspid valve. The aortic valve prevents regurgitation of blood from the aorta back into the left ventricle and the pulmonary valve prevents regurgitation of blood from the pulmonary artery back into the right ventricle.
76. **C.** The cricopharyngeus muscle prevents swallowing air at the pharyngeal end of the esophagus.
77. **A.** The pancreas is enveloped at its head by the first part of the duodenum.
78. **A.** The bile canaliculi drain bile to interlobular ducts. The interlobular ducts form right and left hepatic ducts. These ducts join to form the common hepatic duct. The gallbladder arises from the common hepatic duct.
79. **C.** The apex of a medullary pyramid in the kidney is called the renal papilla. The cortex is the outer layer of the kidney. The medulla is the inner layer. Minor calyces receive secretions from the renal papillae. Several minor calyces join to form a major calyx.
80. **D.** Ureters travel inferiorly just below the parietal peritoneum of the posterior body wall. They pass anterior to the common iliac arteries as they enter the pelvis.
81. **A.** The lumen of the gastrointestinal tract is lined with mucosa. The rest of the choices are in order from lumen out. Fibrosa and adventitia are synonymous.
82. **A.** Gut-associated lymphoid tissue (GALT) produces secretory IgA.
83. **B.** The muscularis externa has a third layer in the stomach. It is an inner oblique layer of smooth muscle. In the rest of the digestive tract, the muscularis externa has two layers; an inner circular layer and an outer longitudinal layer.
84. **C.** The thin segment of Henle's loop contains squamous epithelial cells. The proximal convoluted tubule, also known as the thick descending limb of Henle's loop, the thick ascending segment of Henle's loop, and the distal convoluted tubule all consist of cuboidal epithelial cells.
85. **E.** The macula densa is a component of the juxtaglomerular apparatus which functions in regulation of blood pressure. The proximal convoluted tubule, distal convoluted tubule, Bowman's capsule, and glomerulus all function in the production of urine.

86. **E.** Urinary filtrate is most hypotonic in the distal convoluted tubule. It is isotonic in the proximal convoluted tubule and thick descending limb of Henle's loop. It becomes hypertonic as it passes through the thin descending limb of Henle's loop, and becomes hypotonic as it passes through the thick ascending segment of Henle's loop. Finally, it becomes increasingly hypotonic as it passes through the distal convoluted tubule.
87. **C.** The inner enamel epithelium in the bell stage differentiates into ameloblasts
88. **B.** The dental lamina arises from neural crest cells.
89. **B.** The correct order of tooth formation is ameloblasts form, odontoblasts form, odontoblasts start to form dentin, ameloblasts start to form enamel.
90. **C.** The auricular hillocks are derived from the first and second branchial arch.
91. **C.** Reduction division occurs during the first stage of meiosis. The second stage mirrors mitosis. There is no third stage of meiosis.
92. **C.** The embryo develops from the embryonic disc. The morula, blastocyst, and trophoblast all include structures of the extraembryonic coelem that will lead to development of the amnion, vitelline sac, and chorion.
93. **C.** Tooth enamel is derived from ectoderm. Dentin and pulp are derived from mesoderm.
94. **C.** The olecranon fossa is located on the posterior surface of the humerus.
95. **D.** The latissimus dorsi muscle is supplied by the thoracodorsal nerve.
96. **C.** The middle trunk of the brachial plexus of nerves arises from C7.
97. **A.** The first rib cannot be palpated.
98. **B.** Odontogenic infections of a mandibular incisor with an apex below the mylohyoid muscle have the potential to spread to the submental space. If the apex is above the mylohyoid muscle, the infection would spread to the sublingual space. Both of these spaces communicate with the submandibular space.
99. **D.** From the retropharyngeal space, i.e. "danger space," odontogenic infections can quickly spread down this space into the thorax (posterior mediastinum) and cause possible death.
100. **E.** The superior, middle, and inferior constrictor muscles all insert into the median pharyngeal raphe (the superior constrictor muscle was the only one listed), however, their origins differ.

Answer Key for Section 2

1. **B.** Cyclo-oxygenase includes isoenzymes of prostaglandin endoperoxidase synthase, which is required for the first step in the synthesis of prostaglandins from arachidonic acid. Phospholipase A_2, which is involved in the synthesis of arachidonic acid, is inhibited by steroidal anti-inflammatory agents.
2. **A.** The initial rate-limiting reaction involves the removal of six carbons from cholesterol and hydroxylation of the steroid nucleus to produce pregnenolone. Pregnenolone can be further isomerized and oxidized to produce the other steroid hormones.
3. **A.** A micelle is a globular structure that forms when the polar heads of an amphipathic molecule (fatty acids) interact with the aqueous external environment and the nonpolar hydrocarbon tails are clustered inside.
4. **B.** A ketose sugar is on that contains a keto group. Glyceraldehyde, mannose, glucose, and galactose are all aldoses since they contain an aldehyde group.
5. **B.** Individuals suffering from mucopolysaccharidoses have normal production of proteoglycans and glycosaminoglycans but, due to genetic defects, lack the enzymes which degrade mucopolysaccharides.
6. **E.** Arginine is an amino acid that is deaminated to form ornithine primarily in the liver as part of the urea cycle. Ornithine, argininosuccinate, aspartate and citrulline are generated in the urea cycle but do not provide free ammonia for urea synthesis.
7. **B.** Both epinephrine and glucagons result in activities which serve to increase (maintain) blood glucose. Activation of glycogen phosphorylase will result in glycogen degradation, ultimately providing a source of glucose. Glycogen synthase inhibition results in decreased synthesis of glycogen.
8. **D.** Unlike in noncompetitive inhibition, the inhibitor competes for the same site as the substrate. It is therefore possible (with increased amounts of substrate) to reach the V_{max}. Apparent K_m is increased since more substrate is required to reach 1/2 V_{max} (the definition of K_m).
9. **C.** NADPH is required as a reducing agent for the synthesis of fatty acids. The hexose monophosphate pathway also produces ribose 5-phosphate for nucleotide synthesis. No ATP or NADH is produced in the pathway. Fructose 1,6-bisphosphate is produced during glycolysis.
10. **D.** Oxidation of fatty acids, glucagon release, and glycogenolysis are all increased to provide energy sources for exercising muscle. The synthesis of lipid (lipogenesis) would be decreased during periods of exercise.
11. **A.** During a fast, catabolism is increased to provide additional sources of energy. This is characterized by increased utilization of fatty acids. When the production of acetyl CoA (produced by enhanced β-oxidation) exceeds the oxidative capacity of the citric acid cycle, ketone bodies are formed. During fasting conditions, glucagon concentrations are increased and glycogenesis is inhibited due to limited energy availability. Acetyl CoA production in the liver is increased due to enhanced β-oxidation.
12. **C.** Glucose 6-phosphate dehydrogenase and 6-phosphogluconate dehydrogenase are irreversible enzymes in the pentose phosphate pathway. Glucokinase is involved with phosphorylation of glucose when hepatic concentrations of glucose are high. Glucose 6-phosphatase hydrolyzes glucose 6-phosphate to form free glucose, as the final step in gluconeogenesis.
13. **B.** Glucose transport in muscle and adipose tissue is under the influence of insulin-sensitive glucose transporters. Although several

metabolic pathways are influenced by insulin, glucose uptake into the liver is not affected by insulin.

14. **D.** Phenylketonuria (PKU) is an inherited disorder of amino acid metabolism in which the affected individual lacks enzymes to metabolize phenylalanine. Albinism is a condition that results in a defect in tyrosine metabolism and the inability to produce melanin. Porphyria is an inherited disorder involving defects in heme synthesis. Homocystinuria is a disorder in the metabolism of homocysteine resulting in high levels of homocysteine and methionine in plasma and urine.
15. **B.** Guanine base pairs with cytosine which, on a molar basis, will also equal 30% of the DNA. If guanine and cytosine constitute a total of 60% of DNA, the remaining percentage (40%) must be equally divided between the base pairs of adenine and thymine (20% + 20%).
16. **A.** Restriction enzymes are also known as restriction endonucleases. These enzymes cleave DNA at specific sites to release fragments of DNA for further analysis and characterization by complementary probes.
17. **B.** Tetrahydrofolic acid is the coenzyme form of folic acid required for the synthesis of nucleic acids and normal cell division and replication.
18. **A.** DNA ligase is required to ligate the fragments together. DNA and RNA polymerases are catalysts that synthesize DNA and RNA in a continuous process. Reverse transcriptase is an enzyme found in viruses that makes DNA by using viral RNA.
19. **C.** RNA synthesis is not required for genetic cloning. All the other enzymes are required to synthesize and splice DNA.
20. **B.** Vitamin K is involved with the posttranslational modification of glutamic acid to form γ-carboxyglutamic acid. This carboxylation permits prothrombin to interact with platelets and ions in the process of clot formation. Hydroxylation of proline requires ascorbic acid and iron.
21. **D.** Chondroitin sulfate is a glucosaminoglycan found in ligaments, tendons, and cartilage. It is the most abundant glucosaminoglycan in the body.
22. **A.** The α chains are polypeptides which characterize the collagen molecule. The most abundant amino acids in collagen are proline and glycine. Proline (due to its imino ring structure), interrupts the α chain, resulting in the bending/twisting of the peptide. Glycine (due to its small size) fits into the smaller spaces of the peptide and is positioned at every third position in the chain.
23. **C.** Although fluoride may be incorporated in mineralized tissues, it is not required for the mineralization process. Matrix vesicles produced by osteoblasts are considered to be the initial site of mineralization. Amelogenins are matrix proteins in enamel that regulate crystallite growth. Phosphoryns are initiator proteins that bind minerals to facilitate nucleation and crystal growth.
24. **E.** The transport of glucose into muscle (and fat) cells is due to the activity of glucose transporters (GLUT-4), which does not require ATP and is independent of any ionic concentration gradient. ATP is required for the activity of all other transport mechanisms listed in the question.
25. **D.** Facilitated diffusion does not require energy and moves down a concentration gradient. Active transport, in addition to utilizing energy, is often coupled to transport ions in both directions across the membrane. Both active transport and facilitated diffusion are carrier-mediated and therefore are influenced by competitive inhibition.
26. **B.** The salivary glands are influenced by both the sympathetic and parasympathetic (glossopharyngeal and facial) branches of the ANS. The oculomotor nerve (CN III) carries parasympathetic fibers to the eye which, when stimulated, produces constriction of the pupil. The parasympathetic system innervates primarily smooth and cardiac muscle, resulting in specific activation and responses.
27. **B.** Regulation of blood flow to skin is under the control of factors acting locally (metabolites) and α-adrenergic receptors. Slowing of the heart and activation of gastrointestinal motility are mediated through the cholinergic system. α–adrenergic receptors produce decreased renal blood flow.
28. **A.** C fibers are the smallest of the sensory and motor fibers. They are postganglionic, unmyelinated, and have the slowest conduction velocity.
29. **A.** Calcium is stored and released from the sarcoplasmic reticulum during excitation-contraction coupling. This provides an extensive reservoir of calcium while permitting intracellular free Ca^{2+} to be low when the muscle fiber is at rest. The release of calcium is due to conformational changes which open Ca^{2+} channels in the sarcoplasmic reticulum.
30. **A.** Calmodulin is a calcium-binding protein in smooth muscle which, when bound to myosin, initiates contraction. Calmodulin activates myosin kinase, which results in myosin–actin crosslinking and contraction of smooth muscle.
31. **B.** A motor unit is composed of a single motor neuron and the muscle fibers it innervates. Since the motor neuron will stimulate all muscle fibers it innervates, "fractions" of a motor unit cannot be stimulated. The number of motor units recruited, the number of muscle fibers contracting, and the frequency of stimulation will all affect the degree of muscle tension produced.
32. **B.** The sum total of the pressures moving fluid *out* of the capillary is P_c (37 mmHg) and π_{if} (1 mmHg) at the arteriolar end and P_c (16 mmHg) and π_{if}

(1 mmHg) at the venular end. The sum total of the pressures moving *into* the capillary is P_{if} (0 mmHg) and π_p (26 mmHg). The net exchange pressure on the arteriolar end leads to ultrafiltration (12 mmHg). On the venular end, reabsorption occurs (9 mmHg). Overall net exchange results in 3 mmHg of fluid loss out of the capillary.

33. **C.** Cardiac output is the volume of blood pumped per minute by each ventricle. This is influenced by cardiac rate and stroke volume (end-diastolic volume – end-systolic volume). The cardiac output for this patient is 70 × 110 mL or 7,700 mL per minute.
34. **B.** The velocity of blood flow is the rate of displacement of blood per unit time. Velocity changes inversely with cross-sectional area (cm^2). The greater the area in the vessels, the lower the velocity. Since blood is always flowing due to the distensability of the arterial tree, velocity is never zero.
35. **D.** Decreasing total peripheral resistance would produce greater reductions in blood pressure. Due to the baroreceptor reflex, cardiac heart rate would increase. Increased stroke volume (due to increased venous return and sympathetic stimulation of cardiac muscle) would also occur. Increased cardiac output would occur due to increased heart rate and stroke volume.
36. **C.** Although some CO_2 is transported unchanged in the plasma and in the red blood cells as carbaminohemoglobin, most is transported in the form of bicarbonate ion in the plasma.
37. **D.** The most potent stimulant of the respiratory center that increases the rate of breathing (hyperventilation) is increased CO_2 tension. CO_2 is permeable to the blood–brain barrier and ultimately produces an increase in H^+ of the cerebral spinal fluid. However, plasma H^+ and HCO_3^- are not permeable and thus have little direct effect on the respiratory center. The respiratory center is not sensitive to oxygen tension, unlike peripheral chemoreceptors.
38. **A.** Hemoglobin is a globular protein responsible for transporting most of the O_2 in the blood. The percent saturation of hemoglobin is a function of the PO_2 of the blood. The relationship of PO_2 and hemoglobin saturation is not linear but, rather, sigmoidal. Percent saturation increases greatly at low PO_2 and less at higher PO_2. Increased PCO_2, temperature, diphosphoglycerate, and H^+ decrease the affinity of hemoglobin for O_2 but do not alter the characteristic sigmoidal nature of the saturation curve.
39. **E.** Renal clearance is the volume of plasma completely cleared of a substance by the kidneys per unit of time. The renal clearance of glucose is usually 0 since, although it is filtered, it is completely reabsorbed when the plasma glucose concentration is within normal levels. In the uncontrolled diabetic, plasma glucose levels exceed the reabsorptive capacity (T_m) and it then appears in the urine. Urea is filtered and passively reabsorbed to a slight degree. Creatinine is both freely filtered and secreted to a slight extent. Sodium and water are filtered and reabsorbed to various degrees due to physiological regulation of aldosterone and ADH.
40. **D.** In the ascending (distal) loop of Henle, active sodium absorption results in an increased osmolarity of the interstitial fluid, which plays a role in the retention of water under conditions of dehydration.
41. **C.** Under conditions of expansion of extracellular volume (long-term hypertension), renin release and aldosterone secretion are reduced. Increasing ADH, angiotensin II, and increasing sympathetic activity would result in an increase in blood pressure.
42. **D.** Potassium is passively (via the cotransport system) secreted from the plasma into the distal and collecting tubules. Under conditions of acidosis, an individual may become hyperkalemic since the kidneys will retain K^+ and secrete H^+. Under conditions of alkalosis, K^+ secretion will be increased and H^+ secretion reduced.
43. **C.** Saliva is formed by a process that first involves the formation of a solution by the acinar cells, which is subsequently modified by the ductile cells to produce a more hypotonic solution (compared to plasma). The modification primarily involves the reabsorption of sodium and chloride and secretion of potassium and bicarbonate. As salivary flow increases, the ductile cells have less time to modify the composition of saliva, which results in greater concentrations of sodium and chloride ions. Bicarbonate concentration increases as salivary flow increases due to the selective stimulation of bicarbonate by the parasympathetic system. The salivary glands are primarily under the regulation of both branches of the autonomic nervous system.
44. **A.** Secretory IgA is an immunoglobulin that is unique to the oral cavity. The secretory component is synthesized by salivary epithelial cells and complexes with IgA to form secretory IgA.
45. **C.** Vitamins are not digested by enzymes from the pancreas; however, digestion of carbohydrates, fats, and proteins may be required to make vitamins available for absorption. The pancreas produces amylase for carbohydrate digestion, lipase for lipid digestion, and several proteolytic enzymes (trypsinogen, chymotrypsinogen, and procarboxypeptidase) for the digestion of protein.
46. **B.** Secretin stimulates bicarbonate secretion from the pancreatic ducts. Cholecystokinin (CCK) is responsible for stimulating pancreatic enzyme secretion and contraction of the gall bladder. Chymotrypsinogen is activated by trypsin in the intestine.

47. **D.** Phospholipase C, activated by a component of the G-protein (Gα) complexed with GTP, catalyzes the production of diacylglycerol and inositol trisphosphate. Diacylglycerol activates protein kinases, which phosphorylate proteins, and inositol trisphosphate produces increased release of calcium from intracellular stores.
48. **D.** Vasopressin, also known as ADH (antidiuretic hormone), is a peptide secreted from the posterior pituitary in response to an increase in serum osmolarity. The other hormones listed are synthesized and secreted from the anterior pituitary.
49. **A.** Estrogen is a steroid hormone and therefore does not require a membrane receptor and the second messenger cAMP. Steroid hormones directly enter the cell and stimulate intracellular receptors. Peptide hormones and those derived from single amino acids are not readily lipid-soluble (characteristic of membranes) and thus require membrane receptors and a second messenger system (cAMP, IP_3, etc.). Many of the effects of epinephrine and norepinephrine and all of the effects of glucagon are mediated by cAMP.
50. **C.** Phosphodiesterases are intracellular enzymes that degrade cyclic nucleotides, thus catalyzing the hydrolysis of cAMP to a metabolite, 5′ AMP, which lacks the second messenger properties of cAMP. Adenylate cyclase is an enzyme that catalyzes the conversion of ATP to cAMP. Monoamine oxidase (MAO) is an enzyme located in presynaptic nerve terminals that degrades dopamine, norepinephrine, and epinephrine to inactive substances. Aspirin inhibits prostaglandin synthesis by inhibiting the cyclooxygenase enzyme.
51. **E.** Heparin, an anticoagulant is unlike the other glycosaminoglycans since it is an extracellular compound. Hyaluronic acid is found in synovial fluid, keratan sulfate in loose connective tissue such as cornea, chondroitin sulfate in cartilage, ligaments and tendons and dermatan sulfate in skin and blood vessels.
52. **D.** In the initial step of the synthesis of porphyrin, succinyl CoA and glycine are condensed in a rate limiting step in the liver.
53. **B.** An essential amino acid is one that cannot be synthesized by human and therefore we require them in the diet from plant or bacterial sources. All of the other amino acids can be synthesized by humans from other compounds and therefore are not classified as "essential."
54. **A.** Aspartame is a peptide derivative composed of aspartic acid and phenylalanine.
55. **B.** Cells degrade purine nucleotides to uric acid. Xanthine is an intermediate in a series of reactions, but the final product in humans is uric acid which is excreted in the urine. Urea is the degradation product of compounds containing amino groups (amino acids).
56. **C.** Acetyl CoA. Malonyl CoA is produced following carboxylation of acetyl CoA in the synthetic process of fatty acids. FAD and NAD+ are involved in fatty acid oxidation but NADPH is the source of reducing agents in the synthesis of fatty acids.
57. **B.** This enzyme catalyzes the phosphorylation of fructose 6-phosphate to fructose 1,6-bisphosphate. This irreversible reaction is inhibited by ATP and citrate (indicators of energy abundance within the cell). The reaction is stimulated by AMP.
58. **C.** Pyridoxal phosphate is the active coenzyme of pyridoxine, which is involved in a number of enzyme systems essential for normal amino acid metabolism. Biotin is required for carboxylation reactions. Tetrahydrofolate, the coenzyme form of folic acid, is required for the synthesis of nucleic acids and porphyrin. Niacin participates in energy metabolism (oxidation-reduction reactions)
59. **D.** Immediately following a meal, energy sources are high. Glycogenolysis (glycogen breakdown) is reduced. Lipolysis and oxidation of free fatty acids are also unnecessary during this time. Glucagon release is inhibited due to elevated glucose. Glycolysis is increased due to elevated intracellular glucose.
60. **A.** In the irreversible oxidative decarboxylation of pyruvate to acetyl CoA by pyruvate dehydrogenase, the five coenzymes listed are required.
61. **B.** Insulin is a polypeptide hormone that promotes energy storage when it is readily available. The lack of insulin would interfere with this process. Therefore, under conditions of reduced insulin, hyperglycemia would result due to increased gluconeogenesis in the liver. Glycogen breakdown would be enhanced and glycogen synthesis decreased. Since insulin promotes amino acid uptake in the liver, lack of insulin would result in decreased uptake.
62. **A.** Following a meal, chylomicrons are synthesized in the intestine to transport lipid to the liver. Acetoacetate (ketone body) is found under conditions of increased β oxidation (fasting). Glucagon is secreted in response to reduced blood sugar, which usually is not present following a meal. Lactate, a product of anaerobic glycolysis, is not elevated under conditions of elevated energy sources in the post-absorptive state.
63. **A.** Insulin is a hormone that is secreted under conditions of increased sources of energy (glucose) and therefore results in increased uptake and storage of glucose in the form of glycogen. In the process, blood glucose is decreased. The transport of glucose into the brain is not affected by the hormone.

64. **D.** RNA polymerase is an enzyme that transcribes DNA into RNA chains. Synthesis is similar to DNA reproduction since it is synthesized $5' \rightarrow 3'$.
65. **B.** A probe is a single strand of DNA synthesized with a radioisotope that is complimentary to a segment of DNA of interest. The radio-labeled complex can be analyzed subsequently on a gel by a technique known as a Southern Blot.
66. **A.** Since DNA is a double stranded molecule, cytosine will always be base paired to guanine and guanine to cytosine. Therefore there will be equal amounts of these compounds. It is unlikely that RNA or mRNA, being a single-stranded molecule, will have equal amounts of these bases.
67. **D.** The backbone of DNA and RNA is composed of sugars (deoxyribose or ribose) joined $3' \rightarrow 5'$.
68. **B.** Translation is the conversion of information from mRNA into a protein. Transduction is the incorporation of genetic information carried by a virus into bacteria.
69. **A.** Ninety-five percent of enamel is inorganic mineral compared with 84% in calculus, 70% in dentin, and 60% in bone.
70. **C.** tRNA is not required for the hydroxylation of collagen since the process occurs after translation of mRNA and synthesis of collagen. Ascorbic acid is required to modify the collagen molecule by hydroxylating proline to permit cross-linking among collagen in tissues.
71. **C.** Substitution of most ions (with the exception of fluoride) will increase the solubility of the crystal structure. The ratio of calcium and phosphate in hydroxyapatite is 1.67:1.
72. **B.** Type II collagen is one of the fibril-forming collagens found in cartilaginous structures. Type I is characterized as having high tensile strength and found in skin, tendon, bone, and dentin. Type III collagen is characteristically more distensible and is found in large blood vessels. Type IV is found in basement membranes.
73. **C.** Amino acids are transported across the luminal surface of the intestine by Na^+ amino acid cotransporters in the apical membrane. This is facilitated by the Na^+ gradient established in the intestinal cells.
74. **D.** Triacylglycerol is not commonly a component of cell membranes since it serves primarily as a molecule for storage and transport of fatty acids. Phospholipids are abundant since they form the bilayer structure characteristic of membranes. Proteins are present and serve various functions as enzymes, receptors, and transporters/carriers. Cholesterol stabilizes the membrane and is responsible for the maintenance of fluidity. Sphingolipids are components of myelin, which insulates membranes in neurons.
75. **C.** Monoamine oxidase is an enzyme located in the presynaptic nerve terminal, which degrades dopamine, norepinephrine, and epinephrine to inactive substances.
76. **B.** The sympathetic postganglionic fibers innervating the heart release norepinephrine. Acetylcholine is neurotransmitter in sympathetic preganglionic fibers, parasympathetic postganglionic fibers, and parasympathetic preganglionic fibers.
77. **B.** The hypothalamus coordinates many activities mediated by the ANS, including food intake, thirst, and temperature regulation. The cerebellum functions to regulate movement and posture. The medulla is responsible for coordinating respiration. The cerebral cortex performs functions of perception, cognition, higher motor functions, memory, and emotion.
78. **B.** In the process of muscle contraction, ATP bound to myosin is cleaved to form ADP and P_i. Myosin is released to bind to a new actin site producing a force-generating stroke. Sodium influx and calcium binding are involved in the excitation-contraction coupling process but do not serve as a source of energy.
79. **A.** Stretching of muscle spindles results in a reflex that is intended to adjust the muscle to its resting length by contracting the muscle in which it is found. The stretching of the spindle increases afferent impulses to the spinal cord and through a monosynaptic reflex stimulates muscle contraction via an alpha motor neuron.
80. **A.** Muscles are innervated by two types of motor neurons (alpha and gamma). The alpha motor neurons innervate voluntary muscle fibers (extrafusal skeletal muscles). The gamma motor neurons innervate the muscle spindles (intrafusal muscle fibers). The muscles of the iris are controlled by both sympathetic innervation (dilation) and parasympathetic innervation (constriction). The pyloric sphincter in the stomach is regulated primarily by the enteric nervous system and regulatory hormones in the GI tract.
81. **B.** Nitric oxide is a molecule produced in endothelial cells that acts directly on smooth muscle to produce relaxation and vasodilatation. Therefore, inhibition of its synthesis would be expected to raise blood pressure. Inhibitors of angiotensin II synthesis should reduce blood pressure since angiotensin II stimulates aldosterone synthesis resulting in increased fluid retention. Angiotensin II is also a potent vasoconstrictor. Blocking vasopressin (also a potent vasoconstrictor) receptors would reduce blood pressure. Stimulation of the baroreceptor would produce a reflex that would reduce cardiac output and peripheral sympathetic tone.
82. **B.** The concentration of potassium ions within cells is approximately 30 times greater than the extracellular fluid; the other ions are in greater concentrations in extracellular fluid compared with values within the cell.

83. **A.** All the other factors will produce vasodilation and hyperemia to increase the exchange of metabolites in the tissue.
84. **D.** Capillary blood flow is proportional to changes in the radius (r^4) of the vessel. Decreasing the radius would produce increased vascular pressure. Viscosity of the blood depends primarily on the hematocrit (percentage of red blood cells) and would not be changed by changes in the radius of the vessels.
85. **D.** Under conditions of increased intracranial pressure, the vasomotor regions of the medulla are stimulated due to localized ischemia resulting in an increase in systemic blood pressure. Ventricular fibrillation is irregular, rapid, uncoordinated contractions of the ventricle that do not result in effecting blood movement. Anaphylactic shock is caused by severe allergic reactions, widespread release of histamine, and subsequent vasodilatation.
86. **A.** Surfactant is synthesized by alveolar cells and functions to reduce the surface tension of the alveoli. This reduction of surface tension increases pulmonary compliance and decreases the work of breathing. It will also decrease the tendency of the lungs to collapse. Lack of surfactant results in neonatal respiratory distress syndrome.
87. **C.** Residual volume is the volume of air remaining after a maximal forced expiration. Tidal volume is the amount of air exchanged (expiration and inspiration) during normal quiet breathing. Functional residual capacity is a combination of the expired reserve volume (forced expiration) plus the residual volume. Vital capacity is the volume of air expired after maximal inspiration.
88. **B.** The regulatory centers for respiration are in the brain stem—specifically, the medulla. The medulla contains three groups of neurons (medullary respiratory center, apneustic center and pneumotaxic center). The cerebral cortex may influence the medullary centers but does not totally control respiration.
89. **A.** Aldosterone secretion is mediated through the renin-angiotensin system. Angiotensin II stimulates the synthesis and release of aldosterone from the adrenal gland. It acts on the distal tubule and collecting ducts to increase sodium reabsorption and potassium secretion.
90. **A.** Net filtration depends on the hydrostatic pressures in the glomerular capillary, the hydrostatic pressures in bowman's space, and the oncotic pressures in the capillary and bowman's capsule. Reducing the plasma protein (reducing the oncotic pressure) will lower the tendency to retain fluid in the capillary. This would result in a net increase in filtration.
91. **B.** Increasing the hydrostatic pressure within the glomerulus would decrease the net ultrafiltration pressure. Reduced plasma protein concentration decreases the oncotic pressure in the plasma which would increase filtration. Vasodilation of the afferent arterioles would increase capillary pressure resulting in increased filtration. Inulin, although used to measure glomerular filtration, does not affect glomerular filtration rate.
92. **C.** Under normal conditions, all glucose is reabsorbed by both secondary active transport systems and facilitated diffusion utilizing GLUT 1 and 2 carriers. Calcium is passively reabsorbed, but its reabsorption is also regulated by parathyroid hormone in the distal tubule. Not all urea is reabsorbed but about half is excreted. Its permeability is altered by changes in vasopressin. Phosphate reabsorption is also regulated by parathyroid hormone.
93. **C.** The movement of the tongue against the palate is the only voluntary process among the four possible answers.
94. **A.** The gastrointestinal tract is regulated by both the sympathetic and parasympathetic branches of the autonomic nervous system. The parasympathetic system is stimulatory and the sympathetic system inhibitory. The CNS does influence motility and secretory activity through the autonomic nervous system. Numerous endocrine factors (secretin, gastrin, cholecystokinin, etc.) are also involved with the regulation of gastrointestinal activity.
95. **C.** The salivary glands are under the influence of both the sympathetic and parasympathetic nervous system. Parasympathetic stimulation results in a more watery secretion compared with sympathetic stimulation, which produces increased amounts of protein with reduced volume. The vagus is parasympathetic, which in general is stimulatory to gastrointestinal tract. In general, sympathetics are inhibitory to the gastrointestinal tract. (The exceptions are salivary glands.)
96. **C.** Fat in the intestine, low pH, and increased osmolarity of intestinal contents will reduce gastric emptying. This reflex is mediated through neuronal and endocrine factors comprising the enterogastric reflex. Saline in the intestine will not affect gastric emptying.
97. **B.** Thyroxine and triiodothyronine are formed by the cleavage of thyroglobulin following stimulation by TSH. Most thyroxine is converted to triiodothyronine in liver and kidney. Thyroglobulin is the storage form of thyroid hormone. TSH (thyroid-stimulating hormone) is produced in the anterior pituitary. It is not a hormone secreted from the thyroid but acts to stimulate the synthesis and secretion of thyroid hormones.
98. **A.** The terminology used is a classical descriptor of the relationship between the hormone source

and target tissue. Paracrine refers to the target tissue as a cell in close proximity to the secreting tissue. Autocrine stimulation refers to cell that releases a factor (hormone) which stimulates the cell from which it was released. Endocrine factors are hormones that have an effect at a distal site in the body.

99. **B.** Progesterone concentration in blood is highest following the surge of LH (leuteinizing hormone) following ovulation. During ovulation, estrogen surges due to positive feedback during the follicular phase. During menstruation there are sharp declines in estrogen and progesterone due to reduced secretion of LH and FSH.

100. **C.** Glucagon is secreted from the pancreas in response to reduced plasma glucose due to fasting and exercise. It functions to mobilize energy stores (glucose) and return blood glucose to normal levels. Glycogen synthesis (glycogenesis) will not occur in response to glucagon.

Answer Key for Section 3

1. **B**. Neutrophils are quick to arrive to the site of infection or injury and are therefore associated with acute inflammation. All of the other cells listed are mediators of chronic inflammation.
2. **C**. Dust cells, along with heart failure cells, are macrophages that are found in the lungs. They are part of the reticuloendothelial system.
3. **E**. Bacteria that are phagocytosed by macrophages are kept in membrane-bound vacuoles called *phagosomes*. A phagosome will fuse with a lysosome, which contains many degradative enzymes, including lysozyme.
4. **C**. Although IgE is the least prevalent immunoglobulin in the body, it is the major antibody mediator of type I hypersensitive reactions. These reactions are caused primarily by prior sensitization and the accumulation of IgE to a specific allergen.
5. **B**. DiGeorge's syndrome is characterized by a deficiency of T cells. It is caused by the failure of the third and fourth brachial pouches to develop normally, resulting in a lack of thymus and parathyroid development.
6. **C**. Intraoral *Streptococcus viridans* is the most common cause of subacute endocarditis. *Staphylococcus aureus* is the most common cause of acute endocarditis.
7. **D**. Aschoff bodies are the classic lesions observed in rheumatic fever. They are areas of focal necrosis surrounded by a dense inflammatory infiltration and may be observed in heart tissues.
8. **A**. Endotoxin or lipopolysaccharide is found in the cell walls of gram-negative bacteria.
9. **D**. Endocarditis is most commonly caused by group B, α-hemolytic streptococci, such as *S. viridans, S. mutans, S. sanguis, and S. salivarius*. All of the other conditions are associated with group A β-hemolytic streptococcal infections, such as *S. pyogenes*.
10. **A**. The only disease listed that is related to an abnormal number of chromosomes is Klinefelter's syndrome. This disease is characterized by two or more X chromosomes and one or more Y chromosome. Typically, those affected have 47 chromosomes with a karyotype of XXY.
11. **C**. Pemphigus is an autoimmune disease wherein autoantibodies against epidermis cells are produced. Histologically, a phenomenon called *acantholysis*, wherein epidermal cells appear to detach and separate from each other, is observed.
12. **E**. Chronic bronchitis predisposes those affected to squamous neoplasia of the bronchial epithelium (i.e., bronchogenic carcinoma).
13. **A**. Chronic granulomatosis results from neutrophils with a defective NAPDH oxidase system. This affects their ability to kill microorganisms, since they are unable to produce superoxide radicals.
14. **B**. Dysplastic cells are abnormal in appearance and organization. The potential to develop into a malignant tumor is present; however, this risk varies.
15. **D**. HIV's envelope contains two glycoproteins, gp120 and gp41. gp120 binds specifically with CD4 surface receptors.
16. **A**. The most common cause of gastroenteritis in children is the rotavirus. It is found in the reovirus family.
17. **B**. Radiographic findings of a cotton-wool appearance is common in patients diagnosed with osteitis deformans or Paget's disease.
18. **B**. Autoclaves function by denaturing proteins. They are effective against spores.
19. **B**. Ehlers-Danlos syndromes are characterized by defects in collagen (i.e., connective tissues).

20. **B.** Increased levels of alkaline phosphatase may be observed in diseases that display extensive bone loss. Osteoporosis is characterized by a decrease in bone mass. There are either normal or decreased levels of alkaline phosphatase in patients diagnosed with this disease.
21. **C.** The leading cause of death for diabetic patients is cardiovascular disease. Other complications include retinopathy, nephropathy, and peripheral neuropathy.
22. **A.** Neuraminidase is found on the surface envelope of influenza viruses. It functions to attach the virus to the host cell.
23. **D.** Actinic keratosis produces dry, scaly plaques with an erythematous base. They may be premalignant. Both compound and intraepidermal nevi are benign. As to nevi, only junctional nevi are considered to be premalignant.
24. **A.** Hepatitis A is spread via oral–anal/fecal contamination. The other hepatitis viruses can be transmitted through blood, sexual contact, and/or perinatally.
25. **E.** Cardiac tamponade is a serious condition caused by accumulation of fluid in the pericardium. This can result in impaired ventricular filling and can rapidly lead to decreased cardiac output and death.
26. **C.** Pyelonephritis is usually caused by gram-negative, rod-shaped bacteria that are part of the normal flora of the enteric tract. It is most commonly caused by *Escherichia coli,* followed by *Proteus*, *Klebsiella*, and *Enterobacter.*
27. **D.** Polycystic kidney disease is characterized by the formation of cysts in kidney. It is commonly associated with berry aneurysms.
28. **D.** Squamous cell carcinoma is the most common oral cancer, occurring in 90% of all cases. It is a cancer of squamous epithelium, specifically a tumor of keratinocytes.
29. **E.** Both *Epidermophyton* and *Trichophyton* can cause tinea pedis.
30. **A.** Stenosis describes fibrotic and thickened valves, resulting in reduced blood flow through the valve.
31. **C.** Cystic fibrosis results from an abnormal chloride channel that affects all exocrine glands.
32. **B.** Trisomy 21, which is also known as *Down syndrome,* is a disorder affecting autosomes. It is generally caused by meiotic nondisjunction in the mother, which results in an extra copy of chromosome 21 (trisomy 21).
33. **D.** These oral findings can be observed in patients with hyperthyroidism. The only endocrine disorder listed that is related to hyperthyroidism is Plummer's disease. It is caused by a nodular growth or adenoma of the thyroid.
34. **D.** Poststreptococcal glomerulonephritis is a classic example of nephritic syndrome, which occurs after a *Streptococcus* infection (e.g., strep throat). It is characterized by all of the symptoms listed except polyuria. A decrease in urination is usually observed.
35. **B.** Osteomyelitis, or an infection of bone, is most commonly caused by *Staphylococcus aureus*. Symptoms include pain and systemic signs of infection (i.e., fever, malaise).
36. **E.** All of the features listed are commonly observed in malignant cells, except a low nuclear– cytoplasmic ratio. Due to the large nuclei present, there is usually a high nuclear-cytoplasmic ratio.
37. **E.** Carcinoma in situ. Although the cells have not yet invaded the basement membrane, the likelihood of invasive growth is presumed to be high.
38. **D.** The Western blot tests for HIV proteins. The ELISA tests for HIV antibodies. When these two tests are used together, a 99% accuracy rate is achieved.
39. **C.** Since 90% of blood transfusion-related hepatitis cases are caused by hepatitis C, and the patient has a history of having had a blood transfusion, the answer is C.
40. **D.** Opportunistic infections are a serious problem with patients infected with HIV. This patient's intraoral thrush is such an infection, which is caused by *Candida albicans*. Treatment for candidiasis includes nystatin.
41. **C.** The HIV is an RNA virus that contains three enzymes: reverse transcriptase, integrase, and protease. Neuraminidase is a protein found on the surface of the influenza virus.
42. **C.** Although all of the microbes listed cause pneumonia, the most common cause of pneumonia in patients with AIDS is *P. jiroveci (carinii).*
43. **A.** McCune-Albright's syndrome is a type of fibrous dysplasia that presents with a triad of symptoms including polyostotic fibrous dysplasia, café au lait spots, and endocrine abnormalities.
44. **B.** Fibrous dysplasia is caused by replacement of normal bone with an irregular bone containing fibrous connective tissue. This gives the radiographs a characteristic ground glass appearance.
45. **B.** Fibrous dysplasia is caused by replacement of normal bone with an irregular bone containing fibrous connective tissue. Therefore, the pathology report usually describes abnormally shaped trabeculae in loosely arranged fibrous tissue.
46. **D.** The partial thromboplastin time (PTT) test measures the intrinsic and common pathways of the coagulation cascade. A prolonged PTT could result from a deficiency of factor V, VIII, IX, X, XI, or XII or of prothrombin or fibrinogen.
47. **C.** Hemophilia A is caused by a deficiency of factor 8 (antihemophilic factor).
48. **C.** Hemophilia A is a hereditary disorder that is X-linked; thus, it only affects males. However, females can be carriers.
49. **B.** The only way to distinguish hemophilia A from hemophilia B is to assay the levels of coagula-

tion factors. Hemophilia A is caused by a deficiency of factor 8, while hemophilia B is caused by a deficiency of factor 9.

50. **C.** Gummas are granulomas that may be seen in tertiary syphilis. Since syphilis is caused by *Treponema pallidum*, the correct answer is C. Granulomas may also be seen in tuberculosis, an infection caused by *Mycobacterium tuberculosis*; however, in this disease, they are known as *tubercles*.
51. **A.** CD8 lymphocytes recognize class I MHC molecules on antigen-presenting cells. CD4 lymphocytes recognize class II MHC molecules on antigen-presenting cells.
52. **E.** IL-5 is released by helper T cells to stimulate B lymphocytes to differentiate into plasma cells. It also activates eosinophils and increases the production of IgA.
53. **B.** Tuberculin reaction (i.e. PPD skin test), is an example of a type IV delayed (cell-mediated) hypersensitivity. Type IV reactions are the only type of hypersensitivity immune reactions that are not mediated by antibodies. They are mainly mediated by T cells.
54. **D.** Mast cells contain dense granules with inflammatory mediators, including histamine and SRS-A, which is a leukotriene.
55. **C.** Symptoms of a myocardial infarction include chest pain, shortness of breath, diaphoresis (sweating), clammy hands, nausea, and vomiting.
56. **B.** A quelling reaction occurs in a laboratory when the polysaccharide capsule of a bacterium swells after being treated with antiserum or antibodies.
57. **E.** Dipicolinic acid is only found in spores. Since *Clostridium* is the only spore-forming microorganism listed, the correct answer is E.
58. **D.** Dextrans consist of glucose molecules linked together. They not only act as the structural component of plaque, but they also contribute to the retention of lactic acid near the tooth. Fructans or levans are also found in plaque; however, they contain fructose.
59. **C.** The most common cause of bacterial meningitis in newborns is *Escherichia coli*. *Haemophilus influenzae* and *Neisseria meningitides* are the most common cause of bacterial meningitis in infants/children or young adults, respectively.
60. **D.** Teichoic acid may be found only in the cell walls of gram-positive bacteria and contain antigenic properties. All of the other answers listed are found in the cell walls of gram-negative bacteria.
61. **B.** The tetanus vaccine consists of tetanus toxoid. It is part of the DPT vaccine and should be given about every 10 years.
62. **A.** IgA is found in mucosal secretions of the genitourinary, intestinal, and respiratory tracts, including tears, saliva and colostrums.
63. **D.** HBeAg is present when there is active viral replication and the carrier is highly infectious.
64. **C.** Opportunistic infections are seen in patients with AIDS. All of the following microbes represent opportunistic organisms except coxsackievirus.
65. **E.** Rheumatoid arthritis is characterized by inflammation of the synovial membrane. Granulation tissue will form in the synovium and expand over the articular cartilage. This causes the destruction of the underlying cartilage and results in fibrotic changes or ankylosis.
66. **A.** The most common form of breast cancer is adenocarcinoma arising from the ductal epithelium.
67. **E.** Both tetracycline and streptomycin, an aminoglycoside, inhibit protein synthesis in bacteria. Streptomycin, however, is bactericidal, not bacteriostatic.
68. **D.** Rickets is a vitamin D deficiency seen in infants and children. Oral findings include a delayed eruption of teeth and abnormal dentin.
69. **D.** 12 hours is required.
70. **C.** Cretinism is hypothyroidism in children. Oral findings include macroglossia, prolonged retention of primary teeth, and delayed eruption of permanent teeth.
71. **A.** In general, plaque is first colonized by gram-positive, cocci bacteria, such as *Streptococci*. They are followed by gram-negative, rod-shaped anaerobes, like *Bacteroides, Fusobacterium, Porphyromonas, Prevotella*, and then filament-type bacteria, such as *Actinomyces*.
72. **A.** Peutz-Jeghers syndrome is a hereditary disease that is transmitted by autosomal dominance.
73. **C.** Although all of the structures listed are common sites for oral cancer, the lower vermilion border of the lip is the most common oral site.
74. **C.** Auer rods are observed in blast cells characteristic of acute myelogenous leukemia.
75. **A.** Complications of Barrett's esophagus include: adenocarcinoma, stricture formation, or hemorrhage (ulceration).
76. **A.** M-protein is an important virulent factor found only in the species *Streptococcus pyogenes*.
77. **D.** An infection by molds, such as mucormycosis, results in the invasion of blood vessel endothelium. This leads to hemorrhagic infarction and tissue necrosis.
78. **D.** Chronic lymphocytic leukemia is characterized by the proliferation of B cells. It is both the most common and least malignant type of leukemia.
79. **B.** Consequences of asbestosis include mesothelioma and bronchogenic carcinoma.
80. **D.** Jaundice is characterized by yellowness of tissues, including skin, eyes, and mucous membranes. It is caused by diseases that increase serum conjugated and/or unconjugated bilirubin. These conditions include liver disease, such as cirrhosis or hepatitis; hemolytic anemias; obstruction of the common bile duct, as caused

by gallstones or cholelithiasis; and carcinoma involving the head of the pancreas.

81. **D.** Asthma is an obstructive lung disease caused by narrowing of the airways. Common symptoms include dyspnea, wheezing on expiration, and a dry cough.
82. **C.** Systemic lupus erythematosus, also known as *lupus*, is considered an autoimmune disease, although the exact cause is unknown. It is characterized by the presence of antinuclear antibodies (ANA). Common ANA findings include anti-DNA, anti-RNA, and anti-Sm antigen.
83. **A.** Due to the excessive levels of serum calcium, osseous changes, such as metastatic calcifications and kidney stones, will occur in patients with hyperparathyroidism.
84. **C.** Osteopetrosis, also known as *Albers-Schönberg disease* or *marble bone disease*, is caused by abnormal osteoclasts. The lack of bone resorption results in defective bone remodeling and increased bone density, which may invade into the bone marrow space.
85. **A.** Whooping cough is caused by *Bordetella pertussis*. All of the factors listed contribute to its virulence except IgA protease. This enzyme is produced by *Haemophilus influenzae*, another gram-negative, rod-shaped bacteria.
86. **E.** Celiac sprue is characterized by malabsorption and mucosal lesions of the small intestines that is caused by an allergy to gluten. A complication of this disease includes T-cell lymphomas.
87. **B.** Tuberculosis is caused by the bacteria *Mycobacterium tuberculosis*. These bacteria cannot be Gram stained due to their waxy cell walls. Therefore, to identify these bacteria, an acid-fast stain must be ordered.
88. **D.** *M. tuberculosis* infects macrophages, which are initially unable to kill the phagocytosed bacteria.
89. **A.** Cord factor is a glycolipid found on the surface of *M. tuberculosis*.
90. **D.** Type IV delayed type hypersensitivity reactions are the only type of hypersensitivity immune reactions that are not mediated by antibodies. They are mainly mediated by T cells.
91. **E.** Treatment for tuberculosis includes a multidrug therapy. Rifampin, isoniazid, and ethambutol are three of the first-line drugs used.
92. **E.** Ghon complex describes the calcified scar that remains following the primary infection. It is usually found in the lung and includes the primary lesion and its regional lymph node.
93. **A.** Given the patient's history of rheumatic fever, the heart murmur is most likely from a dysfunctioning mitral valve. Rheumatic fever most commonly affects the mitral valve, resulting in mitral valve stenosis, regurgitation, or both.
94. **B.** Rheumatic fever is usually preceded by a group A streptococcus respiratory infection (e.g., strep throat or pharyngitis).
95. **A.** The most common cause of subacute endocarditis is *Streptococcus viridans*. *S. viridans* is a α-hemolytic streptococci, representing incomplete lysis of red blood cells in laboratory cultures.
96. **E.** During subacute endocarditis, vegetations, or thrombi, form on previously damaged heart valves. Complications can arise if the thrombus embolizes, (i.e. when a fragment separates and enters the circulation), causing septic infarcts. Other complications include valvular dysfunction or abscess formation.
97. **C.** Aminoglycosides block the 30S ribosomal subunit to inhibit protein synthesis.
98. **C.** Burkitt's lymphoma is an aggressive lymphoma that affects B lymphocytes.
99. **E.** Histologic evaluation of Burkitt's lymphoma reveals a characteristic "starry-sky" appearance, which results from the lighter-colored macrophages present.
100. **A.** Epstein-Barr virus is responsible for causing mononucleosis, a disease that also affects B lymphocytes.

Answer Key for Section 4

1. **C.** Universal tooth numbering system for primary dentition, A though T.
2. **A.** Said to be the most atypical of human molars.
3. **C.** A, Smaller in all dimensions; B, All roots seen from buccal aspect; D, roots nearly the same length.
4. **D.** *Mesial aspect:* A, Pronounced convexity present; B, Curvature in an occlusal direction; C, Cervical third greater occlusal third; D, Mesiolingual cusp longer and sharper than mesiobuccal cusp.
5. **D.** *Lingual aspect:* D, Well-defined developmental groove separating ML and DL cusps. A, ML cusp large and well-developed; B, DL cusp well-developed, more so than that of the primary first molar; C, There is a supplemental cusp apical to the ML cusp, but poorly developed.
6. **D.** A developmental depression but not a groove divides the two buccal cusps. A, It does not resemble other primary teeth; B, It has a rhomboidal outline from the occlusal aspect; C, The mesial buccal cusp is larger.
7. **A.** The MB, DB, and distal (D) cusps are almost equal in size, whereas the D cusp of the permanent molar is smaller. B, The primary molar crown is *narrower*, not wider BL; C, The primary molar outline is somewhat rectangular; D, The ratio of crown/root not the same.
8. **B.** Comparatively, roots of primary anterior teeth are narrower and longer. A, Crowns of anterior primary teeth are *wider*, not narrower; C, Cervical ridges of primary anterior teeth *more* prominent; D, B, and L surfaces are *more flat,* not less flat.
9. **B.** The overall average length of the primary mandibular central incisor is 14 mm (Black GV, cited by Ash and Nelson, 2003); 16 mm (Woelfel and Scheid, 2002); 14 mm (Kraus et al., 1969). The anwer is 14 to 16 mm, not 16 to 17 mm.
10. **A.** Greater MD diameter relative to crown height than permanent teeth. B, Squat appearance, not elongated appearance; C, Crowns are a milky white, not translucent white; D, There is no root trunk.
11. **C.** Chronologies from textbooks vary so that age of eruption for the primary mandibular central incisor may be given as 6 months (Woelfel and Scheid, 2002); 6.5 months (Kraus et al., 1969); 7.5 months (Charlick et al.); or 8 (6 to 10) months (Ash and Nelson, 2003).
12. **C.** The most favorable sequence for prevention of malocclusion.
13. **B.** Textbook chronologies indicate that the maxillary primary second molar is most commonly the last to erupt: 24 months (Woelfel and Scheid, 2002); 20 to 30 months (Kraus et al., 1969); 25 to 33 months (Ash and Nelson, 2003).
14. **C.** The length of the primary maxillary central incisor is 16 mm (Black GV, cited by Ash and Nelson, 2003); 16 mm (Kraus et al., 1969) or 17.2 mm (Woelfel and Scheid, 2002). The permanent maxillary incisor is 23.6 mm (Ash and Nelson, 2003); 23.5 mm (Kraus et al., 1969); 23.6 mm (Woelfel and Scheid, 2002). 16/23.5 = 0.68 or 68%; 17.2/23.6 = 0.73 or 73%. The answer is about 70%.
15. **C.** The correct answer for A would be about *1.5 months or 6 weeks;* B, About *4 to 5 years;* C, About *2.5 months or 10 weeks;* D, About *4 to 5 years.*
16. **A.** (Ash and Nelson, 2003; Woelfel and Schied, 2002).
17. **C.** No, or almost never does the mesial marginal developmental groove cross the mesial marginal ridge.
18. **B.** M_1: DB height equals MB height; M_2: DB cusp height slightly less than MB cusp height; M_3: DB cusp height much shorter than MB cusp height.
19. **D.** Marked *asymmetry* of mesial and distal halves.
20. **D.** From MD aspect, all posterior teeth have a trapezoidal outline with shortest uneven side toward the occlusal surface. A, Present prima-

rily on first premolar; B, Exceptions may be the DB root of the maxillary second molar; C, From mesial and distal aspect, all posterior mandibular teeth, not maxillary posterior teeth, have a rhomboidal outline.

21. **C.** Below the apices, 63% of the time.
22. **C.** Greater than 5% (even up to 40%) in populations with Mongolian traits. A, Does not exceed 4.2% in Caucasians; B, Less than 5% in Eurasian and Asian populations; D, Less than 3% in African populations.
23. **D.** Generally a jaw-closing muscle. May stabilize and act with lateral jaw movements.
24. **B.** In the earliest phase, the condyle moves forward *in concert* with the disc, *not before.*
25. **D.** Occlusal contact relations do *not* interfere with jaw opening, but TMJ and muscle disorders may.
26. **C.** Mediotrusive contact, but may be called a nonworking (balancing) contact.
27. **D.** Temporomandibular (TMJ) (Ash and Nelson, 2003); craniomandibular (Woelfel and Scheid, 2002).
28. **A.** Vertical component not seen on horizontal tracing.
29. **C.** Height of contour on lingual surfaces of molars and premolars is at the cervical or middle third.
30. **C.** Transverse ridge connecting MB and ML cusps.
31. **B.** Mandibular first premolar is most likely to have a single pulp horn.
32. **A.** Bifurcated roots are not a normal feature of mandibular incisors.
33. **D.** Height of contour on distal surface of permanent mandibular central incisors is at the incisal third).
34. **C.** The dimension of the permanent maxillary canine at the widest MD diameter is 7.5 mm (7.5 mm (Ash and Nelson, 2003); 7.6 mm [6.3 to 9.5 mm (Woelfel and Scheid, 2002)]).
35. **B.** DB developmental groove is *not* found on mandibular second molars.
36. **D.** Y-shaped central developmental groove is found on the mandibular second premolar.
37. **D.** In the cusp–embrasure occlusal relationship, the maxillary first premolar is most likely to articulate with the first and second premolars.
38. **C.** Equal bilateral contraction of the lateral pterygoid muscles results in protrusion of the mandible.
39. **D.** Molecular tests like the polymerase chain reaction have a fast, not slow, turnaround time.
40. **A.** Rifampin causes orange, not green, urine, tears, and sweat.
41. **B.** The drugs binds tightly only to *prokaryotic* RNA polymerase. D, Rifampin *induces* activity of hepatic mixed oxidases.
42. **C.** Naproxen (naprosyn) has not been reported to exacerbate bruxism.
43. **C.** The mechanisms of the two types of headaches are quite different. A, B, and D are considered true.
44. **B.** β-amyloid deposits are a component of Alzheimer disease but not of migraine headaches.
45. **A.** (Montgomery et al., 1996)
46. **B.** Infection is most likely to involve the submaxillary space, considering the clinical findings.
47. **A.** Given the clinical findings and the involved molar position, it is the lateral upper deep cervical node group that would most likely be the first involved with lymph drainage.
48. **B.** Oral TB most often involves the *tongue.*
49. **B.** Langerhans' giant cells, epitheliod cells, and caseous necrotic areas are highly suggestive of TB; however, special stains for acid-fast bacilli (AFB) and isolation of *M. tuberculosis* may be necesary, keeping in mind that staining may not differentiate TB from other mycobacterial infections. Other molecular tests may be indicated.
50. **D.** There is no evidence of a connection between myositis and bruxing.
51. **C.** The anticoagulant effect of warfarin is inhibited by rifampin. A, Rifampin *decreases* the anticoagulation effect of warfarin; B, Rifampin *interferes* with cyclic conversion; D, Rifampin *increases* the metabolic clearance.
52. **B.** Combination name for joining buccal and lingual cusp triangular ridges.
53. **B, C, D.** For A, the crown outline converges only *lingually*; B, The small transverse ridge has been called an oblique ridge.
54. **D.** A, The *mesiolingual* cusp is most prominent; B, The *distolingual* cusp is poorly defined; C, The *distobuccal* cusp *may be seen* because it is longer.
55. **C.** The central groove is well-defined. A, The primary maxillary second molar *does* have a well-defined mesial triangular fossa; B, The oblique ridge is *prominent*; D, The supplementary cusp is *not* well-developed.
56. **A.** B, It has *four* well-developed cusps; C, It has only *one* supplementary cusp; D, It has a *well-developed* mesial triangular fossa.
57. **A.** B, The outline of the crown converges *distally*; C, The three buccal cusps are *similar* in size; D, *Well-defined* triangular ridges extend from the cusp tips.
58. **C.** A, Enamel cap *thinner* and *more* consistent in depth; B, Comparatively *greater* thickness; D, Pulp horns are *higher* in primary molars.
59. **D.** A, Enamel rods slope *occlusally*, not gingivally, in the primary molars; B, Enamel rods at cervix slope *gingivally*, not occlusally, in permanent molars; C, The buccal cervical ridge is *more* pronounced.
60. **B.** The total of average overall mesiodistal diameters of primary maxillary crowns is 68.2 mm

(Black GV, cited by Ash and Nelson, 2003); 76.8 mm (Woelfel and Scheid, 2002).

61. **A.** On average, the height of curvature is 3.5 mm on the mesial and 2.5 mm on the distal of the maxillary central incisor; it is 3.0 mm on the mesial and 2.0 mm on the distal of the mandibular central incisor.
62. **D.** The width and depth of arch are more or less constant after 9 months of age. However, a substantial increase in the anterior-posterior distance occurs for permanent molars.
63. **C.** These are the most common sequences of eruption.
64. **A.** First evidence of the maxillary central incisor calcification is given as 14 (13 to 16) weeks by Kraus and Jordon, 1965 and by Ash and Nelson, 2003; this is given as 4 months by Woelfel and Scheid, p. 111.
65. **B.** (Kraus et al., 1969)
66. **A.** The correct answer (7 to 8 years) is based on chronologies in Ash and Nelson, 2003 and Woelfel and Scheid, 2002, which are based on original chronologies by Schour and Massler, modified for permanent dentition by Kronfeld (Bur) and by Kronfeld and Schour (1939) for deciduous teeth. Also, with slight modifications, by McCall and Schour (cited by Orban, 1981).
67. **B.** The permanent maxillary first premolar usually has two roots but they are buccal and lingual, not mesial and distal.
68. **D.** (Ash and Nelson, 2003)
69. **C.** The labiolingual diameter of crown near the cervix is *greater* than in mandibular canine.
70. **D.** The labial, mesioincisal angle of tooth 8 and 9 (central incisors) is a sharp, right angle, not slightly rounded. The labial, mesioincisal angle of tooth 7 and 10 (lateral incisors) is slightly rounded, not a sharp right angle.
71. **C.** Distal to the second premolar, 56%.
72. **A.** (McCauley, 1945; Ash and Nelson, 2003)
73. **D.** Internal aponeuroses *do* move and deform.
74. **A.** B, Tooth grinding in sleep bruxism lasts up to 5 minutes, not 20 minutes; C, Sleep bruxism often coincides with passage from deeper to lighter sleep, not lighter to deep sleep; D, Sleep bruxism occurs approximately every 90 minutes, not every 20 minutes in the sleep cycle.
75. **A.** Bruxism is now thought to be mainly regulated centrally, not peripherally.
76. **D.** Mandibular supporting cusps are buccal cusps.
77. **A.** To measure horizontal overlap, measure from labial of mandibular central incisor to labial of maxillary central incisor
78. **B.** (Ash and Nelson, 2003)
79. **A.** The auriculotemporal nerve provides primary innervation to the TMJ.
80. **D.** The DL cusp is smallest on a five-lobed mandibular second premolar.
81. **D.** The primary mandibular first molar typically has four pulp horns.
82. **D.** Clinically in relation to interocclusal space
83. **C.** (Ash and Nelson, 2003)
84. **B.** Root bifurcation is more likely in the mandibular canine.
85. **D.** All posterior teeth viewed from distal aspect have a rhomboidal outline.
86. **A.** A distinct developmental groove, prominent buccal triangular ridge, two cusps, and distinct mesial and distal occlusal pits are most characteristic of the mandibular first premolar.
87. **A.** From the incisal aspect, the maxillary central incisor has a greater MD diameter (8.5 mm) than FL diameter (7.0 mm). B, The MD diameter is 7.5 mm and the FL diameter is 8.0 mm; C, The MD diameter is 7.0 mm and the FL diameter is 7.5 mm; D, The MD diameter is 5.5 mm and the FL diameter is 6.0 mm.
88. **A.** Maximum condylar rotation takes place with maximum jaw opening.
89. **D.** Use of the formula indicates on the basis of ± 6 months that the ADF is 2 to 3 years.
90. **C.** A and B are correct. D is per the manufacturerís recommendations on product, 2005.
91. **B.** Systemic etiologic factors for hypoplasia are thought to occur possibly after birth and before 6 years of age.
92. **C.** Measles is not known to cause enamel hypoplasia.
93. **D.** Intermediate filament is a smooth muscle filament. Connectin is another name for titin. Statements relative to A, B, and C are true and refer to *skeletal* muscle filaments.
94. **D.** Masseter muscles provide most of the force between molar teeth with clenching in the intercuspal position.
95. **D.** Individuals who brux during the day do not necessarily brux at night.
96. **D.** Sequential changes from autonomic cardiac/brain cortical acrivities *precede* SB-related jaw motor activity.
97. **D.** Malocclusion has not been suggested as causing or aggravating bruxism.
98. **D.** Fluorosis versus NF opacities may be difficult to diagnose clinically.
99. **B.** Thick and thin filaments do not change in length.
100. **C.** SHLP helps stabilize the head and condyle against the eminence in clenching; A, B, and D are true.

Sample Exam Answer Key

1. **D.** Mandibular supporting cusps are buccal cusps.
2. **A.** The inferior head of the lateral pterygoid muscle attaches to the lateral surface of the lateral pterygoid plate of sphenoid bone. Its superior head attaches to the infratemporal crest of the greater wing of sphenoid bone. The deep fibers of the medial pterygoid muscle attaches to the medial surface of the lateral pterygoid plate.
3. **B.** Combination name for joining buccal and lingual cusp traingular ridges.
4. **B.** Consequences of asbestosis include mesothelioma and bronchogenic carcinoma.
5. **C.** Under normal conditions, all glucose is reabsorbed by both secondary active transport systems and facilitated diffusion utilizing GLUT 1 and 2 carriers. Calcium is passively reabsorbed, but its reabsorption is also regulated by parathyroid hormone in the distal tubule. Not all urea is reabsorbed but about half is excreted. Its permeability is altered by changes in vasopressin. Phosphate reabsorption is also regulated by parathyroid hormone.
6. **C.** Although IgE is the least prevalent immunoglobulin in the body, it is the major antibody mediator of type I hypersensitive reactions. These reactions are caused primarily by prior sensitization and the accumulation of IgE to a specific allergen.
7. **A.** Since DNA is a double stranded molecule, cytosine will always be base paired to guanine and guanine to cytosine. Therefore there will be equal amounts of these compounds. It is unlikely that RNA or mRNA, being a single-stranded molecule, will have equal amounts of these bases.
8. **B.** The branchial arches disappear when the second arch grows down to contact the fifth branchial arch.
9. **C.** Glucagon is secreted from the pancreas in response to reduced plasma glucose due to fasting and exercise. It functions to mobilize energy stores (glucose) and return blood glucose to normal levels. Glycogen synthesis (glycogenesis) will not occur in response to glucagon.
10. **D.** Unlike in noncompetitive inhibition, the inhibitor competes for the same site as the substrate. It is therefore possible (with increased amounts of substrate) to reach the V_{max}. Apparent Km is increased since more substrate is required to reach 1/2 V_{max} (the definition of Km).
11. **D.** The primary mandibular first molar typically has four pulp horns.
12. **C.** Burkitt's lymphoma is an aggressive lymphoma that affects B lymphocytes.
13. **E.** Histologic evaluation of Burkitt's lymphoma reveals a characteristic "starry-sky" appearance, which results from the lighter-colored macrophages present.
14. **A.** Epstein-Barr virus is responsible for causing mononucleosis, a disease that also affects B lymphocytes.
15. **A.** To measure horizontal overlap, measure from labial of mandibular central incisor to labial of maxillary central incisor (Ash and Nelson, 2003; Woelfel and Scheid, 2002).
16. **D.** Capillary blood flow is proportional to changes in the radius (r4) of the vessel. Decreasing the radius would produce increased vascular pressure. Viscosity of the blood depends primarily on the hematocrit (percentage of red blood cells) and would not be changed by changes in the radius of the vessels.
17. **D.** The facial nerve supplies special sensory (taste) to the anterior two thirds of the tongue, via one of its branches, the chorda tympani. The chorda tympani branches from the facial nerve, carrying both sensory fibers for taste and preganglionic parasympathetic fibers. It exits from of

the temporal bone to join the lingual nerve (a branch of CN V3), as it courses inferiorly toward the submandibular ganglion (Fig. 1-19). Postganglionic parasympathetic fibers emerge from the ganglion and continue toward the sublingual and submandibular glands (Fig. 1-20). Sensory fibers also branch from the nerve and provide taste sensation to the anterior two thirds of the tongue.

18. **C.** The labiolingual diameter of crown near the cervix is *greater* than in mandibular canine (Kraus et al., 1969).
19. **A.** The gastrointestinal tract is regulated by both the sympathetic and parasympathetic branches of the autonomic nervous system. The parasympathetic system is stimulatory and the sympathetic system inhibitory. The CNS does influence motility and secretory activity through the autonomic nervous system. Numerous endocrine factors (secretin, gastrin, cholecystokinin, etc.) are also involved with the regulation of gastrointestinal activity.
20. **C.** Although all of the structures listed are common sites for oral cancer, the lower vermilion border of the lip is the most common oral site.
21. **A.** Vertical component not seen on horizontal tracing.
22. **D.** The palatopharyngeus forms the posterior tonsillar pillar. It also functions to close off the nasopharynx and larynx during swallowing. The anterior tonsillar pillar is formed by the palatoglossus.
23. **D.** Decreasing total peripheral resistance would produce greater reductions in blood pressure. Due to the baroreceptor reflex, cardiac heart rate would increase. Increased stroke volume (due to increased venous return and sympathetic stimulation of cardiac muscle) would also occur. Increased cardiac output would occur due to increased heart rate and stroke volume.
24. **B.** Insulin is a polypeptide hormone that promotes energy storage when it is readily available. The lack of insulin would interfere with this process. Therefore, under conditions of reduced insulin, hyperglycemia would result due to increased gluconeogenesis in the liver. Glycogen breakdown would be enhanced and glycogen synthesis decreased. Since insulin promotes amino acid uptake in the liver, lack of insulin would result in decreased uptake.
25. **D.** 12 hours is required.
26. **C.** The roof of the orbit consists of lesser wing of the sphenoid bone and the orbital plate of the frontal bone (not listed).
27. **C.** The dimension of the permanent maxillary canine at the widest MD diameter is 7.5 mm (7.5 mm, Ash and Nelson, 2003; 7.6 mm [6.3 to 9.5 mm] Woelfel and Scheid, 2002).
28. **D.** Facilitated diffusion does not require energy and moves down a concentration gradient. Active transport, in addition to utilizing energy, is often coupled to transport ions in both directions across the membrane. Both active transport and facilitated diffusion are carrier-mediated and therefore are influenced by competitive inhibition.
29. **A.** In general, plaque is first colonized by gram-positive, cocci bacteria, such as *Streptococci.* They are followed by gram-negative, rod-shaped anaerobes, like *Bacteroides, Fusobacterium, Porphyromonas, Prevotella,* and then filament-type bacteria, such as *Actinomyces.*
30. **D.** Triacylglycerol is not commonly a component of cell membranes since it serves primarily as a molecule for storage and transport of fatty acids. Phospholipids are abundant since they form the bilayer structure characteristic of membranes. Proteins are present and serve various functions as enzymes, receptors, and transporters/carriers. Cholesterol stabilizes the membrane and is responsible for the maintenance of fluidity. Sphingolipids are components of myelin, which insulates membranes in neurons.
31. **A.** Lateral cricoarytenoid. The oblique and transverse arytenoids and thyroarytenoid also adduct the vocal folds. The posterior cricoarytenoids abducts the vocal cords. The cricothyroid muscle raises the cricoid cartilage and tenses the vocal cords.
32. **E.** Carcinoma in situ. Although the cells have not yet invaded the basement membrane, the likelihood of invasive growth is presumed to be high.
33. **D.** The rectus abdominus muscle of the anterolateral abdominal wall is described as being beltor strap-like. The remaining three muscles of the anterolateral abdominal wall (external oblique muscle, internal oblique muscle, and transverses abdominus muscle) are all described as sheet-like. The quadratus lumborum muscle is part of the posterior abdominal wall.
34. **D.** A, Enamel rods slope *occlusally*, not gingivally, in the primary molars; B, Enamel rods at cervix slope *gingivally*, not occlusally, in permanent molars; C, The buccal cervical ridge is *more* pronounced.
35. **A.** McCune-Albright's syndrome is a type of fibrous dysplasia that presents with a triad of symptoms including polyostotic fibrous dysplasia, café au lait spots, and endocrine abnormalities.
36. **B.** Fibrous dysplasia is caused by replacement of normal bone with an irregular bone containing fibrous connective tissue. This gives the radiographs a characteristic ground glass appearance.
37. **B.** Fibrous dysplasia is caused by replacement of normal bone with an irregular bone containing fibrous connective tissue. Therefore, the pathology report usually describes abnormally shaped trabeculae in loosely arranged fibrous tissue.

38. **B.** The overall average length of the primary mandibular central incisor is 14 mm (Black GV, cited by Ash and Nelson, 2003); 16 mm (Woelfel and Scheid, 2002); 14 mm (Kraus et al., 1969). The answer is 14 to 16 mm, not 16 to 17 mm.
39. **A.** Stenosis describes fibrotic and thickened valves, resulting in reduced blood flow through the valve.
40. **A.** B, It has *four* well-developed cusps; C, Tt has only *one* supplementary cusp; D, It has a *well-developed* mesial triangular fossa.
41. **A.** All the other factors will produce vasodilation and hyperemia to increase the exchange of metabolites in the tissue.
42. **C.** The inferior aspect of the diaphragm is supplied with blood by the inferior phrenic arteries. The median sacral artery supplies the anterior aspect of the sacral area, and the lumbar arteries supply the lower abdominal wall. The celiac trunk and superior mesenteric arteries are both unpaired branches to the gut and associated glands.
43. **C.** Pyridoxal phosphate is the active coenzyme of pyridoxine, which is involved in a number of enzyme systems essential for normal amino acid metabolism. Biotin is required for carboxylation reactions. Tetrahydrofolate, the coenzyme form of folic acid, is required for the synthesis of nucleic acids and porphyrin. Niacin participates in energy metabolism (oxidation-reduction reactions)
44. **C.** Equal bilateral contraction of the lateral pterygoid muscles results in protrusion of the mandible.
45. **D.** Oligodendrocytes produce the myelin sheath around myelinated axons in the central nervous system. Schwann cells make up the myelin sheath around myelinated axons in the parasympathetic nervous system.
46. **A.** Ninety-five percent of enamel is inorganic mineral compared with 84% in calculus, 70% in dentin, and 60% in bone.
47. **D.** Poststreptococcal glomerulonephritis is a classic example of nephritic syndrome, which occurs after a *Streptococcus* infection (e.g., strep throat). It is characterized by all of the symptoms listed except polyuria. A decrease in urination is usually observed.
48. **D.** In the cusp–embrasure occlusal relationship, the maxillary first premolar is most likely to articulate with the first and second premolars.
49. **C.** Universal tooth numbering system for primary dentition, A though T.
50. **B.** Oblique alveolodental fibers resist occlusal forces that occur along the long axis of the tooth. The rest of the alveolodental (PDL) fibers listed provide resistance against forces which pull the tooth in an occlusal direction (i.e., forces that try to pull the tooth from its socket).
51. **A.** When pulpal nerves are stimulated, they can only transmit one signal: pain.
52. **C.** The mylohyoid muscle forms the floor of the mouth. Relaxation of this muscle would help the dentist push the film down, to help ensure that the apical root is captured on the radiograph.
53. **B.** Fibers of the lateral pterygoid muscle are attached to the anterior end of the disc. Contraction of this muscle pulls the disc in an anterior and medial direction.
54. **B.** The sensory distribution for the maxillary nerve (CN V2) includes the cheek and upper lip, and lower eyelid, upper lip, nasopharynx, tonsils, palate, and maxillary teeth. The sensory distribution for the long buccal also includes the (lower) cheek; however, it does not include the upper lip. The long buccal is a branch of the mandibular nerve (CN V3) and provides sensory nerves to the cheek, buccal gingiva of the posterior mandibular teeth, and buccal mucosa.
55. **A.** The inferior alveolar nerve (IAN) courses between the sphenomandibular ligament and the ramus of the mandible before entering the mandibular foramen. The sphenomandibular ligament may therefore be damaged during the administration of an IAN block.
56. **D.** Polycystic kidney disease is characterized by the formation of cysts in kidney. It is commonly associated with berry aneurysms.
57. **B.** The oropharynx is lined by stratified squamous epithelium. This type of epithelium also lines the oral cavity, laryngopharynx, esophagus, vaginal canal and anal canal.
58. **C.** Phosphodiesterases are intracellular enzymes that degrade cyclic nucleotides, thus catalyzing the hydrolysis of cAMP to a metabolite, 5' AMP, which lacks the second messenger properties of cAMP. Adenylate cyclase is an enzyme that catalyzes the conversion of ATP to cAMP. Monoamine oxidase (MAO) is an enzyme located in presynaptic nerve terminals that degrades dopamine, norepinephrine, and epinephrine to inactive substances. Aspirin inhibits prostaglandin synthesis by inhibiting the cyclooxygenase enzyme.
59. **A.** Said to be the most atypical of human molars.
60. **B.** Osteomyelitis, or an infection of bone, is most commonly caused by *Staphylococcus aureus*. Symptoms include pain and systemic signs of infection (i.e., fever, malaise).
61. **C.** Intercalated discs are only found in cardiac muscle. Multiple, peripherally positioned nuclei are found in the fibers of skeletal muscle. Smooth muscle cells are spindle-shaped.
62. **D.** The DL cusp is smallest on a five-lobed mandibular second premolar.
63. **C.** Although fluoride may be incorporated in mineralized tissues, it is not required for the mineralization process. Matrix vesicles produced by

osteoblasts are considered to be the initial site of mineralization. Amelogenins are matrix proteins in enamel that regulate crystallite growth. Phosphoryns are initiator proteins that bind minerals to facilitate nucleation and crystal growth.

64. **E.** Celiac sprue is characterized by malabsorption and mucosal lesions of the small intestines that is caused by an allergy to gluten. A complication of this disease includes T-cell lymphomas.
65. **E.** Renal clearance is the volume of plasma completely cleared of a substance by the kidneys per unit of time. The renal clearance of glucose is usually 0 since, although it is filtered, it is completely reabsorbed when the plasma glucose concentration is within normal levels. In the uncontrolled diabetic, plasma glucose levels exceed the reabsorptive capacity (Tm) and it then appears in the urine. Urea is filtered and passively reabsorbed to a slight degree. Creatinine is both freely filtered and secreted to a slight extent. Sodium and water are filtered and reabsorbed to various degrees due to physiological regulation of aldosterone and ADH.
66. **B.** DiGeorge's syndrome is characterized by a deficiency of T cells. It is caused by the failure of the third and fourth brachial pouches to develop normally, resulting in a lack of thymus and parathyroid development.
67. **A.** Restriction enzymes are also known as restriction endonucleases. These enzymes cleave DNA at specific sites to release fragments of DNA for further analysis and characterization by complementary probes.
68. **A.** The bile canaliculi drain bile to interlobular ducts. The interlobular ducts form right and left hepatic ducts. These ducts join to form the common hepatic duct. The gallbladder arises from the common hepatic duct.
69. **D.** There is no evidence of a connection between myositis and bruxing.
70. **E.** The superior and inferior ophthalmic veins drain into the facial vein and cavernous sinus.
71. **D.** The partial thromboplastin time (PTT) test measures the intrinsic and common pathways of the coagulation cascade. A prolonged PTT could result from a deficiency of factor V, VIII, IX, X, XI, or XII or of prothrombin or fibrinogen.
72. **C.** Hemophilia A is caused by a deficiency of factor 8 (antihemophilic factor).
73. **C.** Hemophilia A is a hereditary disorder that is X-linked; thus, it only affects males. However, females can be carriers.
74. **B.** The only way to distinguish hemophilia A from hemophilia B is to assay the levels of coagulation factors. Hemophilia A is caused by a deficiency of factor 8, while hemophilia B is caused by a deficiency of factor 9.
75. **E.** Arginine is an amino acid that is deaminated to form ornithine primarily in the liver as part of the urea cycle. Ornithine, argininosuccinate, aspartate and citrulline are generated in the urea cycle but do not provide free ammonia for urea synthesis.
76. **E.** The superior, middle and inferior constrictor muscles all insert into the median pharyngeal raphe (the superior constrictor muscle was the only one listed), however, their origins differ.
77. **C.** The most favorable sequence for prevention of malocclusion.
78. **D.** Immediately following a meal, energy sources are high. Glycogenolysis (glycogen breakdown) is reduced. Lipolysis and oxidation of free fatty acids are also unnecessary during this time. Glucagon release is inhibited due to elevated glucose. Glycolysis is increased due to elevated intracellular glucose.
79. **A.** Hepatitis A is spread via oral–anal/fecal contamination. The other hepatitis viruses can be transmitted through blood, sexual contact, and/or perinatally.
80. **B.** Guanine base pairs with cytosine which, on a molar basis, will also equal 30% of the DNA. If guanine and cytosine constitute a total of 60% of DNA, the remaining percentage (40%) must be equally divided between the base pairs of adenine and thymine (20% + 20%).
81. **B.** The muscularis externa has a third layer in the stomach. It is an inner oblique layer of smooth muscle. In the rest of the digestive tract, the muscularis externa has two layers; an inner circular layer and an outer longitudinal layer.
82. **C.** Gummas are granulomas that may be seen in tertiary syphilis. Since syphilis is caused by *Treponema pallidum*, the correct answer is C. Granulomas may also be seen in tuberculosis, an infection caused by *Mycobacterium tuberculosis*; however, in this disease, they are known as *tubercles*.
83. **A.** The medulla of the thymus contains Hassall's corpuscles, which consist of epithelial cells with keratohyaline granules. The medulla is the lighter-staining (less dense) central area of the gland, where T cells maturation occurs.
84. **C.** The masseter originates from the inferior border of the zygomatic arch; specifically, its superficial head and deep head originate from the anterior two thirds or posterior one third of the inferior border, respectively. Its superficial head inserts into the lateral surface of the angle of the mandible; its deep head inserts into the ramus and body of the mandible.
85. **D.** The width and depth of arch are more or less constant after 9 months of age. However, a substantial increase in the anterior-posterior distance occurs for permanent molars.
86. **A.** Hemoglobin is a globular protein responsible for transporting most of the O_2 in the blood. The percent saturation of hemoglobin is a function of the PO_2 of the blood. The relationship of PO_2 and

hemoglobin saturation is not linear but, rather, sigmoidal. Percent saturation increases greatly at low PO_2 and less at higher PO_2. Increased PCO_2, temperature, diphosphoglycerate, and H^+ decrease the affinity of hemoglobin for O_2 but do not alter the characteristic sigmoidal nature of the saturation curve.

87. **A.** On average, the height of curvature is 3.5 mm on the mesial and 2.5 mm on the distal of the maxillary central incisor; it is 3.0 mm on the mesial and 2.0 mm on the distal of the mandibular central incisor.
88. **B.** Dysplastic cells are abnormal in appearance and organization. The potential to develop into a malignant tumor is present; however, this risk varies.
89. **D.** Generally a jaw-closing muscle. May stabilize and act with lateral jaw movements.
90. **D.** An infection by molds, such as mucormycosis, results in the invasion of blood vessel endothelium. This leads to hemorrhagic infarction and tissue necrosis.
91. **A.** The first rib cannot be palpated.
92. **D.** Mast cells contain dense granules with inflammatory mediators, including histamine and SRSA, which is a leukotriene.
93. **B.** The hypothalamus coordinates many activities mediated by the ANS, including food intake, thirst, and temperature regulation. The cerebellum functions to regulate movement and posture. The medulla is responsible for coordinating respiration. The cerebral cortex performs functions of perception, cognition, higher motor functions, memory, and emotion.
94. **E.** Chronic bronchitis predisposes those affected to squamous neoplasia of the bronchial epithelium (i.e., bronchogenic carcinoma).
95. **A.** The MB, DB, and distal (D) cusps are almost equal in size, whereas the D cusp of the permanent molar is smaller. B, The primary molar crown is *narrower*, not wider BL; C, The primary molar outline is somewhat rectangular; D, The ratio of crown/root not the same.
96. **B.** In smooth muscle, the binding of calcium to calmondulin will activate the enzyme myosin light chain kinase. This enzyme phosphorylates myosin, allowing it to bind to actin, and the muscle contracts. For contraction in skeletal and cardiac muscle, calcium binds to troponin C.
97. **A.** Estrogen is a steroid hormone and therefore does not require a membrane receptor and the second messenger cAMP. Steroid hormones directly enter the cell and stimulate intracellular receptors. Peptide hormones and those derived from single amino acids are not readily lipid-soluble (characteristic of membranes) and thus require membrane receptors and a second messenger system (cAMP, IP3, etc.). Many of the effects of epinephrine and norepinephrine and all of the effects of glucagon are mediated by cAMP.
98. **D.** The Western blot tests for HIV proteins. The ELISA tests for HIV antibodies. When these two tests are used together, a 99% accuracy rate is achieved.
99. **C.** Since 90% of blood transfusion-related hepatitis cases are caused by hepatitis C, and the patient has a history of having had a blood transfusion, the answer is C.
100. **D.** Opportunistic infections are a serious problem with patients infected with HIV. This patient's intraoral thrush is such an infection, which is caused by *Candida albicans*. Treatment for candidiasis includes nystatin.
101. **C.** The HIV is an RNA virus that contains three enzymes: reverse transcriptase, integrase, and protease. Neuraminidase is a protein found on the surface of the influenza virus.
102. **C.** Although all of the microbes listed cause pneu monia, the most common cause of pneumonia in patients with AIDS is *P. jiroveci (carinii)*.
103. **C.** A, Smaller in all dimensions; B, All roots seen from buccal aspect; D, roots nearly the same length.
104. **B.** Cells degrade purine nucleotides to uric acid. Xanthine is an intermediate in a series of reactions, but the final product in humans is uric acid which is excreted in the urine. Urea is the degradation product of compounds containing amino groups (amino acids).
105. **B.** An essential amino acid is one that cannot be synthesized by human and therefore we require them in the diet from plant or bacterial sources. All of the other amino acids can be synthesized by humans from other compounds and therefore are not classified as "essential."
106. **B.** The fovea centralis only contains cone cells. It is located approximately 2.5 mm lateral to the optic disc in an yellow-pigmented area (macula luna). Vision is most acute from this area.
107. **C.** The middle trunk of the brachial plexus of nerves arises from C7.
108. **E.** Both *Epidermophyton* and *Trichophyton* can cause tinea pedis.
109. **B.** Comparatively, roots of primary anterior teeth are narrower and longer. A, Crowns of anterior primary teeth are *wider*, not narrower; C, Cervical ridges of primary anterior teeth *more* prominent; D, B, and L surfaces are *more flat*, not less flat.
110. **C.** Cystic fibrosis results from an abnormal chloride channel that affects all exocrine glands.
111. **A.** The site of cell division (mitosis) occurs in the stratum basale (basal layer, stratum germinativum) of oral epithelium.
112. **A.** IgA is found in mucosal secretions of the genitourinary, intestinal, and respiratory tracts, including tears, saliva and colostrums.
113. **A.** Chronic granulomatosis results from neutrophils with a defective NAPDH oxidase system. This affects their ability to kill microorganisms, since they are unable to produce superoxide radicals.

114. **B.** Tetrahydrofolic acid is the coenzyme form of folic acid required for the synthesis of nucleic acids and normal cell division and replication.
115. **D.** Phenylketonuria (PKU) is an inherited disorder of amino acid metabolism in which the affected individual lacks enzymes to metabolize phenylalanine. Albinism is a condition that results in a defect in tyrosine metabolism and the inability to produce melanin. Porphyria is an inherited disorder involving defects in heme synthesis. Homocystinuria is a disorder in the metabolism of homocysteine resulting in high levels of homocysteine and methionine in plasma and urine.
116. **D.** Molecular tests like the polymerase chain reaction have a fast, not slow, turnaround time.
117. **A.** Rifampin causes orange, not green, urine, tears, and sweat.
118. **B.** The drugs binds tightly only to *prokaryotic* RNA polymerase. D, Rifampin *induces* activity of hepatic mixed oxidases.
119. **C.** Naproxen (naprosyn) has not been reported to exacerbate bruxism. For A, refer to Romanelli et al., 1996; B, Refer to Gerber and Lynd, 1998; D, Refer to Milosevic et al., 1999.
120. **C.** The mechanisms of the two types of headaches are quite different. A, B, and D are considered true.
121. **B.** β-amyloid deposits are a component of Alzheimer disease but not of migraine headaches.
122. **A.** (Montgomery et al., 1996).
123. **B.** Infection is most likely to involve the submaxillary space, considering the clinical findings.
124. **A.** Given the clinical findings and the involved molar position, it is the lateral upper deep cervical node group that would most likely be the first involved with lymph drainage (Shafer et al., 1983).
125. **B.** Oral TB most often involves the *tongue*.
126. **B.** Langerhans giant cells, epitheliod cells, and caseous necrotic areas are highly suggestive of TB; however, special stains for acid-fast bacilli (AFB) and isolation of *M. tuberculosis* may be necesary, keeping in mind that staining may not differentiate TB from other mycobacterial infections. Other molecular tests may be indicated.
127. **C.** The anticoagulant effect of warfarin is inhibited by rifampin. A, Rifampin *decreases* the anticoagulation effect of warfarin; B, Rifampin *interferes* with cyclic conversion; D, Rifampin *increases* the metabolic clearance.
128. **A.** Gut-associated lymphoid tissue (GALT) produces secretory IgA.
129. **C.** Systemic lupus erythematosus, also known as *lupus*, is considered an autoimmune disease, although the exact cause is unknown. It is characterized by the presence of antinuclear antibodies (ANA). Common ANA findings include anti-DNA, anti-RNA, and anti-Sm antigen.
130. **D.** The backbone of DNA and RNA is composed of sugars (deoxyribose or ribose) joined $3' \rightarrow 5'$.
131. **C.** The hypoglossal (CN XII) nerve is not found in the posterior triangle; it is, however, present in the submandibular triangle. Contents of the posterior triangle include the external jugular and subclavian vein and their tributaries, the subclavian artery and its branches, branches of the cervical plexus, CN XI, nerves to the upper limb and muscles of the triangle floor, the phrenic nerve, and the brachial plexus.
132. **A.** The α-chains are polypeptides which characterize the collagen molecule. The most abundant amino acids in collagen are proline and glycine. Proline (due to its amino ring structure), interrupts the α-chain, resulting in the bending/twisting of the peptide. Glycine (due to its small size) fits into the smaller spaces of the peptide and is positioned at every third position in the chain.
133. **B.** Increasing the hydrostatic pressure within the glomerulus would decrease the net ultrafiltration pressure. Reduced plasma protein concentration decreases the oncotic pressure in the plasma which would increase filtration. Vasodilation of the afferent arterioles would increase capillary pressure resulting in increased filtration. Inulin, although used to measure glomerular filtration, does not affect glomerular filtration rate.
134. **A.** The most common form of breast cancer is adenocarcinoma arising from the ductal epithelium.
135. **D.** The labial, mesioincisal angle of tooth #8 and #9 (central incisors) is a sharp, right angle, not slightly rounded. The labial, mesioincisal angle of tooth #7 and #10 (lateral incisors) is slightly rounded, not a sharp right angle.
136. **C.** The apex of a medullary pyramid in the kidney is called the renal papilla. The cortex is the outer layer of the kidney. The medulla is the inner layer. Minor calyces receive secretions from the renal papillae. Several minor calyces join to form a major calyx.
137. **D.** Endocarditis is most commonly caused by group B, α-hemolytic streptococci, such as *S. viridans, S. mutans, S. sanguis, and S. salivarius*. All of the other conditions are associated with group A β-hemolytic streptococcal infections, such as *S. pyogenes*.
138. **D.** After branching from the mandibular nerve (CN V3), the auriculotemporal nerve travels posteriorly and encircles the middle meningeal artery, remaining posterior and medial to the condyle. It then continues up towards the TMJ, external ear, and temporal region, passing through the parotid gland and traveling with the superficial temporal artery and vein.
139. **A.** Given the patient's history of rheumatic fever, the heart murmur is most likely from a dysfunctioning mitral valve. Rheumatic fever most commonly affects the mitral valve, resulting in mitral valve stenosis, regurgitation, or both.
140. **B.** Rheumatic fever is usually preceded by a group A streptococcus respiratory infection (e.g., strep throat or pharyngitis).

141. **A.** The most common cause of subacute endocarditis is *Streptococcus viridans*. *S. viridans* is a α-hemolytic streptococci, representing incomplete lysis of red blood cells in laboratory cultures.

142. **E.** During subacute endocarditis, vegetations, or thrombi, form on previously damaged heart valves. Complications can arise if the thrombus embolizes, (i.e. when a fragment separates and enters the circulation), causing septic infarcts. Other complications include valvular dysfunction or abscess formation.

143. **C.** Aminoglycosides block the 30S ribosomal subunit to inhibit protein synthesis.

144. **B.** Translation is the conversion of information from mRNA into a protein. Transduction is the incorporation of genetic information carried by a virus into bacteria.

145. **A.** Maximum condylar rotation takes place with maximum jaw opening.

146. **B.** The right subclavian artery arises from the brachiocephalic artery, and the left subclavian artery arises from the aortic arch. The subclavian artery becomes the axillary artery upon crossing the first rib. The axillary artery becomes the brachial artery when it leaves the axilla.

147. **D.** Clinically in relation to interocclusal space.

148. **B.** The concentration of potassium ions within cells is approximately 30 times greater than the extracellular fluid; the other ions are in greater concentrations in extracellular fluid compared with values within the cell.

149. **B.** Neutrophils are quick to arrive to the site of infection or injury and are therefore associated with acute inflammation. All of the other cells listed are mediators of chronic inflammation.

150. **A.** The correct answer (7 to 8 years) is based on chronologies in Ash and Nelson, 2003 and Woelfel and Scheid, 2002, which are based on original chronologies by Schour and Massler, modified for permanent dentition by Kronfeld (Bur) and by Kronfeld and Schour (1939) for deciduous teeth. Also, with slight modifications, by McCall and Schour (cited by Orban, 1981).

151. **E.** Heparin, an anticoagulant is unlike the other glycosaminoglycans since it is an extracellular compound. Hyaluronic acid is found in synovial fluid, keratan sulfate in loose connective tissue such as cornea, chondroitin sulfate in cartilage, ligaments and tendons and dermatan sulfate in skin and blood vessels.

152. **A.** The pancreas is enveloped at its head by the first part of the duodenum.

153. **B.** Individuals suffering from mucopolysaccharidoses have normal production of proteoglycans and glycosaminoglycans but, due to genetic defects, lack the enzymes which degrade mucopolysaccharides.

154. **A.** The terminology used is a classical descriptor of the relationship between the hormone source and target tissue. Paracrine refers to the target tissue as a cell in close proximity to the secreting tissue. Autocrine stimulation refers to cell that releases a factor (hormone) which stimulates the cell from which it was released. Endocrine factors are hormones that have an effect at a distal site in the body.

155. **C.** Pyelonephritis is usually caused by gram-negative, rod-shaped bacteria that are part of the normal flora of the enteric tract. It is most commonly caused by *Escherichia coli,* followed by *Proteus*, *Klebsiella*, and *Enterobacter*.

156. **C.** The salivary glands are lined by simple cuboidal epithelium. This type of epithelium also lines the bronchioles, thyroid gland, and ovary capsule.

157. **E.** The macula densa is a component of the juxtaglomerular apparatus which functions in regulation of blood pressure. The proximal convoluted tubule, distal convoluted tubule, Bowman's capsule, and glomerulus all function in the production of urine.

158. **D.** Internal aponeuroses *do* move and deform.

159. **C.** The cricopharyngeus muscle prevents swallowing air at the pharyngeal end of the esophagus.

160. **C.** The most common cause of bacterial meningitis in newborns is *Escherichia coli. Haemophilus influenzae* and *Neisseria meningitides* are the most common cause of bacterial meningitis in infants/children or young adults, respectively.

161. **B.** Glucose transport in muscle and adipose tissue is under the influence of insulin-sensitive glucose transporters. Although several metabolic pathways are influenced by insulin, glucose uptake into the liver is not affected by insulin.

162. **C.** Deoxygenated blood from the transverse sinus drains to the sigmoid sinus, which empties into the internal jugular veins. The transverse sinuses receive blood from the confluence of sinuses, which is located in the posterior cranium.

163. **C.** The central groove is well-defined. A, The primary maxillary second molar *does* have a well-defined mesial triangular fossa; B, The oblique ridge is *prominent*; D, The supplementary cusp is *not* well-developed.

164. **B.** Facial nerves are derived from the second branchial arch. The trigeminal nerve is derived from the first branchial arch.

165. **B.** A probe is a single strand of DNA synthesized with a radioisotope that is complimentary to a segment of DNA of interest. The radio-labeled complex can be analyzed subsequently on a gel by a technique known as a Southern Blot.

166. **A.** B, The outline of the crown converges *distally*; C, The three buccal cusps are *similar* in size; D, *Well-defined* triangular ridges extend from the cusp tips.

167. **B.** M1: DB height equals MB height; M2: DB cusp height slightly less than MB cusp height; M3: DB cusp height much shorter than MB cusp height.
168. **B.** Radiographic findings of a cotton-wool appearance is common in patients diagnosed with osteitis deformans or Paget's disease.
169. **B.** In the process of muscle contraction, ATP bound to myosin is cleaved to form ADP and Pi. Myosin is released to bind to a new actin site producing a force-generating stroke. Sodium influx and calcium binding are involved in the excitation-contraction coupling process but do not serve as a source of energy.
170. **A.** C fibers are the smallest of the sensory and motor fibers. They are postganglionic, unmyelinated, and have the slowest conduction velocity.
171. **B.** The tendon of the tensor tympani is attached to the handle of the malleus in the middle ear. Loud sounds cause the tensor tympani to contract, pulling the malleus and tympanic membrane inward to reduce vibrations and prevent damage.
172. **B.** Increased levels of alkaline phosphatase may be observed in diseases that display extensive bone loss. Osteoporosis is characterized by a decrease in bone mass. There are either normal or decreased levels of alkaline phosphatase in patients diagnosed with this disease.
173. **A.** Peutz-Jeghers syndrome is a hereditary disease that is transmitted by autosomal dominance.
174. **D.** Temporomandibular (TMJ) (Ash and Nelson, 2003); craniomandibular (Woelfel and Scheid, 2002).
175. **B.** Tuberculosis is caused by the bacteria *Mycobacterium tuberculosis*. These bacteria cannot be Gram stained due to their waxy cell walls. Therefore, to identify these bacteria, an acid-fast stain must be ordered.
176. **D.** *M. tuberculosis* infects macrophages, which are initially unable to kill the phagocytosed bacteria.
177. **A.** Cord factor is a glycolipid found on the surface of *M. tuberculosis*.
178. **D.** Type IV delayed type hypersensitivity reactions are the only type of hypersensitivity immune reactions that are not mediated by antibodies. They are mainly mediated by T cells.
179. **E.** Treatment for tuberculosis includes a multi-drug therapy. Rifampin, isoniazid, and ethambutol are three of the first-line drugs used.
180. **E.** Ghon complex describes the calcified scar that remains following the primary infection. It is usually found in the lung and includes the primary lesion and its regional lymph node.
181. **B.** Odontogenic infections of a mandibular incisor with an apex below the mylohyoid muscle have the potential to spread to the submental space. If the apex is above the mylohyoid muscle, the infection would spread to the sublingual space. Both of these spaces communicate with the submandibular space.
182. **D.** Phospholipase C, activated by a component of the G-protein (Gα) complexed with GTP, catalyzes the production of diacylglycerol and inositol trisphosphate. Diacylglycerol activates protein kinases, which phosphorylates proteins, and inositol trisphosphate produces increased release of calcium from intracellular stores.
183. **E.** IL-5 is released by helper T cells to stimulate B lymphocytes to differentiate into plasma cells. It also activates eosinophils and increases the production of IgA.
184. **B.** The salivary glands are influenced by both the sympathetic and parasympathetic (glossopharyngeal and facial) branches of the ANS. The oculomotor nerve (CN III) carries parasympathetic fibers to the eye which, when stimulated, produces constriction of the pupil. The parasympathetic system innervates primarily smooth and cardiac muscle, resulting in specific activation and responses.
185. **A.** From the incisal aspect, the maxillary central incisor has a greater MD diameter (8.5 mm) than FL diameter (7.0 mm). B, The MD diameter is 7.5 mm and the FL diameter is 8.0 mm; C, The MD diameter is 7.0 mm and the FL diameter is 7.5 mm; D, The MD diameter is 5.5 mm and the FL diameter is 6.0 mm.
186. **A.** The vestigial cleft of Rathke's pouch is located between the anterior and posterior lobes—specifically, between the pars intermedia and anterior lobe. It consists of cyst-like spaces (Rathke's cysts) and represents the vestigial lumen of Rathke's pouch.
187. **C.** A, Enamel cap *thinner* and *more* consistent in depth; B, Comparatively *greater* thickness; D, Pulp horns are *higher* in primary molars.
188. **B.** The regulatory centers for respiration are in the brain stem—specifically, the medulla. The medulla contains three groups of neurons (medullary respiratory center, apneustic center and pneumotaxic center). The cerebral cortex may influence the medullary centers but does not totally control respiration.
189. **D.** The brachial plexus of nerves arises from five roots from the anterior primary rami of spinal nerves C5 through C8 and T1.
190. **D.** Aschoff bodies are the classic lesions observed in rheumatic fever. They are areas of focal necrosis surrounded by a dense inflammatory infiltration and may be observed in heart tissues.
191. **B.** Cyclo-oxygenase includes isoenzymes of prostaglandin endoperoxidase synthase, which is required for the first step in the synthesis of prostaglandins from arachidonic acid. Phospholipase A2, which is involved in the synthesis of arachidonic acid, is inhibited by steroidal anti-inflammatory agents.
192. **B.** Terminal bronchioles are characterized by ciliated cuboidal cells.

193. **C.** Greater than 5% (even up to 40%) in populations with Mongolian traits. A, Does not exceed 4.2% in Caucasians; B, Less than 5% in Eurasian and Asian populations; D, Less than 3% in African populations.
194. **C.** The salivary glands are under the influence of both the sympathetic and parasympathetic nervous system. Parasympathetic stimulation results in a more watery secretion compared with sympathetic stimulation, which produces increased amounts of protein with reduced volume. The vagus is parasympathetic, which in general is stimulatory to gastrointestinal tract. In general, sympathetics are inhibitory to the gastrointestinal tract. (The exceptions are salivary glands).
195. **C.** Transverse ridge connecting MB and ML cusps.
196. **D.** Jaundice is characterized by yellowness of tissues, including skin, eyes, and mucous membranes. It is caused by diseases that increase serum conjugated and/or unconjugated bilirubin. These conditions include liver disease, such as cirrhosis or hepatitis; hemolytic anemias; obstruction of the common bile duct, as caused by gallstones or cholelithiasis; and carcinoma involving the head of the pancreas.
197. **B.** Arteriovenous anastomoses in deeper skin are important in thermoregulation.
198. **A.** Complications of Barrett's esophagus include: adenocarcinoma, stricture formation, or hemorrhage (ulceration).
199. **D.** The elongation and overgrowth of filiform papillae results in hairy tongue. Filiform papillae are thin, pointy projections that make up the most numerous papillae and gives the tongue's dorsal surface its characteristic rough texture. Note: a loss of filiform papillae results in glossitus.
200. **B.** Tertiary dentin, or reactive/reparative dentin, is dentin that is formed in localized areas in response to trauma or other stimuli, such as caries, tooth wear or dental work. Histologically, its consistency and organization varies; it has no defined dentinal tubule pattern.
201. **E.** Innervation to the maxillary second molar, as well as the palatal and distobuccal root of the maxillary first molar and the maxillary sinus, is provided by the Posterior superior alveolar nerve. The nerve is a branch of the maxillary nerve (CN V2).
202. **D.** The suprarenal glands secrete epinephrine. Specifically, chromaffin cells of the the adrenal medulla, which act as modified postganglionic sympathetic neurons that synthesize, store and secrete catecholamines, produce epinephrine. It also produces norepinephrine.
203. **A.** The most common cause of gastroenteritis in children is the rotavirus. It is found in the reovirus family.
204. **C.** (Ash and Nelson, 2003.)
205. **D.** Ureters travel inferiorly just below the parietal peritoneum of the posterior body wall. They pass anterior to the common iliac arteries as they enter the pelvis.
206. **A.** Aspartame is a peptide derivative composed of aspartic acid and phenylalanine.
207. **E.** The abducens nerve (CN VI) provides innervation to the lateral rectus muscle, which moves the eyeball laterally, i.e. abducts the eye. The medial rectus muscle, which is innervated by the oculomotor nerve (CN III), is responsible for adduction of the eyeball.
208. **D.** Potassium is passively (via the cotransport system) secreted from the plasma into the distal and collecting tubules. Under conditions of acidosis, an individual may become hyperkalemic since the kidneys will retain K and secrete H. Under conditions of alkalosis, K secretion will be increased and H secretion reduced.
209. **B.** Epiphyseal closure marks the end of growth in length of long bones.
210. **A.** M-protein is an important virulent factor found only in the species *Streptococcus pyogenes*.
211. **A.** The initial rate-limiting reaction involves the removal of six carbons from cholesterol and hydroxylation of the steroid nucleus to produce pregnenolone. Pregnenolone can be further isomerized and oxidized to produce the other steroid hormones.
212. **D.** Use of the formula indicates on the basis of ± 6 months that the ADF is 2 to 3 years.
213. **C.** A and B are correct. D is per the manufacturer's recommendations on product, 2005.
214. **B.** Systemic etiologic factors for hypoplasia are thought to occur possibly after birth and before 6 years of age.
215. **C.** Measles is not known to cause enamel hypoplasia.
216. **D.** Intermediate filament is a smooth muscle filament. Connectin is another name for titin. Statements relative to A, B, and C are true and refer to *skeletal* muscle filaments.
217. **D.** Masseter muscles provide most of the force between molar teeth with clenching in the intercuspal position.
218. **D.** Individuals who brux during the day do not necessarily brux at night.
219. **D.** Sequential changes from autonomic cardiac/brain cortical acrivities *precede* SB-related jaw motor activity.
220. **D.** Malocclusion has not been suggested as causing or aggravating bruxism.
221. **D.** Fluorosis versus NF opacities may be difficult to diagnose clinically.
222. **B.** Thick and thin filaments do not change in length.
223. **C.** SHLP helps stabilize the head and condyle against the eminence in clenching; A, B, and D are true.
224. **D.** In the ascending (distal) loop of Henle, active sodium absorption results in an increased osmolarity of the interstitial fluid, which plays a

role in the retention of water under conditions of dehydration.

225. **C.** Under conditions of expansion of extracellular volume (long-term hypertension), renin release and aldosterone secretion are reduced. Increasing ADH, angiotensin II, and increasing sympathetic activity would result in an increase in blood pressure.

226. **E.** The most superficial layer of the epidermis is the stratum corneum. From deep to superficial, the layers are basale, spinosum, granulosum, lucidum, and corneum.

227. **D.** Calcitonin is secreted by parafollicular cells (clear cells) that are located at the periphery of thyroid follicles in the thyroid gland. Calcitonin plays an important role in the regulation of calcium and phosphates. It suppresses bone reabsorption, resulting in decreased calcium and phosphate release.

228. **C.** The ratio of inorganic to organic matter in mature dentin is approximately 70:30. In enamel and cementum, it is approximately 96:4 and 50:50, respectively.

229. **B.** Tuberculin reaction (i.e. PPD skin test), is an example of a type IV delayed (cell-mediated) hypersensitivity. Type IV reactions are the only type of hypersensitivity immune reactions that are not mediated by antibodies. They are mainly mediated by T cells.

230. **C.** Vitamins are not digested by enzymes from the pancreas; however, digestion of carbohydrates, fats, and proteins may be required to make vitamins available for absorption. The pancreas produces amylase for carbohydrate digestion, lipase for lipid digestion, and several proteolytic enzymes (trypsinogen, chymotrypsinogen, and procarboxypeptidase) for the digestion of protein.

231. **C.** The mesencephalic nucleus contain the nuclei of the trigeminal sensory nerves (CN V) involved in proprioception and the jaw jerk reflex, including periodontal ligament fibers involved in the reflex. It is located in the midbrain and pons.

232. **A.** Aldosterone secretion is mediated through the renin-angiotensin system. Angiotensin II stimulates the synthesis and release of aldosterone from the adrenal gland. It acts on the distal tubule and collecting ducts to increase sodium reabsorption and potassium secretion.

233. **A.** First evidence of the maxillary central incisor calcification is given as 14 (13 to 16) weeks by Kraus and Jordon, 1965, and by Ash and Nelson, 2003; this is given as 4 months by Woelfel and Scheid, 2003.

234. **D.** *Lingual aspect:* D, Well-defined developmental groove separating ML and DL cusps. A, ML cusp large and well-developed; B, DL cusp well-developed, more so than that of the primary first molar; C, There is a supplemental cusp apical to the ML cusp, but poorly developed.

235. **B.** Cretinism is hypothyroidism in children. Oral findings include macroglossia, prolonged retention of primary teeth, and delayed eruption of permanent teeth.

236. **A.** Surfactant is synthesized by alveolar cells and functions to reduce the surface tension of the alveoli. This reduction of surface tension increases pulmonary compliance and decreases the work of breathing. It will also decrease the tendency of the lungs to collapse. Lack of surfactant results in neonatal respiratory distress syndrome.

237. **D.** The red pulp of the spleen consists of cords, containing numerous macrophages, and venous sinusoids. It is the site of blood filtration. The white pulp of the spleen contains numerous T and B lymphocytes.

238. **B.** The velocity of blood flow is the rate of displacement of blood per unit time. Velocity changes inversely with cross-sectional area (cm^2). The greater the area in the vessels, the lower the velocity. Since blood is always flowing due to the distensability of the arterial tree, velocity is never zero.

239. **A.** Neuraminidase is found on the surface envelope of influenza viruses. It functions to attach the virus to the host cell.

240. **C.** These are the most common sequences of eruption.

241. **E.** All of the features listed are commonly observed in malignant cells, except a low nuclear–cytoplasmic ratio. Due to the large nuclei present, there is usually a high nuclear-cytoplasmic ratio.

242. **B.** The two vertebral arteries join together at the border of the pons to form the basilar artery. Branches of the basilar provide blood supply to the pons.

243. **C.** RNA synthesis is not required for genetic cloning. All the other enzymes are required to synthesize and splice DNA.

244. **D.** The most potent stimulant of the respiratory center that increases the rate of breathing (hyperventilation) is increased CO_2 tension. CO_2 is permeable to the blood–brain barrier and ultimately produces an increase in H^+ of the cerebral spinal fluid. However, plasma H^+ and HCO_3^- are not permeable and thus have little direct effect on the respiratory center. The respiratory center is not sensitive to oxygen tension, unlike peripheral chemoreceptors.

245. **D.** It is a branch of the maxillary (CN V2) nerve. The maxillary nerve branches from the trigeminal ganglion and exits the skull through the foramen rotundum. When it reaches the pterygopalatine ganglion, it terminates as the infraorbital and zygomatic nerves.

246. **B.** Root bifurcation is more likely in the mandibular canine.

247. **B.** A ketose sugar is on that contains a keto group. Glyceraldehyde, mannose, glucose, and galac-

tose are all aldoses since they contain an aldehyde group.

248. **E.** Both tetracycline and streptomycin, an aminoglycoside, inhibit protein synthesis in bacteria. Streptomycin, however, is bactericidal, not bacteriostatic.
249. **C.** The auricular hillocks are derived from the first and second branchial arch.
250. **C.** The length of the primary maxillary central incisor is 16 mm (Black GV, cited in Ash and Nelson, 2003); 16 mm (Kraus et al., 1969); or 17.2 mm (Woelfel and Scheid, 2002). The permanent maxillary incisor is 23.6 mm (Ash and Nelson, 2003); 23.5 mm (Kraus et al., 1969); 23.6 mm (Woelfel and Scheid, 2002). 16/23.5 = 0.68 or 68%; 17.2/23.6 = 0.73 or 73%. The answer is about 70%.
251. **B.** Ehlers-Danlos syndromes are characterized by defects in collagen (i.e., connective tissues).
252. **C.** Acetyl CoA. Malonyl CoA is produced following carboxylation of acetyl CoA in the synthetic process of fatty acids. FAD and NAD are involved in fatty acid oxidation but NADPH is the source of reducing agents in the synthesis of fatty acids.
253. **A.** Insulin is a hormone that is secreted under conditions of increased sources of energy (glucose) and therefore results in increased uptake and storage of glucose in the form of glycogen. In the process, blood glucose is decreased. The transport of glucose into the brain is not affected by the hormone.
254. **B.** Osteocytes are found in lacunae in mature bone.
255. **D.** From MD aspect, all posterior teeth have a trapezoidal outline with shortest uneven side toward the occlusal surface. A, Present primarily on first premolar; B, Exceptions may be the DB root of the maxillary second molar; C, From mesial and distal aspect, all posterior mandibular teeth, not maxillary posterior teeth, have a rhomboidal outline.
256. **A.** Due to the excessive levels of serum calcium, osseous changes, such as metastatic calcifications and kidney stones, will occur in patients with hyperparathyroidism.
257. **B.** This enzyme catalyzes the phosphorylation of fructose 6-phosphate to fructose 1,6-bisphosphate. This irreversible reaction is inhibited by ATP and citrate (indicators of energy abundance within the cell). The reaction is stimulated by AMP.
258. **B.** Type II collagen is one of the fibril-forming collagens found in cartilaginous structures. Type I is characterized as having high tensile strength and found in skin, tendon, bone, and dentin. Type III collagen is characteristically more distensible and is found in large blood vessels. Type IV is found in basement membranes.
259. **B.** (Kraus et al., 1969.)
260. **D.** From the retropharyngeal space, i.e. "danger space," odontogenic infections can quickly spread down this space into the thorax (posterior mediastinum) and cause possible death.
261. **B.** Trisomy 21, which is also known as *Down syndrome,* is a disorder affecting autosomes. It is generally caused by meiotic nondisjunction in the mother, which results in an extra copy of chromosome 21 (trisomy 21).
262. **A.** Type I collagen is the predominant collagen found in cementum. Type III collagen may be present during the formation of cementum, but it is largely reduced during maturation.
263. **A.** Net filtration depends on the hydrostatic pressures in the glomerular capillary, the hydrostatic pressures in bowman's space, and the oncotic pressures in the capillary and bowman's capsule. Reducing the plasma protein (reducing the oncotic pressure) will lower the tendency to retain fluid in the capillary. This would result in a net increase in filtration.
264. **C.** Auer rods are observed in blast cells characteristic of acute myelogenous leukemia.
265. **D.** Vasopressin, also known as ADH (antidiuretic hormone), is a peptide secreted from the posterior pituitary in response to an increase in serum osmolarity. The other hormones listed are synthesized and secreted from the anterior pituitary.
266. **A.** Secretory IgA is an immunoglobulin that is unique to the oral cavity. The secretory component is synthesized by salivary epithelial cells and complexes with IgA to form secretory IgA.
267. **D.** Marked *asymmetry* of mesial and distal halves.
268. **D.** Oxidation of fatty acids, glucagon release, and glycogenolysis are all increased to provide energy sources for exercising muscle. The synthesis of lipid (lipogenesis) would be decreased during periods of exercise.
269. **B.** The thymus is active at birth and increases in size until puberty (around age 12), after which it gradually atrophies and is replaced by fatty tissue.
270. **C.** Monoamine oxidase is an enzyme located in the presynaptic nerve terminal, which degrades dopamine, norepinephrine, and epinephrine to inactive substances.
271. **A.** B, Tooth grinding in sleep bruxism lasts up to 5 minutes, not 20 minutes; C, Sleep bruxism often coincides with passage from deeper to lighter sleep, not lighter to deep sleep; D, Sleep bruxism occurs approximately every 90 minutes, not every 20 minutes in the sleep cycle.
272. **D.** These oral findings can be observed in patients with hyperthyroidism. The only endocrine disorder listed that is related to hyperthyroidism is Plummer's disease. It is caused by a nodular growth or adenoma of the thyroid.
273. **C.** Fat in the intestine, low pH, and increased osmolarity of intestinal contents will reduce gastric emptying. This reflex is mediated through neuronal and endocrine factors comprising the

enterogastric reflex. Saline in the intestine will not affect gastric emptying.

274. **D.** Occlusal contact relations do *not* interfere with jaw opening, but TMJ and muscle disorders may.
275. **C.** The olecranon fossa is located on the posterior surface of the humerus.
276. **D.** Chronic lymphocytic leukemia is characterized by the proliferation of B cells. It is both the most common and least malignant type of leukemia.
277. **C.** tRNA is not required for the hydroxylation of collagen since the process occurs after translation of mRNA and synthesis of collagen. Ascorbic acid is required to modify the collagen molecule by hydroxylating proline to permit cross-linking among collagen in tissues.
278. **C.** Distal to the second premolar, 56%.
279. **D.** A, The *mesiolingual* cusp is most prominent; B, The *distolingual* cusp is poorly defined; C, The *distobuccal* cusp *may be seen* because it is longer.
280. **D.** The posterior and anterior vagal trunks pass through the diaphragm through the esophageal opening. The aorta enters the diaphragm through the median arch, the inferior vena cava through its own opening in the central tendon, the azygos vein through the right crus, and the splanchnic nerves through the crura.
281. **B.** The sympathetic postganglionic fibers innervating the heart release norepinephrine. Acetylcholine is neurotransmitter in sympathetic preganglionic fibers, parasympathetic postganglionic fibers, and parasympathetic preganglionic fibers.
282. **C.** Osteopetrosis, also known as *Albers-Schönberg disease* or *marble bone disease*, is caused by abnormal osteoclasts. The lack of bone resorption results in defective bone remodeling and increased bone density, which may invade into the bone marrow space.
283. **D.** Langerhans cells are located primarily in stratum spinosum.
284. **B.** Nitric oxide is a molecule produced in endothelial cells that acts directly on smooth muscle to produce relaxation and vasodilatation. Therefore, inhibition of its synthesis would be expected to raise blood pressure. Inhibitors of angiotensin II synthesis should reduce blood pressure since angiotensin II stimulates aldosterone synthesis resulting in increased fluid retention. Angiotensin II is also a potent vasoconstrictor. Blocking vasopressin (also a potent vasoconstrictor) receptors would reduce blood pressure. Stimulation of the baroreceptor would produce a reflex that would reduce cardiac output and peripheral sympathetic tone.
285. **A.** (Ash and Nelson, 2003; Woelfel and Scheid, 2002.)
286. **C.** The movement of the tongue against the palate is the only voluntary process among the four possible answers.
287. **A.** CD8 lymphocytes recognize class I MHC molecules on antigen-presenting cells. CD4 lymphocytes recognize class II MHC molecules on antigen-presenting cells.
288. **A.** Bifurcated roots are not a normal feature of mandibular incisors.
289. **C.** The inner enamel epithelium in the bell stage differentiates into ameloblasts
290. **D.** The cartilage of the trachea is covered by a perichondrium. The mucosa is covered with respiratory epithelium. Hyaline cartilage rings lie deep to the submucosa. The open end of the cartilage faces the posterior. Smooth muscle extends across the open end of each cartilage.
291. **C.** Pemphigus is an autoimmune disease wherein autoantibodies against epidermis cells are produced. Histologically, a phenomenon called *acantholysis*, wherein epidermal cells appear to detach and separate from each other, is observed.
292. **A.** Following a meal, chylomicrons are synthesized in the intestine to transport lipid to the liver. Acetoacetate (ketone body) is found under conditions of increased β oxidation (fasting). Glucagon is secreted in response to reduced blood sugar, which usually is not present following a meal. Lactate, a product of anaerobic glycolysis, is not elevated under conditions of elevated energy sources in the post-absorptive state.
293. **A.** Bruxism is now thought to be mainly regulated centrally, not peripherally.
294. **A.** A distinct developmental groove, prominent buccal triangular ridge, two cusps, and distinct mesial and distal occlusal pits are most characteristic of the mandibular first premolar.
295. **B.** Autoclaves function by denaturing proteins. It is effective against spores.
296. **D.** In the initial step of the synthesis of porphyrin, succinyl CoA and glycine are condensed in a rate limiting step in the liver.
297. **B.** The dental lamina arises from neural crest cells.
298. **A.** The only disease listed that is related to an abnormal number of chromosomes is Klinefelter's syndrome. This disease is characterized by two or more X chromosomes and one or more Y chromosome. Typically, those affected have 47 chromosomes with a karyotype of XXY.
299. **A.** Stretching of muscle spindles results in a reflex that is intended to adjust the muscle to its resting length by contracting the muscle in which it is found. The stretching of the spindle increases afferent impulses to the spinal cord and through a monosynaptic reflex stimulates muscle contraction via an alpha motor neuron.
300. **C.** Below the apices, 63% of the time.

301. **E.** Urinary filtrate is most hypotonic in the distal convoluted tubule. It is isotonic in the proximal convoluted tubule and thick descending limb of Henle's loop. It becomes hypertonic as it passes through the thin descending limb of Henle's loop, and becomes hypotonic as it passes through the thick ascending segment of Henle's loop. Finally, it becomes increasingly hypotonic as it passes through the distal convoluted tubule.
302. **C.** There are seven pairs of true ribs, meaning they attach directly to the sternum via costal cartilages. The remaining five pairs are called false ribs because they attach indirectly to the sternum via costal cartilages. The last pair does not attach at all.
303. **B.** The total of average overall mesiodistal diameters of primary maxillary crowns is 68.2 mm (Black GV, cited by Ash and Nelson, 2003); 76.8 mm (Woelfel and Scheid, 2002).
304. **C.** Symptoms of a myocardial infarction include chest pain, shortness of breath, diaphoresis (sweating), clammy hands, nausea, and vomiting.
305. **C.** Amino acids are transported across the luminal surface of the intestine by Na^+ amino acid cotransporters in the apical membrane. This is facilitated by the Na^+ gradient established in the intestinal cells.
306. **A.** Of the cell types listed, only smooth muscle cells are capable of cell division.
307. **B.** Vitamin K is involved with the posttranslational modification of glutamic acid to form γ-carboxyglutamic acid. This carboxylation permits prothrombin to interact with platelets and ions in the process of clot formation. Hydroxylation of proline requires ascorbic acid and iron.
308. **D.** Squamous cell carcinoma is the most common oral cancer, occurring in 90% of all cases. It is a cancer of squamous epithelium, specifically a tumor of keratinocytes.
309. **B.** The permanent maxillary first premolar usually has two roots but they are buccal and lingual, not mesial and distal.
310. **D.** Actinic keratosis produces dry, scaly plaques with an erythematous base. They may be premalignant. Both compound and intraepidermal nevi are benign. Only junctional nevi are considered to be premalignant.
311. **B.** Secretin stimulates bicarbonate secretion from the pancreatic ducts. Cholecystokinin (CCK) is responsible for stimulating pancreatic enzyme secretion and contraction of the gall bladder. Chymotrypsinogen is activated by trypsin in the intestine.
312. **B.** Textbook chronologies indicate that the maxillary primary second molar is most commonly the last to erupt: 24 months (Woelfel and Scheid, 2002); 20 to 30 months (Kraus et al., 1969); 25 to 33 months (Ash and Nelson, 2003).
313. **D.** The latissimus dorsi muscle is supplied by the thoracodorsal nerve.
314. **B.** Regulation of blood flow to skin is under the control of factors acting locally (metabolites) and α-adrenergic receptors. Slowing of the heart and activation of gastrointestinal motility are mediated through the cholinergic system. α-adrenergic receptors produce decreased renal blood flow.
315. **A.** The auriculotemporal nerve provides primary innervation to the TMJ.
316. **B.** The submental artery is a branch of the facial artery. Branches of the mandibular division of the maxillary artery include the inferior alveolar, deep auricular, anterior tympanic, mylohyoid, incisive, mental and middle meningeal arteries.
317. **E.** Rheumatoid arthritis is characterized by inflammation of the synovial membrane. Granulation tissue will form in the synovium and expand over the articular cartilage. This causes the destruction of the underlying cartilage and results in fibrotic changes or ankylosis.
318. **D.** (Ash and Nelson, 2003.)
319. **C.** The trapezius muscle is supplied by CN XI. Latissimus dorsi is supplied by the thoracodorsal nerve, levator scapulae is supplied by the dorsal scapular nerve, and the major and minor rhomboid muscles are supplied by the dorsal scapular nerve.
320. **B.** A quelling reaction occurs in a laboratory when the polysaccharide capsule of a bacterium swells after being treated with antiserum or antibodies.
321. **D.** Under conditions of increased intracranial pressure, the vasomotor regions of the medulla are stimulated due to localized ischemia resulting in an increase in systemic blood pressure. Ventricular fibrillation is irregular, rapid, uncoordinated contractions of the ventricle that do not result in effecting blood movement. Anaphylactic shock is caused by severe allergic reactions, widespread release of histamine, and subsequent vasodilatation.
322. **D.** Teichoic acid may be found only in the cell walls of gram-positive bacteria and contain antigenic properties. All of the other answers listed are found in the cell walls of gram-negative bacteria.
323. **A.** The articulating surfaces of the TMJ are covered with fibrocartilage, directly overlying periosteum. The non-articulating surfaces of the TMJ are covered with periosteum. The articulating surfaces of diarthrodial joints are covered with hyaline cartilage.
324. **B.** Both epinephrine and glucagons result in activities which serve to increase (maintain) blood glucose. Activation of glycogen phosphorylase will result in glycogen degradation, ultimately providing a source of glucose. Glycogen synthase inhibition results in decreased synthesis of glycogen.

325. **C.** Mediotrusive contact, but may be called a nonworking (balancing) contact.
326. **C.** The internal carotid artery is joined to the posterior cerebral artery via the posterior communicating artery, which is part of the circle of Willis.
327. **E.** The transport of glucose into muscle (and fat) cells is due to the activity of glucose transporters (GLUT-4), which does not require ATP and is independent of any ionic concentration gradient. ATP is required for the activity of all other transport mechanisms listed in the question.
328. **C.** Opportunistic infections are seen in patients with AIDS. All of the following microbes represent opportunistic organisms except coxsackievirus.
329. **C.** No, or almost never does the mesial marginal developmental groove cross the mesial marginal ridge.
330. **D.** All posterior teeth viewed from distal aspect have a rhomboidal outline.
331. **D.** Dextrans consist of glucose molecules linked together. They not only act as the structural component of plaque, but they also contribute to the retention of lactic acid near the tooth. Fructans or levans are also found in plaque; however, they contain fructose.
332. **C.** Substitution of most ions (with the exception of fluoride) will increase the solubility of the crystal structure. The ratio of calcium and phosphate in hydroxyapatite is 1.67:1.
333. **C.** Tooth enamel is derived from ectoderm. Dentin and pulp are derived from mesoderm.
334. **C.** The thin segment of Henle's loop contains squamous epithelial cells. The proximal convoluted tubule, also known as the thick descending limb of Henle's loop, the thick ascending segment of Henle's loop, and the distal convoluted tubule all consist of cuboidal epithelial cells.
335. **C.** Glucose 6-phosphate dehydrogenase and 6-phosphogluconate dehydrogenase are irreversible enzymes in the pentose phosphate pathway. Glucokinase is involved with phosphorylation of glucose when hepatic concentrations of glucose are high. Glucose 6-phosphatase hydrolyzes glucose 6-phosphate to form free glucose, as the final step in gluconeogenesis.
336. **D.** Height of contour on distal surface of permanent mandibular central incisors is at the incisal third.
337. **E.** Cardiac tamponade is a serious condition caused by accumulation of fluid in the pericardium. This can result in impaired ventricular filling and can rapidly lead to decreased cardiac output and death.
338. **B.** The correct order of tooth formation is ameloblasts form, odontoblasts form, odontoblasts start to form dentin, ameloblasts start to form enamel.
339. **C.** Reduction division occurs during the first stage of meiosis. The second stage mirrors mitosis. There is no third stage of meiosis.
340. **A.** Whooping cough is caused by *Bordetella pertussis*. All of the factors listed contribute to its virulence except IgA protease. This enzyme is produced by *Haemophilus influenzae*, another gram-negative, rod-shaped bacteria.
341. **C.** Residual volume is the volume of air remaining after a maximal forced expiration. Tidal volume is the amount of air exchanged (expiration and inspiration) during normal quiet breathing. Functional residual capacity is a combination of the expired reserve volume (forced expiration) plus the residual volume. Vital capacity is the volume of air expired after maximal inspiration.
342. **D.** *Mesial aspect:* A, Pronounced convexity present (Ash and Nelson, 2003); B, Curvature in an occlusal direction; C, Cervical third greater occlusal third; D, Mesiolingual cusp longer and sharper than mesiobuccal cusp.
343. **C.** The embryo develops from the embryonic disc. The morula, blastocyst, and trophoblast all include structures of the extraembryonic coelem that will lead to development of the amnion, vitelline sac, and chorion.
344. **C.** Chronologies from textbooks vary so that age of eruption for the primary mandibular central incisor may be given as 6 months (Woelfel and Scheid, 2002); 6.5 months (Kraus et al., 1969); 7.5 months (Charlick et al.,); or 8 (6 to 10) months (Ash and Nelson, 2003).
345. **B.** Progesterone concentration in blood is highest following the surge of LH (leuteinizing hormone) following ovulation. During ovulation, estrogen surges due to positive feedback during the follicular phase. During menstruation there are sharp declines in estrogen and progesterone due to reduced secretion of LH and FSH.
346. **B.** The left atrioventricular valve of the heart is also known as the mitral valve. The right atrioventricular valve of the heart is also known as the tricuspid valve. The aortic valve prevents regurgitation of blood from the aorta back into the left ventricle and the pulmonary valve prevents regurgitation of blood from the pulmonary artery back into the right ventricle.
347. **C.** The leading cause of death for diabetic patients is cardiovascular disease. Other complications include retinopathy, nephropathy, and peripheral neuropathy.
348. **C.** The correct answer for A would be about *1.5 months or 6 weeks;* B, About *4 to 5 years;* C, About *2.5 months or 10 weeks;* D, About *4 to 5 years.*
349. **D.** Y-shaped central developmental groove is found on the mandibular second premolar.
350. **B.** The sternal angle between the manubrium and the sternum marks the position of the second rib. From this location ribs can be counted externally. This is important, because the first rib cannot be palpated.

351. **C.** NADPH is required as a reducing agent for the synthesis of fatty acids. The hexose monophosphate pathway also produces ribose 5-phosphate for nucleotide synthesis. No ATP or NADH is produced in the pathway. Fructose 1,6-bisphosphate is produced during glycolysis.
352. **C.** Intraoral *Streptococcus viridans* is the most common cause of subacute endocarditis. *Staphylococcus aureus* is the most common cause of acute endocarditis.
353. **B, C, D.** For A, the crown outline converges only *lingually*; B, The small transverse ridge has been called an oblique ridge.
354. **B.** The mandibular incisors, as well as the lower lip, floor of the mouth, tip of the tongue and chin, primarily drain into the submental nodes. The rest of the mandibular teeth (premolars and molars) mainly drain into the submandibular nodes.
355. **D.** Rickets is a vitamin D deficiency seen in infants and children. Oral findings include a delayed eruption of teeth and abnormal dentin.
356. **A.** In the irreversible oxidative decarboxylation of pyruvate to acetyl CoA by pyruvate dehydrogenase, the five coenzymes listed are required.
357. **D.** A developmental depression but not a groove divides the two buccal cusps. A, It does not resemble other primary teeth; B, It has a rhomboidal outline from the occlusal aspect; C, The mesial buccal cusp is larger.
358. **D.** Fibers of the superior head of the lateral pterygoid muscle attach to the anterior end of the disc, which helps to balance and stabilize the disc during mouth closure.
359. **B.** (Ash and Nelson, 2003.)
360. **D.** HBeAg is present when there is active viral replication and the carrier is highly infectious.
361. **C.** Saliva is formed by a process that first involves the formation of a solution by the acinar cells, which is subsequently modified by the ductile cells to produce a more hypotonic solution (compared to plasma). The modification primarily involves the reabsorption of sodium and chloride and secretion of potassium and bicarbonate. As salivary flow increases, the ductile cells have less time to modify the composition of saliva, which results in greater concentrations of sodium and chloride ions. Bicarbonate concentration increases as salivary flow increases due to the selective stimulation of bicarbonate by the parasympathetic system. The salivary glands are primarily under the regulation of both branches of the autonomic nervous system.
362. **B.** The pulmonary vein of the lung carries oxygenated blood from the lungs to the left atrium of the heart. The pulmonary artery carries unoxygenated blood from the right ventricle of the heart to the lungs.
363. **B.** Thoracic vertebrae are characterized by a heart-shaped body.
364. **A.** A micelle is a globular structure that forms when the polar heads of an amphipathic molecule (fatty acids) interact with the aqueous external environment and the nonpolar hydrocarbon tails are clustered inside.
365. **D.** HIV's envelope contains two glycoproteins, gp120 and gp41. gp120 binds specifically with CD4 surface receptors.
366. **A.** (McCauley, 1945; Ash and Nelson, 2003.)
367. **B.** In the earliest phase, the condyle moves forward *in concert* with the disc, *not before*.
368. **A.** Endotoxin or lipopolysaccharide is found in the cell walls of gram-negative bacteria.
369. **A.** The trochlea of the humerus articulates with the ulna of the forearm. The capitulum of the humerus bone articulates with the radius of the forearm. The coronoid fossa, located just superior to the trochlea, fits the coronoid process of the ulna of the forearm. The olecranon fossa of the humerus fits the olecranon of the ulna of the forearm. The medial epicondyle is on the humerus itself and serves as an attachment site for muscles.
370. **A.** During a fast, catabolism is increased to provide additional sources of energy. This is characterized by increased utilization of fatty acids. When the production of acetyl CoA (produced by enhanced β-oxidation) exceeds the oxidative capacity of the citric acid cycle, ketone bodies are formed. During fasting conditions, glucagon concentrations are increased and glycogenesis is inhibited due to limited energy availability. Acetyl CoA production in the liver is increased due to enhanced β-oxidation.
371. **D.** The nucleus ambiguus is found in the medulla of the brainstem. It contains the cell bodies of motor neurons for CN IX, X and XI. The cell bodies of CN VII, IX and X's sensory neurons are contained in the nucleus of the solitary tract.
372. **A.** Calcium is stored and released from the sarcoplasmic reticulum during excitation-contraction coupling. This provides an extensive reservoir of calcium while permitting intracellular free Ca^{2+} to be low when the muscle fiber is at rest. The release of calcium is due to conformational changes which opens Ca^{2+} channels in the sarcoplasmic reticulum.
373. **B.** The tetanus vaccine consists of tetanus toxoid. It is part of the DPT vaccine and should be given about every 10 years.
374. **C.** Height of contour on lingual surfaces of molars and premolars is at the cervical or middle third.
375. **A.** Muscles are innervated by two types of motor neurons (alpha and gamma). The alpha motor neurons innervate voluntary muscle fibers (extrafusal skeletal muscles). The gamma motor neurons innervate the muscle spindles (intrafusal muscle fibers). The muscles of the iris are controlled by both sympathetic innervation (dilation) and parasympathetic innervation (con-

striction). The pyloric sphincter in the stomach is regulated primarily by the enteric nervous system and regulatory hormones in the GI tract.

376. **E.** The mitochondria is surrounded by a double (inner and outer) membrane. The nuclear membrane (not listed), which surrounds the nucleus, also consists of a double (inner and outer) membrane.
377. **A.** Calmodulin is a calcium-binding protein in smooth muscle which, when bound to myosin, initiates contraction. Calmodulin activates myosin kinase, which results in myosin–actin crosslinking and contraction of smooth muscle.
378. **A.** The lumen of the gastrointestinal tract is lined with mucosa. The rest of the choices are in order from lumen out. Fibrosa and adventitia are synonymous.
379. **B.** DB developmental groove is *not* found on mandibular second molars.
380. **E.** Bacteria that are phagocytosed by macrophages are kept in membrane-bound vacuoles called *phagosomes*. A phagosome will fuse with a lysosome, which contains many degradative enzymes, including lysozyme.
381. **B.** During metaphase, mitotic spindles form. Chromosomes attach to these spindles, with their centromeres aligned with the equator of the cell.
382. **A.** DNA ligase is required to ligate the fragments together. DNA and RNA polymerases are catalysts that synthesize DNA and RNA in a continuous process. Reverse transcriptase is an enzyme found in viruses that makes DNA by using viral RNA.
383. **D.** The maxillary nerve (CN V2) exits the skull through the foramen rotundum. It then passes through the pterygopalatine fossa, where it communicates with the pterygopalatine ganglion. Contents of the superior orbital fissure include CN III, IV, V1 and VI and the ophthalmic veins. CN VII and VIII pass through the internal acoustic meatus and CN V3 (the mandibular nerve) passes through the foramen ovale. The foramen spinosum is not associated with any cranial nerves; it contains the middle meningeal vessels.
384. **D.** Asthma is an obstructive lung disease caused by narrowing of the airways. Common symptoms include dyspnea, wheezing on expiration, and a dry cough.
385. **A.** Greater MD diameter relative to crown height than permanent teeth. B, Squat appearance, not elongated appearance; C, Crowns are a milky white, not translucent white; D, There is no root trunk.
386. **D.** The teres major muscle is a shoulder muscle, however, it is not a rotator muscle. All of the other four listed in this question are rotator cuff muscles.
387. **B.** A motor unit is composed of a single motor neuron and the muscle fibers it innervates. Since the motor neuron will stimulate all muscle fibers it innervates, "fractions" of a motor unit cannot be stimulated. The number of motor units recruited, the number of muscle fibers contracting, and the frequency of stimulation will all affect the degree of muscle tension produced.
388. **E.** In the liver, smooth endoplasmic reticulum is involved in glycogen metabolism and detoxification of various drugs and alcohols; it therefore, contains P450 enzymes, which are cytochromes that are important in the detoxification process.
389. **C.** Cardiac output is the volume of blood pumped per minute by each ventricle. This is influenced by cardiac rate and stroke volume (end-diastolic volume – end-systolic volume). The cardiac output for this patient is 70×110 mL or 7700 mL per minute.
390. **B.** Mandibular first premolar is most likely to have a single pulp horn.
391. **E.** Dipicolinic acid is only found in spores. Since *Clostridium* is the only spore-forming microorganism listed, the correct answer is E.
392. **D.** RNA polymerase is an enzyme that transcribes DNA into RNA chains. Synthesis is similar to DNA reproduction since it is synthesized $5' \rightarrow 3'$.
393. **C.** The frontal bone of the skull is formed by intramembranous ossification. The humerus, vertebrae, ribs, and clavicle all are formed by endochondral ossification.
394. **B.** The sum total of the pressures moving fluid *out* of the capillary is P_c (37 mmHg) and π_{if} (1 mmHg) at the arteriolar end and P_c (16 mmHg) and π_{if} (1 mmHg) at the venular end. The sum total of the pressures moving *into* the capillary is P_{if} (0 mmHg) and π_p (26 mmHg). The net exchange pressure on the arteriolar end leads to ultrafiltration (12 mmHg). On the venular end, reabsorption occurs (9 mmHg). Overall net exchange results in 3 mmHg of fluid loss out of the capillary.
395. **B.** Thyroxine and triiodothyronine are formed by the cleavage of thyroglobulin following stimulation by TSH. Most thyroxine is converted to triiodothyronine in liver and kidney. Thyroglobulin is the storage form of thyroid hormone. TSH (thyroid-stimulating hormone) is produced in the anterior pituitary. It is not a hormone secreted from the thyroid but acts to stimulate the synthesis and secretion of thyroid hormones.
396. **C.** Dust cells, along with heart fail cells, are macrophages that are found in the lungs. They are part of the reticuloendothelial system.
397. **C.** The lateral thoracic wall of the axilla is covered by the serratus anterior muscle. The

anterior wall is covered by pectoralis major and pectoralis minor. Latissimus dorsi contributes to the inferior aspect of the posterior wall.

398. **C.** Although some CO_2 is transported unchanged in the plasma and in the red blood cells as carbaminohemoglobin, most is transported in the form of bicarbonate ion in the plasma.

399. **D.** Oral epithelium is composed of nonkeratinized, stratified, squamous epithelium.

400. **D.** Chondroitin sulfate is a glucosaminoglycan found in ligaments, tendons, and cartilage. It is the most abundant glucosaminoglycan in the body.

Index

Note: Page numbers followed by f refer to figures; page numbers followed by t refer to tables; page numbers followed by b refer to boxes.